LUNG CANCER
Standards of Care

Goetz Kloecker MD, MBA, MSPH, FACP
Professor of Medicine
Division of Hematology/Medical Oncology
Director of Thoracic Oncology
University of Louisville
James Graham Brown Cancer Center
Louisville, Kentucky

Susanne M. Arnold, MD
Professor of Medicine, Division of Medical Oncology
University of Kentucky College of Medicine
Associate Director of Clinical Translation
Markey Cancer Center
Lexington, Kentucky

Mostafa M. Fraig, MD, MBA
William M. Christopherson Professor of Pathology and Laboratory Medicine
Vice Chair and Director of Anatomic Pathology
University of Louisville School of Medicine
Louisville, Kentucky

Cesar A. Perez, MD
Associate Professor (cand), Department of Internal Medicine
Associate Director, Experimental Therapeutics Program
Co-Leader, Head and Neck Group
Medical Director of Utilization
Division of Medical Oncology, Sylvester Comprehensive Cancer Center
University of Miami Miller School of Medicine Miami, Florida

New York   Chicago   San Francisco   Athens   London   Madrid   Mexico City
Milan   New Delhi   Singapore   Sydney   Toronto

Lung Cancer: Standards of Care

1 2 3 4 5 6 7 8 9   DSS   25 24 23 22 21 20

ISBN 978-1-260-13620-3
MHID 1-260-13620-5

This book was set in Minion Pro by Cenveo® Publisher Services.
The editors were Karen Edmonson and Harriet Lebowitz.
The production supervisor was Catherine H. Saggese.
The text designer was Mary McKeon.
Project management was provided by Revathi Viswanathan, Cenveo Publisher Services.

Library of Congress Cataloging-in-Publication Data

Names: Kloecker, Goetz, editor. | Fraig, Mostafa M., editor. | Arnold,
  Susanne Markesbery, editor. | Perez, Cesar A., 1980- editor.
Title: Lung cancer : standards of care / [edited by] Goetz Kloecker,
  Mostafa M. Fraig, Susanne Markesbery Arnold, Cesar A. Perez.
Other titles: Lung cancer (Kloecker)
Description: New York : McGraw Hill, [2021] | Includes bibliographical
  references and index. | Summary: "Covers the new standards of care and
  helps you to remain current on lung cancer for practice, board review,
  and re-certification in a very easy-to-read, concise and quick to digest
  format. The fast-changing paradigms of care are presented in print,
  e-book and the on line access will be updated annually"—Provided by
  publisher.
Identifiers: LCCN 2020018840 | ISBN 9781260136203 (paperback) | ISBN
  9781260136210 (ebook)
Subjects: MESH: Lung Neoplasms
Classification: LCC RC280.L8 | NLM WF 658 | DDC 616.99/424—dc23
LC record available at https://lccn.loc.gov/2020018840

For Leni and Vincent Klöcker

CONTENTS

CONTRIBUTORS

Jonathan S. Alexander, MD
Department of Internal Medicine
University of Louisville
School of Medicine
Louisville, Kentucky

Andrea Anampa-Guzmán
Medical Student
San Fernando Faculty of Human Medicine
Universidad Nacional Mayor de San Marcos
Lima, Peru

Susanne Markesbery Arnold, MD
Professor of Medicine, Division of
    Medical Oncology
University of Kentucky College of Medicine
Associate Director of Clinical Translation
Markey Cancer Center
Lexington, Kentucky

Shruti Bhandari, MD
Hematology and Medical Oncology
University of Louisville
Department of Medicine
School of Medicine
Louisville, Kentucky

Christine Fillmore Brainson, PhD
Assistant Professor, Toxicology and
    Cancer Biology
University of Kentucky College of Medicine
Markey Cancer Center
Lexington, Kentucky

Michael J. Carr, MD, MS
Hiram C. Polk Jr., MD Department of
    Surgery
University of Louisville School of Medicine
Louisville, Kentucky

Douglas M. Coldwell, MD, PhD
Professor of Radiology and Bioengineering
Vice Chair, Radiology
University of Louisville
School of Medicine
Louisville, Kentucky

Jennifer Cudris, MD
Section Chief, Hematology and Oncology
Miami VA Healthcare system
Miami, Florida

Brian Dong, MD
Hematology and Medical Oncology
Department of Medicine
University of Louisville
School of Medicine
Louisville, Kentucky

Neal E. Dunlap, MD
Professor and Vice Chairman
Residency Director
Department of Radiation Oncology
University of Louisville
School of Medicine
Louisville, Kentucky

Matthew Fox, MD
Assistant Professor of Cardiovascular and
    Thoracic Surgery
University of Louisville
School of Medicine
Louisville, Kentucky

Mostafa M. Fraig, MD, MBA
William M. Christopherson Professor of
*   Pathology and Laboratory Medicine*
Vice Chair, Director of Anatomic Pathology
Director of Pulmonary Pathology
Adjunct Professor of Medicine
Division of Pulmonary Medicine
School of Medicine
University of Louisville
Louisville, Kentucky

Umair Gauhar, MBBS
Associate Professor of Medicine
Director, Interventional Pulmonary Program
Division of Pulmonary, Critical Care, and
*   Sleep Disorders Medicine*
Department of Medicine
University of Louisville
School of Medicine
Louisville, Kentucky

Ignacio Gil-Bazo, MD, PhD
Chairman, Department of Oncology
Co-Director, Lung Cancer Unit
Associate Professor, School of Medicine
Principal Investigator, Program of Solid
*   Tumors and Biomarkers*
Clínica Universidad de Navarra—Center for
*   Applied Medical Research*
Pamplona, Spain

Amitoj Gill, MD
Hematology and Oncology
Columbus Regional Hospital
Columbus, Indiana

Rahul Gosain, MD
Co-Founder and President, Learn From Apps
Division of Hematology and Oncology
Guthrie–Corning Cancer Center
Corning, New York

Moises Harari Turquie, MD
Hematology and Oncology Fellow
University of New Mexico Comprehensive
*   Cancer Center*
Albuquerque, New Mexico

Hamza Hashmi, MD
Assistant Professor
Department of Medicine
Division of Hematology/Oncology
Medical University of South Carolina
Charleston, South Carolina

Muhammad Husnain, MD
Assistant Professor of Medicine
Division of Hematology and Medical Oncology
Department of Medicine
University of Arizona
Tucson, Arizona

Bilal Athar Jalil, MD
Assistant Professor
Division of Pulmonary, Critical Care and
*   Sleep Disorders Medicine*
Department of Medicine
University of Louisville
College of Medicine
Louisville, Kentucky

Emily Jonczak, MD
Hematology and Medical Oncology
Jackson Memorial Hospital
University of Miami/Sylvester
*   Comprehensive Cancer Center*
Miami, Florida

Alden Klarer, MD, PhD
Department of Radiation Oncology
University of Louisville
School of Medicine
Louisville, Kentucky

Goetz Kloecker, MD, MBA, MSPH, FACP
Professor of Medicine
Division of Hematology and Medical
*   Oncology*
Director of Thoracic Oncology
Director of the Fellowship Program
Department of Medicine
Adjunct Faculty Epidemiology and Public
*   Health*
University of Louisville School of Medicine
James Graham Brown Cancer Center
Louisville, Kentucky

Rohit Kumar, MD
Hematology and Medical Oncology
James Graham Brown Cancer Center
University of Louisville
School of Medicine
Louisville, Kentucky

Steven Mandish, MD
Department of Radiation Oncology
University of Louisville
School of Medicine
Louisville, Kentucky

Katy Alyse Marino, MD
Assistant Professor of Surgery
University of Arkansas for Medical Sciences
Winthrop P. Rockefeller Cancer Institute
Little Rock, Arkansas

Michael May, MD
Department of Radiation Oncology
University of Louisville
School of Medicine
Louisville, Kentucky

Raja Mudad, MD, FACP
Associate Professor of Medicine
Florida Precision Oncology
Aventura, Florida

Phuong T. Ngo, MD
Assistant Professor
Department of Internal Medicine
Division Hematology and Oncology
University of Louisville
School of Medicine
Louisville, Kentucky

Chandler Park, MD, MSc, FACP
President, Kentucky Society of Clinical
*   Oncology (Kentucky ASCO chapter)*
CME Faculty ASCO
Clinical Assistant Professor
University of Kentucky
Co-director GU Oncology Trials
Norton Cancer Institute
Louisville, Kentucky

Cesar A. Perez, MD
Associate Professor (cand)
Department of Internal Medicine
Associate Director, Experimental
*   Therapeutics Program*
Co-Leader, Head and Neck Group
Medical Director of Utilization
Division of Medical Oncology
Sylvester Comprehensive Cancer Center
University of Miami Miller School of
*   Medicine Miami, Florida*

Dhan Pham, MD
Assistant Professor
Department of Medicine
Section of Hematology/Oncology
West Virginia University
School of Medicine
Morgantown, West Virginia

Jose Pinto-Llerena, MD, FACP
Clinical Associate Professor,
*   Faculty of Medicine*
Gastrointestinal Cancer Unit
National Cancer Institute of Panama
HOPE Clinic, Pacifica Salud
University of Panama
Columbus University
Panama City, Panama

Luis E. Raez, MD, FACP, FCCP
President, Florida Society of Clinical
*   Oncology (FLASCO)*
Chief Scientific Officer and Medical Director
Memorial Cancer Institute/Memorial
*   Health Care System*
Clinical Professor of Medicine
Herbert Wertheim College of Medicine
Florida International University
Miami, Florida

Samuel Reynolds, MD
Chief Medicine Resident, Internal Medicine
Department of Medicine
University of Louisville
School of Medicine
Louisville, Kentucky

Jonathan Rice, MD, PhD
Research Fellow in Cardiovascular and
*   Thoracic Surgery*
University of Louisville
School of Medicine
Louisville, Kentucky

Jorge A. Rios, MD
Co-Chair, Medical Advisory Board
State of Ohio Cancer Control Program
Medical Oncology
Zangmeister Cancer Center
Columbus, Ohio

Edgardo S. Santos, MD, FACP
Founding Partner, Florida Precision
*   Oncology R&C*
Thoracic and Head/Neck Cancer Programs
Clinical Associate Professor
Charles E. Schmidt College of Medicine
Florida Atlantic University
Boca Raton, Florida

Diana Saravia, MD
Hematology and Medical Oncology
Jackson Memorial Hospital
University of Miami/Sylvester
*   Comprehensive Cancer Center*
Miami, Florida

Susan Ansley Smith, MD
Surgery
Hiram C. Polk Jr, MD, Department of
*   General Surgery*
University of Louisville
School of Medicine
Louisville, Kentucky

Andrew Tumen, MD, MS
Surgery
Hiram C. Polk Jr, MD, Department of
*   General Surgery*
University of Louisville
School of Medicine
Louisville, Kentucky

Victor van Berkel, MD, PhD
Associate Professor of Cardiovascular and
*   Thoracic Surgery*
Division Chief, Thoracic Surgery
University of Louisville
School of Medicine
Louisville, Kentucky

William M. Whited, MD
Surgery
Hiram C. Polk Jr, MD, Department of
*   General Surgery*
University of Louisville
School of Medicine
Louisville, Kentucky

Celeste T. Worth, MCHES
Director of the LuCa National Training
*   Network*
Tobacco Treatment Specialist
University of Louisville
Louisville, Kentucky

Mehran Yusuf, MD
Department of Radiation Oncology
University of Louisville
School of Medicine
Louisville, Kentucky

Omar Safi Zuberi, DO
Fellow in Vascular and
*   Interventional Radiology*
University of Texas/MD Anderson
*   Cancer Center*
Houston, Texas

PREFACE

The readers of *Lung Cancer: Standards of Care* will not be surprised to hear—again—that lung cancer is still the deadliest cancer in absolute numbers worldwide. And yet, it's a cancer that is mostly due to behavioral and environmental factors. One hundred years ago, lung cancer was among the rarest seen. It took decades to realize its main cause—tobacco—and still, decades later, tobacco's addictiveness is the major challenge for its users. It's a major roadblock for countries and global organizations trying to control the use and sale of tobacco and reduce the addiction to it.

For the longest time, lung cancer patients were shamed, and their physicians dealt them fatalism and not hope. In that same era, many other cancers became success stories. Lung cancer was labeled a treatment-refractory disease when other common cancers became curable, preventable, or turned into chronic conditions with well-preserved quality of life.

The new standards of care for lung cancer are never to accept it as an inevitable part of life or to expect that diagnosis leads only to a grave prognosis. Public health measures over the last decades have bent the curve in mortality rate for both men and women. The decrease in lung cancer mortality in the last decade, in the economically more advanced nations, is a tribute to the science of epidemiology and to modern medicine, advocacy groups, and prudent policy.

Our understanding of lung cancer's etiology and biology, of its molecular machinery, and of its dependence on host-related and environmental factors has led to breakthroughs in survival that were not imaginable a few years ago. A cancer that was until very recently simplified as either "small or non–small cell" histology has become a cancer with many genomic variants, dynamic in its molecular and histologic evolution and staged to its anatomical extent. We track it by new imaging modalities and new techniques of tissue sampling, using interventional radiology and interventional pulmonary techniques. New surgical modalities that are minimally invasive, and new radiation modalities, allow curative intent with minimal risk and side effects. Inhibiting oncogenes and activating hosts' immune defenses have both added a new dimension in cancer care, with the promise of more breakthroughs to come.

This book is intended for a broad audience and is meant to highlight the most important points and new principles of lung cancer management, still allowing the reader to go into more detail, especially in terms of etiology, diagnosis, and therapy.

In a field that is rapidly evolving, the organization of the book and the intent of the authors are to give the readers a practical and efficient way to familiarize themselves with the newest developments in the field. The bibliography will allow the interested reader to see the data of numerous studies and trials that are behind the new developments, such as immunotherapy and oncogene inhibition, and newer concepts, such as the stem cell concept of lung cancer.

The rapidly changing landscape, with ever-increasing options available in diagnostics and therapeutics, makes any attempt to capture in print the oncoming waves of recommendations a Sisyphean task.

The hope and intent of the authors are to give the readers a solid foundation of the new principles approaching this disease. Many contributors from a wide range of disciplines provide the reader with practice-changing information that can be applied in patient care today.

Moreover, this book may give the readers a glimpse of a future where lung cancer will no longer be accepted as a common and natural cause of death.

ACKNOWLEDGMENTS

For the image of lung cancer cells, we thank Levi J. Beverly, PhD, associate professor and co-leader of the Experimental Therapeutics Program, James Graham Brown Cancer Center, Department of Medicine, University of Louisville.

For his help with the bibliography, we also thank John Chenault, PhD, associate professor and medical librarian, Kornhauser Health Sciences Library, University of Louisville.

Goetz Kloecker, MD, MBA, MSPH, FACP
Susanne Markesbery Arnold, MD
Mostafa M. Fraig, MD, MBA
Cesar A. Perez, MD

PART I

Background

HISTORY OF LUNG CANCER

Goetz Kloecker, MD, MBA, MSPH, FACP

A medical student reading about lung cancer notices that the number of lung cancer deaths has steadily increased worldwide.

She asks when lung cancer was first described in the medical literature and how it was treated in the past. She wonders, how the frequency of deaths due to lung cancer compares to the frequency of deaths due to other cancers.

Learning Objectives:
1. Who described cancers within the chest for the first time?
2. How was lung cancer diagnosed and treated in the last 200 years?
3. For how long has lung cancer been the most common cause of cancer deaths globally?

FIRST DESCRIPTION OF LUNG CANCER

In 1912, Isaac Adler published the first literature review about lung cancer.[1] He listed the known 374 cases mentioned in several European registries over the preceding 50 years. Most physicians at the time thought of lung cancer as an extremely rare disease, and Dr. Adler suspected that lung cancer was underdiagnosed. Not all cases were diagnosed by microscopy, but the number of reported cases had been rising since the mid-1800s.[2]

The concept of cancers arising in the lung has been a rather recent development in medical history. In the 1800s, Dr. René Laennec at the Hopital Necar in Paris started a new practice of combining postmortem pathology with clinical observation. Dr. Laennec also is known for his invention of the stethoscope. He was a keen clinical observer and well-published writer. The lesions that Dr. Laennec described based on his autopsies were unlike the well-known tuberculosis cases in the 1800s. He described these lesions as encephaloid (cerebral) or medullary tumors due to the visual appearance, which was similar to brain tissue. Dr. Laennec was the first author to describe them as cancers arising from the lung. Dr. Laennec's work was soon translated into English by John Forbes in 1821 and reached a wider audience, who became aware of this new entity of cancer arising in the chest.[3] New medical journals, such as the *Lancet Journal* (launched in 1823), promoted the practice of autopsies and helped their readers identify lung cancer as a diagnosis apart from the widespread tuberculosis.[2]

The paradigm of cancer's cellular origin was slowly evolving in the middle of the 1800s based on microscopic work by Theodor Schwann, Johannes Mueller, and Matthias Schleiden.[4] Microscopes, as well as new histological staining and fixing techniques, helped decipher the nature of cell growth. In 1858, Dr. Rudolf Virchow published his book on cellular pathology.[5] He lectured on cellular pathology in the 1860s and the new cellular pathology replaced the theory of humoral imbalances which has been the pathological concept explaining diseases since ancient times.

LUNG CANCER IN THE NINETEENTH CENTURY

The lung cancers in the 19th century were often called fungiform and encephaloid tumors following Laennec's terminology. The diagnosis was mainly based on history and autopsy and not always on histopathology. The identification and terminology were evolving faster in the case of breast cancer because of the better surgical access to breast cancer than to the interthoracic lung cancer.

Since the tumor was not easily accessible and microscopic examination of tissue was not routinely done, it took until the development of chest x-rays and bronchoscopy in the early 20th century to diagnose lung cancer more frequently and reliably.

The epidemiology of lung cancer in the 19th century is therefore difficult to assess. Medical statistics was not commonly used. The field started with Pierre Charles Alexandre Louis (concerning debunking bloodletting) in the early 19th century and was further pioneered by John Snow (concerning the cholera epidemic) and Florence Nightingale (concerning sanitation). Cancer, however, was not the main interest of epidemiologists in the 19th century; rather, the focus was on diseases such as gout, congestive heart failure, and tuberculosis. In the late 19th century, cancer was increasingly mentioned in registries.[2] A registry in Frankfurt, Germany, listed all cancer deaths in the city, and lung cancer was found to involve less than 1% of the deaths.

FIRST BREAKTHROUGHS IN LUNG CANCER TREATMENT

The surgical resection of lung cancer evolved in the first part of the 20th century. Surgery within the chest was mainly driven by trying to treat tuberculosis. Another reason why thoracic surgery became more standard was the treatment of war casualties, often involving the chest, during the World War I (WWI). It is important to know that surgery in the early 20th century was done in spontaneously breathing patients.

At the time, surgery was limited to the collapse of the lungs when opening the chest cavity. To circumvent this problem, Dr. Ernst Ferdinand Sauerbruch developed the negative-pressure chamber, in which the operating field was within a negative-pressure chamber.[6] At the same time, Dr. Morristan Davies, a young surgeon in the United Kingdom, started active intubation; however, this was performed without anesthesia. Dr. Davies is also credited for doing the first lobectomy in 1912 on a young man with lung cancer. The patient unfortunately succumbed to postoperative empyema. Dr. Ivan Magill developed artificial ventilation in the 1920s, which made chest surgery more feasible by intubating one lung while doing surgery on the other lung. This technique became standard of care after the 1940s.[7]

Dr. Evarts Graham accomplished the first curative resection of lung cancer. In 1933, he performed a successful pneumonectomy at Barnes Hospital in St. Louis, Missouri. The patient was an obstetrician who received anesthesia with nitrous oxide and oxygen and was intubated. He had a central left upper lobe mass, and a left pneumonectomy was performed, with cauterization of the stump by silver nitrate. Radon seeds were left in the chest cavity to irradiate tumor cells.[8] The ribs of the right chest wall were removed to allow the collapse onto the stump. This was the first published patient cured of lung cancer. Incidentally, the patient survived his surgeon, Dr. Graham, who died in 1957 of lung cancer himself.[9]

Over the course of the next 20 years, surgeons were resecting lung cancers more routinely. X-rays and bronchoscopy also were more commonly used.[10] In the 1950s, radiation therapy of lung cancer became a more standard option as well in patients unable to undergo surgery.

Despite the early advances, the mortality of lung cancer remained very high. Studies in the 1950s compared radiation therapy to surgery in lung cancer; both modalities continued to have dismal results, with mortalities more than 80%.[2]

Chemotherapy had its first clinical breakthrough in the 1940s for patients with leukemia. It was soon tried in solid cancers, and in the late 1950s chemotherapy, such as cyclophosphamide and busulfan, was tested in lung cancer, with disappointing results[11] (**Figure 1-1**).

THE CHALLENGE OF LUNG CANCER AND ITS GLOBAL EPIDEMIC

By the 1970s, lung cancer has turned into one of the most common causes of death. Few patients with lung cancer were referred to surgery in Great Britain and rarely cured. Often, the patients were not told that they had lung cancer, and many of the patients dying of lung cancer died at home in agonizing pain and distress. Possibly related to the frequency, fatality, and high symptom burden of lung cancer in the 1970s, the hospice movement started in the United Kingdom.[2]

Due to the poor outcomes treating lung cancer, increased efforts were undertaken to prevent lung cancer. Antismoking campaigners were increasingly politically active, and the media presented more and more of the rest of the Marlboro story. These campaigns helped in the stigmatization of smoking. Several decades after the initial scientific connection between tobacco and lung cancer was published, the public discussion about tobacco's use and risks started to become louder and more influential.

Once smoking was more and more negatively stigmatized, doctors and professionals were the first to stop smoking. In 1980, the consumption of cigarettes was almost half compared to consumption in the 1950s[12] (**Figure 1-2**). Smoking was increasingly associated with socioeconomic biases in the late 1970s, and smokers were increasingly thought of as social misfits.

Also adding to the stigma, more research in the 1980s showed the risk of passive smoking (secondhand smoking, environmental tobacco exposure). Studies, initially from Japan, clearly demonstrated the risk of passive smoking. The finding of passive smoking as a risk factor was a major contributor to the change of policies and the approach toward the tobacco industry.[13]

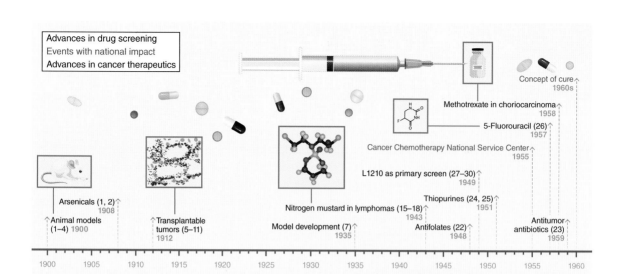

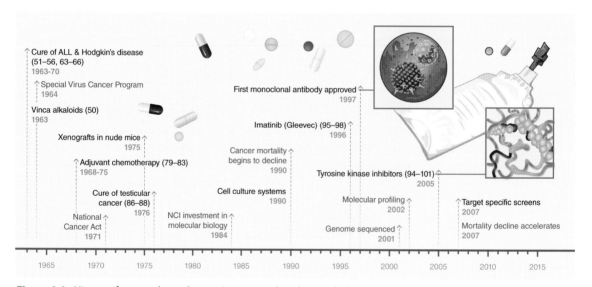

Figure 1-1. History of cancer chemotherapy (ALL, acute lymphocytic leukemia; NCI, National Cancer Institute). (Reproduced with permission from DeVita VT Jr, Chu E. A history of cancer chemotherapy. *Cancer Res.* 2008;68(21): 8643-53.)

In the 1950s, the idea arose that lung cancer could be found by chest x-rays in an early stage. The idea was based on positive experience in cervical cancer screening outcomes, and the intent was to find lung cancer early in its asymptomatic stage and to have a better chance of curing it. However, none of these large studies in the United States and Europe using chest x-rays alone showed any benefit in screening to improve survival despite finding more cancers by using chest x-rays.

Only in recent years have large screening trials using chest computed tomography (CT) (NLST, NELSON) been successful in shifting the stage of lung cancer to an earlier, curable stage.

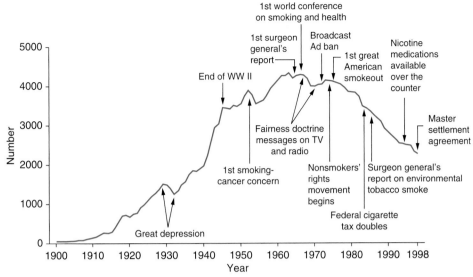

Figure 1-2. Cigarette consumption per capita in the United States in the 20th century. (Reproduced with permission from Centers for Disease Control and Prevention. Achievements in public health 1900-1999, tobacco use—United States 1900-1999. *MMWR Morb Mortal Wkly Rep.* 1999;48(43):986-93.)

In the 1970s, medical oncology was established as a specialty. Based on experience in other cancers (eg, lymphoma, testicular cancer), attempts to treat lung cancer with chemotherapy again were initiated.[14] Small cell lung cancer, which was described as its own entity in 1959, had in fact impressive, but short-lived, responses to chemotherapy.[15,16] However, in non–small cell lung cancer no significant responses to the prevailing alkylating chemotherapy regimens were seen, and it took until the 1990s for chemotherapy to find a role in the treatment of non–small cell lung cancer.

While the treatment of lung cancer was not advancing, prognostication of lung cancer was slowly adapting lung cancer staging based on tumor size, lymph-node involvement, and metastasis (TNM) at time of diagnosis. The TNM staging system was first introduced in 1943 by Dr. Paul Denoix, a breast surgeon at the Institute Gustave Roussy in Paris.[17] The American Joint Commission on Cancer announced in 1968 the adaptation of the TNM system. The arrival of CT scans in the 1970s made TNM staging of lung cancer more practical. The International Association for the Study of Lung Cancer (IASLC) proposed the TNM staging system that was based on Dr. Clifton Mountain's for a few thousand patients at MD Anderson Cancer Center.[18] Since then, the IASLC has systematically expanded the database worldwide to more than 100,000 patients, with periodic updates refining its criteria of stage classifications.

CLINICAL PEARL: It was only in the 1990s that the benefit of systemic chemotherapy in non–small lung cancer was demonstrated in randomized trials, first in stage III disease (Dillman trial, 1990)[19] and later in stage IV lung cancer (ELVIS [Elderly Lung Cancer Vinorelbine Italian Study] trial, 2001).[20]

In the past 20 years, systemic therapy of lung cancer has made major breakthroughs in all stages of lung cancer. At the same time, local therapies have advanced to be minimally invasive, selecting the patients who benefit the most from them. Improved imaging technologies, molecular testing, and innovative treatments targeting oncogenes and tumor environment have led to survival rates in lung cancer in all patient populations.

REFERENCES

1. Adler I. *Primary Malignant Growths of the Lung and Bronchi.* New York, NY: Longmans, Green; 1912.
2. Timmermann C. *A History of Lung Cancer—The Recalcitrant Disease.* London, UK: Palgrave Macmillan; 2014.
3. Laennec RTH. *A Treatise on the Diseases of the Chest and on Mediate Auscultation.* New York, NY: Samuel S. and William Wood; 1838.
4. Ribatti D. An historical note on the cell theory. *Exp Cell Res.* 2018;364(1):1-4. Epub 2018/02/03. doi:10.1016/j.yexcr.2018.01.038.
5. Virchow R. *Cellular Pathology. Physiological and Pathological Histology.* London, UK: Churchill; 1859:486.
6. Vossschulte K. [Thoracic surgery: history and present status (author's transl)]. *Langenbecks Arch Surg.* 1975;339:599-612. Epub 1975/11/01.
7. Meade Richard HE. *A History of Thoracic Surgery.* Springfield, IL: Thomas, Bannerstone House; 1961.
8. D'Amico TA. Historical perspectives of the American Association for Thoracic Surgery: Evarts A. Graham (1883-1957). *J Thorac Cardiovasc Surg.* 2011;142(4):735-739. Epub 2011/08/09. doi:10.1016/j.jtcvs.2011.06.028.
9. Horn L, Johnson DH. Evarts A. Graham and the first pneumonectomy for lung cancer. *J Clin Oncol.* 2008;26(19):3268-3275. Epub 2008/07/02. doi:10.1200/jco.2008.16.8260.
10. Mountain CF. The evolution of the surgical treatment of lung cancer. *Chest Surgery Clin N Am.* 2000;10(1): 83-104. Epub 2000/02/26.
11. DeVita VT Jr, Chu E. A history of cancer chemotherapy. *Cancer Res.* 2008;68(21):8643-8653. Epub 2008/11/01. doi:10.1158/0008-5472.Can-07-6611.
12. Centers for Disease Control and Prevention. Achievements in public health 1900-1999, tobacco use—United States 1900-1999. *MMWR Morb Mortal Wkly Rep.* 1999;48(43):986-993.
13. Allan BM. *The Cigarette Century.* New York, NY: Basic Books; 2007.
14. Burchenal JH. The historical development of cancer chemotherapy. *Semin Oncol.* 1977;4(2):135-146. Epub 1977/06/01.
15. Azzopardi JG. Oat-cell carcinoma of the bronchus. *J Pathol Bacteriol.* 1959;78:513-519. Epub 1959/10/01.
16. Haddadin S, Perry MC. History of small-cell lung cancer. *Clin Lung Cancer.* 2011;12(2):87-93. Epub 2011/05/10.
17. Harmer M, Denoix P, Hamperl H. The TNM-system. *Aktuelle Probl Chir.* 1970;14:25-36. Epub 1970/01/01.
18. Carr DT, Mountain CF. The staging of lung cancer. *Semin Oncol.* 1974;1(3):229-334. Epub 1974/09/01.
19. Dillman RO, Seagren SL, Propert KJ, Guerra J, Eaton WL, Perry MC, et al. A randomized trial of induction chemotherapy plus high-dose radiation versus radiation alone in stage III non-small-cell lung cancer. *N Engl J Med.* 1990;323(14):940-945.
20. Gridelli C, Perrone F, Gallo C, De Marinis F, Ianniello G, Cigolari S, et al. Vinorelbine is well tolerated and active in the treatment of elderly patients with advanced non-small cell lung cancer. A two-stage phase II study. *Eur J Cancer.* 1997;33(3):392-397.

EPIDEMIOLOGY OF LUNG CANCER

Goetz Kloecker, MD, MBA, MSPH, FACP

You are director of the World Health Organization and ask your global experts which cancer should receive the most attention to prevent its incidence and mortality and consequently decrease the burden of cancer mortality worldwide the most.

Learning Objectives:
1. What is the overall cancer mortality worldwide?
2. What are the cancers that cause the highest number of cancer deaths?
3. How has the lung cancer mortality rate changed over the last century?
4. Which parts of the world have the highest lung cancer mortality?

GLOBAL LUNG CANCER MORTALITY

It is estimated that in 2018 worldwide 18.1 million people were diagnosed with cancer, and 9.6 million died of cancer. Non-communicable diseases are now the cause for most deaths globally; cancer is expected to be the leading cause of deaths in the 21st century.[1]

In 2018, the global incidence of lung cancer was 2,093,876 (11.6% of all cancers), and global deaths by lung cancer were 1,761,007. Of all cancer deaths, 18.4% were due to lung cancer.[1] In 2012, the lung cancer incidence rates were lower, 1.8 million, which demonstrates the expanding epidemic of lung cancer worldwide.[2,3]

Lung cancer is the leading cause of deaths caused by cancer in men and women in high-income countries based on registry data collected by the International Agency for Research on Cancer (IARC) and published by GLOBOCAN (Global Cancer Registry provided by the UICC (Union for International Cancer Control)) and the World Health Organization (WHO) (**Figure 2-1**). Smoking is the main reason for the high incidence of lung cancer. WHO estimated that 100 million people died of tobacco's effect in the 20th century, and for the 21st century, WHO predicted that 1 billion could die due to smoking.[4]

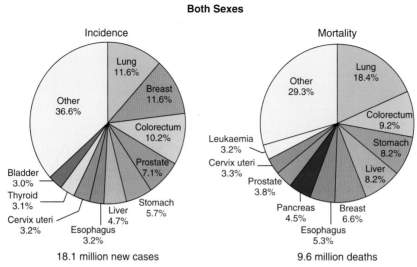

Figure 2-1. Estimated new cancer cases and deaths worldwide. (Reproduced with permission from Bray F, Ferlay J, Soerjomataram I, Siegel RL, Torre LA, Jemal A. Global cancer statistics 2018: GLOBOCAN estimates of incidence and mortality worldwide for 36 cancers in 185 countries. *CA Cancer J Clin.* 2018;68(6):394-424. © 2018 American Cancer Society.)

The incidence rate of lung cancer varies significantly by country following the country's usage of tobacco in the population (**Figures 2-2 and 2-3**).

The highest mortality rates in males were in Central and Eastern Europe and China, 44-47/100,000, and the lowest rates were in Central America and Africa (4-14/100,000). The highest lung cancer mortality rates for women were in the United States (23.5/100,000) and Northern Europe (19/100,000).[2,5,6]

In countries that had an early peak of the tobacco epidemic in the 1950s and 1960s, lung cancer has been decreasing (United States, Western Europe), while for those countries with a recent uptake of general tobacco consumption (China, India, Indonesia, Africa) lung cancer has been on the rise later, decreasing later or continuing to rise in some countries (**Figure 2-4**).

Half of the lung cancer cases in the world occur presently in developing countries, and the overall number of lung cancer deaths globally has increased by 51% since 1985.[7] Despite the overall trend of improving incidence rates in high-income countries, lung cancer is the leading cause of cancer death in many countries.

LUNG CANCER IN THE UNITED STATES

Lung cancer incidence rates have declined in men and women in the United States over the last 10 years. Lung cancer death rates declined in men by 4% and in women by 2.3% from 2009 to 2015. In 2018, in the United States 135,720 people were estimated to die from lung cancer, 72,500 men and 63,220 women.[8]

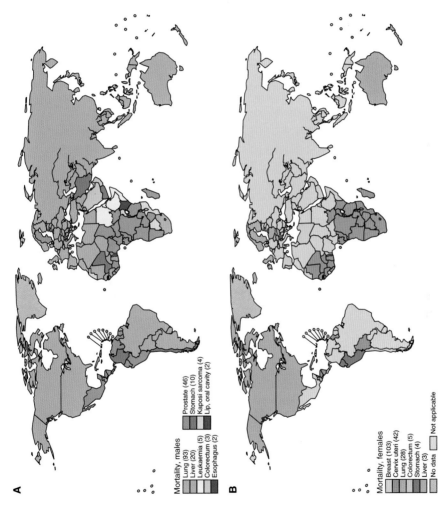

Figure 2-2. Cancer mortality by country. (From Bray F, Ferlay J, Soerjomataram I, Siegel RL, Torre LA, Jemal A. Global cancer statistics 2018: GLOBOCAN estimates of incidence and mortality worldwide for 36 cancers in 185 countries. *CA Cancer J Clin.* 2018;68(6):394-424. Reproduced with permission from World Health Organization. © WHO 2018. All rights reserved.)

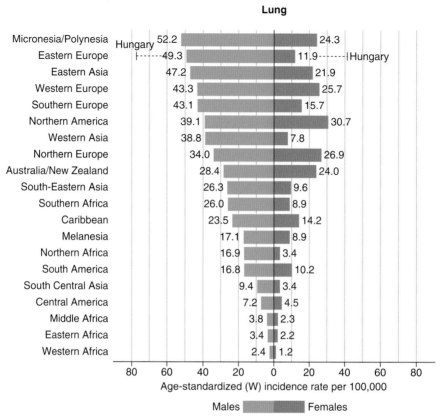

Figure 2-3. Lung cancer incidence by region and gender. (Reproduced with permission from Bray F, Ferlay J, Soerjomataram I, Siegel RL, Torre LA, Jemal A. Global cancer statistics 2018: GLOBOCAN estimates of incidence and mortality worldwide for 36 cancers in 185 countries. *CA Cancer J Clin.* 2018;68(6):394-424. © 2018 American Cancer Society.)

In the United States, there are as many deaths due to lung cancer as there are combined deaths due to colon cancer (50,630), breast cancer (41,400), prostate cancer (29,430), lymphomas (20,960), and kidney cancers (14,970) (**Figure 2-5**).[9]

The mortality in the United States varies by gender and ethnicity. The highest mortality is seen in black men (66.9/100,000) and the lowest in Hispanic women (13.3/100,000) (**Table 2-1**).[9]

LUNG CANCER IN EUROPE

In 2012, there were 3.45 million new cases of cancer in Europe's 40 countries, and there were 1.75 million cancer deaths. The most common causes of cancer deaths were lung (353,000), colorectal (215,000), breast (131,000), and stomach (107,000). Lung cancer killed 254,000 European men and 99,000 European women. The data are based on the European Network of Cancer Registries (ENRC) in collaboration with the IARC[10] (**Figure 2-6**).

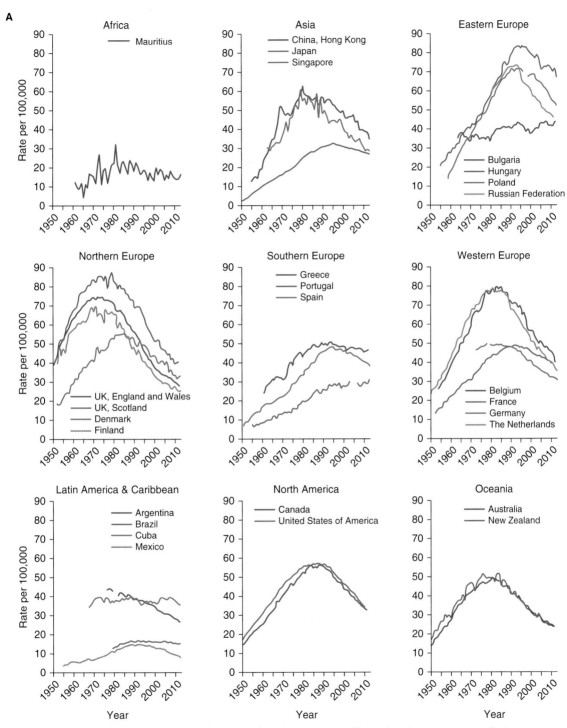

Figure 2-4. (A) Trends in lung cancer mortality in men for select countries; (B) trends in lung cancer mortality in women for select countries. (Reproduced with permission from Islami F, Torre LA, Jemal A. Global trends of lung cancer mortality and smoking prevalence. *Transl Lung Cancer Res.* 2015;4(4):327-338.)

B

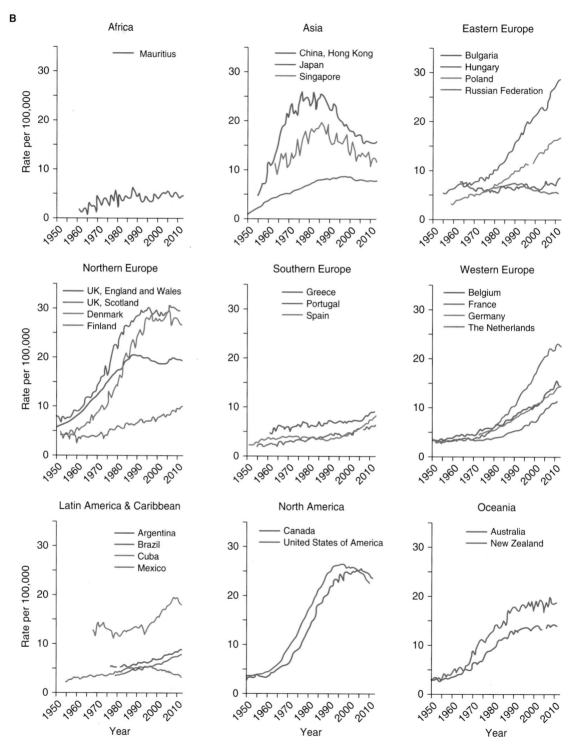

Figure 2-4. (Continued)

Estimated New Cases

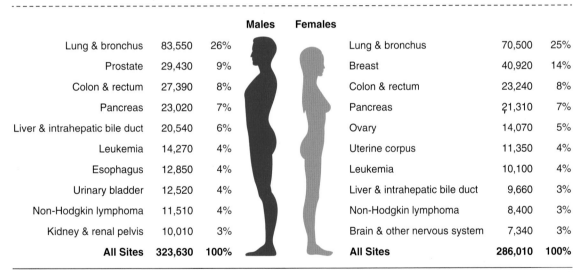

	Males			Females	
Prostate	164,690	19%	Breast	266,120	30%
Lung & bronchus	121,680	14%	Lung & bronchus	112,350	13%
Colon & rectum	75,610	9%	Colon & rectum	64,640	7%
Urinary bladder	62,380	7%	Uterine corpus	63,230	7%
Melanoma of the skin	55,150	6%	Thyroid	40,900	5%
Kidney & renal pelvis	42,680	5%	Melanoma of the skin	36,120	4%
Non-Hodgkin lymphoma	41,730	5%	Non-Hodgkin lymphoma	32,950	4%
Oral cavity & pharynx	37,160	4%	Pancreas	26,240	3%
Leukemia	35,030	4%	Leukemia	25,270	3%
Liver & intrahepatic bile duct	30,610	4%	Kidney & renal pelvis	22,660	3%
All Sites	**856,370**	**100%**	**All Sites**	**878,980**	**100%**

Estimated Deaths

	Males			Females	
Lung & bronchus	83,550	26%	Lung & bronchus	70,500	25%
Prostate	29,430	9%	Breast	40,920	14%
Colon & rectum	27,390	8%	Colon & rectum	23,240	8%
Pancreas	23,020	7%	Pancreas	21,310	7%
Liver & intrahepatic bile duct	20,540	6%	Ovary	14,070	5%
Leukemia	14,270	4%	Uterine corpus	11,350	4%
Esophagus	12,850	4%	Leukemia	10,100	4%
Urinary bladder	12,520	4%	Liver & intrahepatic bile duct	9,660	3%
Non-Hodgkin lymphoma	11,510	4%	Non-Hodgkin lymphoma	8,400	3%
Kidney & renal pelvis	10,010	3%	Brain & other nervous system	7,340	3%
All Sites	**323,630**	**100%**	**All Sites**	**286,010**	**100%**

Figure 2-5. Ten leading cancer incidence and death rates in the United States by gender from 1930 to 2015. (Reproduced with permission from Siegel RL, Miller KD, Jemal A. Cancer statistics, 2018. *CA Cancer J Clin.* 2018;68(1):7-30. © 2018 American Cancer Society.)

TABLE 2-1	Lung Cancer Mortality by Gender and Ethnicity, United States, 2015					
	ALL	WHITE	BLACK	ASIAN	AMERICAN NATIVE	HISPANIC
Men	53.8	56.3	66.9	31.0	45.0	26.4
Women	35.4	39.0	34.4	17.7	30.6	13.3

Data from Siegel RL, Miller KD, Jemal A. Cancer statistics, 2018. *CA Cancer J Clin.* 2018;68(1):7-30.

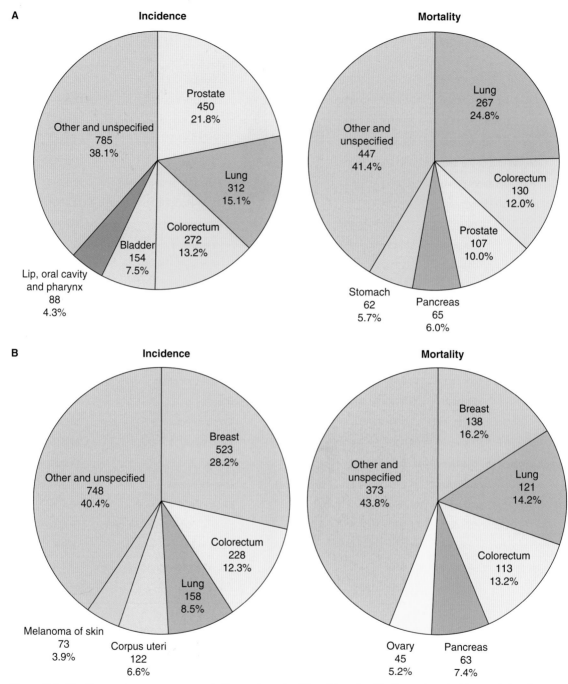

Figure 2-6. The five most common cancers in Europe in males (A) and females (B). (Reproduced with permission from Ferlay J, Steliarova-Foucher E, Lortet-Tieulent J, et al. Cancer incidence and mortality patterns in Europe: estimates for 40 countries in 2012. *Eur J Cancer.* 2013;49(6):1374-403. Copyright © Elsevier.)

REFERENCES

1. Bray F, Ferlay J, Soerjomataram I, Siegel RL, Torre LA, Jemal A. Global cancer statistics 2018: GLOBOCAN estimates of incidence and mortality worldwide for 36 cancers in 185 countries. *CA Cancer Journal Clin.* 2018;68(6):394-424. Epub 2018/09/13. doi:10.3322/caac.21492.
2. Torre LA, Bray F, Siegel RL, Ferlay J, Lortet-Tieulent J, Jemal A. Global cancer statistics, 2012. *CA Cancer J Clin.* 2015;65(2):87-108. Epub 2015/02/06. doi:10.3322/caac.21262.
3. Torre LA, Siegel RL, Ward EM, Jemal A. Global cancer incidence and mortality rates and trends—an update. *Cancer Epidemiol Biomarkers Prev.* 2016;25(1):16-27. Epub 2015/12/17. doi:10.1158/1055-9965.Epi-15-0578.
4. World Health Organization (WHO). *WHO Report on the Global Tobacco Epidemic, 2008.* Geneva, Switzerland: World Health Organization; 2008.
5. Ezzati M, Riboli E. Behavioral and dietary risk factors for noncommunicable diseases. *N Engl J Med.* 2013;369(10):954-964. Epub 2013/09/06. doi:10.1056/NEJMra1203528.
6. Islami F, Torre LA, Jemal A. Global trends of lung cancer mortality and smoking prevalence. *Transl Lung Cancer Res.* 2015;4(4):327-338. Epub 2015/09/18. doi:10.3978/j.issn.2218-6751.2015.08.04.
7. Dela Cruz CS, Tanoue LT, Matthay RA. Lung cancer: epidemiology, etiology, and prevention. *Clin Chest Medic.* 2011;32(4):605-644. Epub 2011/11/08. doi:10.1016/j.ccm.2011.09.001.
8. Siegel RL, Miller KD, Jemal A. Cancer statistics, 2020. *CA Cancer J Clin.* 2020;70(1):7-30. doi: 10.3322/caac.21590. Epub 2020 Jan 8.
9. Siegel RL, Miller KD, Jemal A. Cancer statistics, 2018. *CA Cancer J Clin.* 2018;68(1):7-30. Epub 2018/01/10. doi:10.3322/caac.21442.
10. Ferlay J, Steliarova-Foucher E, Lortet-Tieulent J, et al. Cancer incidence and mortality patterns in Europe: estimates for 40 countries in 2012. *Eur J Cancer.* 2013;49(6):1374-1403. Epub 2013/03/15. doi:10.1016/j.ejca.2012.12.027.

3

ETIOLOGY OF LUNG CANCER

Goetz Kloecker, MD, MBA, MSPH, FACP • Brian Dong, MD • Rohit Kumar, MD

Your 60-year-old female patient with metastatic non-small cell lung cancer never smoked.

She has been healthy all her life, and her social, family, and professional history is noncontributory.

She asks you why she has lung cancer.

Learning Objectives:
1. What are the risk factors for lung cancer?
2. What is the second most common cause of lung cancer?
3. How frequently does asbestos cause lung cancer?
4. What professional exposures are risk factors?

RISK FACTORS

Tobacco

Tobacco smoking accounts for 80%-90% of all lung cancer incidence, with a reported 20- to 30-fold increased risk in smokers compared to non-smokers. This is by far the most thoroughly established causal relationship in medical literature. There is a lag period of approximately 20 years between the exposure and disease occurrence.[1]

The widespread use of tobacco in the form of cigarette smoking started after the invention of the cigarette-rolling machine in the late 19th century. In the mid-20th century, 2 large epidemiological studies established a definite etiologic role of tobacco smoking in lung cancer.[2,3] This led to the US surgeon general issuing a public safety warning in 1964 regarding the potential harmful effects of tobacco smoking and then reemphasizing its stance in 2004.[4] A combined effort has led to a significant decline in tobacco smoking: from 42.4% of the adult population in 1965 to 14.0% of all adults in 2017 (15.8% of men, 12.2% of women smokers).[5]

Since the 1950s, the cigarette has significantly evolved, with a shift to its filtered use. There has also been a decrease in the tar and nicotine contents as per machine-measured yields. Unfortunately, these changes have not resulted in a decrease in lung cancer risk or mortality, as evident by the results of the Cancer Prevention Studies (CPSs). In CPS-1 follow-up period 1960-1972, lung cancer mortality risk was compared based on tar yield of the products. The mortality in the low- and medium-yield group was 20% lower than that in the high-yield group. In CPS-2 follow-up period 1980-1986, with the composition of cigarettes changing, it was expected that there would be a decrease in mortality. To the contrary, the mortality was higher in CPS-2 (**Figure 3-1**).

It has been suggested that the change in smoking habits or more smoking as low-yield products were thought to be "safer" may have dampened any benefits of the low-yield cigarettes. Overall, there has been no benefit of changing cigarette design and composition.[1]

Tobacco contains a psychoactive compound called nicotine that causes addiction but itself is not carcinogenic. It is an acetylcholine agonist that causes release of endorphins and neurotransmitters into the bloodstream, leading to dependence. It has also been associated with progression of a preexisting lung tumor.[6-8] Menthol is a frequent additive to tobacco products to make cigarettes more palatable with mint flavor and reduced mucosal irritation. These products were specially targeted to females, African Americans, and young adults. Besides its soothing effects, menthol upregulates cholinergic receptors and their binding to nicotine, enhancing the addictive effects. It also promotes aggressive smoking habits. Regulatory authorities have proposed a ban on menthol additive altogether.[9,10]

The International Agency for Research on Cancer (IARC) has identified at least 50 carcinogens in tobacco smoke. Mainstream smoke contains many potential carcinogens, including polycyclic aromatic hydrocarbons (PAHs), aromatic amines, N-nitrosamines, and other organic and inorganic compounds (eg, benzene, vinyl chloride, arsenic, and chromium). Of particular importance are the N-nitrosamines, especially 4-(methylnitrosamino)-1(3-pyridyl)-1-butanone (NNK), which has been shown to induce adenocarcinoma in animal models.[9,11]

Tobacco smoking can cause all histologic subtypes of lung cancer. In the last 50 years, there has been a shift in histologic characteristics, with adenocarcinoma taking over squamous cell carcinoma to become the most common subtype. The adenocarcinoma tends to arise more peripherally and squamous cell carcinoma more centrally. This shift is thought to be due to introduction of low-tar filter cigarettes and changes in smoking topography that have increased exposure of peripheral lung tissue to the carcinogens.[11]

The cumulative incidence of lung cancer was 31.7% in male and 15.3% in female heavy smokers compared to 0.9% in male and 0.5% in female non-smokers.[12]

The duration of smoking is a much stronger risk factor than the quantity smoked. For example, a 3-fold increase in quantity of tobacco smoking is associated with a 3-fold increase in lung cancer risk, while an increase in duration of exposure by 3 times has a 100-fold increase in the risk.[13] Approximately 90% of all lung cancer mortality is attributable to tobacco smoking.[14] Smoking cessation significantly decreases (up to 90%) lung cancer risk but remains higher than never-smokers even after more than 50 years of abstinence.[11,15]

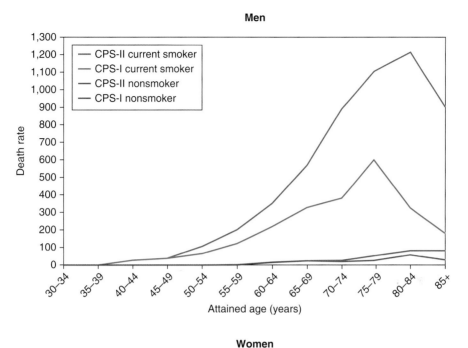

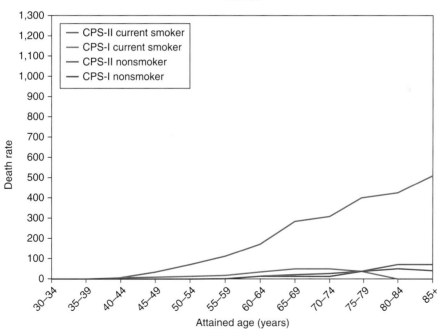

Rate per 100,000 person-years.

Figure 3-1. Age-specific death rates from lung cancer among current cigarette smokers and lifelong never-smokers. (Reproduced with permission from Alberg AJ, Samet JM. Epidemiology of lung cancer. *Chest.* 2003;123(1)(suppl):21s-49s; Adapted from Burns DM, Garfinkel L, Samet JM, eds. Changes in Cigarette Related Disease Risks and Their Implications for Prevention and Control. Bethesda, MD: US Government Printing Office; 1997: 317.)

Other forms of tobacco smoking like cigars and pipes are also associated with lung cancer risk but to a lesser extent compared to cigarette smoking. This likely is due to less smoking frequency and depth of inhalation. On average, smoking 5 cigars a day is equivalent to 1 pack a day of cigarettes.[11,13]

Passive Smoking

Passive or secondhand smoking can also contribute to increased lung cancer risk. Various carcinogens, like benzene, benzo[a]pyrene, and 4-(methylnitrosamino)-1-(13-pyridyl-1-butanone), have been identified in environmental tobacco smoke (ETS).[13] The US Environmental Protection Agency (EPA) and the IARC have identified that ETS contains lung carcinogen. In an analysis of 37 published epidemiological studies, the authors found that the excess risk of lung cancer was 24% (95% CI 13%-36%, $p < .001$) in lifelong non-smokers who were exposed to secondhand smoke. The dose-response relation of the risk of lung cancer with both the number of cigarettes smoked by the spouse and the duration of exposure was significant.[16] It has been estimated that lung cancer deaths attributable to ETS is comparable to that of radon or asbestos.[17]

Electronic Cigarettes

Electronic cigarettes (e-cigs) are battery-operated nicotine delivery systems. The system consists of a heating element and replaceable cartridges filled with liquid nicotine, propylene glycol or glycerol, and flavorings. There may be other carcinogenic metals and organic compounds. The heating coil produces vapors from the liquid that are inhaled by the user. E-cigs were introduced to the US market in 2007 and have been largely unregulated except for mandated age checks. In 2016, the US Food and Drug Administration (FDA) claimed jurisdiction and regulatory authority over the manufacture, promotion, sale, and distribution, although compliance is yet to be enforced and may not include all manufacturers.[18]

Although advertised as the "safer option," potential long-term side effects are not yet known. Use of e-cigs has been shown to be more effective than traditional nicotine replacement therapy. In a recently published randomized control trial of 886 participants, the 1-year abstinence rate was higher in the e-cig group compared to 9.9% for the nicotine replacement group (18.0% vs 9.9%) and had a relative risk (RR) of 1.83 (95% CI 1.30-2.58).[19] The contents of e-cig vapors are different from tobacco smoke, but prolonged exposure to organic compounds, trace metals, and reactive oxygen species can cause chronic inflammation of the respiratory epithelium.

Overall, 15.3% of adults aged 18 years or older has ever used an e-cig, and 3.2% currently used e-cigs in 2016. Adults aged 18-24 years were the most likely to have ever used an e-cig (23.8%).[20] There have been growing concerns regarding the rapid increase in use of e-cigs in adolescents and young adults who were previous non-smokers of traditional tobacco. Furthermore, recent studies have shown initiation of traditional tobacco smoking in previous non-smokers who start using e-cig.[21]

Current Centers for Disease Control and Prevention (CDC) recommendations are that e-cigs have the potential to benefit adult smokers who are not pregnant if used as a complete substitute for regular cigarettes and other smoked tobacco products. E-cigarettes are not safe for youth, young adults, pregnant women, or adults who do not currently use tobacco products.[22]

Cannabis

Marijuana is the most commonly used illicit drug in the United States.[23] The landscape of marijuana use is rapidly changing with the increase in its legalization for recreational use. Cannabis contains a psychoactive substance known as tetrahydrocannabinol or THC that, like nicotine, has addictive properties but has not been directly associated with carcinogenesis. Approximately 9% of those who experiment with marijuana will become dependent.[24] Similar to tobacco smoke, marijuana smoke has several potent carcinogens. Furthermore, the latter may be even more cytotoxic and mutagenic.[25] The tar and PAH content of marijuana smoke is also higher than that of tobacco.[9,26] The smoking technique of marijuana is significantly different from tobacco, involving deep inhalation and longer breath-holding times, and it is frequently used without filters. In addition, experimental studies employing bronchial biopsies have demonstrated that marijuana users manifest not only airway inflammation, but also histopathological or molecular changes indicative of precancerous bronchial activity.[27,28]

Even though there are several experimental studies that provide biological evidence of increased lung cancer risk associated with marijuana, the epidemiological studies of this association have been inconsistent. This is partly due to a small sample size, previous illegal status of marijuana, and several confounding effects of tobacco smoking, including tobacco mixing with marijuana in some regions. In a Swedish 40-year cohort study of military conscripts, there was no significant increased risk of lung cancer in "ever" versus "never" marijuana smokers after adjustment for baseline tobacco use, alcohol use, respiratory conditions, and socioeconomic status. In the subset of heavy cannabis smokers (>50 times), there was a 2-fold increase in risk of lung cancer (adjusted hazard ratio [HR] 2.12, 95% CI 1.08-4.14) over the 40-year follow-up period.[29] The cohort study on lung cancer reported an increased risk for marijuana use with a dose-response evaluation for the number of times used in a lifetime, but "lifetime" use was assessed only up to the ages of 18 to 20 years, with no information on subsequent use over the 40-year follow-up period and no dose-response evaluation for frequency. In a pooled analysis of 6 case-controlled studies from the United States, Canada, United Kingdom, and New Zealand, data on 2,159 lung cancer cases and 2,985 controls analyzed by Zhang et al. The overall pooled odds ratio (OR) for habitual versus non-habitual or never users was 0.96 (95% CI, 0.66-1.38).[30] There is currently no consensus on whether marijuana use is directly associated with increased lung cancer risk, but there are data supporting increased tobacco use associated with marijuana smoking in adolescents and young adults.[31,32]

ENVIRONMENTAL AND OCCUPATIONAL FACTORS

Air (Outdoor) Pollution

With the industrialization of major cities throughout the world in the mid- to late 1900s, an increase in lung cancer incidence raised the question of pollution as a risk factor for developing lung cancer. Particulate matter, in regard to air pollution, is a term used to describe the mixture of small, solid particles and liquid droplets in the air that comes from sources such as power plants and automobiles. In the United States, the awareness was first raised when the Clean Air Act Amendments in 1977 required the EPA review scientific criteria for ambient air pollution to identify air quality standards.

A report from the EPA analyzed size differences in different particles to determine which inhaled particle sizes were the most detrimental to human health. The report showed that there were 2 necessary cutoffs for inhalable particles, 15 and 2.5 μm. Particles greater than 15 μm were retained in the upper respiratory tract and had minimal lower respiratory tract penetration.[33] Particles less than 2.5 μm were classified as fine particles and penetrated deeper into the respiratory tract. The major components of fine particles are sulfate, ammonium, and nitrate ions as well as more carcinogenic compounds, such as arsenic and selenium.[34]

One large study in the United States followed 8,111 adults in 6 different cities for over 14 years and found air pollution to be positively associated with increased death from lung cancer and cardiovascular death.[35] In 2013, a large prospective analysis of 17 European populations called the European Study of Cohorts for Air Pollution Effects (ESCAPE) followed over 300,000 people for an average of 12.8 years and analyzed associations with exposure to different size particulate matter.[36] The risk for lung cancer with particulate matter less than 10 μm was HR 1.22, 95% CI 1.03-1.45 per 10 μg/m³; for particles less than 2.5 μm, the HR was 1.18 (0.96-1.46) per 5 μg/m³.[36] In an another study, a 10-μg/m³ change in fine particles measuring less than 2.5 μm has been associated with an 8% increase in lung cancer mortality after adjusting for various factors, including smoking status.[37] The risk of lung cancer from pollution is further increased with tobacco smoking.

With an overwhelming amount of data confirming associations between particulate matter and lung cancer, the World Health Organization (WHO) in conjunction with the IARC officially declared particulate matter as carcinogenic to humans.[38] In the year 2015, ambient air pollution was attributable for 4.4 (95% CI 2.7-6.1) age-adjusted lung cancer deaths per 100,000 people worldwide.[39]

Indoor Pollution

In many developing countries, fossil and plant-based fuels have been the primary source of domestic energy for heating and cooking. Indoor pollution due to burning of these fuels, along with poor ventilation, has been associated with lung cancer risk. In a case-control study of rural China, the OR for lung cancer associated with coal use compared with that for biomass (crop residues, wood, sticks, and twigs) in the house of longest residence was 1.29 (95% CI 1.03-1.61), adjusted for smoking and socioeconomic status. The risk for lung cancer increased relative to the percentage of time that coal was used over the past 30 years ($p = .02$).[40] In a pooled analysis from International Lung Cancer Consortium, predominant coal users (OR = 1.64, 95% CI 1.49-1.81)—particularly coal users in Asia (OR = 4.93, 95% CI 3.73-6.52)—and predominant wood users in North American and European countries (OR = 1.21; 95% CI 1.06-1.38) experienced a higher risk of lung cancer when compared to non–solid fuel user (oil, gas, electricity).[41]

The IARC has classified indoor emissions from household coal combustion as human carcinogens.

Asbestos

Asbestos is a term used to refer to a collection of naturally occurring minerals that share a fibrous nature in their composition. It is the most common occupational cause of lung cancer. It consists of 2 subtypes: serpentine (chrysotile) and amphibole (amosite, crocidolite, and tremolites). Asbestos materials are largely inert and non-flammable and have a tensile strength stronger than steel. These properties have led to it being incorporated into over 3,000 products, from brake pad lining in car manufacturing to insulation and cement products for the construction industry.

Asbestos exposure can cause both pleural and pulmonary disease. Asbestos-induced interstitial lung disease is referred to as asbestosis. The pathogenesis of asbestos-associated disorders was believed to be due to inspiration of fiber complexes that penetrated deep into the lungs. Several studies in the 1970s explored the response of mesothelial cells, macrophages, and alveoli to deposition of various asbestos fibers.[42,43] More recent research has shed more light on asbestosis-mediating mesothelial cells, leading to release of reactive oxygen species that lead to translocation of high-mobility group box 1 (HMGB-1) protein, a driving force of oncogenesis. HMGB-1 has served as an important focus of malignant mesothelioma and has been proposed as a possible biomarker for diagnosis and a target for treatment.[44]

Several asbestosis-related diseases have been noted, such as benign pleural effusions, interstitial lung disease pattern secondary to asbestos, bronchogenic carcinoma, and mesothelioma.[13] The risk appears to be higher for workers exposed to amphibole fibers than chrysotile fibers. The question of whether asbestos exposure alone or asbestosis represents the risk factor for lung cancer remains an area of debate, although the latter has been shown to be more important.[45] In a prospective cohort study, asbestos exposure had an RR of 3.49 (95% CI 1.69-7.18) compared to the non-exposed group after adjusting for several factors, including age, smoking, and other occupational exposures.[46] Asbestos and cigarette smoking are both independent causes of lung cancer but in combination have a multiplicative effect. There is also a dose- and duration-dependent increase in lung cancer risk to asbestos exposure.[11] The RRs for lung cancer with asbestos exposure alone and cigarette smoking alone are 6-fold and 11-fold, respectively, but with exposure to both, the risk is increased 59-fold.[47]

The United States has taken extensive measures over the last 50 years to limit any use of asbestos given the increasing knowledge about its adverse health effects. The Occupational Safety and Health Act of 1970 was the first US congressional act to regulate and limit work exposures to asbestos. This regulatory power was extended by the EPA in 1976 with the Toxic Substances Control Act, allowing the EPA to monitor how chemicals were manufactured and used in various products. Additionally, asbestosis is listed as a type of air pollution in the Clean Air Act given concern for airborne fibers that can lead to respiratory issues. In the Asbestos Hazard Emergency Response Act (AHERA) of 1986, Congress forced schools to have regulations for limiting asbestos materials given unintended exposures to children. To date, there is no full ban on asbestos products. Most states have their own legislation on asbestos regulation, and most follow recommendations from the EPA's National Emission Standards for Hazardous Air Pollutants. Such regulations include how to dispose of asbestos-containing products when doing residential demolition or renovations and how to handle asbestos-contaminated materials.

Radon

The radon 222 is a gaseous decay product of elements (radium 226 and uranium 238) found ubiquitously in soil and rocks. Radon can accumulate in enclosed areas, such as mines or houses, and dissolve in groundwater. Radon is an established human lung carcinogen. It emits alpha particles that cause DNA damage in respiratory epithelium.[48,49]

Although radon exposure in uranium mine workers led to our understanding of its association with lung cancer, there are significant differences between the conditions of exposure in mines and those in houses. These differences include the relative proportion of radon itself to its decay products, respiratory rate, and particle size distributions.[13,50] These differences may complicate extrapolation data from miners' radon lung cancer risks to residential settings, but there have been studies that confirm generalizability of data from miners to the general population.

In a combined analysis of 7 case-control studies from North America, the estimated risk of lung cancer was 11% higher after exposure to residential radon. The estimated OR after exposure to radon at a concentration of 100 Bq/m^3 (2.7 pCi/L) in the exposure time window 5 to 30 years before the index date was 1.11 (95% CI 1.00-1.28). Among cases, 38% were diagnosed with adenocarcinoma, 22% with squamous cell carcinoma, and 16% with small/oat cell carcinoma.[51] These findings were similar to the meta-analysis of 13 European studies.[52] The RR was found to be time dependent and decreased when more time had elapsed since the last exposure. Long-term exposure yielded a greater risk than did short-term exposure, irrespective of the rate of exposure.[53]

The National Research Council has estimated that residential radon may account for 10% to 15% of the lung cancer burden in the United States. The average level of radon in homes in the United States is 1.3 pCi/L, and the average level outside is 0.4 pCi/L. Radon is potentially harmful in poorly ventilated structures. The EPA estimates that exposure to a radon level of 4 pCi/L has the lifetime risk of lung cancer death of 7 per 1,000 in never-smokers compared with 62 per 1,000 for ever-smokers. Approximately, 15,000 to 22,000 annual lung cancer deaths in the United States are related to radon, but only 10% of deaths occur among non-smokers.[54] A map of high-radon areas in the United States is shown in **Figure 3-2.**

The EPA recommends taking action to remediate the residential radon level at or above 4 pCi/L and to consider remediation for levels between 2 and 4 pCi/L. An estimated 1 in 15 US homes has radon levels at or above this EPA action level. Lowering radon levels below the EPA action level has been estimated to decrease 2%-4% of lung cancer mortality.[54] The cost-effectiveness analyses of radon control strategies in the United States have been shown to reach the threshold level only if residential high-risk patients like smokers are engaged in testing and remediation.[50]

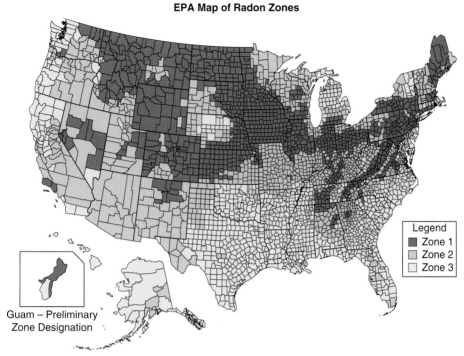

EPA Map of Radon Zones

Legend
- ■ Zone 1
- ▨ Zone 2
- □ Zone 3

Guam – Preliminary
Zone Designation

The Map of Radon Zones was developed in 1993 to identify areas of the U.S. with the potential for elevated indoor radon levels. The map is intended to help governments and other organizations target risk reduction activities and resources. The Map of Radon Zones should not be used to determine if individual homes need to be tested. No matter where you live, test your home for radon—it's easy and inexpensive. Fix your home if your radon level is 4 picocuries per liter (pCi/L) or higher. Consider fixing if your level is between 2 and 4 pCi/L.

The Map of Radon Zones was developed using data on indoor radon measurements, geology, aerial radioactivity, soil parameters, and foundation types. EPA recommends that this map be supplemented with any available local data in order to further understand and predict the radon potential for a specific area.

Figure 3-2. Radon distribution in the United States, US Geological Society. Generalized radon potential of United States. (United States Geological Survey; 1995. https://www.epa.gov/radon/find-information-about-local-radon-zones-and-state-contact-information. Accessed August 21, 2020.)

Other Occupational Exposures

Silica is the most abundant mineral on Earth. It exists in amorphous and crystalline forms. The latter is associated with various pulmonary diseases referred to as silicosis. The IARC classified crystalline silica as a human carcinogen in 1997. In the largest meta-analysis of 85 studies, the pooled standardized mortality ratio (SMR) and standardized incidence ratio (SIR) were 2.32 (95% CI 1.91-2.81) and 2.49 (95% CI 1.87-3.33), respectively, in silicosis and 1.78 (95% CI 1.07-2.96) and 1.18 (95% CI 0.86-1.62), in non-silicosis patients, respectively. A positive exposure-response relation was found between cumulative silica exposure and risk of lung cancer.[55] Based on this evidence, the US Occupational Safety and Health Administration (OSHA) lowered the occupational exposure limit for crystalline silica from 0.1 to 0.05 mg/m^3. Concomitant smoking has an additive effect on lung cancer risk from silica exposure. In a large cohort study, risk of lung cancer death among smokers exposed to silica (HR 5.07, 95% CI 3.41-7.52) was higher compared to non-smokers (HR 1.60, 95% CI 1.01-2.55) when exposed to the same cumulative dose of silica (>1.12 mg/m³).[56]

Occupational exposures to several metals, like arsenic, beryllium, cadmium, chromium, and nickel, are also known to increase lung cancer risk.[57]

DIETARY

Several previously published observational studies have reported beneficial effects of the dietary factor on lung cancer. For example, antioxidants like vitamins A, C, and E are shown to have cancer-protective effects. Unfortunately, these effects were not observed in several randomized controlled trials. In a prospective epidemiological study in 1954, the dietary intake of beta-carotene was associated with a lower 19-year incidence of lung cancer in middle-aged men.[58] In a case-control study, the RRs by vitamin A intake quartiles (lowest to highest) were 1.8, 1.8, 1.0, 1.0 (*p* for trend = .001) for men. The effect was not statistically significant for women.[59] At least 2 large randomized double-blind control trials, Beta-Carotene and Retinol Efficacy Trial (CARET) and Alpha-Tocopherol, Beta Carotene Cancer Prevention (ATBC), failed to show such a beneficial effect. Unexpectedly, the mortality rate and incidence of lung cancer in the experimental arm was higher.[60-62]

A large cohort study from the Netherlands has reported the protective effect of a diet rich in fruits and vegetables on lung cancer incidence. Protective effects of fruits and vegetables were stronger in current than in former smokers.[63] In the National Institutes of Health–AARP Diet and Health Study, total fruit and vegetable intake was not associated with lung cancer incidence, although higher consumption of certain botanical subgroups (rosaceae, convolvulaceae, and umbelliferae) had a significant inverse relation to cancer risk in men only.[64] There are reports of other dietary items, like saturated fats, dairy products, and smoked and salted meats, increasing the risk of lung cancer.[65-67]

Despite the inconsistent results of trials and epidemiological studies, the current recommendation by the American Cancer Society https://www.cancer.org/cancer/lung-cancer/causes-risks-prevention/prevention.html is to have a balanced dietary intake and avoid overindulgence in vitamins and other dietary supplements.

INFECTION

The role of infection as a risk factor for lung cancer remains debatable. Lung cancer is the most common non–AIDS-defining malignancy in patients with HIV infection. With the introduction of highly active antiretroviral therapy (HAART), AIDS-related mortality has significantly dropped, but there has been an accompanying increase in lung cancer–related deaths, accounting for 30% of all cancer deaths and 10% of all non–HIV-related deaths.[68] There is no evidence that HAART therapy directly led to this increased risk. Although smoking is more prevalent among individuals with HIV, the risk of lung cancer remains significantly high even after adjusting for smoking status.[69] Among 2,086 AIDS patients, HIV infection was associated with increased lung cancer risk (HR 3.6, 95% CI 1.6-7.9) after adjusting for age, sex, smoking status, and calendar period.[70] Although the not well established but frequent co-infection with oncogenic viruses (Epstein-Barr virus, human herpesvirus, or human papilloma virus [HPV]), the direct effect of HIV virus or prolonged immunosuppression may be the cause of the excess risk of lung cancer in this population.[13] Lung cancer in an individual with HIV/AIDS tends to present in younger patients, more advanced stage, and has significantly reduced overall survival.[68,71]

HPV has been implicated in various cancers, such as genital, anal, and oropharyngeal cancers, but studies regarding its etiologic role in lung cancer have been inconsistent. The possible involvement of HPV in bronchial squamous cell lesions was first suggested in 1979 by Syrjanen, who described epithelial changes in bronchial carcinomas closely resembling those of established HPV lesions in the genital tract, such as exophytic and flat condyloma.[72] The highly oncogenic HPV types associated with lung cancer include 16, 18, 31, 33, and 35. There is inconsistency in the reported prevalence of infection by HPV in patients with lung cancer in different countries, with racial and geographic variations.

One study on lung biopsies from Taiwanese patients showed a significant difference between HPV 16 and HPV 18 infection in lung cancer versus non-cancerous samples (54.6% vs 26.7%).[73] A study in patients from Wuhan showed a different incidence (27.7% vs 5.9%) for HPV 16 and HPV 18 in cancerous and non-cancerous lung samples.[74] On the other hand, in Western Europe, studies with a large number of patients failed to show an etiologic role for HPV in lung cancer.[75,76] Variability in the reported number of HPV-positive lung cancer may be explained by several factors, such as environmental variables, high-risk behavior, genetic susceptibility, and methodologic approaches with varying sensitivity and specificity for HPV identification.[77] In a recently published meta-analysis, HPV infection was associated with cancer of lung; the pooled OR was 3.64 (95% CI 2.60-5.08).[78] It would be interesting to see if the HPV vaccine has had any impact on the incidence of lung cancer.

CHRONIC LUNG AND AIRWAY DISEASE

There is some evidence that certain chronic non-malignant lung diseases may be independent risk factors for lung cancer. Chronic obstructive pulmonary disease (COPD) has been reported to have the strongest risk factor for lung cancer. Although tobacco is the primary cause for both COPD and lung cancer, studies have shown increased lung cancer risk in patients with COPD independent of smoking status. One study showed a significantly higher prevalence of COPD in patients with lung cancer (50% vs 8%) compared to those in a randomly recruited control group (OR 11.6, $p < .0001$) after adjustment for age, sex, and smoking exposure.[79] COPD has been suggested to be an independent risk factor for lung cancer by increasing oxidative stress, chronic inflammation, defective DNA repair mechanisms, and increased cellular proliferation.[80] A large retrospective study has shown cancer-protective effects of inhaled corticosteroids in patients with COPD, which further supports the theory of chronic inflammation leading to lung cancer.[81]

Patients with idiopathic pulmonary fibrosis (IPF), regardless of smoking status, have been reported to have up to an 8-fold increase in risk of cancer compared to controls.[82] The mechanism of this increased risk remains unclear. A study from the United Kingdom compared 1,064 patients with IPF to 4,238 matched controls found a significant in increase in the incidence of lung cancer (rate ratio 4.96; 95% CI 3.00-8.18) after adjusting for age, gender, and smoking status.[83] Besides the confounding effects of smoking, the fibrosis might itself lead to carcinogenesis by the occurrence of atypical or dysplastic epithelial changes.[82,84]

In a case-control study, α1-antitrypsin deficiency carriers had a higher risk of lung cancer when compared to unrelated non-carriers (OR 1.7, 95% CI 1.2-2.4) after adjusting for tobacco use and COPD diagnosis.[85]

GENETIC RISK FACTORS

The genetic risk factors for lung cancer are poorly elucidated. This is supported by the fact that only a fraction of tobacco smokers develop lung cancer, and positive family history is an independent risk factor. In a meta-analysis of 41 published cohort and case-control studies, an affected family member led to a significantly higher risk of lung cancer (RR 1.72, 95% CI 1.56-1.88). The association was only slightly weaker among non-smokers (OR 1.4, 95% CI 1.17-1.68). A positive family history of lung cancer in 2 or more relatives was associated with higher risk (OR 3.6, 95% CI 1.56-8.31).[86] In a retrospective study of lung cancer patients who were never smokers, 18% of the patients had a family history of lung cancer. In a subgroup of patients with lung cancer that has an *EGFR* mutation or ALK translocation, 23% and 12% of the patients had a family history of lung cancer, respectively.[87] The familial incidence of lung cancer may be caused by similar environmental factors or an inherited susceptibility, but teasing out the independent effect of the latter may be difficult.

The genetic factors associated with tobacco-induced lung cancer have been extensively investigated. Large-scale genome-wide association (GWA) studies have identified several lung cancer–susceptible genes. Some of the notable genes are on chromosome 5p15.33, 6p21, and 15q24-25.1. The 15q25 region contains 3 nicotine acetylcholine receptor subunit genes, and its polymorphism has been associated with nicotine dependence. The 5p15.33 region is associated with risks specifically for lung adenocarcinoma. The 6q23-25 and 13q31.3 regions were also identified by GWA studies as being associated with risk for lung cancer, particularly in never-smokers.[88,89] Further studies are required to understand the individual risk of lung cancer based on genetic factors.

RADIATION

Radiation can cause detrimental effects to the exposed tissue by direct damage, generation of free radicals, and inflammation. Radiation therapy (RT) for other cancers like breast cancer and Hodgkin lymphoma increases the risk of secondary lung cancer. In an observational study, breast cancer treated with RT had a higher risk of a second primary lung cancer (2.25% vs 0.23%) compared to patients who did not receive RT (HR 10.078, 95% CI 3.713-27.351).[90] One study of long-term complications of Hodgkin lymphoma reported a mean RR of 2.6-7.0.[91] With improvement in radiation techniques, the risk of second primary lung cancer may not be this prominent.

In the analysis of the Italian COSMOS lung cancer screening trial, an estimated lifetime attributable risk of lung cancer ranged from 5.5 to 1.4 per 10,000 people after 10 years of low-dose computed tomographic screening.[92] This risk has been deemed acceptable as a trade-off to significant reduction in lung cancer mortality in high-risk patients who are currently recommended for lung cancer screening.

TABLE 3-1	Causes of Lung Cancer, Estimates of Relative Risk
TOBACCO SMOKERS	78% (In women) and 92% (In men) (RR 40)
Radon	3%-15% (RR 2-10)
Environmental tobacco smoke	2%-3% (RR 1.7)
Asbestos	1%-2% (RR 1.96)
Vitamin-poor diet	1%-2% (RR 1.3)
Air pollution	1%-2% (RR 1.3-2.3)
Silicosis	0.5%-1% (RR 1.45)
Genetic	1%-3% (RR 1.3-4.0)

RR = relative risk.

Reproduced with permission from Sethi, TK, El-Ghamry MN, Kloecker GH, Radon and lung cancer. Clin Adv Hematol Oncol. 2012;10(3):157-64.

There is evidence for increased lung cancer risk in industrial radiation workers, especially those who process plutonium and may inhale radioactive particles. There does not seem to be an increased risk of lung cancer in health care workers who perform fluoroscopic procedures.[93]

A list of common causes of lung cancer is shown in **Table 3-1**.

REFERENCES

1. Alberg AJ, Samet JM. Epidemiology of lung cancer. *Chest.* 2003;123(1 Suppl):21s-49s. Epub 2003/01/16.
2. Doll R, Hill AB. Smoking and carcinoma of the lung: preliminary report. *Br Med J.* 1950;2(4682):739-748. Epub 1950/09/30. doi:10.1136/*bmj*.2.4682.739.
3. Wynder EL, Graham EA. Etiologic factors in bronchiogenic carcinoma with special reference to industrial exposures; report of eight hundred fifty-seven proved cases. *AMA Arch Ind Hyg Occup Med.* 1951;4(3):221-235. Epub 1951/09/01.
4. US Department of Health and Human Services PHS, Centers for Disease Control and Prevention. *The Health Consequences of Smoking: A Report of the Surgeon General.* Vol. 7829. Washington, DC: CDC; 2004.
5. Centers for Disease Control and Prevention. Smoking and tobacco use. https://www.cdc.gov/tobacco/data_statistics/fact_sheets/index.htm. Accessed May 25, 2019.
6. Benowitz NL. Clinical pharmacology of nicotine: implications for understanding, preventing, and treating tobacco addiction. *Clin Pharmacol Ther.* 2008;83(4):531-541. Epub 2008/02/29. doi:10.1038/clpt.2008.3.
7. Saccone SF, Hinrichs AL, Saccone NL, et al. Cholinergic nicotinic receptor genes implicated in a nicotine dependence association study targeting 348 candidate genes with 3713 SNPs. *Hum Mol Genet.* 2007;16(1):36-49. Epub 2006/12/01. doi:10.1093/hmg/ddl438.
8. Costa F, Soares R. Nicotine: a pro-angiogenic factor. *Life Sci.* 2009;84(23-24):785-790. Epub 2009/03/19. doi:10.1016/j.lfs.2009.03.002.
9. de Groot PM, Wu CC, Carter BW, Munden RF. The epidemiology of lung cancer. *Transl Lung Cancer Res.* 2018;7(3):220-233. Epub 2018/07/28. doi:10.21037/tlcr.2018.05.06.
10. Kabbani N. Not so Cool? Menthol's discovered actions on the nicotinic receptor and its implications for nicotine addiction. *Front Pharmacol.* 2013;4:95. Epub 2013/07/31. doi:10.3389/fphar.2013.00095.
11. Alberg AJ, Brock MV, Ford JG, Samet JM, Spivack SD. Epidemiology of lung cancer: diagnosis and management of lung cancer, 3rd ed: American College of Chest Physicians evidence-based clinical practice guidelines. *Chest.* 2013;143(5)(suppl):e1S-e29S. Epub 2013/05/10. doi:10.1378/chest.12-2345.
12. Samet JM, Wiggins CL, Humble CG, Pathak DR. Cigarette smoking and lung cancer in New Mexico. *Am Rev Respir Dis.* 1988;137(5):1110-1113. Epub 1988/05/01. doi:10.1164/ajrccm/137.5.1110.
13. Dela Cruz CS, Tanoue LT, Matthay RA. Lung cancer: epidemiology, etiology, and prevention. *Clini Chest Med.* 2011;32(4):605-644. Epub 2011/11/08. doi:10.1016/j.ccm.2011.09.001.

14. *The Health Consequences of Smoking—50 Years of Progress: A Report of the Surgeon General.* Atlanta, GA; 2014.

15. Peto R, Darby S, Deo H, Silcocks P, Whitley E, Doll R. Smoking, smoking cessation, and lung cancer in the UK since 1950: combination of national statistics with two case-control studies. *BMJ.* 2000;321(7257):323-329. Epub 2000/08/05.

16. Hackshaw AK, Law MR, Wald NJ. The accumulated evidence on lung cancer and environmental tobacco smoke. *BMJ.* 1997;315(7114):980-88. Epub 1997/11/20.

17. Beckett WS. Epidemiology and etiology of lung cancer. *Clin Chest Med.* 1993;14(1):1-15. Epub 1993/03/01.

18. FDA Enforcement Priorities for Electronic Nicotine Delivery Systems (ENDS) April 2020. https://www.fda.gov/media/133880/download.

19. Hajek P, Phillips-Waller A, Przulj D, et al. A randomized trial of e-cigarettes versus nicotinereplacement therapy. *N Engl J Med.* 2019;380(7):629-637. Epub 2019/01/31. doi:10.1056/NEJMoa1808779.

20. QuickStats: percentage of adults who ever used an e-cigarette and percentage who currently use e-cigarettes, by age group—National Health Interview Survey, United States, 2016. *MMWR Morb Mortal Wkly Rep.* 2017;66:892. http://dx.doi.org/10.15585/mmwr.mm6633a6External.

21. Leventhal AM, Strong DR, Kirkpatrick MG, et al. Association of electronic cigarette use with initiation of combustible tobacco product smoking in early adolescence. *JAMA.* 2015;314(7):700-7. Epub 2015/08/19. doi:10.1001/jama.2015.8950.

22. Centers for Disease Control and Prevention. About electronic cigarettes (e-cigarettes). https://www.cdc.gov/tobacco/basic_information/e-cigarettes/about-e-cigarettes.html. Accessed May 25, 2019.

23. Substance Abuse and Mental Health Services Administration. Results from the 2015 National Survey on Drug Use and Health: Detailed tables, SAMHSA, CBHSQ. https://www.samhsa.gov/data/sites/default/files/NSDUH-DetTabs-2015/NSDUH-DetTabs-2015/NSDUH-DetTabs-2015.htm. Accessed May 25, 2019.

24. Lopez-Quintero C, Perez de los Cobos J, Hasin DS, et al. Probability and predictors of transition from first use to dependence on nicotine, alcohol, cannabis, and cocaine: results of the National Epidemiologic Survey on Alcohol and Related Conditions (NESARC). *Drug Alcohol Depend.* 2011;115(1-2):120-130. Epub 2010/12/15. doi:10.1016/j.drugalcdep.2010.11.004.

25. Maertens RM, White PA, Rickert W, et al. The genotoxicity of mainstream and sidestream marijuana and tobacco smoke condensates. *Chem Res Toxicol.* 2009;22(8):1406-14. Epub 2009/12/02. doi:10.1021/tx9000286.

26. Rickert WS, Robinson JC, Rogers B. A comparison of tar, carbon monoxide and pH levels in smoke from marihuana and tobacco cigarettes. *Can J Public Health.* 1982;73(6):386-391. Epub 1982/11/01.

27. Barsky SH, Roth MD, Kleerup EC, Simmons M, Tashkin DP. Histopathologic and molecular alterations in bronchial epithelium in habitual smokers of marijuana, cocaine, and/or tobacco. *J Natl Cancer Inst.* 1998;90(16):1198-1205. Epub 1998/08/27. doi:10.1093/jnci/90.16.1198.

28. Roth MD, Arora A, Barsky SH, Kleerup EC, Simmons M, Tashkin DP. Airway inflammation in young marijuana and tobacco smokers. *Am J Respir Crit Care Med.* 1998;157(3, pt 1):928-937. Epub 1998/03/28. doi:10.1164/ajrccm.157.3.9701026.

29. Callaghan RC, Allebeck P, Sidorchuk A. Marijuana use and risk of lung cancer: a 40-year cohort study. *Cancer Causes Control.* 2013;24(10):1811-1820. Epub 2013/07/13. doi:10.1007/s10552-013-0259-0.

30. Zhang LR, Morgenstern H, Greenland S, et al. Cannabis smoking and lung cancer risk: pooled analysis in the International Lung Cancer Consortium. *Int J Cancer.* 2015;136(4):894-903. Epub 2014/06/21. doi:10.1002/ijc.29036.

31. Hindocha C, Shaban ND, Freeman TP, et al. Associations between cigarette smoking and cannabis dependence: a longitudinal study of young cannabis users in the United Kingdom. *Drug Alcohol Depend.* 2015;148:165-171. Epub 2015/01/28. doi:10.1016/j.drugalcdep.2015.01.004.

32. Ramo DE, Liu H, Prochaska JJ. Tobacco and marijuana use among adolescents and young adults: a systematic review of their co-use. *Clin Psychol Rev.* 2012;32(2):105-21. Epub 2012/01/17. doi:10.1016/j.cpr.2011.12.002.

33. Miller FJ, Gardner DE, Graham JA, Lee RE, Wilson WE, Bachmann JD. Size considerations for establishing a standard for inhalable particles. *J Air Pollut Control Assoc.* 1979;29(6):610-615. doi:10.1080/00022470.1979.10470831.

34. Natusch DF, Wallace JR. Urban aerosol toxicity: the influence of particle size. *Science.* 1974;186(4165):695-699. Epub 1974/11/22.

35. Dockery DW, Pope CA 3rd, Xu X, et al. An association between air pollution and mortality in six US cities. *N Engl J Med.* 1993;329(24):1753-1759. Epub 1993/12/09. doi:10.1056/NEJM199312093292401.

36. Raaschou-Nielsen O, Andersen ZJ, Beelen R, et al. Air pollution and lung cancer incidence in 17 European cohorts: prospective analyses from the European Study of Cohorts for Air Pollution Effects (ESCAPE). *Lancet Oncol.* 2013;14(9):813-822. Epub 2013/07/16. doi:10.1016/s1470-2045(13)70279-1.

37. Pope CA 3rd, Burnett RT, Thun MJ, et al. Lung cancer, cardiopulmonary mortality, and long-term exposure to fine particulate air pollution. *JAMA.* 2002;287(9):1132-1141. Epub 2002/03/07.

38. Loomis D, Huang W, Chen G. The International Agency for Research on Cancer (IARC) evaluation of the carcinogenicity of outdoor air pollution: focus on China. *Chin J Cancer*. 2014;33(4):189-196. Epub 2014/04/04. doi:10.5732/cjc.014.10028.

39. Cohen AJ, Brauer M, Burnett R, et al. Estimates and 25-year trends of the global burden of disease attributable to ambient air pollution: an analysis of data from the Global Burden of Diseases Study 2015. *Lancet*. 2017;389(10082):1907-1918. Epub 2017/04/15. doi:10.1016/s0140-6736(17)30505-6.

40. Kleinerman RA, Wang Z, Wang L, et al. Lung cancer and indoor exposure to coal and biomass in rural China. *J Occup Environ Med*. 2002;44(4):338-44. Epub 2002/04/30.

41. Hosgood HD 3rd, Boffetta P, Greenland S, et al. In-home coal and wood use and lung cancer risk: a pooled analysis of the International Lung Cancer Consortium. *Environ Health Perspect*. 2010;118(12):1743-1747. Epub 2010/09/18. doi:10.1289/ehp.1002217.

42. Jaurand MC, Bignon J, Sebastien P, Goni J. Leaching of chrysotile asbestos in human lungs. Correlation with in vitro studies using rabbit alveolar macrophages. *Environ Res*. 1977;14(2):245-254. Epub 1977/10/01.

43. Jaurand MC, Kaplan H, Thiollet J, Pinchon MC, Bernaudin JF, Bignon J. Phagocytosis of chrysotile fibers by pleural mesothelial cells in culture. *Am J Pathol*. 1979;94(3):529-538. Epub 1979/03/01.

44. Wang Y, Jiang Z, Yan J, Ying S. HMGB1 as a potential biomarker and therapeutic target for malignant mesothelioma. *Dis Markers*. 2019;2019:4183157. Epub 2019/03/21. doi:10.1155/2019/4183157.

45. Weiss W. Asbestosis: a marker for the increased risk of lung cancer among workers exposed to asbestos. *Chest*. 1999;115(2):536-549. Epub 1999/02/23. doi:10.1378/chest.115.2.536.

46. van Loon AJ, Kant IJ, Swaen GM, Goldbohm RA, Kremer AM, van den Brandt PA. Occupational exposure to carcinogens and risk of lung cancer: results from the Netherlands cohort study. *Occup Environ Med*. 1997;54(11):817-824. Epub 1998/04/16. doi:10.1136/oem.54.11.817.

47. Hammond EC, Selikoff IJ, Seidman H. Asbestos exposure, cigarette smoking and death rates. *Ann N Y Acad Sci*. 1979;330:473-490. Epub 1979/01/01.

48. Darby S, Hill D, Doll R. Radon: a likely carcinogen at all exposures. *Ann Oncol*. 2001;12(10):1341-1351. Epub 2002/01/05. doi:10.1023/a:1012518223463.

49. Frumkin H, Samet JM. Radon. *CA Cancer J Clin*. 2001;51(6):337-344, 22; quiz 45-48. Epub 2002/01/05.

50. Lantz PM, Mendez D, Philbert MA. Radon, smoking, and lung cancer: the need to refocus radon control policy. *Am J Public Health*. 2013;103(3):443-447. Epub 2013/01/19. doi:10.2105/AJPH.2012.300926.

51. Krewski D, Lubin JH, Zielinski JM, et al. Residential radon and risk of lung cancer: a combined analysis of 7 North American case-control studies. *Epidemiology*. 2005;16(2):137-145. Epub 2005/02/11.

52. Darby S, Hill D, Auvinen A, et al. Radon in homes and risk of lung cancer: collaborative analysis of individual data from 13 European case-control studies. *BMJ*. 2005;330(7485):223. Epub 2004/12/23. doi:10.1136/bmj.38308.477650.63.

53. Lubin JH, Boice JD Jr, Edling C, et al. Lung cancer in radon-exposed miners and estimation of risk from indoor exposure. *J Natl Cancer Inst*. 1995;87(11):817-827. Epub 1995/06/07. doi:10.1093/jnci/87.11.817.

54. US Environmental Protection Agency. Radon. https://www.epa.gov/radon. Accessed May 25, 2019.

55. Poinen-Rughooputh S, Rughooputh MS, Guo Y, Rong Y, Chen W. Occupational exposure to silica dust and risk of lung cancer: an updated meta-analysis of epidemiological studies. *BMC Public Health*. 2016;16(1):1137. Epub 2016/11/07. doi:10.1186/s12889-016-3791-5.

56. Liu Y, Steenland K, Rong Y, et al. Exposure-response analysis and risk assessment for lung cancer in relationship to silica exposure: a 44-year cohort study of 34,018 workers. *Am J Epidemiol*. 2013;178(9):1424-1433. Epub 2013/09/18. doi:10.1093/aje/kwt139.

57. Straif K, Benbrahim-Tallaa L, Baan R, et al; WHO International Agency for Research on Cancer Monograph Working Group. A review of human carcinogens—part C: metals, arsenic, dusts, and fibres. *Lancet Oncol*. 2009;10(5):453-454. Epub 2009/05/07.

58. Shekelle RB, Lepper M, Liu S, et al. Dietary vitamin A and risk of cancer in the Western Electric study. *Lancet*. 1981;2(8257):1185-1190. Epub 1981/11/28.

59. Byers TE, Graham S, Haughey BP, Marshall JR, Swanson MK. Diet and lung cancer risk: findings from the Western New York Diet Study. *Am J Epidemiol*. 1987;125(3):351-363. Epub 1987/03/01. doi:10.1093/oxfordjournals.aje.a114542.

60. Goodman GE, Thornquist MD, Balmes J, et al. The Beta-Carotene and Retinol Efficacy Trial: incidence of lung cancer and cardiovascular disease mortality during 6-year follow-up after stopping beta-carotene and retinol supplements. *J Natl Cancer Inst*. 2004;96(23):1743-1750. Epub 2004/12/02. doi:10.1093/jnci/djh320.

61. Omenn GS, Goodman GE, Thornquist MD, et al. Risk factors for lung cancer and for intervention effects in CARET, the Beta-Carotene and Retinol Efficacy Trial. *J Natl Cancer Inst*. 1996;88(21):1550-1559. Epub 1996/11/06. doi:10.1093/jnci/88.21.1550.

62. Omenn GS, Goodman GE, Thornquist MD, et al. Effects of a combination of beta carotene and vitamin A on lung cancer and cardiovascular disease. *N Engl J Med*. 1996;334(18):1150-1155. Epub 1996/05/02. doi:10.1056/NEJM199605023341802.

63. Voorrips LE, Goldbohm RA, Verhoeven DT, et al. Vegetable and fruit consumption and lung cancer risk in the Netherlands Cohort Study on diet and cancer. *Cancer Causes Control*. 2000;11(2):101-15. Epub 2000/03/10.

64. Wright ME, Park Y, Subar AF, et al. Intakes of fruit, vegetables, and specific botanical groups in relation to lung cancer risk in the NIH-AARP Diet and Health Study. *Am J Epidemiol*. 2008;168(9):1024-1034. Epub 2008/09/16. doi:10.1093/aje/kwn212.

65. Swanson CA, Brown CC, Sinha R, Kulldorff M, Brownson RC, Alavanja MC. Dietary fats and lung cancer risk among women: the Missouri Women's Health Study (United States). *Cancer Causes Control*. 1997;8(6):883-893. Epub 1998/01/14.

66. Hecht SS. Approaches to cancer prevention based on an understanding of *N*-nitrosamine carcinogenesis. *Proc Soc Exp Biol Med*. 1997;216(2):181-191. Epub 1998/02/12.

67. Goodman MT, Kolonel LN, Yoshizawa CN, Hankin JH. The effect of dietary cholesterol and fat on the risk of lung cancer in Hawaii. *Am J Epidemiol*. 1988;128(6):1241-1255. Epub 1988/12/01. doi:10.1093/oxfordjournals.aje.a115078.

68. Winstone TA, Man SFP, Hull M, Montaner JS, Sin DD. Epidemic of lung cancer in patients with HIV infection. *Chest*. 2013;143(2):305-314. Epub 2013/02/06. doi:10.1378/chest.12-1699.

69. Mdodo R, Frazier EL, Dube SR, et al. Cigarette smoking prevalence among adults with HIV compared with the general adult population in the United States: cross-sectional surveys. *Ann Intern Med*. 2015;162(5):335-344. Epub 2015/03/04. doi:10.7326/M14-0954.

70. Kirk GD, Merlo C, O'Driscoll P, et al. HIV infection is associated with an increased risk for lung cancer, independent of smoking. *Clin Infect Dis*. 2007;45(1):103-110. Epub 2007/06/08. doi:10.1086/518606.

71. Pakkala S, Chen Z, Rimland D, et al. Human immunodeficiency virus-associated lung cancer in the era of highly active antiretroviral therapy. *Cancer*. 2012;118(1):164-172. Epub 2011/06/30. doi:10.1002/cncr.26242.

72. Syrjanen KJ. Bronchial squamous cell carcinomas associated with epithelial changes identical to condylomatous lesions of the uterine cervix. *Lung*. 1980;158(3):131-142. Epub 1980/01/01.

73. Cheng YW, Chiou HL, Sheu GT, et al. The association of human papillomavirus 16/18 infection with lung cancer among nonsmoking Taiwanese women. *Cancer Res*. 2001;61(7):2799-2803. Epub 2001/04/18.

74. Fei Y, Yang J, Hsieh WC, et al. Different human papillomavirus 16/18 infection in Chinese non-small cell lung cancer patients living in Wuhan, China. *Jpn J Clin Oncol*. 2006;36(5):274-279. Epub 2006/05/13. doi:10.1093/jjco/hyl017.

75. Coissard CJ, Besson G, Polette MC, Monteau M, Birembaut PL, Clavel CE. Prevalence of human papillomaviruses in lung carcinomas: a study of 218 cases. *Mod Pathol*. 2005;18(12):1606-1609. Epub 2005/08/02. doi:10.1038/modpathol.3800472.

76. Ciotti M, Giuliani L, Ambrogi V, et al. Detection and expression of human papillomavirus oncogenes in non-small cell lung cancer. *Oncol Rep*. 2006;16(1):183-189. Epub 2006/06/21.

77. Rezazadeh A, Laber DA, Ghim SJ, Jenson AB, Kloecker G. The role of human papilloma virus in lung cancer: a review of the evidence. *Am J Med Sci*. 2009;338(1):64-67. Epub 2009/07/14. doi:10.1097/MAJ.0b013e3181a393ba.

78. Xiong WM, Xu QP, Li X, Xiao RD, Cai L, He F. The association between human papillomavirus infection and lung cancer: a system review and meta-analysis. *Oncotarget*. 2017;8(56):96419-96432. Epub 2017/12/10. doi:10.18632/oncotarget.21682.

79. Young RP, Hopkins RJ, Christmas T, Black PN, Metcalf P, Gamble GD. COPD prevalence is increased in lung cancer, independent of age, sex and smoking history. *Eur Respir J*. 2009;34(2):380-386. Epub 2009/02/07. doi:10.1183/09031936.00144208.

80. Durham AL, Adcock IM. The relationship between COPD and lung cancer. *Lung Cancer*. 2015;90(2):121-127. Epub 2015/09/14. doi:10.1016/j.lungcan.2015.08.017.

81. Parimon T, Chien JW, Bryson CL, McDonell MB, Udris EM, Au DH. Inhaled corticosteroids and risk of lung cancer among patients with chronic obstructive pulmonary disease. *Am J Respir Crit Care Med*. 2007;175(7):712-719. Epub 2006/12/23. doi:10.1164/rccm.200608-1125OC.

82. Hubbard R, Venn A, Lewis S, Britton J. Lung cancer and cryptogenic fibrosing alveolitis. A population-based cohort study. *Am J Respir Crit Care Med*. 2000;161(1):5-8. Epub 2000/01/05. doi:10.1164/ajrccm.161.1.9906062.

83. Le Jeune I, Gribbin J, West J, Smith C, Cullinan P, Hubbard R. The incidence of cancer in patients with idiopathic pulmonary fibrosis and sarcoidosis in the UK. *Respir Med*. 2007;101(12):2534-2540. Epub 2007/09/18. doi:10.1016/j.rmed.2007.07.012.

84. Fraire AE, Greenberg SD. Carcinoma and diffuse interstitial fibrosis of lung. *Cancer*. 1973;31(5):1078-1086. Epub 1973/05/01.

85. Yang P, Sun Z, Krowka MJ, et al. Alpha1-antitrypsin deficiency carriers, tobacco smoke, chronic obstructive pulmonary disease, and lung cancer risk. *Arch Intern Med.* 2008;168(10):1097-1103. Epub 2008/05/28. doi:10.1001/archinte.168.10.1097.

86. Lissowska J, Foretova L, Dabek J, et al. Family history and lung cancer risk: international multicentre case-control study in Eastern and Central Europe and meta-analyses. *Cancer Causes Control.* 2010;21(7):1091-1104. Epub 2010/03/23. doi:10.1007/s10552-010-9537-2.

87. Gaughan EM, Cryer SK, Yeap BY, Jackman DM, Costa DB. Family history of lung cancer in never smokers with non-small-cell lung cancer and its association with tumors harboring EGFR mutations. *Lung Cancer.* 2013;79(3):193-197. Epub 2013/01/01. doi:10.1016/j.lungcan.2012.12.002.

88. Yokota J, Shiraishi K, Kohno T. Genetic basis for susceptibility to lung cancer: Recent progress and future directions. *Adv Cancer Res.* 2010;109:51-72. Epub 2010/11/13. doi:10.1016/B978-0-12-380890-5.00002-8.

89. Kanwal M, Ding XJ, Cao Y. Familial risk for lung cancer. *Oncol Lett.* 2017;13(2):535-542. Epub 2017/03/31. doi:10.3892/ol.2016.5518.

90. Huang YJ, Huang TW, Lin FH, Chung CH, Tsao CH, Chien WC. Radiation therapy for invasive breast cancer increases the risk of second primary lung cancer: a nationwide population-based cohort analysis. *J Thorac Oncol.* 2017;12(5):782-790. Epub 2017/02/20. doi:10.1016/j.jtho.2017.01.021.

91. Lorigan P, Radford J, Howell A, Thatcher N. Lung cancer after treatment for Hodgkin's lymphoma: a systematic review. *Lancet Oncol.* 2005;6(10):773-779. Epub 2005/10/04. doi:10.1016/S1470-2045(05)70387-9.

92. Rampinelli C, De Marco P, Origgi D, et al. Exposure to low dose computed tomography for lung cancer screening and risk of cancer: secondary analysis of trial data and risk-benefit analysis. *BMJ.* 2017;356:j347. Epub 2017/02/10. doi:10.1136/*bmj*.j347.

93. Deas SD, Huprikar N, Skabelund A. Radiation exposure and lung disease in today's nuclear world. *Curr Opin Pulm Med.* 2017;23(2):167-172. Epub 2016/12/03. doi:10.1097/MCP.0000000000000349.

4

TOBACCO AND LUNG CANCER

Goetz Kloecker, MD, MBA, MSPH, FACP • Celeste T. Worth, MCHES • Samuel Reynolds, MD

HISTORY OF TOBACCO

Goetz Kloecker, MD, MBA, MSPH, FACP

Learning Objectives:

1. How did worldwide cigarette consumption change over the last 100 years?
2. Has the risk of lung cancer due to cigarette smoking changed over the last 50 years?

Tobacco is the single most preventable risk to health worldwide according to the World Health Organization.[1] The tobacco plant, *Nicotiana tabacum/rustica*, was first cultivated more than 3,000 years ago in Central America.[2] The Spanish conquistadores brought tobacco to Europe. In 1559, it was planted in "Los Cigarrales", Spain, from where it acquired its modern names *cigars* and *cigarettes*.

Tobacco was very important for the economy of the US colonies. The agricultural needs of planting and harvesting tobacco determined much of the economy of the early colonies and is mentioned as a reason for slavery at that time.[3]

Tobacco was used up the late 19th century mainly in pipes, cigars, and chewable form. A change in curing the tobacco allowed more tobacco to be better tolerated when inhaled. Also, the invention of the safety match facilitated the increased use of cigarettes.

The mass production of cigarettes started in the late 1800s after James Albert Bonsack (1859-1924) patented the cigarette-rolling machine in 1880. The cigarette-rolling machine was able to produce cigarettes 100-fold faster than manual cigarette rolling at that time (**Figure 4-1**).

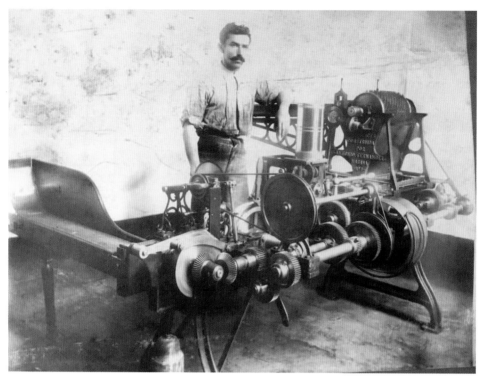

Figure 4-1. Bonsack's machine for cigarette mass production (1882).

Industrial mass production, helped by an effective marketing method, led to several tobacco producer monopolies. The US American Tobacco Company (ATC) combined several US companies, with Buck Duke as chairman, in 1889. The ATC then combined forces with the United Kingdom's Imperial Tobacco to form British American Tobacco (BAT). BAT now is based in the United Kingdom and has the widest international network. Philip Morris started as a cigarette shop in the 1850s in London and transformed into multinational Altria, now among the largest tobacco companies, next to BAT, Japan Tobacco Industry, and state monopolies, such as China Tobacco.

Cigarette consumption increased after 1900 and peaked in 1960 in the United States. There is a significant difference in tobacco use epidemiology between men and women and societies of different economic wealth[4,5] (**Figure 4-2**).

PREVALENCE OF SMOKING

In the 20th century, tobacco caused the death of 100 million and is predicted to cause the death of a billion people in the 21st century.[1,6] In 1949, Ernest Wynder and Evarts Graham published a case-control study in *JAMA* pointing at tobacco as a possible risk factor for lung cancer. In 1951 the *British Medical Journal* published a large epidemiologic study confirming tobacco as a significant risk factor for lung cancer.

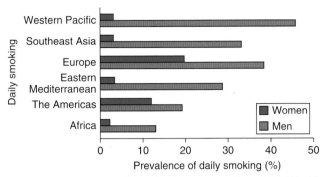

Figure 4-2. Prevalence of daily tobacco smoking. (Adapted with permission from World Health Organization (WHO). *Global Status Report on Noncommunicable Diseases 2010.* Geneva, Switzerland: World Health Organization; 2011. Copyright © World Health Organization 2011.)

In 1964, Surgeon General Luther K. Terry published the first report on smoking warning about its risk.[7] Over the following decades, more evidence was collected that smoking harms the secondhand smoker as well. In 1986, the surgeon general reported on the risk to secondhand smokers.[8] In the 1990s, a master settlement enforced a penalty of billions of dollars on the tobacco industry.

Despite all the educational efforts and regulatory barriers, tobacco consumption has significantly increased worldwide. Especially, countries and continents in the southern hemisphere have increased tobacco consumption and smoking by 300% to 1,400%.[5] The major tobacco producers worldwide are presently China, 3 million tons per year; Brazil, 860,000 tons; India, 700,000 tons; and the United States, 400,000 tons in 2014.

According to the Centers for Disease Control and Prevention (CDC), presently 15.5% of the adult US population smokes, and 16 million live with smoking-related diseases. Tobacco causes half a million deaths per year in the United States, of which 41,000 are due to secondhand smoking. Smokers on average died 10 years earlier than non-smokers. The US economic costs are approximately $300 billion. The average state tax in 2018 for a pack of cigarettes was $1.75. The smoking health costs and lost productivity per pack equals $19.16.[9]

A map of lung cancer mortality in the United States between 1980 in 2014 shows a significant variation in lung cancer deaths. The majority of lung cancer deaths occur in the Southeast and Midwest. Amazingly, in the last 30 years the death rate due to lung cancer has increased by up to 100% in some of these regions.[10]

There have been changes over time in the annual death rates from lung cancer and chronic obstructive pulmonary disease (COPD). Since 1964, at the time of the first surgeon general's warning about smoking, there have been more than 20 million premature deaths attributable to smoking and secondhand smoke. Despite declines in the prevalence of current smoking, the annual burden of smoking-attributable mortality in the United States has remained above 400,000 for more than a decade and currently is estimated to be about 480,000, with millions more living with smoking-related diseases. The risk of dying of lung cancer per pack of cigarettes has doubled over the last 50 years **(Figure 4-3)**.

A Lung Cancer

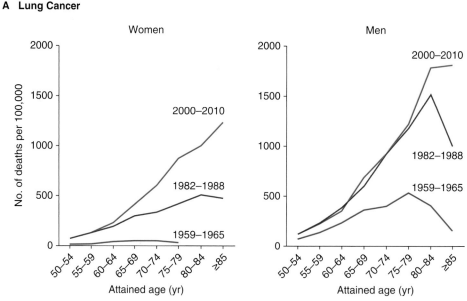

Figure 4-3. The increase in death rate of lung cancer in the last 40 years. (Reproduced with permission from US Department of Health and Human Services. *The Health Consequences of Smoking—50 Years of Progress: A Report of the Surgeon General.* Atlanta, GA: US Department of Health and Human Services, Centers for Disease Control and Prevention, National Center for Chronic Disease Prevention and Health Promotion, Office on Smoking and Health; 2014.)

SURGEON GENERAL REPORT 2014

The annual burden of smoking-attributable mortality is expected to be at high levels for decades into the future, and 5.6 million youth are projected to die prematurely from a smoking-related illness. Smoking-attributable economic costs in the United States estimated for the years 2009-2012 were between $289 and $332.5 billion annually. This takes into account $132.5-$175.9 billion for direct medical care of adults and $151 billion for lost productivity due to premature death estimated from 2005 to 2009 and $5.6 billion (in 2006) for lost productivity due to exposure to secondhand smoke. Smoking remains the leading preventable cause of premature death in the United States and worldwide.[11]

In 1992, the Environmental Protection Agency (EPA) made tobacco a class A human lung carcinogen. This led to an effort to a ban smoking at the work place.[8]

CONTROL OF TOBACCO
Celeste T. Worth, MCHES, Samuel Reynolds, MD

A 55-year-old smoker of two packs a day asks you about smoking cessation.

He has a history of seizures, COPD, and coronary artery disease (CAD).

He has tried to quit smoking many times and never has been able to stop for more than 1 month.

Learning Objectives:

1. What are the most efficient and effective ways to briefly address patients' tobacco use?
2. What are the lesser-known aspects of over-the-counter (OTC) cessation pharmacotherapy product use?
3. What are the recommended approaches for those patients unwilling to quit smoking?
4. How do patients already diagnosed with lung cancer most benefit from cessation prior to or during treatment?
5. Which oncology treatment therapeutics are most affected by tobacco use and how?
6. Which resources are available to assist patients during their quit attempt?

INTERNATIONAL TOBACCO CONTROL

Luther L. Terry, MD, was the surgeon general of the US Public Health Service in 1964, and, perhaps unbeknownst to him or to many Americans at the time, he would become a critical figure in the history of both tobacco and lung cancer. Through the Surgeon General's Advisory Committee on Smoking and Health, he released what is considered the first formal public report on the association between lung cancer and tobacco use on January 11, 1964. As per the CDC, this report was based on over 7,000 thousand articles that had already been published.[12]

The ramifications stemming from this report cannot be overstated. The National Clearinghouse for Smoking and Health was established less than 2 years later in September 1965 and would later be succeeded by the Centers for Disease Control and Prevention's Office on Smoking and Health, with 29 additional reports on the health outcomes of cigarette smoking. In the political arena, the Federal Cigarette Labeling and Advertising Act and the Public Health Cigarette Smoking Act were adopted by the United States in 1965 and 1969, respectively. Laws were subsequently enacted that

1. Banned the use of advertising for cigarettes in broadcasting media
2. Requested annual reports on the consequences of smoking on health
3. Made a requirement for health warnings on cigarette packaging

The history and study of tobacco and its association with lung cancer is not limited the United States or to the 20th century; in fact, there have been studies by countries all over the world. In the present day, for instance, data from the Swiss National Institute for Cancer Epidemiology and Registration (NICER) were extracted for gender- and age-specific rates of incidence for diagnosed cancers affecting the trachea, bronchi, and lungs between 1990 and 2014, along with smoking prevalence. Rates of cancer were decreased in men aged 40 to 44, 45 to 49, and 50 to 54, with a tendency toward decreasing rates in older cohorts. Authors conversely identified a higher smoking prevalence in younger as compared to older men born in the mid-1950s and 1960s. In women, cancer rates were increasing for those born from 1935 to the 1950s; increased smoking prevalence was seen in younger as compared to older women born in the mid-1960s. The authors concluded that an increasing incidence of lung cancer in young women was reflective of an evolving smoking epidemic and called for prevention strategies targeting young women.[13]

A modern application of these guidelines was summarized in a 2014 report by the surgeon general, which concluded that the risk of developing lung adenocarcinoma from smoking had increased since the 1960s, and that this increased risk was attributable to the changing composition and design of cigarettes. Speaking to this last point, the report further discussed that it was unclear which design changes had been responsible for this increased risk, but that increased tobacco-specific nitrosamines and ventilated filters were role players. Last, the report indicated that a decline in squamous cell carcinoma was correlated with a decline in the prevalence of smoking.[14]

Other countries are looking to the future in predictive analysis models. In August 2018, a group in South America published the results of an age-period-cohort analysis of patients in the National Cancer Registry of Uruguay between 1990 and 2014. A 70% risk reduction was seen in new cases of lung cancer in men born in 1970 compared to the early 1940s. In women, however, new diagnoses of lung cancer increased between 1991 and 2014, with specific increases in those born between 1940 and 1960. These trends were used to extrapolate data that predicted rates of new lung cancer diagnoses, which were calculated at 8% reduction in men but a 69% increase in females by 2035.[15]

Going forward, it is expected that studies similar to those performed in Switzerland and Uruguay will be expanded to other countries as researchers and public health entities around the world seek not only to explore the relationship between tobacco and lung cancer but also to reduce the global burden of cigarette smoking in the first place.

TYPES OF TOBACCO AND E-CIGARETTES

The sustainment of tobacco use, and, as stated previously, increase of tobacco use in some populations is perhaps partially attributable to the various delivery systems that provide consumers with ease of use and even a sense of social belonging. It is not clear which of the numerous tobacco products that have emerged in more recent years may contribute more than others to lung cancer risk. But, since it is reasonable to consider all combustible forms of tobacco as sharing much of the same risk that is already well established with cigarette smoking, tobacco use by patients in any form should be determined.

1. *Cigarettes.* Although tobacco has been grown for consumption for centuries, a major milestone in the history of tobacco product manufacturing was the invention of a cigarette-rolling machine by James Bonsack in the late 19th century. In 1884, James Buchanan Duke would obtain the rights to this machine and, in the same year, began using it to manufacture cigarettes in Durham, North Carolina. Approximately 20 years later, in 1906, Duke convinced the US Congress to exclude tobacco from the Food and Drug Act. The Bonsack machine was capable of producing 120,000 cigarettes per day. By a comparison to modern times, the Hauni cigarette machine is currently capable of 20,000 cigarettes per minute.[16] Today, almost 140 years later, the cigarette remains the most classic and recognizable form of tobacco use.

2. *Cigars/cigarillos.* Cigars are defined by the CDC as a rolled collection of tobacco wrapped within another tobacco-containing substance, such as a tobacco leaf. In the

United States, cigar types are divided into large cigars, which contain approximately as much tobacco as a pack of cigarettes; cigarillos, which are 3-4 inches in length and do not traditionally have filters; and little cigars, which have filters and are similar in size to cigarettes. Of the cigar market share, 95% as of 2015 was occupied by large cigars and cigarillos. The cigar industry's youth marketing focus increased in the 1990s, contributing to the nearly 8% of high school students who smoked cigars in 2017. In 2016, approximately 5% of US adults smoked cigars.[17]

3. *Pipes.* Pipe smoking is another form of tobacco use that is often compared to cigarette smoking in terms of safety. Seeking to answer this question, two researchers (Aage Tverdal and Kjell Bjartveit) conducted a prospective cohort study consisting of 16,932 men, age 20 to 29, across three Norwegian counties. These men were either exclusive users of pipe tobacco or had switched from exclusive cigarettes to exclusive pipe use. The authors found no significant difference in overall survival between exclusive cigarette and exclusive pipe users or in those who had transitioned from exclusive cigarette to exclusive pipe use.[18]

4. *Hookah.* Perhaps an even more well-known tobacco delivery system is the hookah, which consists of a head, long body, water bowl, and a mouthpiece connected to a hose, through which tobacco smoke is inhaled. Commonly used in small groups, the hookah is popular among youth. A 2010 study reported that, from a population of students in their final year of high school in the United States, 15% of girls and 17% of boys had used a hookah within a year of being surveyed. The percentage of college-aged students using a hookah was even higher, at 22%-40%.[19] These statistics are unfortunate not only because of the high number of young users but also because of the physical amount of smoking involved in hookah smoking. To compare, approximately 500-600 mL smoke are inhaled over 20 puffs taken in smoking a single cigarette, while 90,000 mL are inhaled over 200 puffs taken in an average hookah session.[20-22]

5. *Bidis, kreteks.* Other forms of tobacco delivery, although low in prevalence, are important to be aware of, as they pose similar health risks to those of cigarettes. Smoking bidis, for example, which are hand-rolled cigarettes imported from India and other parts of Southeast Asia, increase the risk of both lung and oral cancer.[23-28] Kreteks, which come from Indonesia and are known as clove cigarettes because they contain cloves as well as additives, have been shown in regular users to increase the risk for either reduced absorption of oxygen or obstruction of airflow by a factor of 13 to 20. By comparison to the traditional US cigarette, kreteks and bidis are both more highly concentrated with carbon monoxide, tar, and nicotine.[23,26,29,30]

6. *Smokeless/spit tobacco.* Smokeless tobacco, such as that which is placed in the buccal mucosa or chewed in the mouth and later disposed of (thus referred to as "chewing tobacco"), has the high potential for nicotine addiction and has been demonstrated to cause oral as well as esophageal cancer.[11,31] As of 2016, approximately 3.4% of persons greater than 18 years old (6.6% of men and 0.5% of women) in the United States were current users of smokeless tobacco. Demographically, American Indians/Alaskan Natives (non-Hispanic) were the most common consumers at 8.4%.[32]

7. *E-cigarettes/vaping devices.* The final category of tobacco delivery systems, electronic cigarettes (e-cigarettes), has gained national attention in the United States in recent years, specifically because of the staggering number of young users. Often referred to as "vaping," electronic cigarettes are small devices that come in various structures that serve to heat a nicotine-containing liquid, which is then aerosolized and inhaled.[33] As of 2018, within 30 days of being surveyed, 20.8% of students in US high schools (generally age 14-18) and 4.9% in middle schools (age 10-14) had used an e-cigarette, amounting to 3.6 million users in these age groups.[34] Another interesting and unfortunate point about e-cigarettes is that, for many persons, their intended utility is to wean off of and eventually quit smoking standard tobacco-containing cigarettes. The issue, however, is that adults attempting this method are often smoking cigarettes concurrently in a practice known as "dual use."[25,26,35,36] Moreover, it is important to note that the US Preventive Services Task Force determined in a 2015 synthesis that there was insufficient evidence in both pregnant women and adults for the use of e-cigarettes in smoking cessation.[37]

US CURRENT SMOKING STATISTICS

According to the CDC, the percentage of adults (meaning age $\geq$ 18 years) in the United States decreased from 20.9% in 2005 to 15.5% in 2016. However, almost 38 million adults are smoking a cigarette at least some days but up to every day.[38]

By state, Kentucky, Louisiana, and West Virginia have the highest prevalence, with 22.9%-26.4% of their population smoking cigarettes. They are closely followed by several other states, whose percentages range between 19.4% and less than 22.9%; these states include Alabama, Alaska, and Ohio.[39,40] A depiction of smoking prevalence across the entire United States is shown in **Figures 4-4** (adults) and **Figure 4-5** (youth).

The high prevalence of cigarette usage in the United States does not reflect a lack of desire or active effort to quit smoking. In 2015, for example, approximately 68% of adults who used cigarettes wanted to engage in smoking cessation, and 54% had attempted smoking cessation within 1 year of being surveyed.[41] Regarding successful quit attempts, researchers from the University of San Diego School of Medicine and Moores Cancer Center reported an annual smoking cessation rate of approximately 4.5% among active American smokers up to 2013-2014. This value increased to 5.6% in 2014-2015, which the authors attributed to a high rate of electronic cigarette use (49.3%) in persons who had recently quit successfully.[42]

TOBACCO'S SYNERGISTIC RISK FOR LUNG CANCER

According to the National Cancer Institute (NCI), "On average, current smokers have approximately 20 times the risk of lung cancer compared with nonsmokers." Tobacco smoking is estimated to cause 90% of lung cancer in males and 78% in females. Cigar and pipe smoking are also associated with increased lung cancer risk.[43]

Occupational carcinogens, including asbestos, radon, tar, and soot (sources of polycyclic aromatic hydrocarbons), and arsenic, chromium, nickel, beryllium, and cadmium are estimated to cause 10% of lung cancers. When cigarette smoking is added to radon or asbestos exposure, the combination interacts synergistically to increase the risk of

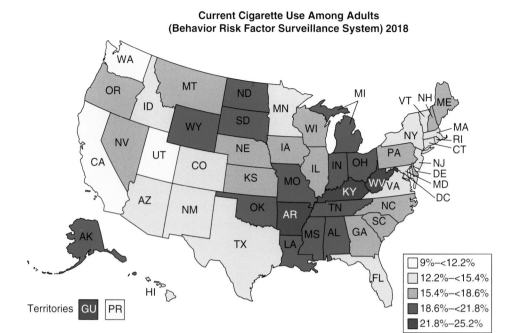

Figure 4-4. Map of the United States, with states differentially shaded by prevalence of cigarette use in adults. (From Centers for Disease Control and Prevention. *Map of Current Cigarette Use Among Adults* 2018. https://www.cdc.gov/statesystem/cigaretteuseadult.html. Accessed April 21, 2019.)

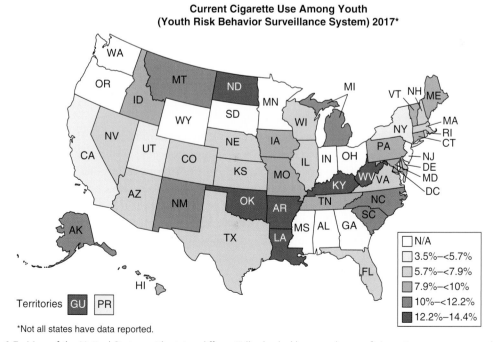

Figure 4-5. Map of the United States, with states differentially shaded by prevalence of cigarette use among youth. (From Centers for Disease Control and Prevention. *Map of Current Cigarette Use Among Youth.* 2018. https://www.cdc.gov/statesystem/cigaretteuseyouth.html. Accessed April 21, 2019.)

lung cancer development, resulting in a risk much higher than the sum of the risks associated with each factor alone.[43,44]

Radon exposure is the leading cause of lung cancer in those who have never smoked cigarettes. A radioactive gas emitted from uranium in the soil, radon can become trapped in homes and other buildings, with the potential for reaching elevated levels equivalent to 200 chest x-rays a year. Since radon is invisible, odorless, and tasteless, the only way to know if there are elevated levels is by employing a test kit from a state radon program or home improvement store; a home can also be tested by a certified radon mitigation contractor. The EPA has categorized radon as a class A carcinogen and considers elevated levels to be those above 4 picocuries/liter of air.[43] Given the possible role radon may have had in the development of lung cancer in a person without a history of tobacco use or significant occupational carcinogen exposure (eg, asbestos), clinicians should recommend radon testing to patients and those living with them. This will prevent further risk not only to the patient but also to others who have been exposed.

LUNG CANCER PREVENTION AND TOBACCO CONTROL

The potential impact of smoking cessation on lung cancer rates has been studied for years across multiple nations. Researchers in the year 2000, for example, published a study in the *British Medical Journal* reporting on smoking and smoking cessation trends in relation to lung cancer in the United Kingdom; the study was based on a summary of studies from 1950 to 1990. Smoking prevalence decreased by 50% from 1950 to 1990 in "early middle age" men, while rate of death in those aged 35 to 54 declined even more significantly. Higher rates of lung cancer were expectedly seen in older men and women who had persistently smoked throughout their adult lives. Assuredly, however, both women and men in 1990 who were designated as former smokers had lower cumulative risk of lung cancer than those who had continually smoked since 1950. Cumulative risk, moreover, declined with increased duration of smoking cessation. Results from this study are depicted in **Figure 4-6**.[6]

In similar research conducted as part of the Singapore Chinese Health Study in 2010, regarding risk of lung cancer, a 28% reduction was observed in patients who had quit smoking relative to current smokers.[45] An even more recent 2015 study examined a US population of nearly 150,000 patients. Relative to never-smokers, the hazard ratio was substantially greater in those whose years since quitting (YSQ) was less than 5 at a hazard ratio of 30.8 than in those whose YSQ was greater than 30 at a 6.4 hazard ratio.[46]

Despite potential for improved lung cancer survival due to recent treatment advances and the ability to detect lung cancer earlier through the use of low-dose computed tomographic (LDCT) scans, smoking cessation still has the ability to prevent more lung cancers and resulting deaths than any other approach. Most smokers are fully aware that smoking is harmful to their health and can cause lung cancer. This points to the fact that knowledge of the risk is not what can make a significant impact on smoking behavior. The reality is that cigarettes are extremely addictive and keep people using a product that in many cases they cognitively and rationally want to stop using.

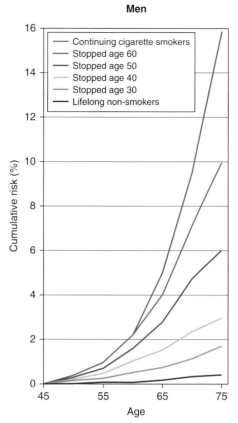

Figure 4-6. Cumulative risk of lung cancer by duration of smoking cessation. (From Inamura K, Ninomiya H, Nomura K, et al. Combined effects of asbestos and cigarette smoke on the development of lung adenocarcinoma: different carcinogens may cause different genomic changes. *Oncol Rep.* 2014;32(2):475-482.)

TOBACCO AND NICOTINE ADDICTION

Nicotine addiction is referred to by experts as a chronic brain disorder.[47] Tobacco use moreover is sometimes cast as a bad or even unsightly habit, which places an unfortunate stigma on cigarette consumers because a major driving force for use is not personal weakness, but rather physiological addiction. Once cigarette smoke is inhaled and carried into the lungs, nicotine enters the pulmonary venous circulation, ultimately leading to the delivery of nicotine to the brain in as few as 11 seconds or less. Here, nicotine binds to acetylcholine receptors, which opens ligand-gated channels to allow for the entry of calcium and sodium into neurons, an action that subsequently releases neurotransmitters into the brain. Among these neurotransmitters is dopamine, which results in a sensation of pleasure.[48] These same nicotinic cholinergic receptors, termed *nicotinic acetylcholine receptors*, or nAChRs, are actually upregulated by cigarette smoking, specifically the α4β2*nAChR subtype. Cigarette smokers with less upregulation of α4β2*nAChR have a higher likelihood of complete smoking cessation.[49]

Neurochemical and related effects include the following:

NEUROTRANSMITTER	EFFECTS
Dopamine	Pleasure, appetite suppression
Norepinephrine	Arousal, appetite suppression
Acetylcholine	Arousal, cognitive enhancement
Glutamate	Learning, memory enhancement
Serotonin	Mood modulation, appetite suppression
β-Endorphin	Reduction of anxiety and tension
GABA (γ-aminobutyric acid)	Reduction of anxiety and tension

These effects collectively provide significant reinforcement for continued tobacco use.[50]

Eighty percent of tobacco users initiate smoking by the age of 18. Of this population, between 20% and 25% of consumers will then become dependent on daily smoking in adulthood. It is common for adolescents to believe that a small amount of tobacco use will not be addicting, that they can quit at any time when ready, and that the long-term consequences of smoking will not befall them. Lung cancer is one of the potential consequences that, when it happens, will likely be decades after smoking initiation, so it is therefore not of much concern to an adolescent. For this reason, some have even considered lung cancer a pediatric disease given when the most predominant cause actually originated for the patient.

Unfortunately, addiction to tobacco is even more common in persons with disorders of substance abuse or general mental health, with such individuals smoking approximately 40% of all cigarettes consumed in the United States.[48,51] The tobacco industry has not missed the opportunity to take advantage of such populations and have in fact crafted directives to specifically target homeless, mentally ill, lesbian, gay, bisexual, and transsexual persons, such as Project Sub Culture Urban Marketing, or SCUM, which in the 1990s was introduced to San Francisco.[51]

Nicotine Replacement Therapy

In relation to other substances, tobacco smoking has been demonstrated to increase craving for both heroin and cocaine, and the research group that reached this conclusion in 2010 suggested that treatment for heroin and cocaine dependence should be conducted in conjunction with tobacco cessation counseling, so as to treat the addictive process itself rather than addiction to individual substances.[52] And fortunately, modern medicine has made tremendous advances in smoking cessation with nicotine replacement therapy (NRT), making tobacco cessation for such patients a distinct and attainable goal. NRT releases small amounts of nicotine into the systemic circulation while removing the tar burden brought forth by smoking tobacco-laden cigarettes. Varenicline serves as a partial $\alpha 4\beta 2^*$nAChR agonist, thus delivering similar effects of nicotine without the harmful effects of inhaled cigarette smoke.[53]

Scientists are now taking the study of tobacco cessation even deeper and have developed the nicotine metabolite ratio, which is a phenotypic index of nicotine metabolism that serves to guide clinicians in selecting the most appropriate form of cessation therapy for their patients. In slow nicotine metabolizers, for example, NRT is most appropriate. Those who metabolize nicotine at a normal rate, however, are better candidates for non–NRTs, such as varenicline.[54] NRT is discussed further in this chapter.

CHALLENGES IN SMOKING CESSATION

The Patient's Challenge

Approximately 70% of patients want to quit smoking when asked, but unfortunately 95% of attempts that are unassisted by supportive counseling and therapies will result in failure. Poor medication adherence is a major cause, as is poor attendance at counseling sessions.[55]

Challenges to Clinician Intervention

Most clinicians have not received substantial, if any, training prior to their medical practice about evidence-based recommendations for treating tobacco use. To address this by providing essential guidance for clinicians in practice, the Public Health Service (PHS) Treating Tobacco Use and Dependence Clinical Practice Guideline (TTUD-CPG) was published in 2008, along with a Quick Reference Guide that provided key recommendations for providers, with these recommendations based on a summary from decades of research and cumulative analysis.[56]

Time is a big limitation for all clinicians, and a common perception is that cessation counseling can be very time consuming. The TTUD-CPG states that clinicians can be effective with patient cessation in as little as 3 minutes. More specifically, the likelihood that a patient will quit is increased by 40% with a 1- to 3-minute intervention. If 30 minutes of counseling is provided, even over multiple visits, that likelihood increases to 90%.[14]

Benefits of Clinician Intervention

Clinician intervention in treating tobacco use and dependence can be powerful and have a significant impact, even more substantial than that of family members. The so-called white coat effect reinforces the influential role of a health care professional.

Adopting use of the TTUD-CPG tool would be of specific benefit to the many clinicians who have attempted counseling but have been unsuccessful in guiding patients to full cessation. Following the guideline's recommendations would also improve efficiency by implementing approaches proven to be effective.

Last, when clinicians do not ask about tobacco use or assist with cessation, the patient can perceive this as their tobacco use not being a priority or posing a significant threat to their health. Since patients are typically aware that smoking is bad for them on some level and that they should quit, if not addressed, they could question the quality of care they are receiving in general.

Engaging Multiple Caregivers

The ideal approach in managing smoking cessation, particularly for providers, involves multiple individuals working together as a comprehensive care team to perform tobacco use assessment, provide counseling and assistance for patients, and ensure follow-up. This team should include nurses, pharmacists, tobacco education specialists (if available), and care coordinators. The team approach serves two purposes, one being the time-saving effect for providers, who can then direct more attention to patient care and counseling, and the other being a reinforcement of important topics by multiple team members, which patients are then likely to interpret as points to commit to memory and to actual practice.

PATIENT COMMUNICATION IN TREATING TOBACCO USE DISORDER

The Five A's Model

The TTUD-CPG recommends using the following five A's for patients, especially those willing to quit:

Ask about all tobacco use

Advise patients to quit

Assess willingness to quit

Assist in developing a quit plan

Arrange for patient follow-up

General Approach to Questioning

Appropriate wording of questions by clinicians can have an impact on the thoroughness and accuracy of patient responses. It is best, for example, to avoid labeling an individual with the term *smoker* and keep wording limited to the behavior alone. Asking about cigarette/tobacco use in the last month/30 days helps to avoid reports of temporary smoking status based on exceptional circumstances, like being sick or having just attempted quitting in the days leading up to the visit.

Assessing Patient Tobacco Use and Dependence: *Ask*

While it is always important for clinicians to have tobacco use documented, a verbal detailed assessment provides a valuable opportunity to discuss various aspects of the patient's tobacco use and for the patient to elaborate on their written response given on a form. A paper-based questionnaire, for example, ideally should ask about all forms of tobacco and/or electronic cigarette use in the prior 30 days, including quantity (ie, how many packs/day), how often, and whether or not any pharmacologic or non-pharmacologic methods of cessation are being utilized. A discussion of use pattern as well as history of attempted cessation should then follow, particularly if the patient is still using tobacco. Electronic medical record systems are also helpful here, as clinicians can enter patients' responses directly into automated programs that prompt the user with related questions. These responses can then be examined at future visits for comparisons and progress updates.

When approaching patients with specific questions about qualitative and quantitative tobacco use, it is best to maintain a neutral, non-judgmental demeanor and to remain as objective as possible. The types of questions discussed next should be included in the initial evaluation of each patient.

Products

First, ask about which type of tobacco or device(s) the patient is currently using or has used since there are many tobacco products other than cigarettes, such as those mentioned previously in this chapter, as well as an array of vaping products, which are considered tobacco products by the Food and Drug Administration (Food and Drug Administration) and may contain nicotine. And interestingly, since tobacco smoke could interact with various therapies (as shown in **Table 4-1**), if the patient is taking any of the medications listed, this potential impact should be explained to the patient as another incentive for cessation. The most significant interactions are highlighted in gray.[57,58]

Quantity

> **CLINICAL PEARL:** Quantifying how much a patient smokes per day is key to prescribing the appropriate amount of cessation medications for adequate withdrawal relief. Furthermore, if the purpose for the question is included when asked, it could help patients to be more forthcoming about the actual amount of tobacco used. Given that this information is most relevant for prescribing if the patient indicates a willingness to quit, at that point the amount given by the patient initially could be revisited with more explanation. Providers can specifically indicate, "I'm asking this so that I can determine the best medication dosage to relieve symptoms you may have since your body is used to a steady supply of nicotine from smoking." This is particularly useful in patients who might be ashamed of their tobacco use or who have had a history of feeling judged by caregivers.

Quantity is also an important figure in determining eligibility for lung cancer screening with LDCT scanning of the chest, which should be performed in adults aged 55-80 who have 30 pack-year or more histories of smoking and who have stopped smoking with the past 15 years. Pack-year calculation is made by taking the average number of packs smoked per day multiplied by the number of years the patient has smoked.

Assessing History of Attempted Smoking Cessation
Rationale

Asking about the patient's quit history can be beneficial for multiple reasons. The discussion itself, for example, provides a neutral opportunity to personally connect with the patient, so even if he or she has indicated that they are not ready or willing to quit, a therapeutic alliance has been established. Assessing quit history can also lead to a better understanding of the patient's perspective about willingness to quit, barriers to doing

TABLE 4-1   Interactions Between Various Medications and Tobacco Smoke

DRUG INTERACTIONS WITH TOBACCO SMOKE

FOR ONCOLOGY SPECIALISTS

There are many known pharmacokinetic interactions between tobacco smoke and therapeutic drugs, the majority of which results from the induction of cytochrome P450 enzymes. Of these enzymes, perhaps the most well-described is CYP1A2. Accordingly, many patients who smoke cigarettes require stronger dosages of medications metabolized as substrates by CYP1A2, so as to achieve the desired clinical effect while continuing to use tobacco. This being said, the quantity of tobacco smoke required to enhance the effects of cytochrome P450 enzymes has not been objectively proven in a clinical setting. Some of the more common medications encountered by both hematologic and oncologic specialists and their associated interactions with tobacco smoke are shown in the following chart.

DRUG NAME (GENERIC)	INTERACTION WITH TOBACCO SMOKE, RECOMMENDED ADJUSTMENT
Bendamustine	CYP1A2 substrate. Bendamustine concentrations and active metabolites are, respectively, decreased and increased when exposed to tobacco smoke. Use with caution advised in patients who smoke.
Clozapine	Metabolism increased through induction of CYP1A2, decreasing circulation drug concentration by an approximate 18%. Accordingly, cessation of smoking may lead to increased plasma levels of clozapine. Clinicians are advised to monitor drug levels closely, including for the presence of agranulocytosis, particularly following smoking cessation.
Erlotinib	Two-fold decrease in trough serum concentrations, with increased drug clearance
Heparin	Smoking generally has a pro-thrombotic effect, although exact mechanism is unknown. Decreased half-life and increased clearance of heparin are likely; consider increasing dosage accordingly.
Irinotecan	Clearance increased upon interaction with tobacco smoke, with subsequent decrease in SN-38 (the active metabolite of irinotecan) through glucuronidation. This effect may minimize hematologic adverse effects, but can also reduce efficacy. Consider dose increase, as tolerated, in patients who smoke.
Nintedanib	Exposure decreased in patients who smoke. A formal dose adjustment is not routinely recommended, but providers should advise patient against tobacco use when taking.
Warfarin	R-enantiomer metabolism is increased through CYP1A2 indication. Effect on INR, however, is unclear. Monitor INR, as with any patient on warfarin therapy, to a goal range that will vary based on underlying pathophysiology.
Inhaled corticosteroids	Patients who smoke cigarettes with concurrent asthma may demonstrate a less clinically significant response to inhaled corticosteroids.
Combined hormonal contraceptives	Women who smoke cigarettes during use have an increased risk of developing comorbid cardiovascular disease, such as myocardial infarction and cerebrovascular accident. Risk of thromboembolism is also increased in this population. Factors that increase this already high risk are age $\geq$35 and daily use of $\geq$15 cigarettes.

Adapted from materials of Rx for Change. Adapted and updated, from Zevin S, Benowitz NL. Drug interactions with tobacco smoking. An update. Clin Pharmacokinet. 1999;36:425–438; and Kroon LA. Drug interactions with smoking. Am J Health-Syst Pharm. 2007;64:1917–1921.

so, and stakeholders who can assist them in cessation. It can also help the clinician and patient to identify triggers to relapse prior to initiating another cessation attempt. If, for example, a patient plays poker once a month where cigarettes are smoked by other players, it would be wise to advise him or her to modify the habits of others at this event (if possible) or to avoid it entirely temporarily.

Number of Attempts

The number of quit attempts can convey why the patient may not feel confident about trying again if the attempts were numerous. For those who have tried quitting five or more times, it can be reassuring to share with them that patients try many times on average before quitting successfully.[57] This information, however, can be discouraging for the patient attempting to quit for the first or second time, so it should be shared selectively. Prior attempts, moreover, should be thought of by patients not as failures but as lessons or learning opportunities, bringing them that much closer to ultimate success.

Dating Prior Attempts

If the patient has only tried to quit in the distant past and was not successful, it is important for clinicians to remind patients that circumstances and many other factors have since changed, including social barriers and medication availability. Reinforcing these changes can reassure patients that a renewed cessation attempt may have a different outcome. The patient should also be asked what his or her longest periods of cessation have been and what did and did not work during this time. This information should be applied to future cessation attempts, and any period of abstinence should be congratulated.

Use of Aids

Patients reluctant to quit may say they have "tried everything." This is not likely since there are seven medications that can be used alone or in combination to achieve abstinence and relieve withdrawal symptoms. A follow-up to this statement should be asking exactly what they have used in prior attempts and how medications were used to determine if inadequate or incorrect use may have contributed. These are common issues for those who relapse while using a medication. If a patient has not tried using a cessation medication with prior attempts, this is an ideal opportunity to provide encouragement and information about the availability of safe and effective medications that could lead to a tobacco-free life.

Causes for Relapse

One of the most common causes cited by patients is a stressful life event. It has also been said that "people don't plan to fail, but fail to plan," which can have tremendous impact on a cessation attempt. If patients expect stress to be a natural occurrence in their lives, however, and know that it could be a trigger to resume tobacco use, they can better plan should such situations arise.

Another commonly reported issue for patients is that the use of even one cigarette after prolonged periods of abstinence often leads to a resumption of prior usage. The pathophysiology here involves the previously formed nicotine receptors at patients' neural synapses, which do not diminish in the setting of abstinence. A single cigarette, therefore, is adequate in delivering nicotine to these receptors and activating the patient's intrinsic reward pathway, which can kick-start a new cycle of tobacco dependence.

Documentation of what is learned through discussions with patients about their tobacco use is important, as tobacco dependence is a chronic condition that often requires multiple interventions over time, often with a variety of caregivers. If the information discussed is in the patient's record, it is there to refresh not only the memory of the clinicians, but also that of patients, as they are the most critical part of the shared decision-making process.

Advising Patients to Quit: *Advise*

Following an assessment of tobacco use and history of attempted cessation, clinicians must then offer advice on quitting. The main purpose of this advice is to indicate the importance and priority of doing so in context with the patient's overall state of health, including existing comorbidities, such as coronary artery disease or type 2 diabetes.

If the clinician does not tell a patient that he or she must attempt to quit tobacco, it can be interpreted by the patient as tacit approval, which is why the TTUD-CPG recommends explicitly stating quitting advice in a clear, strong, and personalized manner. This advice should precede any discussion regarding willingness to quit as that decision does not affect the advice every patient using tobacco should receive.

Assessing Willingness to Quit in the Short Term: *Assess*

After advising the patient to quit smoking, the clinician should assess his or her willingness to quit within the next 2 weeks, which should be accompanied by an offer of assistance. One recommended way of wording this offer is to ask, "With my help, would you be willing to *try* quitting in the next 2 weeks?"

The 2-week time frame helps to determine if the patient not only is truly serious about a current quit attempt but also is key for certain pharmacotherapies that should be initiated 1 to 2 weeks prior to the quit date. In addition, asking the patient to "try" quitting is less intimidating and more manageable than making a commitment that perhaps they have made multiple times in the past and have subsequently not achieved. If the patient is not yet ready to set a quit date, their interest in cutting down while on NRT should be assessed.

Counseling and Cessation Planning: *Assist*

For patients willing to quit in the short term (ie, within 2 weeks), brief counseling will need to be conducted, which will include additional assessment of the patient's smoking behavior, allowing providers to personalize a treatment plan.

Behavior-Based Approach

Tobacco treatment requires a two-prong approach: addressing physical addiction and withdrawal and examining the behavioral component. For many patients, smoking has become a part of their identity and is closely connected with their social interactions, daily activities, and perceived stress management. It is not uncommon, therefore, for patients to continue smoking out of routine, even unconsciously.

General Planning for Cessation

Once a patient has expressed a willingness to quit, it is important for providers to act on that motivation expeditiously, and the first step in doing so is to have the patient choose a quit date or at least a reduction date. The benefit of establishing a set date is not only having a documented date of initiation for the cessation attempt but also being able to allow the patient to choose timing that would work best for them, to plan and prepare for what will be a life-altering effort.

Also, since some cessation pharmacotherapy should be initiated prior to the quit date, advanced planning provides adequate timing for administering prescription medications. Some of the key questions that will assist in anticipation of triggers and challenges include the following:

What are your biggest triggers to smoke?

When and where do you most want to smoke?

Do you live with others who smoke?

Do you smoke at work?

If you have previously quit smoking but restarted, what were the factors contributing to resumption?

Anticipating Challenges

If the patient has a prepared action plan for when a smoking craving arises, his or her chances of success are increased. Home-based situations for patients to be aware of include those discussed next.

Persons in the Household Who Smoke

Patients should be advised to preemptively speak about their efforts to quit smoking with the individuals in the household who smoke. Other household members can either simultaneously participate in cessation or be asked to smoke outside. If possible, an offer to help others in the home with quitting could be very beneficial since they may not have a clinician to provide this assistance. The patient should understand that continuing to have someone smoking around them in the home will make this process much more difficult and could greatly impede success.

Surroundings

All tobacco products, including lighters and ashtrays, should be removed from the household in order to reduce temptation.

Workplace smoking policies that limit the opportunities to smoke can be helpful to individuals attempting cessation. But for many employees, their break times pose the biggest challenge as a long-standing routine of smoking with coworkers. This can be a difficult social time at work to avoid, but patients should understand that at least for the initial several weeks, they should avoid being with others who are smoking and have another activity planned for this time.

Relapse Prevention

Cravings while quitting can be extremely intense, but patients will likely be comforted by the fact that they typically only last several minutes. Suggested activities/distractions for getting through this time are

1. Calling/texting family or friends
2. Exercising
3. Eating or drinking a healthy food item
4. Watching television or a movie
5. Utilizing online support groups

   Suggest patients change as much as possible about their daily routine since it is likely closely tied to their smoking. They could sit at a different place at the table to eat, have tea instead of coffee, drive a different route to work, and so on. These changes will be a part of affecting the cycle of their nicotine addiction. Exercise should be strongly encouraged as it actually helps reduce the desire to smoke and withdrawal symptoms.[59]

   Certain routines in particular should be avoided:

Alcohol usage: Patients should be advised not to drink alcohol while attempting to quit smoking, particularly in the first several weeks, as it affects will power, is associated with smoking for many, and commonly increases desire to smoke.

Proximity to others: Being around family or coworkers who are still using cigarettes can make it challenging for patients to quit themselves, as discussed previously.

   Once past the most vulnerable time for relapse, patients will eventually be able to be around former triggers to smoke without as much difficulty. But, the first month, at least, will require planning and exceptional changes to increase their odds for success.

Cessation Pharmacotherapy

The TTUD-CPG recommends that all patients be offered the benefit of pharmacotherapy except in rare cases of contraindications. Cessation attempts without medication are more likely to result in relapse and future lack of confidence for willingness to attempt again.

   There are seven FDA-approved medications for tobacco cessation that have been shown to double quit rates[47]:

   Five are NRT products: Nicotine patch (extended release), lozenge, gum, nasal spray, and oral inhaler (short-term release). Two are non-nicotine prescription medications: sustained-release bupropion (Zyban®) and varenicline (Chantix®). The brand names, precautions, dosing, adverse effects, advantages, disadvantages, and cost per day are shown in **Table 4-2**.[57]

   Since nicotine is the addictive substance in tobacco, NRT provides some of the nicotine the patient is used to getting from their tobacco without the harmful effects of smoking; withdrawal is eased, allowing the patient to focus on modifying the behavioral aspects of smoking, as discussed previously.

   As shown in **Figure 4-7**, clinicians should be aware that there is a significant difference in the nicotine received from tobacco products versus that in NRT products. The downside to this difference is that the much lower amount of nicotine received

TABLE 4-2 Cessation Pharmacotherapy Guide

FIRST-LINE FDA-APPROVED TOBACCO CESSATION MEDICATIONS[a]

MEDICATION	PRECAUTIONS[c]	ADVERSE EFFECTS	DOSAGE	USE	AVAILABILITY	COST/DAY[b]
Nicotine Gum	• Pregnancy (Category D) and breastfeeding • Recent (≤2 weeks) myocardial infarction • Serious underlying arrhythmias • Serious/worsening angina pectoris • Temporomandibular joint disease • Caution with dentures • Adolescents (<18 years) • Do not eat or drink 15 min before or during use.	• Mouth/jaw soreness • Dyspepsia • Hiccups • Hypersalivation • Effects associated with incorrect chewing technique: - Lightheadedness - Nausea/vomiting - Throat and mouth irritation	• 1st cigarette ≤30 min after waking: 4 mg • 1st cigarette >30 min after waking: 2 mg • Use 1 piece every 1-2 hours • Maximum, 24 pieces/day • Park between cheek and gum upon tingling sensation (15-30 chews). • Repeat when tingle fades. Park on other side.	• Up to 12 weeks • Longer if desired, with provider approval.	Nicorette®, Nicorette Mint®, generic products (OTC only) 2 mg, 4 mg Original, Mint, Cinnamon, and Fruit	2 mg or 4 mg: $1.90–$3.70 (9 pieces)

Nicotine Replacement Therapy (NRT) Formulations

Over the Counter (OTC)

(Continued)

57

TABLE 4-2 Cessation Pharmacotherapy Guide (Continued)

FIRST-LINE FDA-APPROVED TOBACCO CESSATION MEDICATIONS[a]

MEDICATION	PRECAUTIONS[c]	ADVERSE EFFECTS	DOSAGE	USE	AVAILABILITY	COST/DAY[b]
Nicotine Lozenge or Mini-Lozenge	• Pregnancy and breastfeeding—not evaluated by the FDA • Recent (≤2 weeks) myocardial infarction • Serious underlying arrhythmias • Serious/worsening angina pectoris • Adolescents (<18 years) • Do not eat or drink 15 minutes before or during use.	• Hiccups • Heartburn • Nausea • Headache (on 4 mg) • Cough (on 4 mg) • Hypertension • Flatulence • Insomnia	• 1st cigarette ≤30 min after waking: 4 mg • 1st cigarette >30 min after waking: 2 mg • Use 1 lozenge every 1-2 hours, 9-20 per day. • Allow to dissolve between cheek and gum. • Do not chew or swallow. Occasionally rotate to different areas of mouth.	• Up to 12 weeks • Longer if desired, with provider approval.	Commit™ Lozenge, Nicorette Mini Lozenge, generic products (OTC) 2 mg, 4 mg Mint, Original, Cherry	2 mg or 4 mg: $3.36–$3.78 (9 pieces)
Nicotine Patch	• Pregnancy (Category D) and breastfeeding • Recent (≤2 weeks) myocardial infarction • Serious underlying arrhythmias • Serious/worsening angina pectoris • Adolescents (<18 years)	• Local skin reaction • Sleep disturbances - Insomnia - Abnormal/vivid dreams • Headache	• One patch per day (hairless site) • If >10 cigs/day: 21 mg 4-6 weeks, 14 mg 2-4 weeks, 7 mg 2-4 weeks • If <10 cigs/day: 14 mg 6 weeks, then 7 mg 2 weeks • Do not cut/trim patch.	• 8-12 weeks • Longer if desired with provider approval. May wear patch for 16 hours if patient experiences sleep disturbances (remove at bedtime).	Nicoderm CQ®, Nicotrol, generic products (Rx and OTC).	$1.52–$3.48 (1 patch)

Over the Counter (OTC) (continued)

Nicotine Replacement Therapy (NRT) Formulations (continued)

	Precautions/Contraindications	Side Effects	Dosing	Duration	Prescription (Rx) only	Cost
Nicotine Nasal Spray	• Severe reactive airway disease • Underlying chronic nasal disorders (rhinitis, nasal polyps, sinusitis) • Pregnancy (Category D) and breastfeeding • Recent (≤2 weeks) myocardial infarction • Serious underlying arrhythmias • Serious/worsening angina pectoris • Adolescents (<18 years)	• Nasal and/or throat irritation (hot, peppery, or burning sensations, typically, only for a few initial days of use) • Rhinitis • Tearing • Sneezing • Cough • Headache	• 1-2 doses/hour (8-40 doses/day) (1 dose = 1 spray per nostril) • Maximum: 5 doses/hour • Patients should not sniff, swallow, or inhale through the nose as the spray is being administered. • On average 100 doses per bottle.	• 3-6 months	Nicotrol NS® (prescription only)	$6.67 (8 doses)
Nicotine Oral Inhaler	• Recent (≤2 weeks) myocardial infarction • Serious underlying arrhythmias • Serious/worsening angina pectoris • Bronchospastic disease (respiratory disease) • Pregnancy (Category D) and breastfeeding • Adolescents (<18 years) • Do not eat or drink 15 min before or during use.	• Local irritation of mouth and throat (typically, for only a few initial days of use) • Cough • Rhinitis • Hiccups • Dyspepsia • Headache	6-16 cartridges/day. Individualize dosing; initially use 1 cartridge q 1-2 hours. Nicotine in cartridge is used up after about 20 min of continuous puffing. Puffing on the inhaler for 5 min at a time will give enough nicotine for 4 uses. Do not inhale into the lungs, but "puff" or suck as if lighting a pipe.	• Up to 6 months • Taper dosage during final 3 months. • Keep in temp of 40° F or higher.	Nicotrol® Inhaler (prescription only) 10 mg cartridge delivers 4 mg inhaled nicotine vapor.	$11.35 (6 cartridges)

(Continued)

60

TABLE 4-2 Cessation Pharmacotherapy Guide (Continued)

FIRST-LINE FDA-APPROVED TOBACCO CESSATION MEDICATIONS[a]

MEDICATION	PRECAUTIONS[c]	ADVERSE EFFECTS	DOSAGE	USE	AVAILABILITY	COST/DAY[b]
Bupropion SR	• Concomitant therapy with medications known to lower the seizure threshold • Hepatic impairment • Pregnancy (Category C) and breastfeeding • Adolescents (<18 years) • Treatment-emergent neuropsychiatric symptoms: Boxed warning removed December 2016[d] Contraindications: • Seizure disorder • Concomitant bupropion (eg, Wellbutrin) therapy • Current or prior diagnosis of bulimia or anorexia nervosa • Simultaneous abrupt discontinuation of alcohol or sedatives/benzodiazepines • MAI inhibitors during preceding 14 days; concurrent use of reversible MAO inhibitors	• Sleep disturbance (vivid dreams, insomnia) • Dry mouth • Rash • Nervousness • Nausea, dizziness • Constipation • Seizures (risk 1/1,000) [0.1%] • Patients should be monitored for potential neuropsychiatric symptoms (rare).	• Days 1-3: 150 mg PO each morning • Days 4-end: 150 mg twice daily • Allow at least 8 hours between doses. • Avoid bedtime dosing to minimize insomnia. • Dose tapering is not necessary. • Can be used safely with NRT.	• Begin treatment 1-2 weeks before quit date. • Use for 7-12 weeks or maintenance up to 6 months. Don't take extra dose to make up for missed dose.	Zyban®, generic SR products (prescription only) 150 mg sustained-release tablet Do not exceed 300 mg/day	$2.58-$7.87 (2 tablets)

Non-Nicotine Medications[e]

Prescription (Rx) only (continued)

	Varenicline			Chantix™ (prescription only) 0.5 mg, 1 mg tablet	$11.86 (2 tablets)

Non-Nicotine Medications[e] (continued)	• Severe renal impairment (dosage adjustment is necessary)
	• Pregnancy (Category C) and breastfeeding
	• Adolescents (<18 years)
	• Treatment-emergent neuropsychiatric symptoms: Boxed warning removed December 2016[d]
		• Nausea/vomiting
		• Sleep disturbances
		  - Insomnia
		  - Abnormal/vivid dreams
		• Constipation
		• Flatulence
		• Seizures
		• Patients should be monitored for potential neuropsychiatric symptoms (rare)
			• Days 1-3: 0.5 mg PO every morning
			• Days 4-7: 0.5 mg twice daily
			• Days 8-end: 1 mg twice daily
			• Take dose after eating with a full glass of water.
			• Dose tapering is not necessary.
				Begin treatment 1 week before quit date. Dosing adjustments are necessary for patients with severe renal impairment. May initiate up to 35 days before target quit date. May reduce smoking over 12-week period of treatment prior to quitting and continue treatment for an additional 12 weeks. Use for 3 months; maintenance up to 6 months.	Prescription (Rx) only (continued)

[a] The information contained in this table is not comprehensive. Please see package insert for additional information.

[b] Cost/day based on prices provided in Smoking Cessation: A Report from the Surgeon General. January 2020. Wholesale acquisition cost from Red Book Online. Thomson Reuters, December 2016.

[c] Quitting smoking, with or without medication, can result in nicotine withdrawal symptoms (such as depressed mood, agitation) or a worsening of underlying psychiatric illness, such as depression. Monitor patients for behavior or mood changes.

[d] In July 2009, FDA mandated that the prescribing information for all bupropion- and varenicline-containing products include a black-boxed warning highlighting the risk of serious neuropsychiatric symptoms, including changes in behavior, hostility, agitation, depressed mood, suicidal thoughts and behavior, and attempted suicide. Clinicians should advise patients to stop taking varenicline or bupropion SR and contact a healthcare provider immediately if they experience agitation, depressed mood, or any changes in behavior that are not typical of nicotine withdrawal, or if they experience suicidal thoughts or behavior. If treatment is stopped due to neuropsychiatric symptoms, patients should be monitored until the symptoms resolve. Based on results of a mandated clinical trial, FDA removed this boxed warning in December 2016.

[e] Other prescription medications, such as nortriptyline or clonidine are not FDA approved for smoking cessation, but may be utilized for this purpose.

Adapted from: Fiore MC, Jaén CR, Baker TB, et al. Treating Tobacco Use and Dependence: 2008 Update. Quick Reference Guide for Clinicians. Rockville, MD: U.S. Department of Health and Human Services. Public Health Service. April 2009. Smoking Cessation: A Report from the Surgeon General Table 6.2. January 2020.

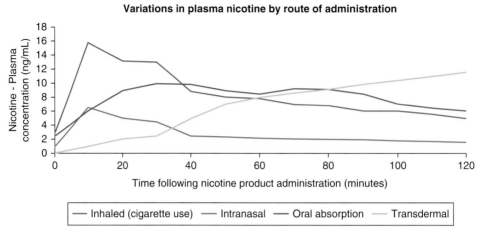

Figure 4-7. Plasma venous nicotine concentrations achieved with the various nicotine delivery systems. (Data from Choi JH, Dresler CM, Norton MR, Strahs KR. Pharmacokinetics of a nicotine polacrilex lozenge. *Nicotine Tob Res.* 2003;5(5):635-644; Fant RV, Henningfield JR, Nelson RA, Pickworth WB. Pharmacokinetics and pharmacodynamics of moist snuff in humans. *Tob Control.* 1999;8(4):387-392; Schneider NG, Olmstead RE, Franzon MA, Lunell E. The nicotine inhaler: clinical pharmacokinetics and comparison with other nicotine treatments. *Clin Pharmacokinet.* 2001;40(9):661-684.)

by a single NRT medication may not be sufficient to alleviate withdrawal symptoms for more nicotine-dependent patients. Nicotine dependence is usually determined by number of cigarettes smoked, on average, per day, or by the time between waking and smoking the first cigarette.[60] Those who smoke within 30 minutes of waking are considered more dependent.[56] The upside to this difference is that it lessens concern regarding nicotine toxicity from increased dosages or combination therapy.

Patient barriers: Often, patients do not have success with medications because of not using enough of the medication or using it incorrectly. The challenge with most NRT medications is counterintuition about their use: One should not chew the gum, suck the lozenge, inhale the inhaler, or sniff the nasal spray. Since these NRTs are not used as a patient would expect, tolerance, compliance, efficacy, and ultimately patient success are variable and can depend on detailed instructions for the chosen medication. Herein lies another issue, whereby patients are not likely to read all of the medication insert, as information may be written at a reading level beyond the patient's literacy.

Pharmacists, anecdotally, have even reported that it is not uncommon for prescribed cessation medications to remain at the pharmacy. This could be due, in part, to patient intimidation and an effort to please clinicians by agreeing to use the medications without definite plans to stop smoking. Another challenge could be concerns that are not being expressed by the patient about using medication or doubts about its benefit. Explaining how medication can affect their desire to smoke, how to use it most effectively with specific verbal instructions on proper use, and its limitations, along with confirming patient understanding can help to reduce barriers to patient medication adherence. It is also important to follow up and make adjustments to nicotine doses based on patient feedback.

The details of each specific NRT are important for both patients and providers to understand. These are discussed next.

Nicotine patch: A major advantage of the nicotine patch is its high compliance rate, likely due to ease of use, once-a-day application, and minimal interference with activities.[47] Patients starting to use the patch should be advised to have a short-term NRT product available to use for help with cravings if he or she completely stops smoking. The reasoning here is that it will take at least several hours for nicotine to reach maximum levels in the body when using the patch. Once withdrawal is achieved, however, the nicotine level remains at a steady state for the remainder of 24 hours. The patch is the only cessation product still available as both a prescription and an over-the-counter (OTC) product; it comes in three strengths (21, 14, and 7 mg) for tapering nicotine levels, although tapering has not increased cessation rates in clinical trials and is optional. Should sleep disturbances occur, which is common, the patch may be removed prior to bedtime.

Nicotine gum, lozenge, and inhaler: Success with the gum is best achieved with the "chew-and-park" technique. After chewing the gum just until the tingling sensation begins, the gum should be placed between the cheek and gum until this sensation fades. The gum should then be revived with a few chews and transitioned to, or "parked," on the other side until the sensation is gone (this process should take 20-30 minutes). The lozenge is similar to the gum, but instead has a "moisten-and-park" technique. The patient should be advised not to bite, chew, or suck hard on the lozenge. In addition to the standard lozenges, there are minilozenges that dissolve faster and are more convenient to carry, but both have a similar effect. The inhaler is plastic, is approximately the size of a cigarette, and has a replaceable nicotine cartridge inside. Describing this product to patients is important, as it does not resemble an asthma inhaler and also requires many short, frequent "puffs." It should not be inhaled into the lungs, as the user would have done with cigarettes. These three forms of NRT are meant to be absorbed in the buccal mucosa, in a basic pH environment. Since acidity in the mouth can limit both absorption and efficacy, patients should be instructed not to eat or drink 15 minutes prior to or during use of these products. If this cannot be avoided, patients should swish with water prior to medication use.[50]

Nicotine nasal spray: For the nicotine nasal spray, nicotine is absorbed through the nasal mucosa, providing the fastest onset but with the risk of nasal irritation. Clinicians should advise patients to tilt their head back when using the spray but not to sniff or inhale while spraying. Patients should also delay blowing the nose to allow for better absorption.

With any of the OTC medications, provide specific recommendations to the patient about which type to purchase since there are many variations (generic vs. brand name, flavors, strengths, etc.), which can be somewhat overwhelming for patients in the retail setting.

Non-nicotine replacement smoking cessation:

a. **Bupropion SR:** This is an oral medication that helps reduce a patient's urge to smoke. The formulation was originally developed as an antidepressant (Wellbutrin®) but was later discovered to aid with cessation. The neurobiological mechanism here is an increase of synaptic dopamine and norepinephrine, in addition to antagonizing some nAChRs.[61] For this indication, it was marketed under another brand name (Zyban®). It can be used in combination with NRT. Dosages are gradually increased over 1-2 weeks to reach full potency by the patient's quit date.

b. **Varenicline:** Varenicline (Chantix) is another oral medication that helps to reduce nicotine withdrawal, urge to smoke, and satisfaction from smoking by partial agonism of nicotine receptors. Dosages are gradually increased to reach full potency by the patient's quit date or can be taken concurrently with cigarette weaning.

c. **Combination therapy:** In general, the combination of the nicotine patch with another form of NRT or with varenicline is both more effective than a single NRT or sustained-release bupropion alone. In addition, research has shown that using the nicotine patch with bupropion was more effective than bupropion alone, while bupropion with combination NRT was seemingly more effective than a combination with NRT alone.[47]

Alternative therapies, such as acupressure, acupuncture, and laser therapy, as per Cochrane analyses, are not associated with sustained (ie, ≥ 6 months) smoking cessation, and the effects of hypnotherapy were not found to effect cessation in randomized clinical trials.[61,62]

Follow-up and Resources: *Arrange*

After establishing a quit plan, it is key also to arrange for a follow-up phone call or visit with the patient 1-2 weeks after the scheduled quit date. This allows time for the patient to adequately determine efficacy and tolerance of their medication(s) and to report any issues that may indicate the need to change dosage or type. Also, if the patient is anticipating a phone call from the clinic or an upcoming appointment, there is more motivation to remain abstinent to report positive results. Perhaps most important, the patient is provided with reassurance that there will be help available going forward as the patient embarks on this challenging process.

Patients should be reminded that pharmacists are a tremendous resource due to their knowledge of both OTC and prescription medications, easy access, and free guidance. Other resources included further in this chapter can provide additional support and follow-up.

Patients Not Ready/Willing to Quit

Often, once a patient indicates he or she is not ready to quit or is not even interested, that tends to end the conversation because clinicians may not be aware of recommended approaches to this situation or do not want to offend or seem pushy about pursuing the topic. At this point in the discussion, after clear, strong, and personalized advice to quit has been given and the patient is not ready to quit, there are questions to foster motivation that may move the patient along the continuum toward contemplating cessation. The PHS guideline recommends the five *R* strategy (relevance, risks, rewards, roadblocks, and repetition). This brief approach involves doing more asking than telling since personally motivating factors originating with the patient can have the most impact.

Relevance: ask how quitting smoking is personally relevant (reasons to quit)

Risks: ask about negative consequences of continued smoking

Rewards: ask about potential benefits of quitting

Roadblocks: ask about barriers to successful quitting and provide potential remedies

Repetition: discussion should be revisited every time the patient returns

If only some of the *R*'s can be addressed due to time constraints, it is still beneficial. The recommended approach for impacting resistance to any behavior is motivational interviewing. While training for this application is ideal, the concept is to ask open-ended questions that do not allow for a yes or no answer and to incorporate reflective listening. These questions help the patient to verbalize, perhaps for the first time, what they perceive as negative about smoking and positive about quitting, which can be very positive reinforcement. One significant negative aspect of tobacco use is the cost. To help motivate the patient, the message can be personalized by asking them how much they spend on a pack of cigarettes and how many packs they smoke a day. Multiplying these amounts by 365 will provide the amount the patient is spending on the smoking each year. This can be surprising and motivating information for the patient, especially since most patients have not wanted to calculate this for themselves.

Perceived stress relief: There are common beliefs and barriers that can hinder patients from taking this important and challenging step. Patients regularly mention the perceived benefit that smoking relieves their stress. It is understandable that they would confuse relief from physical withdrawal symptoms such as irritability and anxiety as "stress relief." It is important for these patients to understand the cycle that has been created by nicotine addiction's effect on brain chemistry and the effects that are both caused and relieved by its routine use.

Fear of failure: Another significant reason for reluctance to quit is due to lack of confidence. Many patients have tried quitting numerous times and have understandably lost hope that another attempt would make any difference. It is important to point out to these patients the clinical assistance they would receive with this attempt versus prior attempts and what can be achieved with adherence to a different medication or combination therapy. These patients could also be reassured that it takes several attempts on average for people to remain a non- smoker for good.

Lack of medication assistance: For those who have quit previously, especially without pharmacotherapy, the experience of withdrawal symptoms can be quite daunting. In addition to previously mentioned symptoms, difficulty concentrating, negative mood, depression, insomnia, restlessness, and increased appetite/weight gain are commonly experienced—discouraging future attempts. Helping patients who have only quit for a matter of hours or a few days to realize that these symptoms are short term and will lessen in both frequency and intensity in a couple of weeks could help them to persist.

Reduce to Quit

> **CLINICAL PEARL:** Last, a pharmacological approach would be to encourage the patient to try NRT, particularly the patch, while continuing to smoke. This will likely lead to the patient smoking less due to the nicotine already in their system, as well as to improved confidence in their ability to cut back or quit altogether.[55]

Lung cancer screening availability with LDCT in recent years has provided an appropriate opportunity to intervene with patients who are currently smoking. In fact, the

Centers for Medicare and Medicaid Services requires shared decision-making prior to screening, which includes tobacco cessation counseling as a component. This is strongly encouraged with every patient who smokes, regardless of insurance coverage.

Following screening, patients with normal scan results should be reminded that an LDCT may not find all lung cancers, and that continued smoking still greatly increases their risk for lung and many other cancers going forward.

Fortunately, reimbursement from Medicare, Medicaid, and private insurance for physician, nurse practitioner, clinical nurse specialist, and physician assistant counseling is better than any time in history. Specific billing codes can be found in resources included at the end of this chapter. In addition, coverage for the various medications has improved. But, patients should be advised to verify with their individual plan which ones are included and if prior authorization or other steps are required for coverage.

Tobacco Treatment After Lung Cancer Diagnosis

About 50% of lung cancer patients are current smokers at the time of diagnosis, and more than 80% of those continue to smoke after diagnosis.[63] For those who continue to smoke, a low proportion report that they were offered or provided assistance in quitting.

After a lung cancer diagnosis, many patients currently smoking and even some providers may take the stance that there is no point in quitting, perceiving that the damage is already done. In fact, current smoking in cancer patients increases the risk for cancer-related mortality and overall mortality by 60% and 50%, respectively. This is compared to a much lower increase of risk in overall mortality by approximately 20% for former smokers, suggesting at least some of the effects from smoking are reversible.[64]

According to the 2014 surgeon general's report,[11] smoking causes adverse outcomes for patients with cancer, and evidence exists that continued smoking may

- Increase risk of cancer recurrence
- Increase the likelihood of a second primary tumor
- Reduce treatment effectiveness
- Worsen side effects of treatment
- Increase treatment-related toxicity
- Increase risk for poor wound healing and for respiratory complications after surgery

Several studies have demonstrated that for patients with lung cancer, tobacco use decreases quality of life and decreases survival. Another study suggested that people who continue to smoke after a diagnosis of early-stage lung cancer almost double their risk of dying. In contrast, data have indicated that outcomes are improved for those cancer patients who quit tobacco use.[63,65]

A meta-analysis of 10 studies highlighted the notable difference between the 5-year survival rate for those who continued to smoke with small cell and non–small cell lung cancer of 29% and 33%, respectively, versus those who quit smoking, whose rates were 63% and 70%, respectively.[63]

There are numerous contributing factors for why structured tobacco treatment services are not well established in all cancer care centers. It is reported that a large portion of oncologists do not feel adequately trained to provide appropriate tobacco cessation assistance and support, contributing to many oncologists not delivering this treatment to their patients who smoke. This is demonstrated by large surveys showing that even though approximately 90% of oncologists ask about tobacco use and 80% advise to quit, only about 40% of oncologists routinely provide recommended assistance to their patients. Contributing to this status could be concern that by focusing on smoking, the existing shame and guilt smokers commonly feel with a cancer diagnosis could just be exacerbated. In turn, due to stigma particularly associated with lung cancer and smoking, patients may understandably be reluctant to answer detailed questions about former or current tobacco use if family members or friends are present.[66,67]

The NCI Cancer Center Cessation Initiative (C3) has been launched with the ultimate goal of ensuring "that all patients with cancer who smoke are provided with cessation support and assistance such as counseling and medication in conjunction with their cancer care."[67]

More time may be needed to provide tobacco treatment to some cancer patients than to others due to factors such as stress, anxiety, and depression. However, a cancer diagnosis also can be highly motivating for cessation. Patients with cancer may be motivated to quit smoking because of awareness of the link between smoking and their diagnosed smoking-related cancer, as well as concern about recurrent disease and the negative effects of smoking on treatment success. Patient motivation based on these factors is highly predicated on their oncology care providers communicating the risks of continued smoking and benefits of quitting as soon as possible after their diagnosis. Discussion about past or current smoking could be more productive if conducted with the patient without family members or friends present. If the subject of blame related to smoking arises from the patient or others, it may be helpful to indicate it is not possible to be certain which factors caused the lung cancer, but that it is very important to focus all energy and effort on survivorship and the steps to successfully treat the cancer moving forward. Patients and family members may also benefit from visiting a behavioral oncologist or psychologist to cope with feelings surrounding the cancer diagnosis.

Resources for Additional Assistance

Certified tobacco treatment specialists (CTTSs): These professionals are highly trained with a focus on tobacco cessation treatment and can provide valuable assistance beyond the clinician visit, throughout the quit attempt. They can spend additional time with the patient that a clinician may not have and can provide in-depth counseling or multiple sessions to increase the likelihood of abstinence. A CTTS may be available for patient referral within the health system or in the community.

Quit line: The quit line sponsored by the NCI (1-800-QUIT-NOW) is staffed with trained coaches who provide assistance, referrals, and resources. The national number is administered by individual states, which offer somewhat different services and call routing is based on the area code of the phone number placing the call. When clinicians refer patients interested in quitting to the quit line for their state through an e-referral, patients will be called proactively; this approach has been shown to double quit rates.

Community classes: These group sessions provide support, education, and possibly some accountability, as those attending share similar experiences and suggestions for coping with cessation challenges. The benefit of this group interaction has been extended to online platforms. Both of these options are available through the American Lung Association's Freedom From Smoking.

Online and other assistance: Several types of resources are available online, including the NCI's live text chat with a specialist, motivational text messages, and information targeted to special populations, such as on smokefree.gov.

Recommended organizations: For additional resources, the following have up-to-date, accurate information for both clinicians and patients:

1. NCI (cancer.gov)
2. American Cancer Society (cancer.org)
3. American Lung Association (lung.org)
4. American Society of Clinical Oncology (asco.org)
5. Rx for Change—Smoking Cessation Leadership Institute (rxforchange.ucsf.edu)
6. GO$_2$ (https://go2foundation.org)
7. LuCa National Training Network (lucatraining.org)
8. Association for the Treatment of Tobacco Use and Dependence (attud.org)

Without assistance, approximately 95% of quit attempts end in failure.[59] Given that tobacco not only is the single greatest preventable cause of death and disease in the United States, but also is responsible for the majority of lung cancers, clinicians should intervene with every patient using tobacco and provide assistance as a top priority in their care.

THE GLOBAL BURDEN OF TOBACCO USE

As a final point in the discussion of tobacco use, it is critical for providers to understand that tobacco consumption is a global issue that is by no means limited to the United States. This is especially important for American-based physicians who care for patients who are traveling from abroad to the United States, as tobacco use greatly impacts their overall state of health. For these patients, a thorough social history should be conducted for each patient, ultimately to better inform the physician of that patient's risk factors for the development of not only lung cancer but also cardiovascular disease and stroke.

In 2017, the World Health Organization released a report on the global epidemic of tobacco use. Included next are some of the key points that highlight the burden of tobacco use worldwide:

- There are approximately 1.1 billion persons in the world who smoke tobacco. Approximately 80% of this population reside in countries of low and middle incomes.
- Over 7 million persons are killed from the effects of tobacco every year. Over 6 million deaths result from direct tobacco use, while approximately 890,000 result from secondhand smoke exposure.
- Only 39% of countries routinely monitor the use of tobacco through youth and adult surveys every 5 years.

- Only 26 countries, representing approximately 33% of the global population, have comprehensive cessation services with either partial or full-cost coverage available on a national level.

- Tobacco advertising in any form has been banned in only 37 countries, comprising a mere 15% of the global population.

For providers, maintaining an awareness of these points is key in screening for tobacco use in *all* patients, in both the pediatric and adult populations. Subsequent treatment of tobacco use disorder, if present, as per the recommendations set forth previously in this chapter will truly be essential in the prevention of lung cancer in patients across the world.[1]

REFERENCES

1. World Health Organization (WHO). *WHO Report on the Global Tobacco Epidemic, 2008*. Geneva, Switzerland: World Health Organization; 2008.
2. Goodman J. *Tobacco in History and Culture: An Encyclopedia*. Detroit, MI: Thompson Gale; 2005.
3. Appleby J. *The Relentless Revolution: A History of Capitalism*. New York, NY: Norton; 2010.
4. Alberg AJ, Shopland DR, Cummings KM. The 2014 surgeon general's report: commemorating the 50th anniversary of the 1964 report of the Advisory Committee to the US surgeon general and updating the evidence on the health consequences of cigarette smoking. *Am J Epidemiol*. 2014;179(4):403-412. Epub 2014/01/18. doi:10.1093/aje/kwt335.
5. Warren G, ed. Tobacco and Lung Cancer. Annual Society of Oncology; 2013; Chicago. DOI: 10.1200/EdBook_AM.2013.33.359.
6. Peto R, Lopez AD. Future worldwide health effects of current smoking patterns. In: Koop CE, Pearson CE, Schwarz MR, eds. *Critical Issues in Global Health*. San Francisco, CA: Wiley (Jossey-Bass); 2001:154-161.
7. General TRotS. General Surgeon Report on "Smoking and Health" 1964. https://profiles.nlm.nih.gov/ps/access/NNBBMR.pdf.
8. Allan BM. *The Cigarette Century*. New York, NY: Basic Books; 2007.
9. Centers for Disease Control and Prevention. Tobacco-related spending 2018. https://www.cdc.gov/tobacco/data_statistics/fact_sheets/economics/econ_facts/index.htm.
10. Mokdad AH, Dwyer-Lindgren L, Fitzmaurice C, et al. Trends and patterns of disparities in cancer mortality among US counties, 1980-2014. *JAMA*. 2017;317(4):388-406. Epub 2017/01/25. doi:10.1001/jama.2016.20324.
11. US Department of Health and Human Services. *The Health Consequences of Smoking—50 Years of Progress: A Report of the Surgeon General*. Atlanta, GA: US Department of Health and Human Services, Centers for Disease Control and Prevention, National Center for Chronic Disease Prevention and Health Promotion, Office on Smoking and Health; 2014. https://www.surgeongeneral.gov/library/reports/50-years-of-progress/full-report.pdf. Accessed April 6, 2019.
12. Centers for Disease Control and Prevention. History of surgeon general's reports on smoking and health. Centers for Disease Control and Prevention; 2006. https://www.cdc.gov/tobacco/data_statistics/sgr/history/index.htm. Accessed April 6, 2019.
13. Mousavi SM, Schmid S, Cerny T, Fruh M. Lung cancer and smoking trends in the young in Switzerland: a study based on data of the National Institute for Cancer Epidemiology and Registration and of the Swiss Health Surveys. *Swiss Med Wkly*. 2018;148:w14708. Epub 2018/12/31. doi:10.4414/smw.2018.14708.
14. US Department of Health and Human Services PHS, Centers for Disease Control and Prevention. *The Health Consequences of Smoking: A Report of the Surgeon General*. Vol. 7829. Washington, DC: CDC; 2004. https://pubmed.ncbi.nlm.nih.gov/20669512/. Accessed April 6, 2019.
15. Alonso R, Pineros M, Laversanne M, et al. Lung cancer incidence trends in Uruguay 1990-2014: an age-period-cohort analysis. *Cancer Epidemiol*. 2018;55:17-22. Epub 2018/05/15. doi:10.1016/j.canep.2018.04.012.
16. Hurt RD. Tobacco and society: How we can make a difference in public policy [Oral presentation]. Mayo Foundation for Medical Education and Research; 2013. https://www.mayo.edu/research/documents/ndep-112013-tobacco-society-hurt/doc-20087324. Accessed April 6, 2019.
17. Centers for Disease Control and Prevention. Smoking and tobacco use: Cigars. 2018. https://www.cdc.gov/tobacco/data_statistics/fact_sheets/tobacco_industry/cigars/index.htm. Accessed April 6, 2019.

18. Tverdal A, Bjartveit K. Health consequences of pipe versus cigarette smoking. *Tob Control*. 2011;20(2):123-130. Epub 2010/10/19. doi:10.1136/tc.2010.036780.

19. National Center for Chronic Disease Prevention and Health Promotion (US) Office on Smoking and Health. *Preventing Tobacco Use Among Youth and Young Adults: A Report of the Surgeon General*. Atlanta, GA: Centers for Disease Control and Prevention; 2012. https://www.surgeongeneral.gov/library/reports/preventing-youth-tobacco-use/full-report.pdf. Accessed April 6, 2019.

20. Cobb C, Ward KD, Maziak W, Shihadeh AL, Eissenberg T. Waterpipe tobacco smoking: an emerging health crisis in the United States. *Am J Health Behav*. 2010;34(3):275-285. Epub 2009/12/17.

21. American Lung Association. *An Emerging Deadly Trend: Waterpipe Tobacco Use*. Tobacco Policy Trend Alert. 2007. https://www.ncbi.nlm.nih.gov/pmc/articles/PMC3215592/. Accessed April 6, 2019.

22. Centers for Disease Control and Prevention. Bidi use among urban youth-Massachusetts, March-April 1999. *MMWR Morbid Mortal Wkly Rep*. 1999;48(36):796-799. https://www.cdc.gov/mmwr/preview/mmwrhtml/mm4836a2.htm. Accessed April 6, 2019.

23. American Lung Association. Hookah smoking: A growing threat to public health. Issue Brief 2011. https://www.lung.org/stop-smoking/tobacco-control-advocacy/reports-resources/cessation-economic-benefits/reports/hookah-policy-brief.pdf. Accessed April 6, 2019.

24. Yen KL, Hechavarria E, Bostwick SB. Bidi cigarettes: An emerging threat to adolescent health. *Arch Pediatr Adolesc Med*. 2000;154(12):1187-1189. Epub 2000/12/15.

25. Rahman M, Fukui T. Bidi smoking and health. *Public Health*. 2000;114(2):123-127. Epub 2000/05/09. doi:10.1038/sj.ph.1900625.

26. Rahman M, Sakamoto J, Fukui T. Bidi smoking and oral cancer: a meta-analysis. *Int J Cancer*. 2003;106(4):600-604. Epub 2003/07/08. doi:10.1002/ijc.11265.

27. Sankaranarayanan R, Duffy SW, Padmakumary G, Nair SM, Day NE, Padmanabhan TK. Risk factors for cancer of the oesophagus in Kerala, India. *Int J Cancer*. 1991;49(4):485-489. Epub 1991/10/21.

28. Gupta PC, Asma S. *Bidi Smoking and Public Health*. New Delhi, India: Ministry of Health and Family Welfare, Government of India. https://www.who.int/tobacco/publications/prod_regulation/bidi_smoking_public_health.pdf. Accessed April 6, 2019.

29. Watson CH, Polzin GM, Calafat AM, Ashley DL. Determination of tar, nicotine, and carbon monoxide yields in the smoke of bidi cigarettes. *Nicotine Tob Research*. 2003;5(5):747-753. Epub 2003/10/28.

30. Malson JL, Lee EM, Murty R, Moolchan ET, Pickworth WB. Clove cigarette smoking: biochemical, physiological, and subjective effects. *Pharmacol Biochem Behav*. 2003;74(3):739-745. Epub 2003/01/25.

31. World Health Organization, Internal Agency for Research of Cancer. *World Health Organization: IARC Monographs on the Evaluation of Carcinogenic Risks to Humans. Volume 89: Smokeless Tobacco and Some Tobacco-Specific N-Nitrosamines*. 2007. https://monographs.iarc.fr/wp-content/uploads/2018/06/mono89.pdf. Accessed April 6, 2019.

32. Center for Behavioral Health Statistics and Quality. *2016 National Survey on Drug Use and Health: Detailed Tables*. 2017. https://www.samhsa.gov/data/sites/default/files/NSDUH-DetTabs-2016/NSDUH-DetTabs-2016.htm#tab2-6B. Accessed April 6, 2019.

33. Centers for Disease Control and Prevention. About electronic cigarettes (e-cigarettes). 2018. https://www.cdc.gov/tobacco/basic_information/e-cigarettes/about-e-cigarettes.html. Accessed April 6, 2019.

34. Cullen KA, Ambrose BK, Gentzke AS, Apelberg BJ, Jamal A, King BA. Notes from the field: use of electronic cigarettes and any tobacco product among middle and high school students—United States, 2011-2018. *MMWR Morb Mortal Wkly Rep*. 2018;67(45):1276-1277. Epub 2018/11/16. doi:10.15585/mmwr.mm6745a5.

35 Caraballo RS, Shafer PR, Patel D, Davis KC, McAfee TA. Quit methods used by US adult cigarette smokers, 2014-2016. *Prev Chronic Dis*. 2017;14:E32. Epub 2017/04/15. doi:10.5888/pcd14.160600.

36. QuickStats: Cigarette smoking status among current adult e-cigarette users, by age group—National Health Interview Survey, United States, 2015. *MMWR Morb Mortal Wkly Rep*. 2016;65(42):1177. Epub 2016/10/28. doi:10.15585/mmwr.mm6542a7.

37. Patnode CD, Henderson JT, Thompson JH, Senger CA, Fortmann SP, Whitlock EP. *Behavioral Counseling and Pharmacotherapy Interventions for Tobacco Cessation in Adults, Including Pregnant Women: A Review of Reviews for the US Preventive Services Task Force*. Rockville, MD: Agency for Healthcare Research and Quality; 2015.

38. Centers for Disease Control and Prevention. Smoking is down, but almost 38 million American adults still smoke. Press release. 2018. https://www.cdc.gov/media/releases/2018/p0118-smoking-rates-declining.html. Accessed April 6, 2019.

39. Centers for Disease Control and Prevention. Map of current cigarette use among adults. 2018. https://www.cdc.gov/statesystem/cigaretteuseadult.html. Accessed April 6, 2019.

40. Centers for Disease Control and Prevention. Map of current cigarette use among youth. 2018. https://www.cdc.gov/statesystem/cigaretteuseyouth.html. Accessed April 6, 2019.

41. Wang TW, Asman K, Gentzke AS, et al. Tobacco product use among adults—United States, 2017. *MMWR Morb Mortal Wkly Rep.* 2018;67(44):1225-1232. Epub 2018/11/09. doi:10.15585/mmwr.mm6744a2.

42. Zhu SH, Zhuang YL, Wong S, Cummins SE, Tedeschi GJ. E-cigarette use and associated changes in population smoking cessation: evidence from US current population surveys. *BMJ.* 2017;358:j3262. Epub 2017/07/28. doi:10.1136/bmj.j3262.

43. National Cancer Institute. *Lung Cancer Prevention (PDQ®)—Health Professional Version.* 2018. https://www.cancer.gov/types/lung/hp/lung-prevention-pdq#_223_toc. Accessed April 7, 2019.

44. Inamura K, Ninomiya H, Nomura K, et al. Combined effects of asbestos and cigarette smoke on the development of lung adenocarcinoma: different carcinogens may cause different genomic changes. *Oncol Rep.* 2014;32(2):475-82. Epub 2014/06/14. doi:10.3892/or.2014.3263.

45. Wong KY, Seow A, Koh WP, Shankar A, Lee HP, Yu MC. Smoking cessation and lung cancer risk in an Asian population: findings from the Singapore Chinese Health Study. *Br J Cancer.* 2010;103(7):1093-1096. Epub 2010/09/16. doi:10.1038/sj.bjc.6605782.

46. Pinsky PF, Zhu CS, Kramer BS. Lung cancer risk by years since quitting in 30+ pack year smokers. *J Med Screening.* 2015;22(3):151-157. Epub 2015/05/01. doi:10.1177/0969141315579119.

47. Prochaska JJ, Benowitz NL. The past, present, and future of nicotine addiction therapy. *Annu Rev Med.* 2016;67:467-486. Epub 2015/09/04. doi:10.1146/annurev-med-111314-033712.

48. Benowitz NL. Nicotine addiction. *N Engl J Med.* 2010;362(24):2295-2303. Epub 2010/06/18. doi:10.1056/NEJMra0809890.

49. Brody AL, Mukhin AG, Mamoun MS, et al. Brain nicotinic acetylcholine receptor availability and response to smoking cessation treatment: a randomized trial. *JAMA Psychiatry.* 2014;71(7):797-805. Epub 2014/05/23. doi:10.1001/jamapsychiatry.2014.138.

50. Henningfield JE, Radzius A, Cooper TM, Clayton RR. Drinking coffee and carbonated beverages blocks absorption of nicotine from nicotine polacrilex gum. *JAMA.* 1990;264(12):1560-1564. Epub 1990/09/26.

51. Centers for Disease Control and Prevention. Tobacco use among adults with mental and substance use disorders. 2019. https://www.cdc.gov/tobacco/disparities/mental-illness-substance-use/index.htm. Accessed April 6, 2019.

52. Epstein DH, Marrone GF, Heishman SJ, Schmittner J, Preston KL. Tobacco, cocaine, and heroin: craving and use during daily life. *Addict Behav.* 2010;35(4):318-324. Epub 2009/11/27. doi:10.1016/j.addbeh.2009.11.003.

53. Allenby CE, Boylan KA, Lerman C, Falcone M. Precision medicine for tobacco dependence: development and validation of the nicotine metabolite ratio. *J Neuroimmune Pharmacol.* 2016;11(3):471-483. Epub 2016/02/14. doi:10.1007/s11481-016-9656-y.

54. Fagerstrom K, Hughes J. Varenicline in the treatment of tobacco dependence. *Neuropsychiatr Dis Treat.* 2008;4(2):353-363. Epub 2008/08/30.

55. Fiore MC, Baker TB. Clinical practice. Treating smokers in the health care setting. *N Engl J Med.* 2011;365(13):1222-1231. Epub 2011/10/14. doi:10.1056/NEJMcp1101512.

56. Tobacco Use and Dependence Guideline Panel. *Treating Tobacco Use and Dependence: 2008 Update.* Rockville, MD: US Department of Health and Human Services; 2008. https://www.ncbi.nlm.nih.gov/books/NBK63952/. Accessed April 6, 2019.

57. Lung Cancer National Training Network. *Drug Interactions With Tobacco Smoke for Oncology Specialists.* Louisville, KY: LuCa National Training Network; 2020. https://lucatraining.org/services/resource-library/drug-interactions-with-tobacco-smoke-for-oncology-specialists.

58. Lung Cancer National Training Network. *First-Line FDA-Approved Medications.* Louisville, KY: LuCa National Training Network; 2020. https://lucatraining.org/services/luca-tools.

59. Jha P CF, Novotny TW, Cohen JC, Yurekli A, Sweanor D, Beyer JD. *Smoking Cessation and Nicotine Replacement Therapies. Tobacco Control in Developing Countries.* New York, NY: Oxford University Press; 2000.

60. Agency for Healthcare Research and Quality. Treating tobacco use and dependence: PHS clinical practice guideline. 2012. https://www.ahrq.gov/professionals/clinicians-providers/guidelines-recommendations/tobacco/systemclin.html. Accessed April 6, 2019.

61. White AR, Rampes H, Liu JP, Stead LF, Campbell J. Acupuncture and related interventions for smoking cessation. *Cochrane Database Syst Rev.* 2014(1):Cd000009. Epub 2014/01/25. doi:10.1002/14651858.CD000009.pub4.

62. Barnes J, Dong CY, McRobbie H, Walker N, Mehta M, Stead LF. Hypnotherapy for smoking cessation. *Cochrane Database Syst Rev.* 2010(10):Cd001008. Epub 2010/10/12. doi:10.1002/14651858.CD001008.pub2.

63. Parsons A, Daley A, Begh R, Aveyard P. Influence of smoking cessation after diagnosis of early stage lung cancer on prognosis: systematic review of observational studies with meta-analysis. *BMJ.* 2010;340:b5569. Epub 2010/01/23. doi:10.1136/bmj.b5569.

64. Warren GW. Cigarette smoking and systemic therapy for lung cancer: considering the evidence to improve cancer care. *J Thorac Oncol.* 2014;9(7):914-916. Epub 2014/06/14. doi:10.1097/jto.0000000000000252.

65. Warren GW, Singh AK. Nicotine and lung cancer. *J Carcinog.* 2013;12:1. Epub 2013/04/20. doi:10.4103/1477-3163.106680.

66. Warren GW, Sobus S, Gritz ER. The biological and clinical effects of smoking by patients with cancer and strategies to implement evidence-based tobacco cessation support. *Lancet Oncol.* 2014;15(12):e568-e580. Epub 2014/12/03. doi:10.1016/s1470-2045(14)70266-70269.

67. Croyle RT, Morgan GD, Fiore MC. Addressing a core gap in cancer care—the NCI Moonshot Program to help oncology patients stop smoking. *N Engl J Med.* 2019;380(6):512-515. Epub 2019/01/03. doi:10.1056/NEJMp1813913.

5

ECONOMICS OF LUNG CANCER

Jorge A. Rios, MD • Shruti Bhandari, MD

Kathy was diagnosed with advanced adenocarcinoma of the left upper lobe metastatic to the bones in January 2016. Within 5 weeks ofer diagnosis, she had low-dose lung computed tomography (CT), a second chest CT scan to confirm the findings, pulmonary function tests, a lung needle biopsy, a positron emission tomography (PET)/CT scan, several blood tests, and next-generation sequencing searching for actionable genetic alterations and was seen by a medical oncologist. Kathy was deemed not a candidate for targeted therapy or immunotherapy up front and began chemotherapy in March 2016. Response to chemotherapy was evaluated with serial CT scans. In May, Kathy was found to have progression of her disease during an emergency room visit and started second-line immunotherapy in June at her doctor's office. The immunotherapy resulted in stable disease and maintained her quality of life, so Kathy continued the treatment and monitoring through the end of the year.

Kathy bought an individual health insurance plan, which started in January 2016, through her state's marketplace. The premium for her plan was $537 per month, but she qualified for tax credits, which helped reduce these costs. Kathy ended up paying $272 per month in premiums. Kathy's highest costs were in January ($3,678) and February ($3,716), when she had multiple diagnostic tests and paid 40% percent co-insurance for imaging tests and scans, in addition to premiums. She met her maximum out-of-pocket limit in February; after that, no cost sharing was required as long as she paid her premiums and received all her care in network. At the end of her plan year, Kathy had paid a total of $3,264 in premiums and $6,850 in cost sharing for her cancer care. The total health care costs for Kathy's lung cancer treatment in 2016 were $210,067. Kathy's insurance plan paid the vast majority of these costs—$203,217. (Adapted from an American Cancer Society Cancer Action Network Report: Singleterry J. *The Cost of Cancer: Addressing Patient Costs*.[1])

Learning Objectives:
1. What are the financial consequences of the improvement in therapies and lung cancer outcomes?
2. What are the factors driving the rising cost of lung cancer care?
3. What is the impact of rising costs on patients and society?
4. What are the instruments and strategies used to evaluate the value of any given lung cancer therapy?
5. What are the current efforts to address these rising costs of lung cancer care?

Lung cancer is the leading cause of cancer-related mortality worldwide.[2,3] The development of new therapies for lung cancer (targeted therapies and immunotherapy), along with an increase in prevention efforts, has resulted in a reduction in the incidence and mortality of lung cancer in some populations (eg, men in Northern Europe and North America). In other groups, however, the incidence and mortality in women have reportedly increased (women in a large part of Europe, South America, and Asia).[4,5] The increase in clinical effectiveness from these new therapies has been accompanied by an increase in the economic burden of cancer care, which in turn could limit patient access to these therapies. Inadequate access to cancer care could have a substantially negative impact on cancer outcomes for those affected individuals.[6,7] Given the increase in the cost of lung cancer care, the challenge for health care providers and health systems is to deliver high-quality cancer care while utilizing the limited economic resources efficiently.

COST OF LUNG CANCER THERAPIES

It has been estimated that in 2017, the United States spent $13.9 billion on lung cancer care, a significant increase from 2010 ($12.1 billion) and 2013 ($12.9 billion).[8] Any discussion regarding the economic impact of lung cancer care must consider the total cost of care (the cost paid by health insurance companies/managed care organizations, employers, patients, and taxpayer-funded programs such as Medicare). Unfortunately, the information available regarding cancer care expenditure and total cost of cancer care is scarce. For instance, the number of articles available in PubMed related to health care expenditure, total cost of care, cost effectiveness, cost analysis, and economics of lung cancer care represent a small fraction (0.74%) of the total number of published lung cancer articles.[9] Furthermore, given the variability among health systems, regulatory agencies, and economic models among countries, attempting a discussion of the economics of lung cancer that would apply to all settings around the globe seems unrealistic. This discussion uses the US society and health system as a framework.

The total cost of cancer care has different components.[10] Direct costs include inpatient care (hospital admissions), emergency room visits, ambulatory care (doctor's visits), radiation, chemotherapy infusions, radiology, and more. These are the most readily measurable. Indirect costs include lost income, child care, mental services, transportation, caregiving costs, and so on. Intangible costs are related to pain, suffering, and grief. All these components of the total cost of care are influenced by multiple factors, such as type of insurance (directly linked to patient out-of-pocket expenses), geographic location, affiliation of health care provided, type of cancer, and more.[3] There is limited

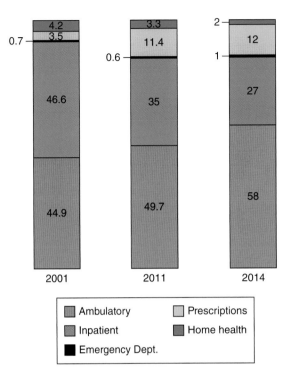

Figure 5-1. Percentage distribution of expenditure for cancer treatment, by type of service. (Agency for Health Care Research and Quality Total expenses and percent distribution selected conditions by source of payment: United States, 2014. Medical Expenditure Panel Survey Household Component Data. 2014. https://meps.ahrq.gov/mepsweb/data_stats/quick_tables_results.jsp?Action=Search&SearchMethod=1&component=1&subcomponent=0&tableSeries=2&year=-1).

information available regarding the fraction of the total cost that each of these components represents.

In the United States, a large-scale survey of individuals, medical providers, and employers conducted yearly since 1996 by the US Department of Health and Human Services has estimated the health care use and expenditure for treating cancer among the US adult civilian population.[11] These estimates have shown variation on the percentage of the cost for each component reported throughout the years (**Figure 5-1**).[11,12] Similar efforts from private entities have also shown variation in the distribution of the health expenditures on cancer care throughout time. For instance, an analysis of claims from a large database containing clinical and health expenditure data from Medicare, Medicaid, and privately insured patients[13] and a sample of 5% of Medicare patients found that health care expenditures for actively treated cancer patients varied between 2004 and 2014, as shown in **Figure 5-2**.[14] Both sources suggested a greater relative increase in the expenditure on ambulatory services and cancer-directed therapy compared to the other components of the total cost.

The total expenditure on cancer care for a single person varies through the course of the disease and is dependent on multiple factors (age at diagnosis, insurance status, insurance carrier, stage at diagnosis, comorbidities).[15] The average spending per patient increases just prior to diagnosis and spikes immediately following diagnosis.[15] The average annualized net costs of cancer care are highest in the last year of life, approximately 30% of the total cost.[8]

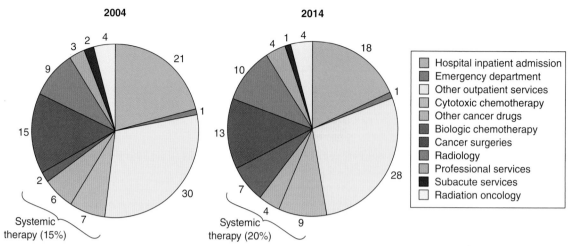

Figure 5-2. Expenditures by type of treatment. (Adapted from Finch KM, Pelizzari PM, Pyenson B. Cost drivers of cancer care: a retrospective analysis of Medicare and commercially insured population claim data 2004-2014. 2016, April 14. https://www.milliman.com/en/insight/cost-drivers-of-cancer-care-a-retrospective-analysis-of-medicare-and-commercially-insured.)

The total expenditure also varies according to the specific cancer diagnosis. A study of the cost to breast, colon, and lung cancer patients and their health plans based on claims from a large database found that spending per patient increased from under $1,000 per month until 2 to 3 months prior to diagnosis, to as high as $25,000 in the period of 2011 to 2014 during the month of diagnosis.[16] In this report, lung cancer was found to have the highest per month spending levels postdiagnosis and throughout the disease course. These findings need to be considered in the context of the subsequent Food and Drug Administration (FDA) approval of immunotherapy drugs for lung cancer, the first of which occurred after the period reported in this study (March 2015).[17] Immunotherapy agents are expected to be a significant component of expenditures of lung cancer care due to their costs.[18]

Moreover, variations in the cost of cancer care across US regions without consistent differences in survival outcomes have been reported. A landmark study showed that high-cost regions had 30% to 40% more inpatient hospitalizations, 70% to 120% more intensive care unit days, and 12% less hospice use without a difference in outcomes compared to lower cost regions.[19]

Impact on Patient and Society

The increased health care expenditure on cancer care can have negative consequences in patients and in the society as a whole[20]:

- The abandonment rate (patient-directed discontinuation) of oral cancer therapy drug has been reported to be around 10% in a nationally representative pharmacy claims database. Higher cost sharing (higher out-of-pocket expenses) and lower income resulted in significantly higher rates of abandonment.[21]

- Recipients of low-income subsidies (financial aid) for patients with Medicare Part D coverage have shown higher adherence to oral cancer therapy compared to those patients who did not qualify for the subsidies, despite the former being of a lower socioeconomic status than the latter.[22]

- In a large claims database analysis, increasing out-of-pockets expenses were associated with decreasing adherence to erlotinib therapy in patient with non–small cell lung cancer (NSCLC) receiving this medication.[23] In a Medicare population sample, it was estimated that an increase of $10 in out-of-pocket expenses per month would result in a 14% increase in the likelihood of discontinuation or delay of therapy with erlotinib in patients with NSCLC receiving this medication.[24]

- A diagnosis of cancer has been associated with a 2.65 times increased risk of bankruptcy.[25] It has been suggested that bankruptcy can in turn have adverse health-related consequences, such as increased mortality, for bankrupted patients compared to those cancer patients who do not file for bankruptcy.[26]

- The lost earnings due to cancer death in the United States were estimated to amount to $94.4 billion in 2015, with the highest loss being in the southern and midwestern states.[27]

Causes of Rising Cancer Costs

Most of the information available and the current discussion on cost of lung cancer care is centered on cancer drug pricing. The likely reasons are multiple. There is a reported increase in the percentage of outpatient cost as a fraction of the total health care expenditures.[11,14] Managed care organizations (private insurance payers) in the United States have recently reported that drug and drug administration represent 26% of the total health care expenditures. They also reported an average of 12% increase in pharmacy benefit cancer drug spending and between 2016 and 2017 an average of 14% increase in medical benefit cancer drug spending.[28]

These findings have likely shaped the perception of the most pressing issues for key stakeholders in cancer care. For instance, when managed care organizations, specialty pharmacies, oncologists, oncology practice managers, and employers in the United States were presented with 14 cancer care issues and asked to rank the top 5 in a large survey, control of cancer specialty drug costs was consistently selected as one of the 3 most pressing 2016 challenges facing cancer care.[29]

There are several factors that are implicated in the acceleration of these rising costs[7]:

- Increase in the rate of introduction of new and expensive FDA-approved drugs

- Slower pace of conversion to generics/biosimilar items and the parallel increase in cost of these generic drugs

- The introduction of expensive drugs for conditions that affect large segments of the population, as opposed to rare conditions as in the past

The last is particularly relevant for lung cancer, for which the current standard treatment for metastatic NSCLC,[30,31] locally advanced NSCLC,[32] and extensive-stage small cell lung cancer[33] now includes immunotherapy in the treatment backbone. Together, these groups represent approximately 65% of all the newly diagnosed cases,[34] which in 2018 was estimated at 234,030 cases.[35]

There are other factors driving escalating costs that are intrinsically related to the complexity of the pharmaceutical market. This is particularly true for the US market, in which the flow of pharmaceutical products from manufacturers to patients evolved separately from the financing mechanisms for those products.[36] Understanding the distribution of drugs and the financing systems provides a vehicle for understanding the complexity of the rise in the cost of cancer therapies (**Figure 5-3**).

Cancer drugs in the United States are delivered from manufacturers to patients through intermediaries: Drug distributors purchase them from manufacturers and then ship them to retailers, where patients obtain their drugs. Financing of the drugs is done through payers, whether public (Medicare) or private (private health insurance carriers, out-of-pocket expenses), as well as through pharmacy benefit managers (PBMs). The vast majority of private health insurance is obtained through employer-based insurance, with most insurances offering drug benefits programs. Many of these payers outsource the management of their drug benefits to PBMs.[36]

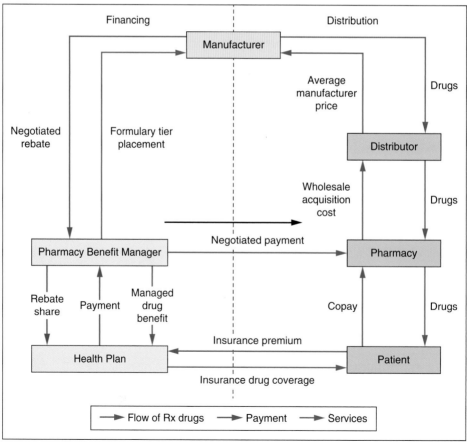

Figure 5-3. Conceptual model of connections between pharmaceuticals, services, costs, and payments. Rx, prescription; Pharmacy, all types of pharmacies, including hospital and mail-order. (Adapted from Congressional Budget Office (CBO). Prescription drug pricing in the private sector. https://www.cbo.gov/publication/18275. January 2007).

The factors attributed to the rising costs in lung cancer care that are related to the pharmaceutical market are abundant. It is beyond the scope of this synopsis to provide a detailed and comprehensive discussion of these factors. The following factors are widely perceived as some of the main drivers of the rising costs:

- In the United States, drug manufacturers are allowed to set the price of their products. In most developed nations with national health systems, drug prices are negotiated or even rejected based on the analysis of its benefit in relation to its cost.[37] In the United Kingdom, for instance, evaluation of a new drug requires that the drug pass a cost-utility threshold (usually between £20,000 and £30,000, or $25,000 and $40,000 per quality-adjusted life-year [QALY]) gained before it is recommended for coverage at a national level.[38]

- It has been estimated that drug prices decline to approximately 52% of brand-name drug prices with two generic manufacturers making the product, 33% with five manufacturers, and 21% with eight manufacturers.[39] However, the process of entry of generic drugs to the market has been deemed excessively slow and plagued with multiple hurdles.[40]

- Market exclusivity of a drug (protection from competition) is granted by the US government through two mechanisms: initial FDA approval (5-7 years for new small molecules[41] and 12 years for new biologics[42]) and patent-related exclusivity (for 20 or more years).[43] The median length of postapproval market exclusivity is 14.5 years for highly innovative, first-in-class drugs.[44] Targeted therapies and immune checkpoint inhibitors are in this category.

- Distributors handle 91% of the overall pharmaceutical sales revenue.[36] Their current business model (distributors are allowed by US law to ask manufacturers to pay them undisclosed vendor fees as a condition to have their drugs listed in the distributor's catalogs) have raised concerns for the possibility of limiting the drug therapy options that hospitals and patients have to a single manufacturer that is the highest bidder, as opposed to the drug with the most value.[45]

- Manufacturers not only offer drug price discounts to distributors and payers (both insurers and PBMs) based on total sales volumes of their products, but also provide cash payments (rebates, charge-backs) as result of complex price negotiations that lack transparency.[46] In 2016, adjustments to revenues and payments from pharmaceutical manufacturers to intermediaries in the market totaled $144 billion.[47]

- Public payers (Medicare and Medicaid) are prohibited by law to negotiate prescription drug prices (such as EGFR TKI inhibitors) or interfere with negotiations between manufacturers and individual Medicaid/Medicare Part D drug distributors or retailers.[48]

Value-Based Therapy in Lung Cancer

Several attempts are in progress to find effective ways to deliver high-quality lung cancer care while utilizing limited economic resources efficiently. Many strategies have been designed, with the common aim to determine the *value* of the available cancer therapies and incorporate this information in treatment decisions.

PHARMACOECONOMICS IN LUNG CANCER

Pharmacoeconomics is a discipline that aims to place a value on a drug or therapy. It describes, measures, and analyzes the consequences (outcomes) of the use of a given drug therapy (clinical benefit, side effects, quality of life) in relation to its cost.[49,50] The *value* of a cancer therapy (as opposed to only the outcomes or only the cost) is then used to determine which therapy provides the best outcomes for the amount of resources invested. Different approaches to this end have been proposed by different organizations and stakeholders around the world.[51-53] This approach is also influenced by the willingness that a given society has to pay a given price for a given treatment.

Perspectives of Pharmacoeconomic Evaluation

The assessment of cost and outcomes of cancer therapies is shaped by, and dependent on, the perspective (patient, provider, payer, society) used to conduct the analysis. For example, evaluating the value of osimertinib as first-line therapy for EGFR-mutant NSCLC from the patient's perspective would consider the clinical benefit over standard of care (8.7 months increase in median progression-free survival [mPFS]),[54] along with a more forgiving safety profile (severe adverse effect rate of 34% vs 45% with standard therapy[54]) and out-of-pocket expenses (copayment, lost wages). In contrast, an evaluation from a different perspective could render a different measure of the value of such therapy. For example, it was reported from the US population's perspective (society), that osimertinib carries an additional cost of over $225,000 for the benefit gained (measured in QALYs) over another TKI agent,[55] an incremental cost that would be considered inefficient by most decision-makers in the United States.[56,57]

Pharmacoeconomics: Methodology and Application

The aim of a pharmacoeconomic evaluation is to compare two alternative therapies by identifying and measuring the value of each of them (costs and outcomes) and comparing those therapies being considered.[58] There are multiple methods used to conduct pharmacoeconomic evaluations, summarized in **Figure 5-4**. The most commonly used for cancer therapy evaluation are cost-effectiveness, cost-minimization, and cost-utility techniques.[59-61] These evaluations are used for different purposes:

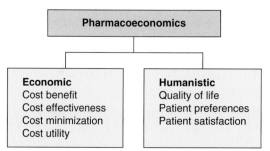

Figure 5-4. Methods to conduct pharmacoeconomic evaluations. (Adapted with permission from DiPiro JT, Talbert RL, Yee GC, Matzke GR, Wells BG, Posey LM. *Pharmacotherapy: A Pathophysiologic Approach.* 8th ed. New York, NY: McGraw Hill; 2011).

- Selection of drugs to be included in pharmacy formularies at a local/regional level.
  - Resource allocation decisions.
  - In some countries (eg, the United Kingdom), these evaluations are used for approval of public reimbursement of cancer drugs.
  - To define the value of cancer therapies using these evaluations as a tool (but not as the only metric of value).

Value-Based Frameworks and Other Cost-Containing Efforts

Due to the political and ethical dilemma of assigning the value of a given therapy based on a monetary amount, many professional societies and organizations have defined the value of a cancer therapy to include cost in the analysis but not relying solely on a pharmacoeconomic evaluation for this purpose. Examples of these are the *value framework* of the American Society of Clinical Oncology[52] and the *magnitude of clinical benefit scale* from the European Society of Medical Oncology.[62]

These efforts are in part driven by the limitations of pharmacoeconomic analysis as the sole means to define value of a given therapy. For example, from the society perspective in France, afatinib was found to improve outcomes (measured in QALYs) compared to gefitinib at an acceptable[56] extra cost of €45,211 (roughly $39,700),[63] despite a modest improvement in mPFS (hazard ratio [HR] 0.73, 11.0 vs 10.9 months),[64] more toxicities (adverse events [AE]) grade 3-4 rate 11% vs 4%), similar response rates, and no difference in overall survival.[65]

Other stakeholders are also currently exploring different strategies to address the rising cost of cancer care. From the payer perspective, both private[66] and public payers[67] are exploring migrating from a fee-for-service payment system to a performance-based or bundled/episode-based system. The oncology care model from the Centers for Medicare and Medicaid Services in the United States is the largest and most ambitious of these efforts.[67]

Multiple potential solutions have been proposed, including improving drug market competition through patent legislation changes, inclusion of pharmacoeconomic evaluations by the US government for decision-making, physician and prescriber education about cost of cancer care, and increased patient and stakeholder involvement. Many efforts are currently underway in each of these areas.

REFERENCES

1. Singleterry J. The cost of cancer: addressing patient costs. American Cancer Society Cancer Action Network. 2017 April. Report No.
2. International Agency for Research on Cancer. New global cancer data: GLOBOCAN 2018. 2018, September 12. https://www.uicc.org/new-global-cancer-data-globocan-2018.
3. World Health Organization. Cancer. 2018, September 12. http://www.who.int/news-room/fact-sheets/detail/cancer.
4. Wong MCS, Lao XQ, Ho KF, Goggins WB, Tse SLA. Incidence and mortality of lung cancer: global trends and association with socioeconomic status. *Sci Rep.* 2017;7(1):14300. Epub 2017/11/01. doi: 10.1038/s41598-017-14513-7.
5. Islami F, Torre LA, Jemal A. Global trends of lung cancer mortality and smoking prevalence. *Transl Lung Cancer Res.* 2015;4(4):327-38. Epub 2015/09/18. doi:10.3978/j.issn.2218-6751.2015.08.04.
6. Albaba H, Lim C, Leighl NB. Economic considerations in the use of novel targeted therapies for lung cancer: review of current literature. *PharmacoEconomics.* 2017;35(12):1195-209. Epub 2017/09/02. doi:10.1007/s40273-017-0563-8.

7. Bach PB. New math on drug cost-effectiveness. *N Engl J Med*. 2015;373(19):1797-99. Epub 2015/11/05. doi:10.1056/NEJMp1512750.

8. Mariotto AB, Yabroff KR, Shao Y, Feuer EJ, Brown ML. Projections of the cost of cancer care in the United States: 2010-2020. *J Natl Cancer Inst*. 2011;103(2):117-28. Epub 2011/01/14. doi:10.1093/jnci/djq495.

9. National Center for Biotechnology Information. PubMed search. June 15, 2019.

10. Schottenfeld D, Fraumeni JF. *Cancer Epidemiology and Prevention*. 3rd ed. New York, NY: Oxford University Press; 2006.

11. Soni A. *Trends in Use and Expenditures for Cancer Treatment Among Adults 18 and Older, US Civilian Noninstitutionalized Population, 2001 and 2011*. Rockville, MD: Agency for Health Care Research and Quality; 2014.

12. Agency for Health Care Research and Quality. Total expenses and percent distribution selected conditions by source of payment: United States, 2014. Medical Expenditure Panel Survey Household Component Data. 2014. https://meps.ahrq.gov/mepsweb/data_stats/quick_tables_results.jsp?Action=Search&SearchMethod=1&component=1&subcomponent=0&tableSeries=2&year=-1

13. IBM. IBM MarketScan Research Databases 2019. https://www.ibm.com/us-en/marketplace/marketscan-research-databases. Accessed July 24, 2019.

14. Finch KM, Pelizzari PM, Pyenson B. Cost drivers of cancer care: a retrospective analysis of Medicare and commercially insured population claim data 2004-2014. 2016, April 14. https://www.milliman.com/en/insight/cost-drivers-of-cancer-care-a-retrospective-analysis-of-medicare-and-commercially-insured

15. Yabroff KR, Lund J, Kepka D, Mariotto A. Economic burden of cancer in the United States: estimates, projections, and future research. *Cancer Epidemiol Biomarkers Prev*. 2011;20(10):2006-14. Epub 2011/10/08. doi:10.1158/1055-9965.

16. Dieguez G, Ferro C, Pyenson BS. A multi-year look at the cost burden of cancer care. 2017, April 10. https://www.milliman.com/en/insight/2017/a-multi-year-look-at-the-cost-burden-of-cancer-care.

17. Food and Drug Administration. Nivolumab BLA approval. Silver Spring, MD: March 2015. https://www.accessdata.fda.gov/drugsatfda_docs/appletter/2015/125527Orig1s000ltr.pdf

18. Kim A, Devine B, Roth JA. Cost-effectiveness of first-line pembrolizumab plus chemotherapy for metastatic squamous non-small cell lung cancer (NSCLC). *J Clin Oncol*. 2019;37(15)(suppl):e20703-e. doi:10.1200/JCO.2019.37.15_suppl.e20703.

19. Brooks GA, Li L, Sharma DB, et al. Regional variation in spending and survival for older adults with advanced cancer. *J Natl Cancer Inst*. 2013;105(9):634-42. Epub 2013/03/14. doi:10.1093/jnci/djt025.

20. Prasad V, De Jesus K, Mailankody S. The high price of anticancer drugs: origins, implications, barriers, solutions. *Nat Rev Clin Oncol*. 2017;146:381-90. Epub 2017/03/16. doi:10.1038/nrclinonc.2017.31.

21. Streeter SB, Schwartzberg L, Husain N, Johnsrud M. Patient and plan characteristics affecting abandonment of oral oncolytic prescriptions. *J Oncol Pract*. 2011;7(3)(suppl):46s-51s. Epub 2011/09/03. doi:10.1200/jop.2011.000316.

22. Biggers A, Shi Y, Charlson J, et al. Medicare D subsidies and racial disparities in persistence and adherence with hormonal therapy. *J Clin Oncol*. 2016;34(36):4398-404. Epub 2016/12/22. doi:10.1200/jco.2016.67.3350.

23. Hess LM, Louder A, Winfree K, Zhu YE, Oton AB, Nair R. Factors associated with adherence to and treatment duration of erlotinib among patients with non-small cell lung cancer. *J Manag Care Spec Pharm*. 2017;23(6):643-52. Epub 2017/05/23. doi:10.18553/jmcp.2017.16389.

24. Kaisaeng N, Harpe SE, Carroll NV. Out-of-pocket costs and oral cancer medication discontinuation in the elderly. *J Manag Care Spec Pharm*. 2014;20(7):669-75. Epub 2014/06/27. doi:10.18553/jmcp.2014.20.7.669.

25. Ramsey S, Blough D, Kirchhoff A, Kreizenbeck K, Fedorenko C, Snell K, Newcomb P, Hollingworth W, Overstreet K. Washington State cancer patients found to be at greater risk for bankruptcy than people without a cancer diagnosis. *Health Aff (Project Hope)*. 2013;32(6):1143-52. Epub 2013/05/17. doi:10.1377/hlthaff.2012.1263.

26. Ramsey SD, Bansal A, Fedorenko CR, et al. Financial insolvency as a risk factor for early mortality among patients with cancer. *J Clin Oncol*. 2016;34(9):980-86. Epub 2016/01/27. doi:10.1200/jco.2015.64.6620.

27. Islami F, Miller KD, Siegel RL, et al. National and state estimates of lost earnings from cancer deaths in the United States. *JAMA Oncol*. 2019;5(9):e191460. Epub 2019/07/04. doi:10.1001/jamaoncol.2019.1460.

28. Genentech. *The 2018 Genentech Oncology Trend Report*. South San Francisco, CA: Genentech; 2018.

29. Genentech. *The 2017 Genentech Oncology Trend Report: Perspectives From Managed Care Organizations, Specialty Pharmacies, Oncologist, Practice Managers and Employers*. South San Francisco, CA: Genentech; 2017.

30. Paz-Ares L, Luft A, Vicente D, et al. Pembrolizumab plus chemotherapy for squamous non-small-cell lung cancer. *N Engl J Med*. 2018;379(21):2040-51. doi:10.1056/NEJMoa1810865.

31. Gandhi L, Rodriguez-Abreu D, Gadgeel S, et al. Pembrolizumab plus chemotherapy in metastatic non-small-cell lung cancer. *N Engl J Med*. 2018;378(22):2078-92. doi:10.1056/NEJMoa1801005.

32. Antonia SJ, Villegas A, Daniel D, et al. Durvalumab after chemoradiotherapy in stage III non-small-cell lung cancer. *N Engl J Med.* 2017;377(20):1919-29. doi:10.1056/NEJMoa1709937.

33. Horn L, Mansfield AS, Szczesna A, et al. First-line atezolizumab plus chemotherapy in extensive-stage small-cell lung cancer. *N Engl J Med.* 2018. Epub 2018/10/04. doi:10.1056/NEJMoa1809064.

34. National Cancer Institute. Online summary of trends in US cancer control measures. Stage at Diagnosis. 2018, February. https://progressreport.cancer.gov/diagnosis/stage.

35. National Cancer Institute SEER Program. Cancer stat facts: lung and bronchus cancer. 2018, November 22. https://seer.cancer.gov/statfacts/html/lungb.html

36. Dabora MC, Turaga N, Schulman KA. Financing and distribution of pharmaceuticals in the United States. *JAMA.* 2017;318(1):21-22. Epub 2017/05/16. doi:10.1001/jama.2017.5607.

37. Kanavos P, Ferrario A, Vandoros S, Anderson GF. Higher US branded drug prices and spending compared to other countries may stem partly from quick uptake of new drugs. *Health Aff (Project Hope).* 2013;32(4):753-61. Epub 2013/04/10. doi:10.1377/hlthaff.2012.0920.

38. Chalkidou K. Comparative effectiveness review within the UK's National Institute for Health and Clinical Excellence. *Issue Brief (Commonw Fund).* 2009;59:1-12. Epub 2009/07/31.

39. Food and Drug Administration. Generic competition and drug prices. 2017, November 28. https://www.fda.gov/media/133509/download

40. Kesselheim AS, Avorn J, Sarpatwari A. The high cost of prescription drugs in the United States: origins and prospects for reform. *JAMA.* 2016;316(8):858-71. Epub 2016/08/24. doi:10.1001/jama.2016.11237.

41. Food and Drug Administration. 21 CFR § 314.108: Code of federal regulations. 2018, April 1.

42. FDA. Regulation of biological products. 42 USC § 262(k)(7)(A). https://www.accessdata.fda.gov/scripts/cdrh/cfdocs/cfcfr/cfrsearch.cfm?fr=314.108

43. Contents and term of patent: provisional rights. 35 USC § 154(a)(2). https://www.govinfo.gov/content/pkg/USCODE-2011-title35/pdf/USCODE-2011-title35-partII-chap14-sec154.pdf

44. Grabowski H, Long G, Mortimer R, Boyo A. Updated trends in US brand-name and generic drug competition. *J Med Econ.* 2016;19(9):836-44. Epub 2016/04/12. doi:10.1080/13696998.2016.1176578.

45. Bruhn WE, Fracica EA, Makary MA. Group purchasing organizations, health care costs, and drug shortages. *JAMA.* 2018;320(18):1859-60. Epub 2018/10/23. doi:10.1001/jama.2018.13604.

46. Schulman KA, Richman BD. The evolving pharmaceutical benefits market. *JAMA.* 2018;319(22):2269-70. doi:10.1001/jama.2018.4269.

47. Quintiles IMS Institute. Outlook for global medicines through 2021. 2016, December. https://morningconsult.com/wp-content/uploads/2016/12/QuintilesIMS-Institute-Global-Outlook-FINAL.pdf.

48. Health insurance for aged and disabled. 42 USC. §1395. https://uscode.house.gov/view.xhtml?path=/prelim@title42/chapter7/subchapter18&edition=prelim

49. Townsend RJ. Postmarketing drug research and development. *Drug Intell Clin Pharm.* 1987;21(1, Pt 2):134-36. Epub 1987/01/01.

50. Mauskopf JA. Why study pharmacoeconomics? *Expert Rev Pharmacoecon Outcomes Res.* 2001;1(1):1-3. doi:10.1586/14737167.1.1.1.

51. Aapro M, Astier A, Audisio R, et al. Identifying critical steps towards improved access to innovation in cancer care: a European CanCer Organisation position paper. *Eur J Cancer.* 2017;82:193-202. Epub 2017/07/12. doi:10.1016/j.ejca.2017.04.014.

52. Schnipper LE, Davidson NE, Wollins DS, et al. Updating the American Society of Clinical Oncology value framework: revisions and reflections in response to comments. *J Clin Oncol.* 2016;34(24):2925-34. doi:10.1200/jco.2016.68.2518.

53. Cheung MC, Chan KK, Sabharwal M, Fields A, Chambers A, Evans WK. Comparing assessment frameworks for cancer drugs between Canada and Europe: What can we learn from the differences? *ESMO Open.* 2016;1(6):e000124. Epub 2017/12/07. doi:10.1136/esmoopen-2016-000124.

54. Soria JC, Ohe Y, Vansteenkiste J, et al. Osimertinib in untreated EGFR-mutated advanced non-small-cell lung cancer. *N Engl J Med.* 2018;3782:113-25. Epub 2017/11/21. doi:10.1056/NEJMoa1713137.

55. Aguiar PN Jr, Haaland B, Park W, San Tan P, del Giglio A, de Lima Lopes G Jr. Cost-effectiveness of osimertinib in the first-line treatment of patients with EGFR-mutated advanced non–small cell lung cancer. *JAMA Oncol.* 2018;4(8):1080-84. doi:10.1001/jamaoncol.2018.1395.

56. Marseille E, Larson B, Kazi DS, Kahn JG, Rosen S. Thresholds for the cost-effectiveness of interventions: alternative approaches. *Bull World Health Organ.* 2015;93(2):118-24. Epub 2015/04/18. doi:10.2471/blt.14.138206.

57. Ubel PA, Hirth RA, Chernew ME, Fendrick AM. What is the price of life and why doesn't it increase at the rate of inflation? *Arch Intern Med.* 2003;163(14):1637-41. Epub 2003/07/30. doi:10.1001/archinte.163.14.1637.

58. Trask LS. Pharmacoeconomics: principles, methods, and applications. In: Joseph T, DiPiro RLT, Yee GC, Matzke GR, Wells BG, Posey M, eds. *Pharmacotherapy: A Pathophysiologic Approach.* 8th ed. New York, NY: McGraw Hill Medical; 2011:1-3.

59. Carlson JJ, Veenstra DL, Ramsey SD. Pharmacoeconomic evaluations in the treatment of non-small cell lung cancer. *Drugs.* 2008;68(8):1105-13. Epub 2008/05/20. doi:10.2165/00003495-200868080-00007.

60. Al-Badriyeh D, Alameri M, Al-Okka R. Cost-effectiveness research in cancer therapy: a systematic review of literature trends, methods and the influence of funding. *BMJ Open.* 2017;7(1):e012648. doi:10.1136/bmjopen-2016-012648.

61. Ma F, Cheng X, Aballéaa S, Toumi M. Current trends in methods of pharmacoeconomic studies of cancer therapies in China. *Value Health.* 2016;19(7):A887. doi:10.1016/j.jval.2016.08.267.

62. Cherny NI, Sullivan R, Dafni U, et al. A standardised, generic, validated approach to stratify the magnitude of clinical benefit that can be anticipated from anti-cancer therapies: the European Society for Medical Oncology Magnitude of Clinical Benefit Scale (ESMO-MCBS). *Ann Oncol.* 2015;26(8):1547-73. Epub 2015/05/31. doi:10.1093/annonc/mdv249.

63. Chouaid C, Luciani L, LeLay K, et al. Cost-effectiveness analysis of afatinib versus gefitinib for first-line treatment of advanced EGFR-mutated advanced non-small cell lung cancers. *J Thorac Oncol.* 2017;12(10):1496-502. doi:10.1016/j.jtho.2017.07.013.

64. Park K, Tan EH, O'Byrne K, et al. Afatinib versus gefitinib as first-line treatment of patients with EGFR mutation-positive non-small-cell lung cancer (LUX-Lung 7): a phase 2B, open-label, randomised controlled trial. *Lancet Oncol.* 2016;17(5):577-89. Epub 2016/04/17. doi:10.1016/s1470-2045(16)30033-x.

65. Paz-Ares L, Tan EH, O'Byrne K, et al. Afatinib versus gefitinib in patients with EGFR mutation-positive advanced non-small-cell lung cancer: overall survival data from the phase IIb LUX-Lung 7 trial. *Ann Oncol.* 2017;28(2):270-7. Epub 2017/04/21. doi:10.1093/annonc/mdw611.

66. United Healthcare. Payment models. 2018. https://www.uhc.com/valuebasedcare/how-value-based-care-benefits-you/for-care-providers/payment-models.

67. Centers for Medicare & Medicaid Services. Oncology Care Model. 2018, October 31. https://innovation.cms.gov/initiatives/oncology-care/.

PART II

Pathobiology

6

PATHOBIOLOGY OF NON–SMALL CELL LUNG CARCINOMA

Mostafa M. Fraig, MD, MBA

A 60–year-old Asian female had a 4-cm lung mass biopsied by core needle biopsy.

She never smoked and has no history of cancer or comorbidities.

What testing do you ask for to confirm the suspicion of lung cancer?

What other histology findings are important if lung cancer is confirmed?

Learning Objectives:
1. What is the new World Health Organization (WHO) classification of lung cancer?
2. What are the markers distinguishing squamous from non-squamous lung cancer?
3. What terminology has replaced the former bronchoalveolar carcinoma?
4. What are scar carcinomas?
5. What are poor prognostic histologies in non-squamous lung cancer?

Historically, the basis of all classifications of lung tumors was based on the sections routinely stained with hematoxylin-eosin (H&E) demonstrating the histomorphologic features of tumor cells: cell size and tumor architecture, cellular differentiation along the known types of histology, and the stage at which arrest of differentiation occurs. The biologic behavior was extensively studied, and clinical outcome was correlated with types and even subtypes of tumors based on some peculiar histomorphologic differences. The introduction of ultrastructural, immunohistochemical markers and lately molecular markers has supplemented but not supplanted the morphologic diagnosis.

To understand how tumors would behave is to understand how they develop and progress from one stage to another based on a multistep progression model that has been studied over decades. Pathologists have observed this process in other organ systems and concluded it is valid in the case of lung tumors.

CLASSIFICATION OF LUNG TUMORS

Lung tumors have been grouped under different major groups with subgroups assigned under those in a branched tree model that not only reserved the broad characteristics but also recognized additional distinctive features. As our understanding of the histogenesis and due to the heterogeneity of tumors, which could create overlapping features and hence confusion, the classification of lung cancer has evolved over the years. The standard classification is the one adopted by WHO, which is meant to be applied worldwide, taking into consideration the variability of practices and differences in the availability of resources in different parts in the world. The last iteration is the one from 2015, and it introduced some transformational improvements based on the revolutionary changes with the advent of targeted therapy and immunotherapy.[1] It not only has altered the classification of resection specimens but also has made recommendations applicable for the diagnosis of small biopsies and cytology specimens.

Lung cancer can be broadly divided into epithelial tumors and mesenchymal tumors. The former includes 4 major groups: adenocarcinoma, squamous cell carcinoma, small cell carcinoma, and large cell carcinoma (**Table 6-1**). Historically, the most important distinction was between small cell carcinoma and non–small cell carcinoma for lack of therapeutic benefit for distinguishing squamous cell carcinoma from adenocarcinoma. A diagnosis of non–small cell carcinoma (not otherwise specified) was frequently used, especially on small biopsies and cytology specimens. Large cell carcinoma served as a wastebasket entity for those tumors with no evident squamous or glandular differentiation.

Since the tumors of 70% of patients are unresectable at the time of diagnosis and with the introduction of new targeted therapies that are dependent on the type of histology, it became imperative to further classify the current broad entities into subsets using ancillary studies that reflexes the patients to further molecular testing. Most lung cancer is first diagnosed by small biopsies and cytology, shifting the emphasis to these type of specimens and how to classify tumors based on them.[2] In the last iteration of the WHO classification system in 2015, new significant changes were introduced. Chief among them[1] are use of immunohistochemistry throughout the classification[2]; integration of molecular testing for personalized strategies for patients with advanced lung cancer[3]; a new classification for small biopsies and cytology[4]; a new classification of lung adenocarcinoma as proposed by the 2011 IASLC/ATS/ERS (International Association for the Study of Lung Cancer/American Thoracic Society/European Respiratory Society)[5]; restriction of the diagnosis of large cell carcinoma only to resected tumors that lack any clear morphologic or immunohistochemical differentiation.

PREINVASIVE LESIONS

The pathology of preinvasive lesions has attracted interest from investigators in recent years. As the importance of early detection of cancer has gained popularity, many of these lesions that used to be an incidental finding and characterized as "field defect" are

TABLE 6-1 Histologic Classification of Lung Cancer	
Preinvasive Lesions	**Squamous Cell Carcinoma**
Squamous dysplasia/carcinoma in situ (CIS)	*Variants*
	Keratinizing
Atypical adenomatous hyperplasia (AIH)	Nonkeratinizing
	Basaloid
Adenocarcinoma in situ (AIS)	**Small Cell Carcinoma**
Diffuse idiopathic neuroendocrine hyperplasia (DIPNECH)	Combined small cell carcinoma
Adenocarcinoma	**Large Cell Carcinoma**
Minimally invasive adenocarcinoma (MIA)	*Variants*
	Large cell neuroendocrine carcinoma (LCNEC)
Tumors < 3.0 cm in size with an invasive component < 5 mm in size	Combined LCNEC
	Adenosquamous Carcinoma
Nonmucinous, mucinous, and nonmucinous/mucinous subtypes	**Sarcomatoid Carcinoma**
Invasive Adenocarcinoma	Pleomorphic carcinoma
Lepidic predominant	Spindle cell carcinoma
Nonmucinous with > 5-mm invasive component.	Giant cell carcinoma
	Carcinosarcoma
Acinar predominant	Pulmonary blastoma
Papillary	**Carcinoid Tumor**
Micropapillary	Typical carcinoid
Solid with mucin	Atypical carcinoid
Variants of Adenocarcinoma	**Carcinoma of Salivary Gland Type**
Invasive mucinous adenocarcinoma	Mucoepidermoid carcinoma
Colloid	Adenoid cystic carcinoma
Fetal (low grade and high grade)	Epimyoepithelial carcinoma
Enteric	Nuclear protein of the testis (NUT) carcinoma

being studied in more detail to understand their impact and provide more understanding in the evolution of cancer.

Early classifications of lung cancer did not provide much detail about those lesions except squamous cell carcinoma in situ (CIS). It was not till 1999 that the WHO classification recognized 2 new lesions: atypical adenomatous hyperplasia (AAH) and diffuse idiopathic pulmonary neuroendocrine cell hyperplasia (DIPNECH). These designations were maintained as three preinvasive lesions in the subsequent classification in 2004. In the latest 2011 and 2015 editions of the WHO classifications, the entity adenocarcinoma in situ (AIS) was added, which used to be called bronchioloalveolar carcinoma (BAC).

Squamous Cell Dysplasia and Carcinoma in Situ

The evolution of lung cancer has been understood to follow a multistep progression from a metaplastic, hyperplastic, and finally dysplastic morphology. The bronchial epithelium would undergo squamous metaplasia, which progressively would acquire basal layer hyperplasia, which will eventually turn dysplastic under the influence of carcinogenic stimulation like that encountered in the cases of smoking.[3]

In the same fashion, multiple molecular "hits" have been reported to occur along this course. Such changes include the allelic loss of the 3p region, which represents an early event in 78% of preinvasive bronchial lesions.[4] Other events are known to follow that, including loss of heterozygosity at 9p21 corresponding to (p16), 17p loss in cases of hyperplasia; telomerase activation and retinoic acid receptor (RAR) B in cases of mild dysplasia; p53 mutation in moderate dysplasia; and bcl-2 and cyclin D and E overexpression in cases of CIS.[5]

Squamous atypia could occur in the setting of severe inflammation and in the cavitary lesion of aspergillosis and should not be overcalled as dysplasia/CIS.

Grading of squamous cell dysplasia has been attempted. Some authors advocated a three-tier system with mild, moderate, and severe dysplasia based on how far the dysplastic features extended within the full thickness of the metaplastic squamous mucosa and dividing the thickness into thirds, with each grade assigned to each third of involvement. The difference between severe dysplasia and CIS was based on the presence of any maturing or flattened layer of squamous cells near the top of the metaplastic layer. If full thickness was involved, a diagnosis of CIS was rendered.

Other authors advocated a two-tier system for dysplasia, eliminating the middle category. However, this system did not provide any clinical utility, and it was difficult to achieve reproducible results as these lesions tend to change their severity from one focus to another, and there is much overlap in features to produce consistent results. Caution must be exercised in areas of prior biopsies and ulceration or squamous metaplasia of the seromucinous glands around the bronchial wall to avoid overcalling these foci as invasive squamous cell carcinoma.

Atypical Adenomatous Hyperplasia and Adenocarcinoma in Situ

Atypical adenomatous hyperplasia (AAH) is a bronchioloalveolar proliferation that resembles, but does not fulfill the criteria, for AIS with a size less than 5 mm. It is usually encountered as an incidental finding in lung resection specimens. The incidence ranges between 5.7% and 21.4% depending on the extent of the search and criteria applied to the diagnosis. It is important to recognize it as a separate lesion and not an intrapulmonary metastatic lesion. It is characterized by a proliferation of atypical cuboidal cells replacing the original alveolar cells, with an abrupt transition from type I pneumocytes to atypical cells, as opposed to the gradual transition that occurs in reactive changes in the alveolar lining in cases of infection and inflammation (**Figure 6-1**). There could be several lesions within the lung, suggesting that this type of lesion represents a "field defect" rather than spread through air spaces (STAS).[6] Several molecular mutations like those encountered in AIS have been detected in these lesions, making them preinvasive lesions.[7] Earlier attempts at grading these proved difficult due to lack of interobserver reproducibility and lack of clinical or therapeutic benefits. There are no data to infer any negative prognostication on patients with AAH when compared with those without.[8]

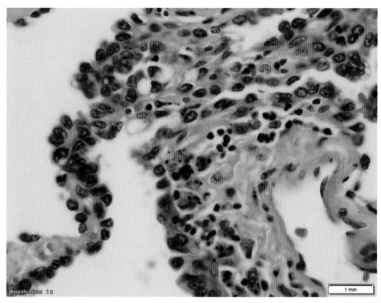

Figure 6-1. Atypical adenomatous hyperplasia shows atypical bronchioloalveolar cell proliferation with large dark nuclei lining alveolar spaces. They are small in size (<5.0 mm).

Adenocarcinoma in Situ

In the current adenocarcinoma classification, AIS is defined as a glandular proliferation measuring less than 3 cm that has a pure lipidic pattern with no invasion (**Figure 6-2**). In most cases, the cells are of the nonmucinous type; rarely, they could represent a mucinous type. These were formerly known as BAC. When they are completely resected, the overall prognosis is 100%. On computed tomographic (CT) scan, they appear as ground glass attenuation if they are of the nonmucinous and as a solid nodule if they are of the mucinous type. In the past classification, the term *BAC* used to cover the nonmucinous type as well as the mucinous type of BAC. It has been recognized that these are two different types of tumors with different biology and different clinical outcomes.

Nonmucinous AIS tends to harbor *EGFR* mutations and could occur in non-smokers and never smokers. Mucinous AIS proved to be very rare in its purist form and usually expresses a *K-ras* mutation similar to those encountered in patients with a history of cigarette smoking. Even rarer is the occurrence of the combination of nonmucinous and mucinous AIS. For a diagnosis to be made, there should be no evidence of invasion, as would be manifested by the presence of thickened stroma, with chronic inflammation as an indication of host response to an invasive carcinoma. In their mucinous form, they show on CT imaging as a pneumonia-like presentation, whereas the nonmucinous type has the morphology of ground glass attenuation.[9]

ADENOCARCINOMA

Adenocarcinoma accounts for 38% of all lung cancers in the United States. The sub-classification of adenocarcinoma of the lung has undergone some transformational change in the last two decades. It started with a somewhat obscure historic controversy

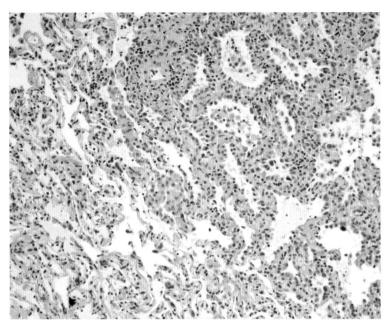

Figure 6-2. Adenocarcinoma in-situ, nonmucinous type. Classically, tumor cells are shown that abruptly stop at the interface with benign lung parenchyma, in contrast to the gradual blending that occurs in reactive lung changes where type II pneumocytes would merge with type I pneumocytes.

surrounding so-called scar carcinoma. One camp of investigators believed that this type of adenocarcinoma usually arises from a preexisting scar from the proliferation of cells within the scar or the surrounding environment. Other authors believed that this was an active fibrotic process representing the host response to the invading carcinoma. Studying those scars diligently led to the recognition that the presence of a scar has an adverse prognostic outcome and, going even further, proved that the size of the scar correlated with the prognosis.[10]

Based on this observation and others, the current classification no longer recognizes BAC diagnostic terminology. The concept of minimally invasive adenocarcinoma (MIA) was introduced, and the mixed subtype was eliminated and replaced by a predominant type and reference to the percentage of tumor subtypes within a heterogeneous adenocarcinoma.

Certain subtypes of adenocarcinoma proved to have worse prognosis than others. For instance, micropapillary and solid adenocarcinoma with mucin have a worse prognosis than the acinar and papillary types of adenocarcinoma.[11] The lipidic pattern is considered as a low-grade type of adenocarcinoma and carries a much better prognosis. It is also the subtype that more likely to harbor *EGFR* mutations and hence respond to the tyrosine kinase inhibitors set of drugs.

Adenocarcinoma Diagnosis in Resected Specimens

Minimally invasive adenocarcinoma is defined as a lipidic-predominant tumor measuring 3 cm or less in maximum dimension, with 5 mm or less of an invasive component. Multiple studies support the notion that the patients with MIA have a near 100% 5-year disease-free survival (DFS). Most of these cases are of the nonmucinous type, but rarely mucinous cases could occur. The presence of a scar is the major criterion separating AIS from MIA. It is very important to carefully sample these tumors to adequately measure the largest dimension at the right plane of sectioning. CT measurement of the solid portion in an otherwise ground glass lesion could be used as a surrogate for the estimation of the invasive portion if the measurement of the lesion proved to be difficult to measure during the gross examination or on the slides.[9]

Invasive Adenocarcinoma

An adenocarcinoma with an invasive component in excess of 5 mm is considered an invasive adenocarcinoma. It should be further subclassified based on the predominance of one component, or if there is more than one component, a percentage of each should be presented in increments of 5%-10%. Since certain subtypes are known to have a worse prognosis, they should be mentioned in the pathology report. Signet ring and clear cell subtypes are now considered cytologic features and do not represent histologic subtypes. Of note, carcinoma with a signet ring feature is the most frequent subtype to express mutations in the *ALK* gene. The recognized subtypes of adenocarcinoma are listed in Table 6-1.

The most recognized pattern is the lipidic pattern, which is basically the AIS component accompanying an invasive component. This is called lipidic-predominant adenocarcinoma (LPA). This used to be called a mixed subtype of adenocarcinoma with a mixture of BAC and acinar types of adenocarcinoma. By CT imaging, the lipidic pattern is represented by ground glass attenuation, and the invasive component shows as a speculated mass within that area.

> **CLINICAL PEARL:** There is a good correlation between CT findings and measurements on the gross specimen in pathologic evaluation.[12]

The other subtypes of adenocarcinoma include acinar (**Figure 6-3**), papillary (**Figure 6-4**), micropapillary (**Figure 6-5**), and solid with mucin-predominant adenocarcinoma. The micropapillary-predominant subtype carries the worst prognosis among all subtypes of adenocarcinoma. It could be encountered in combination with other subtypes and should be reported semiquantitatively for that reason.

Adenocarcinoma Variants

One of the variants of adenocarcinoma consists of invasive mucinous adenocarcinoma (formerly mucinous BAC) (**Figure 6-6**). This type of adenocarcinoma could present with several imaging patterns. One is a multifocal pattern called the "Cheerios pattern" with a lucent center where mucin accumulates and surrounded by tumor cells. Another pattern is a pneumonia-like pattern with a geographic outline and ground glass attenuation and consolidation.[13] Patients with this type of adenocarcinoma usually expectorate copious amount of mucin (bronchorrhea) with a salty taste.[14] They are associated with *kras* mutation, which is mutually exclusive of *EGFR* mutation. They also lack thyroid transcription factor-1 (TTF-1) expression by immunohistochemistry, and for that reason and because of their tendency to be multifocal, exclusion of metastatic adenocarcinoma from other sites is important.

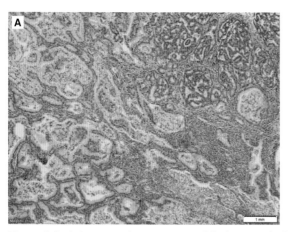 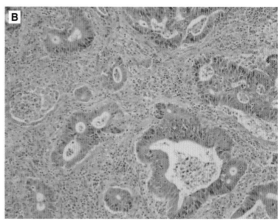

Figure 6-3. A. Invasive adenocarcinoma of the lung can be heterogeneous, presenting glandular differentiation ranging from an enteric type of glands (right side) to a mucinous type reminiscent of the endocervical type (left side). B. Glands or acini of tumor cells are seen embedded in a scar formed by fibrosis and chronic inflammatory infiltrate forming the host response to the invading carcinoma.

Other patterns include colloid adenocarcinoma, fetal adenocarcinoma, and enteric adenocarcinoma. These types share the presence of mucinous cells with apical mucin and extracellular mucin secretion.

The prognosis of adenocarcinoma subtypes in resected specimens follows several studies with criteria similar to those in the current classification reporting 100% DFS for patient with AIS and near 100% for patients with MIA. Since grading of adenocarcinoma is still not standardized, a convention of rules has been introduced in several

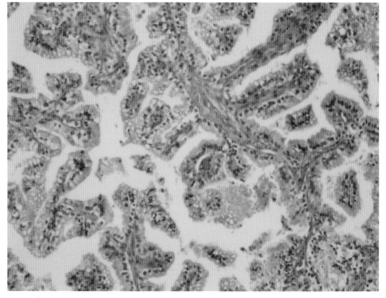

Figure 6-4. Papillary adenocarcinoma is characterized by glandular differentiation with papillary fronds covering distinct fibrovascular cores. The cells could be either columnar or cuboidal in shape.

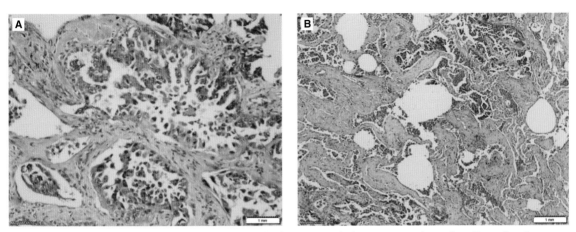

Figure 6-5. Micropapillary adenocarcinoma is a glandular formation with characteristic tufting of small papillary formations devoid of fibrovascular cores shown in A. It tends to spread in surrounding air spaces and in lymphatics, making them very aggressive in their invasive behavior as in image B.

studies, recognizing AIS and MIA as low-grade tumors, with lipidic-, acinar-, and papillary-predominant subtypes as intermediate grade. Mucinous, colloid, micropapillary, and solid are considered high grade tumors. There is a stepwise grading of the 5-year DFS among these groups, which is correlated with the histologic grade based on the subtypes rather than cytologic features or complexity of glandular formation as applied in other organs.

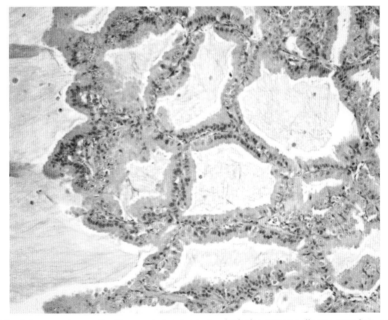

Figure 6-6. Adenocarcinoma in situ, mucinous type, in which the tumor cells are seen lining the alveolar spaces with columnar cytoplasm and basally located nuclei. Mucin is present in the alveolar spaces, seen here as an eosinophilic material.

The impact of the classification system on the TNF staging could occur through two major ways. The first one is by reporting the distribution of percentages of histologic components within a given tumor, one should be able to compare two tumors to assess whether they represent two synchronous or metachronous primaries or intrapulmonary metastases. This has been shown to correlate highly with molecular and clinical findings in making that distinction. The second way is by reporting the size of the scar. As was mentioned previously, the size of the invasive component has proven to be an independent prognostic predictor. Based on that, future studies might reveal that the size of the invasive component, not the size of the whole tumor, is the predictor of the clinical outcome.

Adenocarcinoma Classification in Small Biopsies and Cytologic Material

As 70% of lung cancers present in a late stage and are unresectable, the main method of diagnosis is through either small biopsy or cytologic material. The impetus to distinguish adenocarcinoma from squamous cell carcinoma changed the practice of obtaining tissue for diagnosis with the emphasis on reaching a more definitive diagnosis and providing enough material for the potential testing that will ensue. Patients with a diagnosis of adenocarcinoma, or non–small cell lung cancer (NSCLC), favor adenocarcinoma, or even NSCLC, not otherwise specified (NSCLC, NOS), could be lumped as non-squamous cell carcinoma, and they are eligible for treatment with pemetrexed- or pevacizumab-based therapy. Those patients should be tested for mutations of *EGFR*, *ALK* overexpression, and *ROSS-1* mutations for potential targeted therapy. On the other hand, patients with a diagnosis of squamous cell carcinoma are at risk of life-threatening hemorrhage if treated with pevacizumab-based therapy and less likely to harbor any of these mutations. Testing for the overexpression of programmed death ligand-1 (PDL-1) is performed in both types of tumors, but it requires more tissue in formalin paraffin-embedded material to be tested by immunohistochemistry. It has been recommended to use a minimal amount of tissue for the purpose of immunohistochemical subclassification of lung cancer in the absence of clear morphologic features that define the tumor as an adenocarcinoma or squamous cell carcinoma.

> **CLINICAL PEARL:** Utilizing just two immunohistochemical stains, TTF-1 and p40, one should be able to classify most cases as either squamous cell carcinoma or adenocarcinoma.

In the absence of immunoreactivity of both markers, a diagnosis of NSCLC, NOS, could be used to mean a "non-squamous cell carcinoma," which will render the patient eligible for molecular testing.

SQUAMOUS CELL CARCINOMA

Squamous cell carcinoma accounts for approximately 20% of lung malignant tumors in the United States. It has always been thought of as a more centrally located tumor related to the main bronchi and proximal branches. However, more recently more

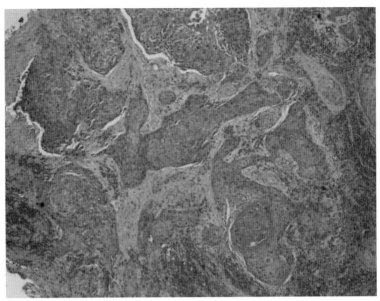

Figure 6-7. Squamous cell carcinoma is characterized by solid sheets of tumor cells with a fair amount of eosinophilic waxy cytoplasm. Intercellular bridges, keratin pearls, and single-cell keratinization are characteristic features on light microscopic evaluation.

than half of the lesions have been reported to be in peripheral location in the lung.[15,16] Squamous epithelium is not normal in the lung, and for cancer to develop, a step involving squamous metaplasia, dysplasia, and squamous cell CIS usually precedes the invasive tumor development. The presence of early mutations that are common in the invasive tumor within the metaplastic squamous epithelium confirms the multistep progression. Squamous differentiation is usually evident by the presence of intercellular bridges, keratin pearls, and single-cell keratinization seen by routine stains and light microscopy (**Figure 6-7**). When any of these features is present, the diagnosis is straightforward. However, the tumor could be poorly differentiated and hard to classify as squamous cell carcinoma. Immunohistochemical stains are helpful in this respect.

> **CLINICAL PEARL:** The most helpful immunohistochemical markers are cytokeratin 5/6, p63, and more recently p40.

The last is being touted as the most sensitive and most specific squamous cell marker.[17]

Squamous cell carcinoma could present with different appearances, including papillary, clear cell, small cell, and basaloid. However, the biologic behavior and the clinical and molecular correlates of these variants are not well studied.[18] The papillary variant, for example, usually is present as an exophytic tumor in the main bronchi. On the other hand, the small cell variant is more akin to the basaloid variant and could be confused with true small cell carcinoma.[19] For that reason, the use of the term *small cell variant of squamous cell carcinoma* should be avoided to preclude its confusion with the true small cell carcinoma. The clear cell type is a cytologic feature but does not represent a clinicopathologic entity. In the latest WHO classification in 2015, only 3 subtypes were recognized: keratinizing, nonkeratinizing, and basaloid. The last two are more aggressive than the first.

Squamous cell carcinoma has a stronger relationship with smoking history and more frequent *kras* mutation than in adenocarcinoma. *EGFR, ALK,* and *ROSS-1* are so infrequent that testing for them is not clinically warranted.

One of the difficulties of diagnosing squamous cell carcinoma in the lung is the separation from metastatic squamous cell carcinoma from elsewhere. Squamous cell carcinoma from the head and neck and esophagus have a strong association with smoking history and can present in the lung prior to finding the primary tumor or sometimes after the fact. Even in patients with known history of squamous cell carcinoma outside the lung, a new separate focus of squamous cell carcinoma could present a difficulty in ascertaining whether it is a metastatic focus or a new primary focus in the lung.

> **CLINICAL PEARL:** Interestingly, the presence of human papilloma virus in squamous cell carcinoma of the head and neck does not help distinguish it from that of the lung.

The morphologic comparison between the two tumors as well as the number of foci in the lung are the only valid correlates to help sort out this controversy. Squamous cell carcinoma can present in combination with other types, including adenocarcinoma and small cell carcinoma. In cases of adenosquamous cell carcinoma, there should be evident morphologic glandular differentiation in excess of 10% of the tumor to receive this designation. Immunohistochemical stains are not needed to document either component. In case of combined squamous cell carcinoma with small cell carcinoma, the 10% cutoff does not apply, and any amount of squamous cell carcinoma in this setting warrants the combined tumor designation.

While the lack of a signature mutation for squamous cell carcinoma excludes it from targeted chemotherapy, the expression of PDL-1 in this type of tumor made many patients eligible for immunotherapy.

LARGE CELL CARCINOMA

Large cell carcinoma represents 3% of all lung cancer and has always been a diagnosis by exclusion. Whenever a tumor did not exhibit notable squamous or glandular differentiation and did not fulfill the criteria for small cell carcinoma, a diagnosis of non–small cell carcinoma NOS or large cell carcinoma was rendered. With the recent emphasis on subtyping lung carcinoma, the proportion of large cell carcinoma is expected to become vanishingly small. In fact, there has been a trend in this direction in the last decade.[20]

Histologically, these tumors usually present as sheets and nests of cells with vesicular nuclei and prominent nucleoli surrounded by a fair amount of cytoplasm (**Figure 6-8**). To separate them from poorly differentiated adenocarcinoma (solid) with mucin, there

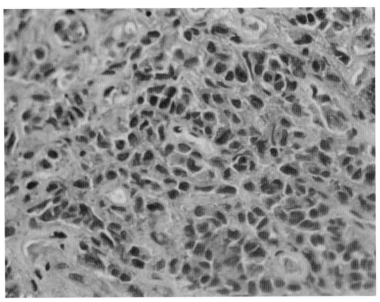

Figure 6-8. Large cell carcinoma is usually composed of sheets and nests of polygonal tumor cells lacking glandular and squamous differentiation by light microscopy. They have larger nuclei and more cytoplasm when compared with small cell carcinoma, which is also poorly differentiated.

have to be at least 5 cells with intracytoplasmic mucin secretion in 2 high-power fields. The diagnosis can only be made on resected specimens and not on small biopsies or on cytologic material. In the last situations, a diagnosis of NSCLC-NOS can be rendered on light microscopy alone. After immunohistochemical evaluation, the tumor could be further categorized as NSCLC, favor adenocarcinoma, or favor squamous cell carcinoma. In a minority of cases, a diagnosis of NSCLC-NOS may be used.

Large cell carcinoma has historically represented a heterogeneous group of tumors that shared the poorly differentiated features mentioned previously under light microscopic evaluation. However, by light microscopic examination and utilizing immunohistochemical studies, some of these tumors demonstrated features similar to those of adenocarcinoma, squamous cell carcinoma, or both. Studies to evaluate the clinical outcome of those tumors that lack the immunophenotype of either adenocarcinoma or squamous carcinoma should help examine the validity of establishing criteria for the diagnosis of large cell carcinoma in the future.

Large cell carcinoma could present in different variants. The WHO classification of 2004 recognized several variants that included a large cell neuroendocrine variant; basaloid, lymphoepithelioma-like variant; clear cell variant; and large cell carcinoma with a rhabdoid phenotype.

REFERENCES

1. Travis WD, Brambilla E, Nicholson AG, et al. The 2015 World Health Organization Classification of Lung Tumors: Impact of Genetic, Clinical and Radiologic Advances Since the 2004 Classification. *J Thorac Oncol.* 2015;10(9):1243-1260. Epub 2015/08/21. doi:10.1097/JTO.0000000000000630.
2. Travis WD, Brambilla E, Van Schil P, et al. Paradigm shifts in lung cancer as defined in the new IASLC/ATS/ERS lung adenocarcinoma classification. *Eur Respir J.* 2011;38(2):239-243. doi:10.1183/09031936.00026711.

3. Lam S, Szabo E. Preinvasive endobronchial lesions: lung cancer precursors and risk markers? *Am J Respir Crit Care Med.* 2015;192(12):1411-1413. Epub 2015/12/17. doi:10.1164/rccm.201508-1668ED.

4. Sundaresan V, Ganly P, Hasleton P, et al. p53 and chromosome 3 abnormalities, characteristic of malignant lung tumours, are detectable in preinvasive lesions of the bronchus. *Oncogene.* 1992;7(10):1989-1997. Epub 1992/10/01.

5. Lantuejoul S, Rouquette I, Brambilla E, Travis WD. [New WHO classification of lung adenocarcinoma and preneoplasia]. *Ann Pathol.* 2016;36(1):5-14. Epub 2016/01/23. doi:10.1016/j.annpat.2015.11.010.

6. Lu S, Tan KS, Kadota K, et al. Spread through air spaces (STAS) is an independent predictor of recurrence and lung cancer-specific death in squamous cell carcinoma. *J Thorac Oncol.* 2017;12(2):223-234. Epub 2016/10/04. doi:10.1016/j.jtho.2016.09.129.

7. Morandi L, Asioli S, Cavazza A, Pession A, Damiani S. Genetic relationship among atypical adenomatous hyperplasia, bronchioloalveolar carcinoma and adenocarcinoma of the lung. *Lung Cancer.* 2007;56(1):35-42. Epub 2007/01/24. doi:10.1016/j.lungcan.2006.11.022.

8. Suzuki K, Nagai K, Yoshida J, et al. The prognosis of resected lung carcinoma associated with atypical adenomatous hyperplasia: a comparison of the prognosis of well-differentiated adenocarcinoma associated with atypical adenomatous hyperplasia and intrapulmonary metastasis. *Cancer.* 1997;79(8):1521-1526. Epub 1997/04/15.

9. Travis WD, Brambilla E, Noguchi M, et al. International association for the study of lung cancer/American Thoracic Society/European Respiratory Society international multidisciplinary classification of lung adenocarcinoma. *J Thorac Oncol.* 2011;6(2):244-285. doi:10.1097/JTO.0b013e318206a221.

10. Borczuk AC, Qian F, Kazeros A, et al. Invasive size is an independent predictor of survival in pulmonary adenocarcinoma. *Am J Surg Pathol.* 2009;33(3):462-469. doi:10.1097/PAS.0b013e318190157c.

11. Tsutsumida H, Nomoto M, Goto M, et al. A micropapillary pattern is predictive of a poor prognosis in lung adenocarcinoma, and reduced surfactant apoprotein A expression in the micropapillary pattern is an excellent indicator of a poor prognosis. *Mod Pathol.* 2007;20(6):638-647. doi:10.1038/modpathol.3800780.

12. Aherne EA, Plodkowski AJ, Montecalvo J, et al. What CT characteristics of lepidic predominant pattern lung adenocarcinomas correlate with invasiveness on pathology? *Lung Cancer.* 2018;118:83-89. Epub 2018/03/25. doi:10.1016/j.lungcan.2018.01.013.

13. Akata S, Fukushima A, Kakizaki D, Abe K, Amino S. CT scanning of bronchioloalveolar carcinoma: specific appearances. *Lung Cancer.* 1995;12(3):221-230. Epub 1995/06/01.

14. Psathakis K, Bostantzoglou K, Sambaziotis D, Tsintiris K. Bronchorrhea in bronchioloalveolar carcinoma. *Respiration.* 2011;82(1):54-55. Epub 2011/05/11. doi:10.1159/000327240.

15. Saijo T, Ishii G, Nagai K, et al. Differences in clinicopathological and biological features between central-type and peripheral-type squamous cell carcinoma of the lung. *Lung Cancer.* 2006;52(1):37-45. Epub 2006/02/25. doi:10.1016/j.lungcan.2005.12.006.

16. Tomashefski JF, Jr., Connors AF, Jr., Rosenthal ES, Hsiue IL. Peripheral vs central squamous cell carcinoma of the lung. A comparison of clinical features, histopathology, and survival. *Arch Pathol Lab Med.* 1990;114(5):468-474. Epub 1990/05/01.

17. Affandi KA, Tizen NMS, Mustangin M, Zin R. p40 immunohistochemistry is an excellent marker in primary lung squamous cell carcinoma. *J Pathol Transl Med.* 2018;52(5):283-289. Epub 2018/09/22. doi:10.4132/jptm.2018.08.14.

18. Yousem SA. Peripheral squamous cell carcinoma of lung: patterns of growth with particular focus on airspace filling. *Hum Pathol.* 2009;40(6):861-867. Epub 2009/03/10. doi:10.1016/j.humpath.2008.11.008.

19. Abe S, Ogura S, Nakajima I, Makimura S, Kawakami Y, Inoue K. Small-cell-type poorly differentiated squamous cell carcinoma of the lung. Cytologic, immunohistochemical and nuclear DNA content analysis. Analytical and quantitative cytology and histology/the International Academy of Cytology [and] American Society of Cytology. *Anal Quant Cytol Histol.* 1990;12(2):73-77. Epub 1990/04/01.

20. Girard N, Ostrovnaya I, Lau C, et al. Genomic and mutational profiling to assess clonal relationships between multiple non-small cell lung cancers. *Clin Cancer Res.* 2009;15(16):5184-5190. Epub 2009/08/13. doi:10.1158/1078-0432.ccr-09-0594.

7

PATHOBIOLOGY OF SMALL CELL CARCINOMA AND OTHER NEUROENDOCRINE TUMORS OF THE LUNG

Mostafa M. Fraig, MD, MBA

A 60-year-old white male had a 6-cm central lung mass biopsied by core needle biopsy.

He smoked two packs of cigarettes per day for 40 years and has had a coronary stent placed.

The magnetic resonance imaging (MRI) of the brain shows 2 subcentimeter metastases.

A positron emission tomographic (PET) scan shows a liver mass and rib lesions.

His serology shows a sodium level of 120 mEq/L.

Learning Objectives:
1. What is the new World Health Organization (WHO) classification for small cell lung cancer?
2. What are the markers distinguishing small cell from non–small cell lung cancer?
3. What are the types of neuroendocrine tumors found in the lung?

Recognition of the distinct biological behavior of small cell carcinoma from that of non–small cell carcinoma has been long established. Therefore, the characterization of small cell carcinoma has proven to be very important as it has therapeutic as well as prognostic implications. However, the presence of other tumors with overlapping morphological, ultrastructural, and immunohistochemical features has complicated this endeavor.

PREINVASIVE LESIONS

Neuroendocrine Hyperplasia and Tumorlets

The spectrum of preinvasive neuroendocrine lesions encompasses conditions of several associations and clinical presentations. However, the histomorphologic features are mostly similar with only a few distinguishing features.

There are conditions that are associated with neuroendocrine cell hyperplasia but the mechanism of action is poorly understood. The chronic conditions of inflammation and fibrosis as in patients with chronic obstructive pulmonary disease have a tendency to harbor small foci of neuroendocrine proliferation. These are usually incidental findings encountered when the lung is sampled for other reasons. In resections for carcinoid tumors, other foci of neuroendocrine proliferation are present and could represent a **"field defect" similar to that of atypical adenomatous hyperplasia (AAH) and adenocarcinoma.** The spectrum of neuroendocrine tumors in their progressive pattern is outlined (**Table 7-1**).

Diffuse Idiopathic Neuroendocrine Cell Hyperplasia

Diffuse idiopathic neuroendocrine cell hyperplasia is an uncommon condition in which the airways are circumferentially involved by a proliferation of neuroendocrine cells underneath the bronchial epithelium (**Figure 7-1**). The origin of these cells is believed to be from Kulchitsky cells, which normally reside as individual cells in this location. In about half of the patients, the neuroendocrine hyperplasia could present in the setting of an interstitial lung disease investigation based on peribronchial fibrosis and inflammation in addition to neuroendocrine cell hyperplasia. In the other half of the patients, it is usually an incidental finding in the course of investigating

TABLE 7-1 Neuroendocrine Proliferations and Tumors of the Lung
1. Neuroendocrine hyperplasia and tumorlets • Neuroendocrine hyperplasia associated with fibrosis and inflammation • Neuroendocrine hyperplasia associated with carcinoid tumors • Diffuse idiopathic neuroendocrine cell hyperplasia • Tumorlets (<5 mm)
2. Tumors with neuroendocrine morphology • Carcinoid tumor • Atypical carcinoid tumor • Large cell neuroendocrine carcinoma (LCNEC): Combined LCNEC • Small cell carcinoma: Combined small cell carcinoma
3. Non–small cell carcinoma with neuroendocrine differentiation
4. Other tumors with neuroendocrine differentiation • Pulmonary blastoma • Desmoplastic round blue cell tumor • Primitive neuroectodermal tumor • Paraganglioma

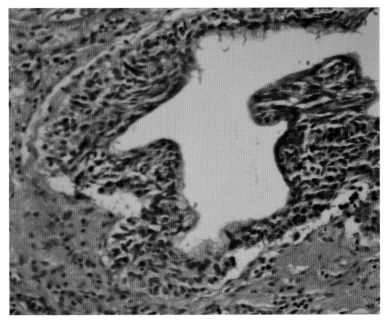

Figure 7-1. Diffuse idiopathic pulmonary neuroendocrine cell hyperplasia (DIPNECH) has a peribronchial pattern with hyperchromatic nuclei and a small amount of cytoplasm compared with the overlying layer of bronchial epithelium.

extrapulmonary malignancies with potential metastasis to the lung.[1] They have a distinctive CT presentation, with pulmonary nodules and centrilobular and peribronchial nodules corresponding to carcinoid tumorlets and carcinoid tumors, respectively.[2]

Because of the coexistence of DIPNECH with carcinoid tumorlets, and the lesions are usually multiple, this led to the belief that they are closely related and represent part of the spectrum in the evolution of other neuroendocrine tumors. DIPNECH present as a layer of darker, more compact cells than those of the overlying bronchial epithelium. They are immunoreactive to the common neuroendocrine markers, such as synaptophysin, chromogranin A, and CD56.

Carcinoid Tumorlets

Carcinoid tumorlets are usually present as nests of neuroendocrine cells separated by the surrounding connective tissue stroma in the peribronchial area. The cells have uniform nuclei with salt-and-pepper chromatin, absent or inconspicuous nucleoli, and granular amphophilic cytoplasm. Mitotic figures are extremely rare, and no necrosis is noted. The overall dimension of the lesion should be **less than 5 mm**; anything beyond this dimension with the same morphology is considered as a typical carcinoid tumor.

CARCINOID TUMORS

Carcinoid tumors account for 1%-2% of all invasive lung malignancies. In about half of the cases, the patients are asymptomatic, and the lesions are discovered incidentally in the course of workup of other conditions. In the other half, nonspecific symptoms such as hemoptysis, postobstructive pneumonia, or dyspnea may manifest themselves. The average age of patients is between 45 and 55 years, but the tumors could occur at any age. They are the most common lung tumors of childhood. They could be associated with a paraneoplastic syndrome, with the most common type Cushing syndrome. The tumor location is usually central with a well-circumscribed or lobulated outline. The tumors could also be peripheral, under the pleural surface. The tumors usually show low uptake by PET scans.

A microscopically typical carcinoid tumor is characterized by an organoid pattern, with tumor cells organized in nests, strips, festoons, papillary, mucinous, or signet ring and pseudoglandular patterns separated by either a delicate or sclerotic stroma. Some tumors could assume enough of spindle cell morphology to be confused with benign or well-differentiated mesenchymal tumors. There is usually peripheral palisading of the nuclei and the presence of rosettes contributes to the organoid pattern. The nuclei are uniform with absent or inconspicuous nucleoli. The chromatin is evenly distributed and could be powdery, imparting the salt-and-pepper quality characteristic of neuroendocrine cells in general. The cytoplasm is faintly granular and amphophilic with a fair amount surrounding the nuclei. The **mitotic activity is very low, with less than 2 mitoses per 2 mm^2** (equal to 10 high-power fields in some microscopes) (**Figure 7-2**). In between 5% and 20% of cases, metastasis to local lymph nodes could occur; however, this should not be used as a criterion for atypical carcinoid (Table 7-1). The treatment of choice is usually surgical resection, with excellent prognosis. Patients rarely die of typical carcinoid tumors.

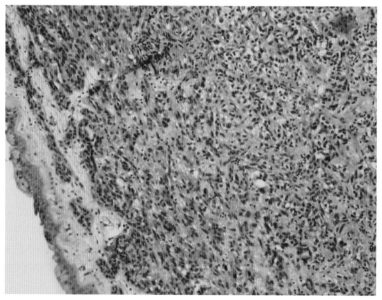

Figure 7-2. Carcinoid tumors could present in different patterns, ranging from nests to sheets, strips, and spindle cells. In the image, the cells have a clear cell pattern, but they share the common features of having uniform nuclei with slightly granular chromatin and inconspicuous nucleoli.

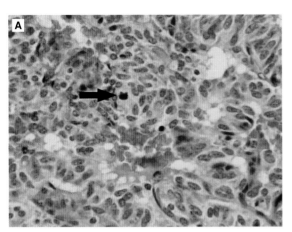
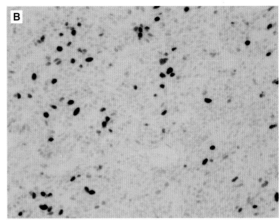

Figure 7-3. Atypical carcinoid tumors demonstrate the cellular features as in a typical carcinoid tumor but with partial loss of architectural organization and the presence of mitotic figures such as seen in the center (arrow) in **A**. As a surrogate for the mitotic activity, immunolabeling for Ki67 shows brisk activity, as illustrated in **B**.

Atypical Carcinoid Tumors

Atypical carcinoid tumors usually share the clinical presentation and most of the microscopic features of carcinoid tumors with few exceptions. The tumors are usually larger in size than typical carcinoid tumors, and they have a higher rate for regional lymph node metastasis, ranging between 40% and 50%. There is partial loss of the organoid pattern, and single-cell necrosis or central punctate necrosis is frequent. **The mitotic activity is between 2 and 10 per 2 mm².** Nuclear pleomorphism and prominent nucleoli are frequently present. The proliferative index as measured by **Ki67 immunolabeling is less than 5% in typical carcinoid tumors and between 5% and 20% for atypical carcinoid tumors.** Large cell neuroendocrine carcinoma (LCNEC) usually has a much higher proliferative index than 20% (**Figure 7-3**). Both types of carcinoid tumors are positive for neuroendocrine markers by immunohistochemistry (IHC). They show positivity for Synaptophysin and CD56, with variable staining for Chromogranin in the case of atypical carcinoid.[3]

SMALL CELL LUNG CARCINOMA

Small cell lung carcinoma (SCLC) comprises 14% of all lung cancers, and as such it presents 30,000 newly diagnosed cases per year in the United States. About two-thirds of these tumors have a prehilar location and are present around the proximal part of the bronchial tree. They circumferentially involve the endobronchial wall, causing compression of the lumen. However, they rarely involve the mucosal surface to cause ulceration or fungating masses within the lumen. Early lymph node and distant metastasis are common at presentation. The tumor is white-tan and friable with extensive necrosis. In about 5% of the cases, the tumor could present as a coin lesion within the lung parenchyma.

Historically, SCLC was classified in three classes: oat cell carcinoma, intermediate cell type, and combined small cell carcinoma with non–small carcinoma.[4] In 1988, the International Association for the Study of Lung Cancer (IASLC) recommended dropping the intermediate cell category for lack of reproducibility among pathologists and lack of significant clinical differences. The category of mixed SCLC and non–small carcinoma was maintained, and a mixed small cell carcinoma/large cell neuroendocrine carcinoma category was added. The last category was subsequently included in the 2004 WHO classification for the same reasons cited for the intermediate cell type.

Clinical Features and Prognosis

Small cell lung carcinoma has very distinctive clinical properties. It has a very aggressive course, and extensive metastasis at the time of presentation is usually expected. **SCLC is frequently associated with paraneoplastic syndrome.** The mediastinal lymphadenopathy could impinge on the superior vena cava and lead to what is known as superior vena cava syndrome.

With combination chemotherapy (etoposide and cisplatin) and radiation chemotherapy to the chest, the median survival for a patient with limited-stage disease is 15 months, and the 5-year survival is 10%. Because of the tendency of SCLC to spread far and fast to other organs, brain radiation and sometimes whole-body radiation are employed in treating this disease, which is very unusual for other lung tumors.[5] The role of surgical excision is not standardized, and some surgeons will resect limited-stage tumors to reduce the tumor burden, with surgery followed by systemic chemotherapy.[6]

Small cell lung carcinoma has very distinctive morphologic features. It is characterized by very **hyperchromatic nuclei with an elliptical or fusiform shape demonstrating nuclear molding and very scant cytoplasm.** The chromatin is granular or is described as "salt and pepper" with absent or inconspicuous nucleoli. The number of mitotic figures is very high, and apoptotic bodies within the cytoplasm are frequent. There are areas of necrosis and crush artifacts due to the fragility of the cells (**Figure 7-4**). The same reasons

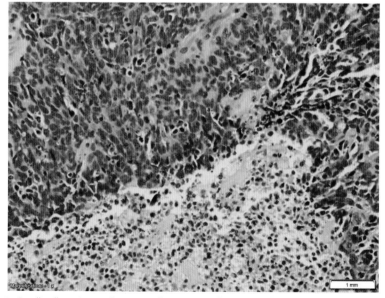

Figure 7-4. Small cell carcinoma (low magnification view) has a very distinct morphology with hyperchromatic nuclei and a scant amount of cytoplasm. There are areas of necrosis among sheets of tumor cells.

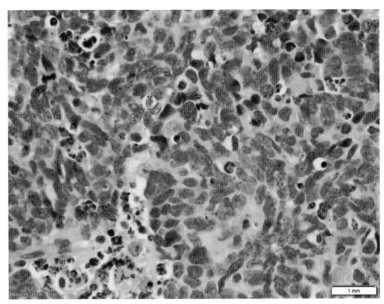

Figure 7-5. Small cell carcinoma, high-magnification view. There is nuclear molding and granular chromatin with absent or faint nucleoli. There are numerous mitotic figures and single-cell apoptosis with areas of necrosis scattered around.

account for the basophilic smearing of adjacent blood vessels by released chromatin, a phenomenon known as the Azzopardi effect. In small forceps-assisted transbronchial biopsies, the crush artifacts could be extensive, so differentiation from peribronchial lymphocytic infiltrate becomes difficult, and resorting to IHC stains becomes inevitable.

Most cases are diagnosed on small biopsies or by cytology. This makes it imperative for pathologists to adhere to the diagnostic criteria as the **diagnosis of SCLC is essentially morphologic.** There are overlapping features as well as IHC reactivity to neuroendocrine markers. Fortunately, the cytomorphologic features are characteristic, with the high cytoplasmic ratio and nuclear molding the easiest features to note. Apoptotic bodies and stringing of chromatin are also evident. In fact, the diagnosis of SCLC on cytologic material is easier than on small biopsies for the experienced cytopathologist (**Figure 7-5**).

Almost 10% of SCLC could be negative for all neuroendocrine markers, and only immunoreactivity to pancytokeratin to exclude hematopoietic and mesenchymal tumors should be relied on to keep the diagnosis as a carcinoma. The positivity of neuroendocrine tumors for pancytokeratin in general, including SCLC, has a characteristic dot-like pattern within the cytoplasm, which could serve as a useful tip-off to the neuroendocrine differentiation in unsuspected cases of poorly differentiated carcinoma. **The histomorphologic features are the key to making a diagnosis in these cases.** Immunoreactivity to thyroid transcription factor-1 (TTF-1) is another peculiar feature found in 70%-80% of cases of SCLC regardless of the tumor site of origin and should not be interpreted as indicative of derivation from a lung primary.

> **CLINICAL PEARL:** As a word of caution, about 10%-20% of non–small cell carcinomas could be positive for one or more neuroendocrine markers.

In addition, combined small cell carcinoma with a component of adenocarcinoma or squamous cell carcinoma could be encountered, and dismissing the small cell component as a poorly differentiated non–small cell lung carcinoma (NSCLC) will be a mistake.[7]

After therapy, a percentage of small cell carcinoma may have a component of NSCLC that is not responsive to the chemotherapy regimen used for SCLC. That does not mean that the initial diagnosis was wrong. Whether this residual carcinoma is a residual portion of a combined SCLC and NSCLC with the latter part being not sampled or too small to be overlooked, or that SCLC underwent some differentiation to produce the NSCLC component subsequent to the treatment.

COMBINED SCLC AND NSCLC

The prevalence of combined SCLC, while depending on the extent of histologic sampling, has been reported to be less than 10% by most studies. Combined SCLC could be a combination of SCLC and squamous carcinoma or adenocarcinoma, in which the proportion of the non–small cell component is not crucial. This combination is usually present in 1%-2% of tumors. However, in case of a combined SCLC and large cell neuroendocrine lung carcinoma (LCNELC), which represents 4%-6% of tumors, there is a cutoff level of 10%. As discussed previously, **the role of IHC should be taken with precaution since not all SCLC are positive for neuroendocrine markers, and not all tumors positive for neuroendocrine markers are SCLC or even neuroendocrine in nature.** SCLC could also be combined with spindle cell carcinoma or giant cell carcinoma, and while these are uncommon, there is no consistent evidence that they affect biologic behavior, response to therapy, or survival of these patients in comparison to those with pure SCLC.

Differential Diagnosis

Since the diagnosis of SCLC is a morphologic one, recognition and adherence to the criteria for diagnosis are important. Separating SCLC from LCNEC are crucial. While they share certain features with neuroendocrine morphology forming nests, rosettes, with peripheral palisading, they have brisk mitotic activity and extensive areas of necrosis. However, they have distinctive features, as summarized in (**Table 7-2**).

Small cell lung carcinoma usually has nuclei that are 2 to 3 times the size of a resting lymphocyte nucleus, and LCNEC has larger and more vesicular nuclei with more prominent nucleoli. There is more of an amphophilic cytoplasm around LCNEC nuclei. This makes the nuclear molding, characteristic of SCLC, less likely in LCNEC. **The mitotic activity percentage based on Ki67 IHC is high (80%-90%) in cases of SCLC as compared with 50%-60% in cases of LCNEC.**

Another frequently overlooked differential diagnosis is basaloid squamous cell carcinoma. The cells could have a high nuclear-to-cytoplasmic ratio and exhibit nuclear molding on cytologic material. IHC should help distinguish these cases by demonstrating the negative staining for neuroendocrine markers, TTF-1, and diffuse staining for p63 or p40. If the keratin staining is negative, one has to be careful with the diagnosis of SCLC and investigate the possibility of chronic inflammation, lymphoma, primitive neuroectodermal tumors, or small round cell sarcoma.

TABLE 7-2	Distinguishing Features Between Small Cell Carcinoma and Large Cell Neuroendocrine Carcinoma Under Light Microscopy	
FEATURE	SMALL CELL CARCINOMA	LARGE CELL NEUROENDOCRINE CARCINOMA
Cell Size	Small (<3 resting lymphocytes)	Larger
Nuclear/cytoplasmic ratio	High	Lower
Nuclear chromatin	Finely granular (salt and pepper)	Clumped and vesicular
Nucleoli	Absent or inconspicuous	Often present
Nuclear molding	Characteristic	Uncommon
Nuclear shape	Fusiform (oat seed)	Polygonal
Cytoplasm	Scant	
Chromatin smearing	Common	Uncommon
Rosetting	Less common	

LARGE CELL NEUROENDOCRINE CARCINOMA

Large cell neuroendocrine carcinoma comprises about 3% of all resected lung cancers. As the name suggests, LCNEC is essentially a non–small carcinoma with neuroendocrine features. It affects patients who are older, with a mean patient age of 62 years and a history of smoking. These patients tend to have a worse prognosis than patients with atypical carcinoid and even non–small carcinoma. The 5-year survival is around 27%, and the 10-year survival was 11% in one study. Most studies failed to show a significant difference between survival of those with SCLC and those with LCNEC.

It fits at the other end of the spectrum from typical carcinoid to atypical carcinoid and finally LCNEC. It retains features of atypical carcinoid with at least a partial organoid pattern with peripheral palisading of nuclei, resetting, and a fair amount of amphophilic granular cytoplasm.[8] It acquires new features in the presence of areas of necrosis, more mitotic activity, and more irregular tumor outline than encountered in carcinoid tumors (**Figures 7-6A-D**). It could be very difficult to recognize the last features on small biopsies or cytologic material. The treatment follows that of non–small cell carcinoma.

Several authors have advocated using a grading system for neuroendocrine tumors and putting SCLC and LCNEC together at the highest grade, with neuroendocrine carcinoma grade 3 and carcinoid grade 1 and with atypical carcinoid grade 2. These attempts have not met much success, especially within the pulmonary pathology community because of the long history of studies that showed a difference in biological behavior and response to treatment.

Also, LCNEC could occur in combination with other non–small cell carcinoma, such as squamous cell carcinoma or adenocarcinoma. The term *large cell carcinoma with neuroendocrine morphology* could be used for tumors lacking neuroendocrine markers of immunoreactivity but demonstrating neuroendocrine features by light microscopy.

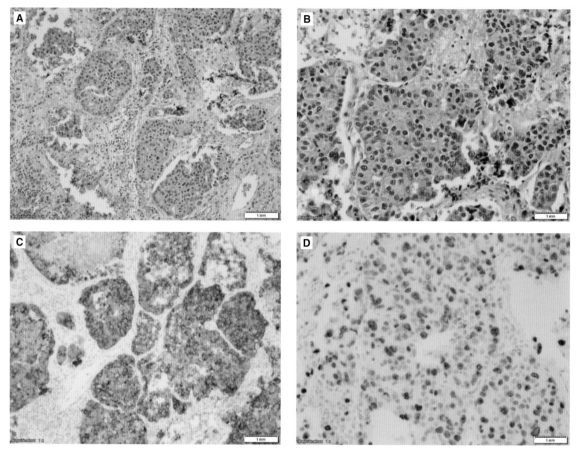

Figure 7-6. Large cell neuroendocrine carcinoma. **A.** A low-magnification view with sheets of tumor cells with peripheral palisading. The nuclei appear to be uniform, surrounded by a fair amount of cytoplasm compared with those in small cell carcinoma. **B.** Resetting of the cells where the cells align in a circle with no lumen in the middle. Occasional nucleoli can be seen in some of the nuclei. **C.** Immunohistochemical stains for synaptophysin decorate the tumor cells, confirming their neuroendocrine differentiation. **D.** The proliferative index as shown by the nuclear staining for Ki67 shows a brisk proliferation in about 50%-60% of the cells.

REFERENCES

1. Mengoli MC, Rossi G, Cavazza A, et al. Diffuse idiopathic pulmonary neuroendocrine cell hyperplasia (DIPNECH) syndrome and carcinoid tumors with/without NECH: a clinicopathologic, radiologic, and immunomolecular comparison study. *Am J Surg Pathol.* 2018;42(5):646-655. Epub 2018/02/14. doi:10.1097/PAS.0000000000001033.

2. Walker CM, Vummidi D, Benditt JO, Godwin JD, Pipavath S. What is DIPNECH? *Clin Imaging.* 2012;36(5):647-649. Epub 2012/08/28. doi:10.1016/j.clinimag.2011.11.011.

3. Travis WD, Gal AA, Colby TV, Klimstra DS, Falk R, Koss MN. Reproducibility of neuroendocrine lung tumor classification. *Hum Pathol.* 1998;29(3):272-279.

4. Hirsch FR, Matthews MJ, Aisner S, et al. Histopathologic classification of small cell lung cancer. Changing concepts and terminology. *Cancer.* 1988;62(5):973-977.

5. Fraire AE, Johnson EH, Yesner R, Zhang XB, Spjut HJ, Greenberg SD. Prognostic significance of histopathologic subtype and stage in small cell lung cancer. *Hum Pathol.* 1992;23(5):520-528.

6. Nicholson SA, Beasley MB, Brambilla E, et al. Small cell lung carcinoma (SCLC): a clinicopathologic study of 100 cases with surgical specimens. *Am J Surg Pathol*. 2002;26(9):1184-1197.

7. Yatabe Y, Dacic S, Borczuk AC, et al. Best practices recommendations for diagnostic immunohistochemistry in lung cancer. *J Thorac Oncol*. 2019;14(3):377-407. doi:10.1016/j.jtho.2018.12.005.

8. Vollmer RT, Ogden L, Crissman JD. Separation of small-cell from non-small-cell lung cancer. The Southeastern Cancer Study Group pathologists' experience. *Arch Pathol Lab Med*. 1984;108(10):792-794.

8

THE CANCER STEM CELL HYPOTHESIS OF LUNG CANCER

Christine Fillmore Brainson, PhD

A 50-year-old heavy smoker was treated for small cell lung cancer, limited stage, with chemotherapy and radiation. The bulky tumor in his chest was no longer seen after the treatment, and he was told he had a complete response.

Two months following the treatment, the cancer recurred and was resistant to any further systemic therapy.

He asks during his last clinic visit before going to hospice, "How did the cancer come back so quickly, and why was it not cured when I had a complete response?"

Learning Objectives:
1. What is meant by the term *cancer stem cells*?
2. How can cancer stem cells (CSCs) explain treatment resistance and recurrence of disease?
3. What are the normal stem cells in the lung that the CSCs may be mimicking?

Lung cancer is a progressive disease arising from accumulation of genetic mutations and natural selection of the genetic clones most fit to continue proliferation. However, even within isogenic cancer cell populations, heterogeneity in phenotypes exists. For example, not every lung cancer cell can grow ex vivo in two-dimensional or three-dimensional culture,[1,2] and it does not appear that every cell has an equal ability to survive chemotherapy, evade the immune system, or metastasize.[3,4] As early as 1858, the idea of "stemness" in cancer was raised by the pathologist Rudolph Virchow,[5] and throughout

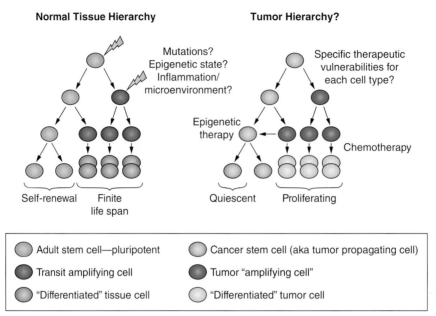

Figure 8-1. Parallels between normal tissue hierarchy and tumor cell hierarchy. Whether cancer stem cells (CSCs) exist within a tumor population depends on extrinsic cues such as inflammation and the microenvironment, as well as cell intrinsic properties. The cell intrinsic properties include the epigenetic state of the cell that acquired sufficient mutations to become malignant and the specific pathways of the mutations. Understanding both the normal lung epithelial hierarchies and hierarchies that exist within the distinct subtypes of lung cancer holds promise to define specific vulnerabilities of both genetic and epigenetic states for lung cancers.

the past century the idea that tumors are driven by a population of stem-like cells has been constantly proposed as the reason for clonal tumor cell heterogeneity. In the past several decades, the idea has been formally termed the *cancer stem cell hypothesis*.[6,7]

The CSC hypothesis proposes that tumors can be hierarchically organized, and that only the cancer cells at the top of the hierarchy have the unique properties of self-renewal and the ability to differentiate into multiple lineages (**Figure 8-1**). In normal tissues, these traits of self-renewal and differentiation allow stem cells to repopulate organs during homeostatic turnover and after tissue injury. In the context of cancer, "**stemness**" implies that these cancer cells have a more **unlimited proliferative potential** than "nonstem" cancer cells and therefore that they are the cells able to drive tumor growth long term. Corollaries **to the CSC hypothesis include that CSCs are relatively resistant to chemotherapies through multiple mechanisms, including relative quiescence; that CSCs drive recurrent disease; and that CSCs are responsible for seeding metastases.**[3,4,8] Whether one or all of these properties of long-term tumor growth, disease resistance to therapy, and metastatic spread of cancer can be attributed to a single subpopulation of cancer cells relies largely on the composition of the tumor, including the mutations present, the polyclonality of the tumor, and the differentiation state of the cells within the tumor.[8] In order to fully appreciate the possible traits of a CSC population, it is first necessary to understand the traits of the normal epithelial differentiation hierarchies that the tumor cells could be mimicking.

In this chapter, the reader will learn about the diverse epithelial cell types from which lung tumors can arise and how tumor cell characteristics may resemble the normal epithelial hierarchies found in lung. **Understanding these hierarchies is key to exploring the CSC hypothesis in lung cancer**, which posits that a rare stem-like population of cells drives tumor growth and recurrence. The reader will learn about possible CSC markers for various subtypes of lung cancer and learn about efforts in the field to target CSCs.

NON–SMALL CELL LUNG CANCER STEM CELLS

Several distinct stem/progenitor cell pools have been identified in the lung, including basal cells, club cell progenitors, alveolar cell progenitors, and bronchioalveolar stem cells[9-12] (**Figure 8-2**). Each of these cell types has some capacity to self-renew and to give rise to other lineages of lung epithelial cells in the contexts of tissue injury and homeostatic turnover. In experimental models, non–small cell lung cancer may arise from any of these stem/progenitor pools, and perhaps other uncharacterized "lineage-negative" cell populations, dependent on the genetic perturbations used.[13-17] As we learn more

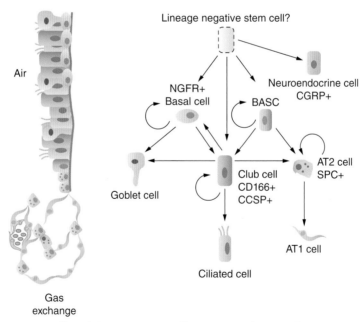

Figure 8-2. Normal progenitor cell pools for cancer stem cells. Numerous distinct cell types exist within the normal lung epithelium. The cells with self-renewal capacity include basal cells of the trachea and upper bronchi that express NGFR and KRT5; secretory club cells that express CD166 and CCSP; and alveolar type II cells that express SPC. Also within the bronchiolar epithelium are innervated CGRP+ neuroendocrine cells, mucus-producing goblet cells, and multiciliated cells. In the murine lung, at the bronchioalveolar duct junction, a cell type that can give rise to both bronchiolar and alveolar lineages is termed the bronchioalveolar stem cell (BASC). Alveolar type I cells are thin cells that perform gas exchange in the distal lung. Each of these cell types has a distinct epigenetic state, and in theory any of these cells can serve as the cell of origin for lung cancer if the proper genetic mutations are accumulated. Many recent reports have suggested a lineage-negative lung epithelial cell may be the most primitive lung cell with the greatest differentiation potential, although further characterization of this elusive cell type is needed.

about the diverse cell types that have regenerative capacity in the adult lung, we will undoubtedly uncover corresponding molecular cell types of non–small cell lung cancer that recapitulate distinct cellular hierarchies. **It is important to remember that due to microenvironmental changes and genetic mutations, CSCs within a tumor may not still resemble the cell from which they arose, but rather may resemble a cell upstream or downstream in the hierarchy due to epigenetic reprogramming.**

The two major subtypes of non–small cell lung cancer are adenocarcinoma and squamous cell carcinoma. Historically, these two major subtypes have been hypothesized to arise from distinct cell populations within the lung due to differences in anatomical location and marker expression retained in the cancers. Adenocarcinomas tend to arise in the more distal airspace and have markers consistent with distal lung cell origin, including proteins expressed by alveolar type II cells such as the homeobox transcription factor NK2 homeobox 1 (NKX2-1) and surfactant protein C (SPC). Some adenocarcinomas are more "bronchiolar" in phenotype and therefore express markers that secretory club cells of the airways express, including club cell secretory protein (CCSP) and the transcription factor SOX2. Supporting the idea that CSCs in adenocarcinoma may be in a more bronchiolar state, **CD166 (also known as ALCAM)** has been shown to mark CSCs in both adenocarcinoma and squamous cell carcinoma xenografts and was shown to enrich for the club cell lineage from human tracheal cell preparations.[18,19] Squamous cell carcinomas tend to arise more proximally, sometimes even connecting physically to the pseudostratified epithelium of the upper airway. However, mixed adenosquamous tumors and peripheral squamous tumors exist in patients as well as in mouse models, and these observations suggest that squamous cell carcinomas can arise from adenocarcinomas or alveolar cells given the correct microenvironment and genetic alterations. Regardless of their genesis, squamous cell carcinomas express markers consistent with basal cells, which are the stem cells of the trachea and upper bronchi, including KRT5, TP63, and NGFR[9,18]; therefore, it is possible that CSCs within these tumors also have basal cell-like characteristics. Indeed, an **NGFR+** cell population was found to have CSC potential by serial orthotopic injections in a mouse model of lung squamous cell carcinoma.[20]

In addition to the lineage markers described, many groups have focused on the known putative CSC markers, including CD133 (prominin), ALDH1 (aldehyde dehydrogenase), and CD44. CD133 was significantly associated with disease recurrence, resistance to therapy, and decreased overall survival.[21,22] ALDH1 also had some prognostic value, being associated with decreased survival, most specifically in the adenocarcinoma subtype.[21] Using primary human lung cancer xenografts, sphere cultures, and established cell lines, several groups have demonstrated **that CD133 is a marker of functional CSCs with the ability to seed tumors in vivo and survive chemotherapy.**[21] Studies of ALDH1 expression in combination with CD133 or CD44 have shown that ALDH1+ cells have an increased ability to seed tumors in serial transplantation assays when compared to the bulk or ALDH1- cells, strongly indicating that cells with these markers could be bona fide adenocarcinoma CSCs.[21,23] Importantly, many of these studies demonstrated that the cells with **functional CSC properties also expressed high levels of NOTCH proteins.**[21,22] As described in material that follows, NOTCH inhibition could be a vulnerability for non–small cell lung cancers.

Due to limitations of primary human tissues, including large interpatient heterogeneity and small sample size, much of what we understand about functional CSCs has been learned in **genetically engineered mouse models** (GEMMs) of lung cancer. GEMMs representing adenocarcinoma, squamous cell carcinoma, and mixed adenosquamous cancer have been established, and new genetic combinations are consistently being produced and assessed for phenotype.[24] Using the mouse adenocarcinoma model driven by oncogenic KRAS and loss of *Tp53*, a population of tumor cells highly enriched for tumorigenic potential was identified to be CD24+/INTGA6+/NOTCH3+; similarly, a population of highly metastatic cells was identified to be CD24+/SCA1+.[25,26] In a mouse model of squamous cell carcinoma driven by biallelic deletion of LKB1 (STK11) and PTEN, the CSC phenotype was SCA1+/NGFR+, and the CSCs were enriched for expression of the immune-evasion marker PD-L1.[20]

As new genetic combinations are tried, it will be very important to compare CSC phenotypes between models, given that a direct comparison of one stem cell marker, SCA1, in several GEMMs demonstrated that **CSCs can differ greatly in phenotype** dependent on genotype.[27] Therefore, going forward the field must start to acknowledge both molecular subtype and genotypes as drivers of CSC phenotypes, and mouse models are an excellent way to control for tumor genotype and produce enough tissue to thoroughly test the CSC hypothesis.

TARGETING CANCER STEM CELLS IN NON–SMALL CELL LUNG CANCER

Due to the heterogeneity of the disease, targeting CSC populations in non–small cell lung cancer will likely require many approaches. Targeting metabolic programs in CSCs, the ability of CSCs to evade the immune system, and the epigenetic state of CSCs addresses viable approaches to prevent disease recurrence that are currently being heavily explored for non–small cell lung cancers. In terms of targeting a signaling protein that CSCs rely on, one promising target that has been validated in several systems is NOTCH3 for lung adenocarcinomas. However, there is not yet a NOTCH3-specific inhibitor, and it is unclear if gamma-secretase inhibition, which targets all forms of NOTCH, would be useful. NOTCH1- and NOTCH2-inactivating mutations are found in both lung squamous cell carcinoma and small cell lung cancer, so it is conceivable that inhibition of all NOTCH receptors would both target the adenocarcinoma CSC pools through NOTCH3 and drive the tumor to "transdifferentiate" to a more squamous or neuroendocrine fate through inhibition of NOTCH1 and NOTCH2. More research on this pathway could allow for a more specific inhibitor that targets only NOTCH3 to be developed.

Targeting epigenetic programs also holds some promise for the field. For example, it was recently identified that inhibition or knockdown of the histone methyltransferases G9A or GLP allows for an expansion of the metastatic CSC pool in KRAS-driven cancers.[28] Therefore, one method to target the CSC pool could be through inhibiting histone d-methylases, which was tested pharmacologically with the inhibitor JIB-01.[28] Inhibition of JIB-01 during establishment of taxane-resistant non–small cell lung cancers was also effective,[29] suggesting that histone demethylase inhibition may be one way forward in lung adenocarcinomas.

SMALL CELL LUNG CANCER STEM CELLS

In the case of small cell lung cancer, it is clear that tumors comprise cells that are neuroendocrine in phenotype. This phenotype is robust and can be validated by several markers specific to the pulmonary neuroendocrine lineage of the lung epithelium, including calcitonin gene-related peptide (CGRP), chromogranin A, and neuron-specific enolase. In the normal lung, neuroendocrine cells reside anatomically at features termed neuroendocrine bodies, which are enervated groups of cells within the bronchiolar epithelium. Study of the genesis of these neuroendocrine bodies in developing lung has suggested that the embryonic alveolar lineage can give rise to these neuroendocrine bodies.[30] This possible lineage relationship between alveolar cells and neuroendocrine cells is further supported by the clinical observation that **EGFR-driven lung adenocarcinomas, which typically resemble alveolar type II cells, can transdifferentiate into small cell lung** during acquired resistance to EGFR tyrosine kinase inhibitors and can return back to the adenocarcinoma fate after the tyrosine kinase inhibitor is removed.[31] However, studies in the adult mouse have suggested that although neuroendocrine cells can serve as progenitor cells to repopulate the club cell lineage,[30,32] they are fully dispensable for proper club cell injury response. Furthermore, genetic ablation of neuroendocrine cells in the adult mouse lung results in a seemingly permanent loss of neuroendocrine cells in the adult mouse lung results in a seemingly permanent loss of neuroendocrine bodies, suggesting that at least in the homeostatic lung, there are not any progenitor cells that can easily differentiate into the neuroendocrine lineage to replace it on loss.[30]

While mouse models of non–small cell lung cancer have been produced with numerous differing genetic perturbations, mouse models of small cell lung cancer appear to require loss of TP53 and RB1.[33,34] Studies using these mouse models have demonstrated that CGRP-expressing pulmonary neuroendocrine cells could give rise to bona fide small cell lung cancers on induction of relevant genetic mutations.[33,34] But, surprisingly, the incidence of tumor formation and extent of disease are always higher in the untargeted cytomegalovirus (CMV)-Cre–infected mice than in mice infected with the CGRP-restricted Cre virus, suggesting a yet uncharacterized cell population that is the major cell of origin of small cell lung cancer.[34,35] Furthermore, although virus restricted to SPC-expressing or CCSP-expressing cells was largely unable to drive small cell lung cancer disease, tumors derived from CMV-Cre, but not CGRP-Cre, were able to express both alveolar and club cell lineage markers.[35] Together, these **data suggest a complex lineage relationship between club cells, alveolar type II cells, and neuroendocrine cells and the possibility that there are distinct types of small cell lung cancer that are derived from neuroendocrine cells or from lineage-negative progenitor cells.** As the field learns more about the normal lung cells and their differentiation potentials, we will be able to define markers, such as expression of NFIB (a chromatin factor that drives widespread chromatin accessibility) as marking distinct tumor types.[36]

Many studies have focused on identifying CSCs through expression of known stem cell markers from other systems. For small cell lung cancer, the markers that have been queried include **CD133** (prominin), **ALDH1** (aldehyde dehydrogenase), and the phenotype associated with epithelial-to-mesenchymal transition (EMT).[2,37,38] In formalin-fixed patient tissues, it was found that CD133 is expressed at low or moderate levels in the majority of tumors assessed, supporting that it could serve as a CSC marker in small cell lung cancer.[38] In contrast, two studies found that expression of ALDH1 is very low in small cell lung cancers, suggesting that it may not serve as a CSC marker as it does in many non–small cell lung cancers.[37,38]

In addition to staining for markers in primary tissues, several researchers have focused on using human small cell lung cancer cell lines to fractionate cell populations based on the cell surface markers. These cells can then be used in a variety of assays, with the gold standard assay being serial orthotopic transplantation at limiting dilution.[8] To date, for small cell lung cancer, the majority of the research has been performed with established cell lines, which are thought to retain some amount of cellular heterogeneity.[39] However, depending on the cell line and the method used, even the same CSC marker, such as CD133, can be ambiguous.[40,41]

One major caveat of cell lines, even those directly from patients, is that there are irreversible changes induced by two-dimensional culture.[42] It is possible that results from a freshly derived cell line, demonstrating CD44(high)/CD90(+) cells from one small cell lung cancer were more EMT-like and clonogenic, could be more representative of the case in primary tumors.[2] Work using freshly isolated circulating tumor cells grown subcutaneously as derived explants is perhaps the most exciting in the field because it allows expansion of tumor material without an in vitro culturing step.[43]

Mouse models of small cell lung cancer have been used for CSC studies, taking advantage of both primary tissue abundance and the robust ability to transplant cells for limiting dilution and serial transplantation assays. Using the *Tp53*-floxed, *Rb*-floxed, *p130*-floxed triple-transgenic mice,[44] researchers found that the subpopulation of neuroendocrine tumor cells that expressed high levels of epithelial cell adhesion molecule (EpCAM) were enriched for tumorigenic potential in subcutaneous serial transplantation assays.[45] These cells were unique from those in the same tumors that were in a more EMT-like state and expressed the highest levels of **CD44** and lacked expression of **EpCAM**. Furthermore, opposing current dogma, the authors found that these EpCAM-positive cells were not intrinsically more resistant to cisplatin,[45] the main chemotherapy used to combat small cell lung cancer. A different study also showed the importance of the EMT-like CD44+ cells within small cell lung cancers, but found that instead of being the CSC population, these EMT-like cells were able to modify the neuroendocrine population to be more tumorigenic and metastatic.[46] In this way, EMT-like cells may serve as a paracrine niche cell that supports CSC, similar to what has been described in breast cancer.[47]

TARGETING CANCER STEM CELLS IN SMALL CELL LUNG CANCER

Targeting small cell lung CSCs remains an important goal for the field. While targeting tyrosine kinases has shown great effects in targeted non–small cell lung cancer populations, small cell lung cancer largely lacks mutations in these targets.[48] However, there are several reports of promising results obtained by targeting the **epigenetic states** that allow small cell lung cancer cells to be stem-like. One such study demonstrated that inhibition of the chromatin reader BRD4 through the drug JQ1 could be used to deplete EpCAM+ CSCs in the mouse model of small cell lung cancer, suggesting that CSCs in this model rely on a certain epigenetic state, which includes MYC expression, to survive.[45]

Using primary small cell lung cancer xenografts known to develop cisplatin resistance, one study found that inhibition of the histone methyltransferase **EZH2** was sufficient to prevent chemoresistance development.[49] Another study demonstrated that inhibition of the histone H3 lysine 4 demethylase called LSD1 decreased in vivo tumor growth of xenografts of human SCLC cell lines and resulted in accumulation of the activating histone H3 lysine 4 methylation mark.[50] One unifying theme of cell lines that responded strongly to LSD1 inhibition was a global DNA hypomethylation signature, which will be explored clinically as a biomarker. These tumors may be similar to the NFIB-overexpressing small cell lung cancers, which were shown to have largely accessible chromatin and were highly metastatic.[36] More recently, the LSD1 inhibitor was demonstrated to allow reactivation of NOTCH1.[51] Likewise, inhibition of the **NOTCH ligand DLL3** by an antibody/drug conjugate in both treatment-naïve and chemotherapy-resistant patient-derived xenografts could effectively kill tumors.[52] Because small cell lung cancers often have NOTCH loss-of-function mutations,[48] this remarkable ability of the DLL3 peptide to work could be in part due to a synthetic lethality. It is hoped these and other novel therapeutics will become clinical realities in the next decade for this notoriously difficult-to-treat disease.

IMPORTANCE OF CANCER STEM CELL HYPOTHESIS

Understanding the cellular origins and molecular determinants of all the diverse subtypes of lung cancer should allow the field to develop more specific and effective treatment options. **Although a universal CSC phenotype may not exist for human lung cancers, there certainly are cells within tumors that behave functionally as CSCs at various stages of disease, including during tumor recurrence and metastatic spread of disease. Understanding the intrinsic and extrinsic cues these cells rely on has the possibility to transform treatment rationales by allowing a better understanding of how cancer begins and evolves.**

FUNDING SUPPORT NOTE

We would like to thank Dr. Dian Yang for critical reading of this work. This work was supported in part by NCI K22 CA201036; Kentucky Lung Cancer Research Program PO2 415 1100000368; V Foundation Scholar Award V2017-010; American Cancer Society Institutional Research Grant IRG-85-001-25; NIGMS P20 GM121327-03; NCI R01 CA237643; American Cancer Society Research Scholar Grant 133123-RSG-19-081-01-TBG; and American Association for Cancer Research Innovation and Discovery Grant (C.F.B.).

REFERENCES

1. Hamburger A, Salmon S. Primary bioassay of human tumor stem cells. *Science.* 1977;197(4302):461-463. doi:10.1126/science.560061.
2. Wang P, Gao Q, Suo Z, et al. Identification and characterization of cells with cancer stem cell properties in human primary lung cancer cell lines. *PloS One.* 2013;8(3):e57020. doi:10.1371/journal.pone.0057020.
3. Sullivan JP, Minna JD, Shay JW. Evidence for self-renewing lung cancer stem cells and their implications in tumor initiation, progression, and targeted therapy. *Cancer Metastasis Rev.* 2010;29(1):61-72. doi:10.1007/s10555-010-9216-5.

4. Visvader JE, Lindeman GJ. Cancer stem cells: current status and evolving complexities. *Cell Stem Cell.* 2012;10(6):717-728. doi:10.1016/j.stem.2012.05.007.

5. Wagner RP. Anecdotal, historical and critical commentaries on genetics. Rudolph Virchow and the genetic basis of somatic ecology. *Genetics.* 1999;151(3):917-920.

6. Reya T, Morrison SJ, Clarke MF, Weissman IL. Stem cells, cancer, and cancer stem cells. *Nature.* 2001;414(6859):105-111. doi:10.1038/35102167.

7. Wicha MS, Liu S, Dontu G. Cancer stem cells: an old idea—a paradigm shift. *Cancer Res.* 2006;66(4): 1883-1890. doi:10.1158/0008-5472.CAN-05-3153.

8. Beck B, Blanpain C. Unravelling cancer stem cell potential. *Nat Rev Cancer.* 2013;13(10):727-738.

9. Rock JR, Onaitis MW, Rawlins EL, et al. Basal cells as stem cells of the mouse trachea and human airway epithelium. *Proc Natl Acad Sci U S A.* 2009;106(31):12771-12775. doi:10.1073/pnas.0906850106.

10. Teisanu RM, Lagasse E, Whitesides JF, Stripp BR. Prospective isolation of bronchiolar stem cells based upon immunophenotypic and autofluorescence characteristics. *Stem Cells.* 2009;27(3):612-622. doi:10.1634/stemcells.2008-0838.

11. Desai TJ, Brownfield DG, Krasnow MA. Alveolar progenitor and stem cells in lung development, renewal and cancer. *Nature.* 2014;507(7491):190-194. doi:10.1038/nature12930.

12. Kim CF, Jackson EL, Woolfenden AE, et al. Identification of bronchioalveolar stem cells in normal lung and lung cancer. *Cell.* 2005;121(6):823-835. doi:10.1016/j.cell.2005.03.032.

13. Sato M, Larsen JE, Lee W, et al. Human lung epithelial cells progressed to malignancy through specific oncogenic manipulations. *Mol Cancer Res.* 2013;11(6):638-650. doi:10.1158/1541-7786.MCR-12-0634-T.

14. Rowbotham SP, Kim CF. Diverse cells at the origin of lung adenocarcinoma. Proceedings of the National Academy of Sciences. 2014. doi:10.1073/pnas.1401955111.

15. Nagaraj AS, Lahtela J, Hemmes A, et al. Cell of origin links histotype spectrum to immune microenvironment diversity in non-small-cell lung cancer driven by mutant kras and loss of Lkb1. *Cell Rep.* 2017;18(3):673-684.

16. Zhang H, Fillmore Brainson C, Koyama S, et al. Lkb1 inactivation drives lung cancer lineage switching governed by polycomb repressive complex 2. *Nat Commun.* 2017;8:14922. doi:10.1038/ncomms14922.

17. Best SA, De Souza DP, Kersbergen A, et al. Synergy between the KEAP1/NRF2 and PI3K pathways drives non-small-cell lung cancer with an altered immune microenvironment. *Cell Metab.* 2018;27(4):935-943.e4. doi:10.1016/j.cmet.2018.02.006.

18. Weeden CE, Chen Y, Ma SB, et al. Lung Basal stem cells rapidly repair DNA damage using the error-prone nonhomologous end-joining pathway. *PLoS Biol.* 2017;15(1):e2000731. doi:10.1371/journal.pbio.2000731.

19. Zhang WC, Shyh-Chang N, Yang H, et al. Glycine decarboxylase activity drives non-small cell lung cancer tumor-initiating cells and tumorigenesis. *Cell.* 2012;148(1-2):259-272. doi:10.1016/j.cell.2011.11.050.

20. Xu C, Fillmore Christine M, Koyama S, et al. Loss of Lkb1 and Pten leads to lung squamous cell carcinoma with elevated PD-L1 expression. *Cancer Cell.* 2014;25(5):590-604. doi:10.1016/j.ccr.2014.

21. Sullivan JP, Spinola M, Dodge M, et al. Aldehyde dehydrogenase activity selects for lung adenocarcinoma stem cells dependent on notch signaling. *Cancer Res.* 2010;70(23):9937-9948. doi:10.1158/0008-5472.can-10-0881.

22. Liu Y-P, Yang C-J, Huang M-S, et al. Cisplatin selects for multidrug-resistant CD133+ cells in lung adenocarcinoma by activating notch signaling. *Cancer Res.* 2013;73(1):406-416. doi:10.1158/0008-5472.can-12-1733.

23. Liu J, Xiao Z, Wong SK-M, et al. Lung cancer tumorigenicity and drug resistance are maintained through ALDH(hi)CD44(hi) tumor initiating cells. *Oncotarget.* 2013;4(10):1698-1711. doi:10.18632/oncotarget.1246.

24. Chen Z, Fillmore CM, Hammerman PS, Kim CF, Wong K-K. Non-small-cell lung cancers: a heterogeneous set of diseases. *Nat Rev Cancer.* 2014;14(8):535-546. doi:10.1038/nrc3775.

25. Zheng Y, de la Cruz CC, Sayles LC, et al. A rare population of CD24+ITGB4+Notchhi cells drives tumor propagation in NSCLC and requires Notch3 for self-renewal. *Cancer Cell.* 2013;24(1):59-74. doi:10.1016/j.ccr.2013.05.021.

26. Lau AN, Curtis SJ, Fillmore CM, et al. Tumor-propagating cells and Yap/Taz activity contribute to lung tumor progression and metastasis. *EMBO J.* 2014;33(5):468-481. doi:10.1002/embj.201386082.

27. Curtis SJ, Sinkevicius KW, Li D, et al. Primary tumor genotype is an important determinant in identification of lung cancer propagating cells. *Cell Stem Cell.* 2010;7(1):127-133. doi:10.1016/j.stem.2010.05.021.

28. Rowbotham SP, Li F, Dost AFM, et al. H3K9 methyltransferases and demethylases control lung tumor-propagating cells and lung cancer progression. *Nat Commun.* 2018;9(1):4559. doi:10.1038/s41467-018-07077-1.

29. Dalvi MP, Wang L, Zhong R, et al. Taxane-platin-resistant lung cancers co-develop hypersensitivity to jumonjiC demethylase inhibitors. *Cell Rep.* 2017;19(8):1669-1684. doi:10.1016/j.celrep.2017.04.077.

30. Song H, Yao E, Lin C, Gacayan R, Chen M-H, Chuang P-T. Functional characterization of pulmonary neuroendocrine cells in lung development, injury, and tumorigenesis. *Proc Natl Acad Sci U S A.* 2012;109(43): 17531-17536. doi:10.1073/pnas.1207238109.

31. Oser MG, Niederst MJ, Sequist LV, Engelman JA. Transformation from non-small-cell lung cancer to small-cell lung cancer: molecular drivers and cells of origin. *Lancet Oncol.* 2015;16(4):e165-172. doi:10.1016/S1470-2045(14)71180-5.

32. Reynolds SD, Giangreco A, Power JHT, Stripp BR. Neuroepithelial bodies of pulmonary airways serve as a reservoir of progenitor cells capable of epithelial regeneration. *Am J Pathol.* 2000;156(1):269-278. doi:http://dx.doi.org/10.1016/S0002-9440(10)64727-X.

33. Park K-S, Liang M-C, Raiser DM, et al. Characterization of the cell of origin for small cell lung cancer. *Cell Cycle.* 2011;10(16):2806-2815.

34. Sutherland KD, Proost N, Brouns I, Adriaensen D, Song J-Y, Berns A. Cell of origin of small cell lung cancer: inactivation of Trp53 and Rb1 in distinct cell types of adult mouse lung. *Cancer Cell.* 2011;19(6):754-764. doi:http://dx.doi.org/10.1016/j.ccr.2011.04.019.

35. Yang D, Denny SK, Greenside PG, et al. Intertumoral heterogeneity in SCLC is influenced by the cell type of origin. *Cancer Discov.* 2018;8(10):1316-1331. doi:10.1158/2159-8290.cd-17-0987.

36. Denny SK, Yang D, Chuang C-H, et al. Nfib promotes metastasis through a widespread increase in chromatin accessibility. *Cell.* 2016;166(2):328-342. Epub 06/30. doi:10.1016/j.cell.2016.05.052.

37. Patel M, Lu L, Zander DS, Sreerama L, Coco D, Moreb JS. ALDH1A1 and ALDH3A1 expression in lung cancers: correlation with histologic type and potential precursors. *Lung Cancer.* 2008;59(3):340-349. doi:10.1016/j.lungcan.2007.08.033.

38. Roudi R, Korourian A, Shariftabrizi A, Madjd Z. Differential expression of cancer stem cell markers ALDH1 and CD133 in various lung cancer subtypes. *Cancer Invest.* 2015;33(7):294-302. doi:10.3109/07357907.2015.1034869.

39. Gazdar AF, Carney DN, Nau MM, Minna JD. Characterization of variant subclasses of cell lines derived from small cell lung cancer having distinctive biochemical, morphological, and growth properties. *Cancer Res.* 1985;45(6):2924-2930.

40. Meng X, Li M, Wang X, Wang Y, Ma D. Both CD133+ and CD133—subpopulations of A549 and H446 cells contain cancer-initiating cells. *Cancer Sci.* 2009;100(6):1040-1046. doi:10.1111/j.1349-7006.2009.01144.x.

41. Sarvi S, Mackinnon AC, Avlonitis N, et al. CD133+ cancer stem-like cells in small cell lung cancer are highly tumorigenic and chemoresistant but sensitive to a novel neuropeptide antagonist. *Cancer Res.* 2014;74(5):1554-1565. doi:10.1158/0008-5472.can-13-1541.

42. Daniel VC, Marchionni L, Hierman JS, et al. A primary xenograft model of small-cell lung cancer reveals irreversible changes in gene expression imposed by culture in vitro. *Cancer Res.* 2009;69(8):3364-3373. doi:10.1158/0008-5472.can-08-4210.

43. Hodgkinson CL, Morrow CJ, Li Y, et al. Tumorigenicity and genetic profiling of circulating tumor cells in small-cell lung cancer. *Nat Med.* 2014;20:897-903. doi:10.1038/nm.3600. https://www.nature.com/articles/nm.3600#supplementary-information.

44. Schaffer BE, Park K-S, Yiu G, et al. Loss of p130 accelerates tumor development in a mouse model for human small-cell lung carcinoma. *Cancer Res.* 2010;70(10):3877-3883. Epub 04/20. doi:10.1158/0008-5472.CAN-09-4228.

45. Jahchan NS, Lim JS, Bola B, et al. Identification and targeting of long-term tumor-propagating cells in small cell lung cancer. *Cell Rep.* 2016;16(3):644-656. Epub 06/30. doi:10.1016/j.celrep.2016.06.021.

46. Calbo J, van Montfort E, Proost N, et al. A functional role for tumor cell heterogeneity in a mouse model of small cell lung cancer. *Cancer Cell.* 2011;19(2):244-256. doi:10.1016/j.ccr.2010.12.021.

47. Fillmore CM, Gupta PB, Rudnick JA, et al. Estrogen expands breast cancer stem-like cells through paracrine FGF/Tbx3 signaling. *Proc Natl Acad Sci U S A.* 2010;107(50):21737-21742. doi:10.1073/pnas.1007863107.

48. George J, Lim JS, Jang SJ, et al. Comprehensive genomic profiles of small cell lung cancer. *Nature.* 2015;524(7563):47-53. doi:10.1038/nature14664.

49. Gardner EE, Lok BH, Schneeberger VE, et al. Chemosensitive relapse in small cell lung cancer proceeds through an EZH2-SLFN11 axis. *Cancer Cell.* 2017;31(2):286-299. doi:10.1016/j.ccell.2017.01.006.

50. Mohammad HP, Smitheman KN, Kamat CD, et al. A DNA hypomethylation signature predicts antitumor activity of LSD1 inhibitors in SCLC. *Cancer Cell.* 2015;28(1):57-69. doi:http://dx.doi.org/10.1016/j.ccell.2015.06.002.

51. Augert A, Eastwood E, Ibrahim AH, et al. Targeting NOTCH activation in small cell lung cancer through LSD1 inhibition. *Sci Signal.* 2019;12(567):eaau2922. doi:10.1126/scisignal.aau2922.

52. Saunders LR, Bankovich AJ, Anderson WC, et al. A DLL3-targeted antibody-drug conjugate eradicates high-grade pulmonary neuroendocrine tumor-initiating cells in vivo. *Sci Transl Med.* 2015;7(302):302ra136. doi:10.1126/scitranslmed.aac9459.

PART III

Prevention and Diagnosis

9

PREVENTION OF LUNG CANCER

Susanne M. Arnold, MD

A 40-year-old African American male with a past medical history of hypertension and myocardial infarction and a 15 pack-year tobacco history presents for a routine health management visit. He has two first-degree relatives with non–small cell lung cancer. He is asymptomatic and has quit smoking, but he requests information on any chemopreventive measures he could utilize to avoid the development of lung cancer. What chemoprevention strategies should be offered to this patient?

Learning Objectives:
1. What are the lifestyle modifications that reduce lung cancer risk?
2. What are the preventable causes of lung cancer?
3. What are the historical chemoprevention strategies that have been utilized in thoracic malignancies?
4. What strategies have improved the prevention of lung cancer?
5. What are the future standards for chemoprevention in thoracic malignancies?

Effective cancer prevention strategies are aimed at reducing the incidence and mortality of that cancer. Primary prevention such as smoking cessation and early screening are covered in other chapters, while lifestyle modification is reviewed here, as well as strategies utilized in both the primary and secondary settings to prevent thoracic cancer. Primary prevention involves interventions in genetic, environmental, biologic, and physical factors that cause cancer. Secondary prevention incorporates strategies to detect cancers in asymptomatic carriers so the treatment can be introduced more promptly. Tertiary prevention refers to prevention of cancers in disease survivors, such as tobacco cessation in lung cancer survivors. Chemoprevention is the use of natural or synthetic compounds to prevent carcinogenesis and the development of cancer.

> **CLINICAL PEARL:** Tobacco smoking is the primary avoidable risk factor for many pulmonary diseases, including lung cancer. Smoking cessation decreases the incidence of lung cancer (primary prevention) and improves overall survival for those diagnosed with lung cancer (tertiary prevention). The prevention of lung cancer is also improved by increasing physical activity and decreasing exposure to radon, nickel, arsenic, chromium, nitrogen mustard, and asbestos, which have also been linked to an increased risk of lung cancer.

LIFESTYLE MODIFICATION

Smoking

The single most important lifestyle modification for the reduction of lung cancer risk is cessation of smoking. Tobacco carcinogenesis and treatment are presented in Chapter 3. All histologic subtypes of lung cancer are caused by cigarette smoking, and cigarettes and tobacco users can benefit at any time by quitting smoking. While lung cancer risk decreases the longer someone is abstinent from smoking, even at greater than 40 years, the risk of former tobacco smokers fails to return to the risk of never-smokers.[1,2] In fact, continued smoking to older age is associated with an exponential increase in the risk of lung cancer compared to people who stop prior to 50. The cumulative risk of death from lung cancer in males who smoke to age 75 is 16%, compared to those who stop by age 50 (6%), and it is even lower if smoking stops by age 30 (2%). This lends credence to targeting youth for smoking cessation and never smoking campaigns by public health officials (**Figure 9-1**).

> **CLINICAL PEARL:** The risk of lung cancer in a daily 1-pack-per-day smoker is over 20 times that of a non-smoker, and in smokers who quit before age 30, the risk falls to 2% cumulative risk of death from lung cancer over their lifetime.[3]

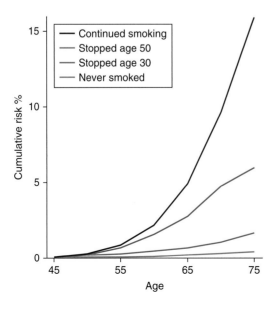

Figure 9-1. Smoking cessation and lifetime risk of lung cancer. (Reproduced with permission from Vineis P, Alavanja M, Buffler P, et al. Tobacco and cancer: recent epidemiological evidence. *J Natl Cancer Inst.* 2004;96(2):99-106. ePub 2004/01/22. Copyright © Oxford University Press.)

Secondhand Smoke

Secondhand smoke exposure has been recognized for over 20 years as a cause of lung cancer among non-smokers. In particular, non-smokers who live with a smoker have up to a 30% increased risk of lung cancer.[4] Children are at highest risk in this scenario because of the developmental effects of tobacco smoke on lung tissue and their smaller lung size per dose of smoke. Local laws to create smoke-free environments have reduced the risk of secondhand smoke exposure in occupations such as the hotel, restaurant, and entertainment industries.[5,6] From a global health perspective, adoption of smoke-free laws is one of the best lifestyle modifications that a community can do to improve the health of its citizens.

Physical Activity and Diet

Diets high in fruits and vegetables have been extensively evaluated as cancer risk reducers, and in 2007, the World Cancer Research Fund (WCRF) recognized a level of evidence of "probable" benefit for fruit consumption and decreased lung cancer risk, with lesser evidence that vegetable consumption is beneficial.[7] Because fruits and vegetables are a major source of antioxidant micronutrients and theoretically can provide detoxification of carcinogens, extensive research has been undertaken concerning the protective effect of antioxidants such as carotenoids in lung cancer. To date, no antioxidant studies have shown a positive benefit in the prevention of lung cancer.

It is well recognized that lifestyle changes to increase aerobic exercise are protective against the development of cancer, as well as improving health during cancer therapy. Data suggest a 13%-30% decrease in lung cancer risk with moderate-to-high levels of physical activity.[8] Clearly, aerobic exercise should be recommended for all people, including those with current or past lung cancer diagnosis. Conversely, a low body mass index (BMI) increases the risk of lung cancer, but this may be related to other lifestyle choices and comorbidities—smoking, alcohol intake, and poor physical fitness—which lead to low BMI. In general, it is accepted to recommend increased physical activity to all cancer patients.

HIGHER RISK HEALTH CONDITIONS

As stated, the primary risk factor for development of lung cancer is smoking; however, other health conditions also increase lung cancer risk. Persons with chronic obstructive pulmonary disease (COPD) have a 2- to 4-fold higher incidence of lung cancer than those who do not have COPD, when controlling for cigarette smoke.[9] Pulmonary fibrosis is also a risk factor for lung cancer. Aside from smoking, radon exposure and asbestos exposure and other less common risk factors for lung cancer include mediastinal or chest wall irradiation (most commonly seen in Hodgkin's lymphoma and breast cancers) and occupational carcinogen exposure (eg, to chromium, arsenic, uranium, nitrogen mustard gas, nickel dust, and polycyclic aromatic hydrocarbons).

Chronic Lung Disease

Persons with COPD and pulmonary fibrosis have higher rates of lung cancer, whether mechanistically related to similar underlying pathophysiology or due to common exposures (tobacco smoke, polycyclic aromatic hydrocarbons, occupational exposure). In fact, persons with chronic obstructive pulmonary disease (COPD) (GOLD class III or IV) have a significantly higher rate of lung cancer development than those without COPD, when controlling for tobacco smoke exposure.[9,10] Part of the risk attributed to airflow obstruction appears to be derived from the presence of radiographic emphysema, which is an important independent risk factor for lung cancer in smokers and never-smokers.[9] Idiopathic pulmonary fibrosis (IPF) also carries a higher risk of lung cancer, ranging from 4.4% to 48%,[11] and is higher in males and people of older age, with a smoking history, and associated emphysema. Squamous cell carcinoma is the most frequent histology, and IPF is correlated with shorter survival compared to those without IPF.[11,12] Connective tissue disease–associated interstitial lung disease (CTD-ILD) is also a risk factor for lung cancer, where approximately 9% of patients develop lung cancer, especially those who have associated emphysema.[10] Computed tomographic (CT) screening of these high-risk groups is becoming more accepted, regardless of smoking history. Aggressive treatment of underlying causes of emphysema and pulmonary fibrosis may help abrogate risk.

Previous Radiation Therapy

Mediastinal, breast[13,14] and chest wall radiation treatments for other malignancies, such as Hodgkin disease,[14] increase the risk of lung cancer. Modern radiation techniques attempt to avoid exposing normal lung tissue to ionizing radiation, but small areas of lung remain in the radiation field in some cases. Scrupulous physics planning and normal tissue protection are critical for radiation of the lung. Lung cancers often develop in the periphery of the lung in these cancer survivors and can occur many years after radiation exposure. While survival is similar to non–radiation-induced lung cancers, smoking cessation is important for primary prevention, and CT screening can help diagnose these cancers earlier.

HIV Infection

Studies of individuals with HIV infection have observed higher rates of lung cancer, albeit almost exclusively in smoking populations, which confounds confirmation of the true risk of HIV infection and pulmonary malignancies. It is generally accepted that HIV adds a relative risk between 2.5 and 3.5 to other risk factors such as smoking.[15,16] As antiretroviral therapy successfully extends life in people with HIV, lung cancer risk, which increases with age, is expected to increase in the HIV-positive population. Lung cancer is now the third most frequent malignancy associated with HIV, highlighting its global importance in this vulnerable population and the need for rigorous CT screening in smokers with HIV. Additionally, aggressive antiretroviral therapy and maintenance of undetectable viral load has potential benefit in cancer prevention, although this has not been confirmed in controlled trials.

Alcohol, Marijuana, and Other Drugs of Abuse

Excessive alcohol abuse has been associated with many forms of cancer, and the American Society of Clinical Oncology (ASCO) recommends limiting alcohol intake to reduce overall cancer risk[17]; however, lung cancer risk reduction related to alcohol is less well understood. While heavy alcohol drinking has been statistically associated with increased lung cancer risk,[18] a study of alcohol consumption in never-smokers was not linked to increased risk,[19] raising the question of tobacco smoke confounding the finding in smokers.[16,17]

Marijuana use has not been proven to be associated with an increase in lung cancer rates because of limited studies and the difficulty of the coadministration of tobacco in most subjects who used daily marijuana.[20] With the widespread legalization of medicinal and recreational marijuana and its expected increased use, it is anticipated that the risk of lung cancer from marijuana exposure will increase. Additionally, a different pattern of lung cancer (histologic and mutational) may emerge. Drugs of abuse, such as cocaine, heroin, and narcotics, have been associated with lung cancer, but less definitively than tobacco.

Genetic Susceptibility

Epidemiologic studies of familial aggregation of lung cancer have suggested a genetic susceptibility in some families. Germline polymorphisms in genes such as cytochrome p450 1A1 and glutathione S transferases Mu-1 and Theta-1, which detoxify tobacco-based carcinogens, have been proposed as possible additive risk factors for lung cancer development in smokers. However, the data are conflicting and not generalizable at the present time. Thus, germline screening cannot identify subjects for increased surveillance or aggressive prevention measures currently. While next-generation sequencing studies have identified multiple potential therapeutic targets for treatment of lung cancer, no common early mutations or germline defects have been discovered that could be applied to chemoprevention. Additionally, there is currently no accepted germline screening for lung cancer, outside of known familial cancer syndromes such as Li Fraumeni, Peutz-Jeager syndrome, and Lynch syndrome. Thus, smoking cessation remains the mainstay of prevention for lung cancer, and chemoprevention for lung cancer is still considered experimental.

ENVIRONMENTAL AND OCCUPATIONAL EXPOSURES

Occupational and environmental toxins have been associated with the development of multiple types of cancer, and lung cancer is the most common cancer associated with occupational exposures. Low–to-moderate levels of many trace elements, including arsenic, cadmium, chromium, and nickel, have been associated with increased incidence of lung cancer in the United States and in developing countries. Well-recognized occupations with higher rates of lung cancer include those that expose the lung to tar and soot (coke oven workers); trace elements or heavy metals such as arsenic, chromium, and nickel (mining); and radiation associated with uranium and radon (mining). Additionally, epidemiologists have identified carcinogens that case a higher rate of lung cancer in populations with groundwater exposure, air particulate exposure, and ingestion of toxic substances. Occupational Safety and Health Administration (OSHA) standards provide excellent primary prevention strategies for occupation-related risk reduction for lung cancer.

Radon

Radon is a naturally occurring, chemically inert gas that develops as a decay product of uranium 238 and radium 226. Radon exposure occurs in occupations such as uranium mining and other underground mining (uranium miners)[21] and in homes via soil and groundwater accumulation. It is thought that between 2% and 10% of lung cancers may be caused by exposure to residential radon. Additionally, the risk of lung cancer in underground miners increases to up to 10 times that of non-smoking miners. The United States Environmental Protection Agency recognizes greater than or equal to 4.0 pCi/L as a level at which corrective measures to reduce radon exposure should be taken; however, no minimum level of radon has been clearly established as safe. The relationship appears to be linear,[22] with the alpha particles of radon thought to damage respiratory epithelium and work alone or synergistically with cigarette smoke.[23] Radon testing in the home is recommended as radon remediation represents an important primary prevention of lung cancer.

Asbestos

Asbestos exposure is directly linked to lung cancer development in multiple industries, including construction, shipping, and others. Asbestos fibers are found in the pulmonary parenchyma of lung cancer patients and may contribute to lung cancer development directly or indirectly through stimulation of inflammation.[24] Asbestos and smoking act synergistically to increase lung cancer risk.[25] Patients with longer exposure times or with associated pulmonary fibrosis are at higher risk of developing lung cancer.[24,26] While the risk of lung cancer is dose dependent, workers exposed to amphibole fibers have a higher risk than those exposed to chrysotile fibers.[26] Prevention of inhalation has been largely effective in reducing fiber exposure, but mesothelioma still occurs despite prevention efforts in the workplace.

Other Environmental Toxins

Many other occupational exposures have been associated with lung cancer. These include exposures to bis-chloromethyl ether, chromium, formaldehyde, ionizing radiation, nickel, polycyclic aromatic hydrocarbons, hard metal dust, and vinyl chloride. As risk reduction strategies in the workplace have changed, some of these exposures have been successfully abrogated. For example, improvement in industrial processes that have eliminated or reduced exposures to chloromethyl ethers and nickel compounds has reduced the risk of lung cancer in some occupations.[27] However, this is not true globally, and continued efforts are needed to decrease occupational exposures worldwide. Given that many of these occupational exposures are synergistic with tobacco smoking, for many workers, the work site may be an important area for intervention in smoking cessation, which still remains the most common cause of lung cancer. Protections for industrial health workers not only should take into account exposure from elemental risks, but also should assess smoking and other airborne health risks when setting occupational exposure standards.

Air Pollution, Fossil Fuels, and Particulate Matter

Urban air pollution is caused by combustion of fossil fuels, leading to polycyclic aromatic hydrocarbons and metals released into the air as well as particulate matter such as sulfur dioxide and nitrogen dioxide. Air pollution can differ across countries, but has been associated with an increased risk of lung cancer of up to 40% in large urban areas of the United States,[28] as well as other countries known for higher rates of air pollution.[16,29] Additionally, occupational exposure to diesel and exhaust fumes is associated with a higher risk of lung cancer in smokers and non-smokers.[30] Air pollution, including exposure to fine particulates, nitrogen dioxide, and ozone, are all linked to higher lung cancer rates. community and international efforts to reduce the causes of these environmental toxins are critical to the reduction in lung cancer risk in future generations.

Indoor air pollution through coal burning,[31] and other solid fuel burning for cooking, as well as indoor wood smoke exposure are associated with lung cancer, most commonly in developing countries. It is estimated that interventions to decrease solid fuel cooking and indoor air pollution exposure would significantly decrease lung cancer risk in these populations.[16]

CHEMOPREVENTION

In addition to tobacco smoke exposure, many other compounds and promoters of carcinogenesis are known to affect lung cancer patients. Chemoprevention uses vitamins, anti-inflammatory agents, hormonal antagonists, antioxidants, and differentiating agents to prevent cancer. Phase III randomized placebo-controlled clinical trials designed to confirm the utility of chemopreventive agents in lung cancer have not yielded positive results, despite excellent preclinical rationale.

Several large phase 3 trials have examined the utility of chemopreventive agents in preventing the development of lung cancer. The Alpha-Tocopherol, Beta Carotene, Cancer Prevention Trial (ATBC) enrolled Finnish male smokers between the ages of 50 and 69 to receive alpha-tocopherol, beta-carotene, both, or placebo in a randomized 2×2 factorial design. Unfortunately, there was an increase in lung cancer incidence and mortality at 6 years in participants receiving beta-carotene. Additionally, there was no protective effect on lung cancer mortality in patients receiving both drugs or alpha-tocopherol alone. Similarly, the Beta-Carotene and Retinol Efficacy Trial (CARET) trial enrolled 17,000 smokers and workers in high-risk occupations related to asbestos. These participants were randomly assigned to receive beta-carotene, retinol, both, or placebo in a 2×2 factorial design. Again, an increase in lung cancer incidence (28%) and in lung cancer–related mortality (17%) were seen in those receiving beta-carotene and retinol or both drugs failed to protect against lung cancer development.

> **CLINICAL PEARL:** The use of beta-carotene or alpha-tocopherol is not recommended in the prevention of non–small cell or small cell lung cancer in smokers.

Over the past three decades, observations that low-dose aspirin and, separately, inhaled corticosteroids are associated with lower incidence of lung cancer have led to several studies of these agents. One provocative result was in the Women's Health Study, a 2×2 design of low-dose aspirin and vitamin E designed to decrease invasive cancer as the primary endpoint.[32] There was a trend toward a decreased incidence of lung cancer (relative risk [RR] = 0.78, 95% CI 0.59–1.03, p = .08) with low-dose aspirin use, and a statistically significant decrease in lung cancer mortality (RR = 0.7, 95% CI 0.50–0.99, p = .04). However, this study has not been replicated, and the use of multiple-endpoint testing is a major criticism; therefore, low-dose aspirin is not currently recommended for prevention of lung cancer in women. A Veterans Affairs analysis of veterans prescribed inhaled corticosteroids who were compliant with this medication revealed a significant reduction in the risk of lung cancer[33]; however, randomized trials have not demonstrated a reduction in lung cancer.

Additionally, multiple smaller studies have yielded negative results in secondary prevention using 13–cis-retinoic acid,[34] fenretinide,[35] beta-carotene,[36] vitamin B$_{12}$, and folate.[37] In a trial studying whether selenium supplementation could decrease skin cancer, selenium was associated with decreased incidence of lung cancer, although this was a secondary endpoint. Additionally, those participants who had a previous history of lung cancer did not receive protective benefit from selenium supplementation.[38]

Hormonal Agents

Data regarding the effect of hormones on lung cancer are conflicting in females. Most studies failed to show an association between long-term estrogen or progesterone intake and increased risk of lung cancer. However, several recent randomized studies have shown an association with lung cancer risk, including the observation in the Women's Health Initiative trial that while treatment with estrogen plus progestin in postmenopausal women did not increase incidence of lung cancer, it did increase the number of deaths from lung cancer.[39] Therefore, for females with a lung cancer diagnosis, it is not recommended to continue or to prescribe estrogen or progesterone.

Anti-inflammatory Agents

Chronic inflammation has been implicated in the development of cancer for many years,[40] and in particular, lung cancer, given that chronic bronchitis, pulmonary fibrosis, alpha-1 antitrypsin deficiency, and chronic exposures to asbestos, silica, tobacco smoke, and other toxins result in a well-described inflammatory response.[41] While no significant anti-inflammatories have been shown to decrease lung cancer risk, the field has discerned inflammatory mediators such as Nod-like receptor protein 3 (NLRP3), which leads to local activation of interleukin 1β in the lung, a process that can lead to both chronic fibrosis and cancer. Thus, inhibition of interleukin 1β might have an adjunctive role in the treatment of cancers that have at least a partial inflammatory basis.[42] In a randomized trial for the prevention of vascular events after myocardial infarction, subjects receiving canakinumab, a human monoclonal antibody targeting interleukin 1β, were found to have less lung cancer incidence in a post hoc analysis.[43] However, this is preliminary work and requires further randomized trials to confirm this result.

In summary, no chemopreventive agents have been definitively proven to reduce lung cancer incidence in the primary or secondary setting. Smoking cessation remains the primary means of reducing lung cancer risk.

REFERENCES

1. Samet JM. The 1990 Report of the Surgeon General: The Health Benefits of Smoking Cessation. *Am Rev Respir Dis*. 1990;142(5):993-994. Epub 1990/11/01. doi:10.1164/ajrccm/142.5.993.

2. McLaughlin JK, Hrubec Z, Blot WJ, Fraumeni JF, Jr. Smoking and cancer mortality among U.S. veterans: a 26-year follow-up. *Int J Cancer*. 1995;60(2):190-193. Epub 1995/01/17.

3. Vineis P, Alavanja M, Buffler P, et al. Tobacco and cancer: recent epidemiological evidence. *J Natl Cancer Inst*. 2004;96(2):99-106. Epub 2004/01/22.

4. Office on Smoking and Health (US). The Health Consequences of Involuntary Exposure to Tobacco Smoke: A Report of the Surgeon General. Atlanta, GA: Centers for Disease Control and Prevention (US); 2006.

5. Hahn EJ, Rayens MK, York N, et al. Effects of a smoke-free law on hair nicotine and respiratory symptoms of restaurant and bar workers. *J Occup Environ Med*. 2006;48(9):906-913. Epub 2006/09/13. doi:10.1097/01.jom.0000215709.09305.01.

6. Hahn EJ, Rayens MK, Wiggins AT, Gan W, Brown HM, Mullett TW. Lung cancer incidence and the strength of municipal smoke-free ordinances. *Cancer*. 2018;124(2):374-380. Epub 2017/12/02. doi:10.1002/cncr.31142.

7. Wiseman M. The second World Cancer Research Fund/American Institute for Cancer Research expert report. Food, nutrition, physical activity, and the prevention of cancer: a global perspective. *Proc Nutr Soc*. 2008;67(3):253-256. Epub 2008/05/03. doi:10.1017/s002966510800712x.

8. Brenner DR, Yannitsos DH, Farris MS, Johansson M, Friedenreich CM. Leisure-time physical activity and lung cancer risk: a systematic review and meta-analysis. *Lung Cancer*. 2016;95:17-27. Epub 2016/04/05. doi:10.1016/j.lungcan.2016.01.021.

9. Mannino DM, Aguayo SM, Petty TL, Redd SC. Low lung function and incident lung cancer in the united states: data from the first national health and nutrition examination survey follow-up. *Arch Intern Med*. 2003;163(12):1475-1480. doi:10.1001/archinte.163.12.1475.

10. Gonzalez J, Marin M, Sanchez-Salcedo P, Zulueta JJ. Lung cancer screening in patients with chronic obstructive pulmonary disease. *Ann transl Med*. 2016;4(8):160. Epub 2016/05/20. doi:10.21037/atm.2016.03.57.

11. Wells C, Mannino DM. Pulmonary fibrosis and lung cancer in the United States: analysis of the multiple cause of death mortality data, 1979 through 1991. *South Med J*. 1996;89(5):505-510. Epub 1996/05/01.

12. Ozawa Y, Suda T, Naito T, et al. Cumulative incidence of and predictive factors for lung cancer in IPF. *Respirology*. 2009;14(5):723-728. Epub 2009/08/08. doi:10.1111/j.1440-1843.2009.01547.x.

13. Huang YJ, Huang TW, Lin FH, Chung CH, Tsao CH, Chien WC. Radiation therapy for invasive breast cancer increases the risk of second primary lung cancer: a nationwide population-based cohort analysis. *J Thorac Oncol*. 2017;12(5):782-790. Epub 2017/02/20. doi:10.1016/j.jtho.2017.01.021.

14. Lorigan P, Radford J, Howell A, Thatcher N. Lung cancer after treatment for Hodgkin's lymphoma: a systematic review. *Lancet Oncol*. 2005;6(10):773-779. Epub 2005/10/04. doi:10.1016/s1470-2045(05)70387-9.

15. Achenbach CJ, Cole SR, Kitahata MM, et al. Mortality after cancer diagnosis in HIV-infected individuals treated with antiretroviral therapy. *AIDS*. 2011;25(5):691-700. Epub 2010/12/17. doi:10.1097/QAD.0b013e3283437f77.

16. Alberg AJ, Brock MV, Ford JG, Samet JM, Spivack SD. Epidemiology of lung cancer: diagnosis and management of lung cancer, 3rd ed: American College of Chest Physicians evidence-based clinical practice guidelines. *Chest*. 2013;143(5 Suppl):e1S-e29S. Epub 2013/05/10. doi:10.1378/chest.12-2345.

17. LoConte NK, Brewster AM, Kaur JS, Merrill JK, Alberg AJ. Alcohol and cancer: a statement of the American Society of Clinical Oncology. *J Clin Oncol*. 2018;36(1):83-93. Epub 2017/11/08. doi:10.1200/jco.2017.76.1155.

18. Chao C. Associations between beer, wine, and liquor consumption and lung cancer risk: a meta-analysis. *Cancer Epidemiol Biomarkers Prev*. 2007;16(11):2436-2447. Epub 2007/11/17. doi:10.1158/1055-9965.epi-07-0386.

19. Thun MJ, Hannan LM, DeLancey JO. Alcohol consumption not associated with lung cancer mortality in lifelong nonsmokers. *Cancer Epidemiol Biomarkers Prev*. 2009;18(8):2269-2272. Epub 2009/08/08. doi:10.1158/1055-9965.epi-09-0361.

20. Jett J, Stone E, Warren G, Cummings KM. Cannabis use, lung cancer, and related issues. *J Thorac Oncol*. 2018;13(4):480-487. Epub 2018/01/29. doi:10.1016/j.jtho.2017.12.013.

21. Grosche B, Kreuzer M, Kreisheimer M, Schnelzer M, Tschense A. Lung cancer risk among German male uranium miners: a cohort study, 1946-1998. *Br J Cancer*. 2006;95(9):1280-1287. Epub 2006/10/18. doi:10.1038/sj.bjc.6603403.

22. Darby S, Hill D, Auvinen A, et al. Radon in homes and risk of lung cancer: collaborative analysis of individual data from 13 European case-control studies. *BMJ*. 2005;330(7485):223. Epub 2004/12/23. doi:10.1136/bmj.38308.477650.63.

23. Field RW, Steck DJ, Smith BJ, et al. Residential radon gas exposure and lung cancer: the Iowa Radon Lung Cancer Study. *Am J Epidemiol.* 2000;151(11):1091-1102. Epub 2000/06/29.

24. Nymark P, Wikman H, Hienonen-Kempas T, Anttila S. Molecular and genetic changes in asbestos-related lung cancer. *Cancer Lett.* 2008;265(1):1-15. Epub 2008/03/28. doi:10.1016/j.canlet.2008.02.043.

25. Ngamwong Y, Tangamornsuksan W, Lohitnavy O, et al. Additive synergism between asbestos and smoking in lung cancer risk: a systematic review and meta-analysis. *PloS One.* 2015;10(8):e0135798. Epub 2015/08/15. doi:10.1371/journal.pone.0135798.

26. Jones RN, Hughes JM, Weill H. Asbestos exposure, asbestosis, and asbestos-attributable lung cancer. *Thorax.* 1996;51(Suppl 2):S9-15. Epub 1996/08/01.

27. Coultas DB, Samet JM. Occupational lung cancer. *Clin Chest Med.* 1992;13(2):341-354. Epub 1992/06/01.

28. Dockery DW, Pope CA, 3rd, Xu X, et al. An association between air pollution and mortality in six U.S. cities. *N Engl J Med.* 1993;329(24):1753-1759. Epub 1993/12/09. doi:10.1056/nejm199312093292401.

29. Hystad P, Demers PA, Johnson KC, Carpiano RM, Brauer M. Long-term residential exposure to air pollution and lung cancer risk. *Epidemiology.* 2013;24(5):762-772. Epub 2013/05/17. doi:10.1097/EDE.0b013e3182949ae7.

30. Olsson AC, Gustavsson P, Kromhout H, et al. Exposure to diesel motor exhaust and lung cancer risk in a pooled analysis from case-control studies in Europe and Canada. *Am J Respir Crit Care Med.* 2011;183(7):941-948. Epub 2010/11/03. doi:10.1164/rccm.201006-0940OC.

31. Barone-Adesi F, Chapman RS, Silverman DT, et al. Risk of lung cancer associated with domestic use of coal in Xuanwei, China: retrospective cohort study. *BMJ.* 2012;345:e5414. Epub 2012/09/01. doi:10.1136/bmj.e5414.

32. Cook NR, Lee IM, Gaziano JM, et al. Low-dose aspirin in the primary prevention of cancer: the Women's Health Study: a randomized controlled trial. *JAMA.* 2005;294(1):47-55. Epub 2005/07/07. doi:10.1001/jama.294.1.47.

33. Parimon T, Chien JW, Bryson CL, McDonell MB, Udris EM, Au DH. Inhaled corticosteroids and risk of lung cancer among patients with chronic obstructive pulmonary disease. *Am J Respir Crit Care Med.* 2007;175(7):712-719. Epub 2006/12/23. doi:10.1164/rccm.200608-1125OC.

34. Kelly K, Kittelson J, Franklin WA, et al. A randomized phase II chemoprevention trial of 13-CIS retinoic acid with or without alpha tocopherol or observation in subjects at high risk for lung cancer. *Cancer Prev Res* (Philadelphia, Pa). 2009;2(5):440-449. Epub 2009/04/30. doi:10.1158/1940-6207.capr-08-0136.

35. Kurie JM, Lee JS, Khuri FR, et al. N-(4-hydroxyphenyl)retinamide in the chemoprevention of squamous metaplasia and dysplasia of the bronchial epithelium. *Clin Cancer Res.* 2000;6(8):2973-2979. Epub 2000/08/24.

36. McLarty JW, Holiday DB, Girard WM, Yanagihara RH, Kummet TD, Greenberg SD. Beta-Carotene, vitamin A, and lung cancer chemoprevention: results of an intermediate endpoint study. *Am J Clin Nutr.* 1995;62(6 Suppl):1431s-1438s. Epub 1995/12/01. doi:10.1093/ajcn/62.6.1431S.

37. Heimburger DC, Alexander CB, Birch R, Butterworth CE, Jr., Bailey WC, Krumdieck CL. Improvement in bronchial squamous metaplasia in smokers treated with folate and vitamin B12. Report of a preliminary randomized, double-blind intervention trial. *JAMA.* 1988;259(10):1525-1530. Epub 1988/03/11.

38. Karp DD, Lee SJ, Keller SM, et al. Randomized, double-blind, placebo-controlled, phase III chemoprevention trial of selenium supplementation in patients with resected stage I non-small-cell lung cancer: ECOG 5597. *J Clin Oncol.* 2013;31(33):4179-4187. Epub 2013/09/05. doi:10.1200/jco.2013.49.2173.

39. Chlebowski RT, Schwartz AG, Wakelee H, et al. Oestrogen plus progestin and lung cancer in postmenopausal women (Women's Health Initiative trial): a post-hoc analysis of a randomised controlled trial. *Lancet.* 2009;374(9697):1243-1251. Epub 2009/09/22. doi:10.1016/s0140-6736(09)61526-9.

40. Grivennikov SI, Greten FR, Karin M. Immunity, inflammation, and cancer. *Cell.* 2010;140(6):883-899. Epub 2010/03/23. doi:10.1016/j.cell.2010.01.025.

41. O'Callaghan DS, O'Donnell D, O'Connell F, O'Byrne KJ. The role of inflammation in the pathogenesis of non-small cell lung cancer. *J Thorac Oncol.* 2010;5(12):2024-2036. Epub 2010/12/16.

42. Dinarello CA, Simon A, van der Meer JW. Treating inflammation by blocking interleukin-1 in a broad spectrum of diseases. *Nat Rev Drug Discov.* 2012;11(8):633-652. Epub 2012/08/02. doi:10.1038/nrd3800.

43. Ridker PM, MacFadyen JG, Thuren T, et al. Effect of interleukin-1β; inhibition with canakinumab on incident lung cancer in patients with atherosclerosis: exploratory results from a randomised, double-blind, placebo-controlled trial. *Lancet.* 2017;390(10105):1833-1842. doi:10.1016/S0140-6736(17)32247-X.

10

EARLY DETECTION OF LUNG CANCER

Shruti Bhandari, MD • Dhan Pham, MD

A 67-year-old man with past medical history of hypertension and chronic obstructive pulmonary disease (COPD) presents for an annual physical. He has no symptoms. He smoked 1 pack a day for 30 years but quit 5 years ago when he was diagnosed with COPD. He is asking about his risk of lung cancer. What screening modality, if any, you can offer this patient?

Learning Objectives:
1. What are the guideline recommendations for lung cancer screening?
2. What are the harms and benefits of lung cancer screening?
3. Is lung cancer screening cost-effective?

Lung cancer is the leading cause of cancer-related mortality worldwide. The 5-year survival rate of lung cancer is only 18% because most cases of lung cancer are diagnosed at an advance stage.[1] Clinical outcomes of lung cancer are related to the stage at diagnosis, ranging from 56% five-year survival rate for stage I to 4% five-year survival rate at stage VI. Therefore, early detection of lung cancer is an important opportunity to decrease mortality.

SCREENING MODALITIES
Chest X-ray and Sputum Cytology
Screening for lung cancer by chest radiograph (CXR) and/or sputum cytology is not recommended. There have been at least six large randomized controlled trials,[2-5] beginning as early as the 1960s, but none of the trials has demonstrated a mortality benefit for CXR screening. However, only the Prostate, Lung, Colorectal, and Ovarian (PLCO) Cancer Screening Trial[5] compared screening with no screening.

In the Memorial Sloan-Kettering[2] and the Johns Hopkins studies,[4] a combined total of 20,427 men were randomized to either an annual CXR alone or a CXR in combination with sputum cytology. No difference was noted in lung cancer incidence or mortality between the 2 groups. In the Mayo Lung Project,[3] 10,993 male smokers underwent a baseline screening with CXR and sputum cytology. If results were negative for cancer, the men were randomized to receive CXR and sputum cytology every 4 months or usual care, which was a recommendation for an annual CXR. After 6 years, the lung cancer mortality rate was not statistically different between the screened and control groups.

The PLCO Cancer Screening Trial[5] is a population-based study of men and women aged 55 to 74 years for several cancers, including lung cancer. A total 154,901 participants were randomly assigned to receive either annual CXR for 4 years or standard of care (no CXR) and were followed up for 12 years. At the end of the study, the two groups demonstrated similar cumulative lung cancer incidences, lung cancer mortality, and stage and histologic findings of detected lung cancers.

Computed Tomographic Screening

Refinement of computed tomographic (CT) scan techniques with evaluation of low-dose CT (LDCT) scan developed interest in CT as screening modality. LDCT refers to a non-contrast study obtained with a multidetector CT scanner during a single maximal inspiratory breath-hold with a scanning time under 25 s and radiation exposure of 1.6 mSv (conventional CT radiation exposure of 7 mSv).

Several observational studies on screening with LDCT demonstrated that LDCT can identify early-stage asymptomatic lung cancer. The larger studies included the Early Lung Cancer Action Program (ELCAP), the International ELCAP (I-ELCAP), the Mayo Clinic CT study, and the Continuous Observation of Smoking (COSMOS) study. These observation studies showed that LDCT detected more lung cancers than did CXR, and the majority of these cancers were detected at an early stage. This led to many randomized trials, but only the National Lung Screening Trial (NLST) and the Dutch Belgian randomized lung cancer screening trial (NELSON Trial) were established to assess the mortality benefit of lung cancer screening.

The NLST,[6] published in 2011, was the first randomized trial to show a mortality benefit to LDCT screening for lung cancer.

- The trial compared annual screening by LDCT to CXR for 3 years in 53,454 people aged 55 to 74; participants had at least 30 pack-years of smoking, including current smokers and former smokers who had quit within 15 years.
- At a median follow-up of 6.5 years, there was a relative mortality reduction of 20% for lung cancer deaths and 6.7% reduction in all-cause mortality in the LDCT group.
- To prevent one lung cancer death, the number needed to screen with LDCT was 320.
- Abnormal screening tests occurred in 24% of the LDCT group and 6.9% of the CXR group, >90% of which were false positives. Most only required additional imaging, but some required invasive procedures. Complications from the diagnostic workup were uncommon, involving about 1.5% of the participants who had abnormal screening tests.

The NELSON trial presented its mortality results at the World Conference on Lung Cancer 2018, showing a 26% reduction in lung cancer mortality in males at 10 years.[7]

- This randomized trial compared screening with LDCT to usual care (no screening) in 15,792 people (87% male) aged 55 to 74 years with more than a 15 pack-year smoking history, including current smokers and former smokers who had quit within 10 years.
- LDCT was performed at baseline, year 1, year 2, year 4, and year 6.5.
- This trial used volume and volume doubling time of nodules rather than nodule diameter.
- In the first and second rounds of screening, 2.6% and 1.8% of the participants, respectively, had a positive test result.[8]

Biomarkers

There is currently no high-quality evidence for biomarkers in early detection of lung cancer. Multiple blood/serum biomarkers are under investigation, but worth mentioning are EarlyCDT-Lung, miR-test, and MSC (Micro-RNA signature classifier) as they have entered phase 4 of development.[9]

1. The EarlyCDT-Lung test is a commercially available blood test based on enzyme-linked immunosorbent assay (ELISA) principles; the test measures a panel of seven tumor-associated autoantibodies: p53, NY-ESO-1, CAGE, GBU4–5, SOX2, HuD, and MAGE A4. EarlyCDT-Lung showed sensitivity, specificity, PPV (positive predictive value), NPV (negative predictive value), and positive likelihood ratio results of 41%, 87%, 11%, 97%, and 3.19, respectively.

2. The miR-test is a serum-based microRNA (miRNA) test that measures a signature of 13 miRNAs: miR-92a-3p, miR-30b-5p, miR-191-5p, miR-484, miR-328-3p, miR-30c-5p, miR-374a-5p, let-7d-5p, miR-331-3p, miR-29a-3p, miR-148a-3p, miR-223-3p, miR-140-5p. The miR-test had sensitivity, specificity, PPV, NPV, and positive likelihood ratio results of 78%, 75%, 10%, 98%, and 3.09, respectively.

3. The MSC is a plasma-based miRNA test that categorizes patients into low, intermediate, or high risk of disease based on predefined positivity for 24 miRNA expression ratios. MSC had sensitivity, specificity, PPV, NPV, and positive likelihood ratio results of 87%, 81%, 27%, 98%, and 4.67, respectively.

CURRENT RECOMMENDATIONS

Multiple medical societies' guidelines recommend annual lung cancer screening with LDCT in high-risk individuals (**Table 10-1**).[10-13] Some guidelines advise patient counseling on the risks and benefits of screening, importance of smoking cessation, and shared decision-making before testing. LDCT screening as a part of a screening program should only be performed when the clinician and patient are committed to pursuing follow-up investigations, including serial imaging and possible surgical lung biopsy and where there is expertise in lung cancer management.

Lung cancer screening with LDCT is covered by most insurance since the Centers for Medicare and Medicaid Services national coverage determination in early 2015.

TABLE 10-1	Current Guideline Recommendations for Lung Cancer Screening			
ORGANIZATION	RECOMMENDS?	AGE	FREQUENCY	SMOKING HISTORY
American Academy of Family Physicians	Neither for or against	—	—	—
American Association of Thoracic Surgery	Yes, since 2012	55-79	Annual	30 pack-year history of smoking Current smoker or quit in last 15 years
American Cancer Society	Yes, since 2013 Shared decision-making before testing	55-74	Annual	30 pack-year history of smoking Current smoker or quit in last 15 years
American College of Chest Physicians	Yes, since 2012 Shared decision-making before testing	55-74	Annual	30 pack-year history of smoking Current smoker or quit in last 15 years
American Society of Clinical Oncology	Yes, since 2012 Shared decision-making before testing	55-74	Annual	30 pack-year history of smoking Current smoker or quit in last 15 years
National Comprehensive Cancer Network	Yes, since 2015	55-74	Annual	≥30 pack-year history of smoking Current smoker or quit in last 15 years
		≥50	Annual	20 pack-year history of smoking with one additional risk factor
US Preventive Services Task Force	Yes, since 2013	55-80	Annual	30 pack-year history of smoking Current smoker or quit in last 15 years

The American College of Radiology (ACR) developed the Lung-RADS (lung imaging reporting and data system) reporting system specifically for the lung cancer screening population in order to provide a standardized reporting and management tool for clinicians. Lung-RADS should be used when interpreting CT findings in an individual who has undergone lung cancer screening. A brief description of Lung-RADS categories is discussed in **Table 10-2**. Lung-RADS has been shown to improve the detection of lung cancer and to decrease the false-positive results by more than 50% as compared to NLST.[14]

In United States, multiple lung cancer screening programs have been established and participate in the Lung Cancer Screening Registry® (LCSR) for quality assurance. As of a 2016 evaluation of LCSR, only 2% of eligible high-risk population is getting screened with LDCT.[15]

TABLE 10-2   Lung-RADS Version 1.0 Assessment Categories

CATEGORY DESCRIPTOR	CATEGORY DESCRIPTOR	PRIMARY CATEGORY	MANAGEMENT
Incomplete	—	0	Additional lung cancer screening CT images and/or comparison to prior chest CT examinations is needed
Negative	No nodules and definitely benign nodules	1	Continue annual screening with LDCT in 12 months
Benign appearance or behavior	Nodules with a very low likelihood of becoming a clinically active cancer due to size or lack of growth	2	
Probably benign	Probably benign finding(s) — short-term follow-up suggested; includes nodules with a low likelihood of becoming a clinically active cancer	3	6-month LDCT
Suspicious	Findings for which additional diagnostic testing and/or tissue sampling is recommended	4A	3-month LDCT; PET/CT may be used when there is a ≥8-mm solid component
		4B	Chest CT with or without contrast, PET/CT and/or tissue sampling depending on the probability of malignancy and comorbidities; PET/CT may be used when there is a ≥8-mm solid component
Significant—other	Other significant findings	S	
Prior lung cancer		C	

PET, positron emission tomography.

LOW-DOSE CT LUNG CANCER SCREENING

Potential Benefits

- Decreased lung cancer mortality: Effective lung cancer screening may prevent more than 12,000 premature lung cancer deaths annually in the United States alone.[16]
- Improved quality of life:
  - Reduction in disease-related morbidity
  - Reduction in treatment-related morbidity
  - Improvement in healthy lifestyles
  - Reduction in anxiety/psychosocial burden
- Discovery of other significant occult health risks (eg, thyroid nodule, severe but silent coronary artery disease, early renal cancer in upper pole of kidney, aortic aneurysm, breast cancer)

Potential Risks

- Futile detection of small aggressive tumors or indolent disease
- Possible distress and anxiety concerning test results. A 2014 systematic review found that LDCT screening may be associated with short-term discomfort but did not affect health-related quality of life.[17]
- Consequences of evaluating abnormal findings:
  - Unnecessary testing and procedures
  - Physical complications from diagnostic workup
- False-positive results
- False-negative results
- Radiation exposure
- Cost
- Incidental lesions

Cost-Effectiveness

Lung cancer screening is cost effective with cost effectiveness ratio of $100,000 (in U.S. dollars) or less per Quality Adjusted Life Years (QALYs) gained for LDCT. Cost-effectiveness is reported by seven separate analyses.[18]

Lung Cancer Screening Outside the United States

Lung cancer screening with LDCT is recommended in high-risk population by most medical society guidelines. It is cost-effective and covered by most insurance. Some medical societies did not recommend LDCT screening as data were based on a single trial (NLST). Now, with updated mortality results from the NELSON trial also showing a mortality benefit of LDCT screening, it is likely to become a globally accepted recommendation.

REFERENCES

1. Siegel RL, Miller KD, Jemal A. Cancer statistics, 2018. *CA Cancer J Clin.* 2018;68(1):7-30. Epub 2018/01/10. doi:10.3322/caac.21442.
2. Melamed MR, Flehinger BJ, Zaman MB, Heelan RT, Perchick WA, Martini N. Screening for early lung cancer. Results of the Memorial Sloan-Kettering study in New York. *Chest.* 1984;86(1):44-53. Epub 1984/07/01.
3. Fontana RS, Sanderson DR, Woolner LB, Taylor WF, Miller WE, Muhm JR. Lung cancer screening: the Mayo program. *J Occup Med.* 1986;28(8):746-750. Epub 1986/08/01.
4. Frost JK, Ball WC, Jr., Levin ML, et al. Early lung cancer detection: results of the initial (prevalence) radiologic and cytologic screening in the Johns Hopkins study. *Am Rev Respir Dis.* 1984;130(4):549-554. Epub 1984/10/01. doi:10.1164/arrd.1984.130.4.549.
5. Oken MM, Hocking WG, Kvale PA, et al. Screening by chest radiograph and lung cancer mortality: the prostate, lung, colorectal, and ovarian (PLCO) randomized trial. *JAMA.* 2011;306(17):1865-1873. Epub 2011/10/28. doi:10.1001/jama.2011.1591.
6. Aberle DR, Adams AM, Berg CD, et al. Reduced lung-cancer mortality with low-dose computed tomographic screening. *N Engl J Med.* 2011;365(5):395-409. Epub 2011/07/01. doi:10.1056/NEJMoa1102873.
7. Harry J. de Koning. PL 02.05—Effects of Volume CT Lung Cancer Screening: Mortality Results of the NELSON Randomised-Controlled Population Based Trial International Association for the Study of Lung Cancer 19th World Conference on Lung Cancer Toronto, Canada, September 2018.
8. van Klaveren RJ, Oudkerk M, Prokop M, et al. Management of lung nodules detected by volume CT scanning. *N Engl J Med.* 2009;361(23):2221-2229. doi:10.1056/NEJMoa0906085.

9. Chu GCW, Lazare K, Sullivan F. Serum and blood based biomarkers for lung cancer screening: a systematic review. *BMC Cancer*. 2018;18(1):181. doi:10.1186/s12885-018-4024-3.

10. Wender R, Fontham ET, Barrera E, Jr., et al. American Cancer Society lung cancer screening guidelines. *CA Cancer J Clin*. 2013;63(2):107-117. Epub 2013/01/15. doi:10.3322/caac.21172.

11. U.S. Preventive Services Task Force Recommendation Statement. Screening for Lung Cancer, 2013.

12. Jaklitsch MT, Jacobson FL, Austin JH, et al. The American Association for Thoracic Surgery guidelines for lung cancer screening using low-dose computed tomography scans for lung cancer survivors and other high-risk groups. *J Thorac Cardiovasc Surg*. 2012;144(1):33-38. Epub 2012/06/20. doi:10.1016/j.jtcvs.2012.05.060.

13. Detterbeck FC, Mazzone PJ, Naidich DP, Bach PB. Screening for lung cancer: diagnosis and management of lung cancer, 3rd ed: American College of Chest Physicians evidence-based clinical practice guidelines. *Chest*. 2013;143(5 Suppl):e78S-e92S. Epub 2013/05/10. doi:10.1378/chest.12-2350.

14. Pinsky PF, Gierada DS, Black W, et al. Performance of Lung-RADS in the National Lung Screening Trial: A Retrospective Assessment. *Ann Intern Med*. 2015;162(7):485-491. doi:10.7326/m14-2086.

15. Pham D, Bhandari S, Oechsli M, Pinkston C, Kloecker G. Lung cancer screening rates: data from the lung cancer screening registry. *J Clin Oncol*. 2018;36(15_suppl):6504.

16. Ma J, Ward EM, Smith R, Jemal A. Annual number of lung cancer deaths potentially avertable by screening in the United States. *Cancer*. 2013;119(7):1381-1385. Epub 2013/02/27. doi:10.1002/cncr.27813.

17. Slatore CG, Sullivan DR, Pappas M, Humphrey LL. Patient-centered outcomes among lung cancer screening recipients with computed tomography: a systematic review. *J Thorac Oncol*. 2014;9(7):927-934. Epub 2014/06/13. doi:10.1097/jto.0000000000000210.

18. Puggina A, Broumas A, Ricciardi W, Boccia S. Cost-effectiveness of screening for lung cancer with low-dose computed tomography: a systematic literature review. *Eur J Public Health*. 2016;26(1):168-175. Epub 2015/09/16. doi:10.1093/eurpub/ckv158.

11

DIAGNOSTICS OF LUNG CANCER

Shruti Bhandari, MD • Umair Gauhar, MBBS • Bilal Athar Jalil, MD • Emily Jonczak, MD • Raja Mudad, MD, FACP • Chandler Park, MD, MSc, FACP • Dhan Pham, MD • Samuel Reynolds, MD

CLINICAL TESTING
Shruti Bhandari, MD, Dhan Pham, MD

A 67-year-old man with past medical history of chronic obstructive pulmonary disease (COPD) presents with complains of cough, shortness of breath, and weight loss for 2 months. He has smoked 1 pack of cigarettes a day for the past 40 years. His primary care doctor obtains a chest radiograph, which shows a mass in the patient's left upper lobe. How will you work up this patient?

Learning Objectives:
1. What are the different symptoms and signs associated with lung cancer?
2. What are the different paraneoplastic syndromes associated with lung cancer?
3. What investigational methods are needed to diagnose lung cancer?

Lung cancer is the leading cause of cancer-related death worldwide.[1] The majority of lung cancer (~80%-85%) includes non–small cell lung cancer (NSCLC) histology, and the remainder is small cell lung cancer (SCLC). It is important to differentiate between NSCLC and SCLC as diagnostic evaluation and management differ.

Most patients with lung cancer are symptomatic at presentation. Some present with a suspicious finding detected on chest imaging done for lung cancer screening, and some can present with an incidental finding on imaging done for other reasons. Lung cancer screening is recommended for early diagnosis in individuals at high risk[2] but has had slow uptake.[3] Of note, the cumulative risk tends to increase with age and with lifetime exposure to cigarette smoke (**Figure 11-1**).

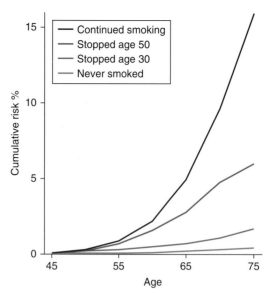

Figure 11-1. Smoking cessation and lung cancer.

The goal of initial evaluation in a patient suspected of having lung cancer is timely diagnosis and staging so appropriate treatment can be administered. In this chapter, we review initial evaluation (history and physical examination) and diagnosis (imaging and pathology) for a patient with suspected lung cancer.

The **general approach** in the diagnosis of lung cancer includes history and physical examination, imaging, biopsy, pathology, staging, and molecular testing.

CLINICAL MANIFESTATIONS
Symptoms

The majority of patients with lung cancer have advanced disease at clinical presentation. Symptoms may result from local effects of the tumor, from regional or distant spread, or from distant effects not related to metastases (paraneoplastic syndromes). Many symptoms are associated with lung cancer and are mostly non-specific.

- Cough: It is the most common symptom and is usually present in 50%-75% of lung cancer patients.[4,5] It is more common in squamous cell and SCLC due to its tendency to involve central airways.
- Dyspnea: The incidence of dyspnea is 25%-50%.[4,5] It can be caused by multiple factors, such as intrinsic or extrinsic compression, pulmonary embolism, pleural effusion, pneumonia, or lymphangitic spread.
- Chest pain: The incidence of chest pain is 30%-50%,[4] usually on the same side of the chest as the primary tumor.
- Hemoptysis: The incidence of hemoptysis is about 20%-50%.[4,5] Bronchitis is the most common cause of hemoptysis.
- Hoarseness: The incidence of hoarseness is about 10%. This is due to malignancy involving the recurrent laryngeal nerve along its course under the arch of the aorta.

- Weight loss: The incidence for weight loss is 36%.
- Community-acquired pneumonia (CAP)[6,7]: Lung cancer can mimic CAP as a differential diagnosis or co-occur with CAP and present with pulmonary infiltrate and cough in about 1%-2% of cases.

Lung cancer can metastasize to any part of the body and present with symptoms related to metastatic disease like bone pain or neurological symptoms (headache, vomiting, seizures, visual disturbances). In a metanalysis, hemoptysis was found to have the greatest diagnostic value for lung cancer, with a diagnostic odds ratio (DOR) of 6.39 (3.32-12.28), followed by dyspnea 2.73 (1.54-4.85), then cough 2.64 (1.24-5.64), and lastly chest pain 2.02 (0.88-4.60).[8]

> **CLINICAL PEARL:** Symptoms in lung cancer are non-specific. Hemoptysis has the greatest diagnostic value (odds ratio [OR] 6.39), but bronchitis is the most common cause of hemoptysis.

Signs

Different signs associated with lung cancer include palpable lymphadenopathy (cervical, supraclavicular area), clubbing, superior vena cava syndrome, and Pancoast syndrome. Clubbing has an incidence of about 20% and a 3.9 likelihood ratio.[9]

Superior vena cava (SVC) syndrome has an incidence of 5%-10%. It is seen more with SCLC compared to NSCLC. Symptoms commonly include a sensation of fullness in the face/head and dyspnea. Physical findings include dilated neck veins, a prominent venous pattern on the chest, facial edema, and a plethoric appearance (**Figure 11-2**).

- SVC syndrome grading system[10]:
  - Grade 0: Asymptomatic—Radiographic SVC obstruction in the absence of symptoms
  - Grade 1: Mild—Edema in head or neck (vascular distention), cyanosis, plethora
  - Grade 2: Moderate—Edema in head or neck with functional impairment (mild dysphagia; cough; mild or moderate impairment of head, jaw, or eyelid movements; visual disturbances caused by ocular edema)
  - Grade 3: Severe—Mild or moderate cerebral edema (headache, dizziness); mild/moderate laryngeal edema; or diminished cardiac reserve (syncope after bending); incidence 10%
  - Grade 4: Life threatening—Significant cerebral edema (confusion, obtundation), significant laryngeal edema (stridor), or significant hemodynamic compromise (syncope without precipitating factors, hypotension, renal insufficiency); incidence 5%

> **CLINICAL PEARL:** Patients who present with life-threatening symptoms (grade 4) secondary to SVC represent a true medical emergency and require immediate intervention (eg, endovenous recanalization with SVC stent placement) to decrease the risk of sudden respiratory failure and death.

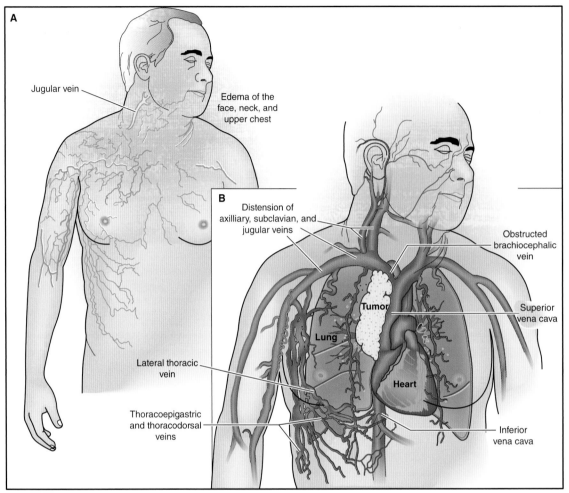

Figure 11-2. Superior vena cava syndrome due to lung cancer causing SVC syndrome. (Adapted from Wilson LD, Detterbeck FC, Yahalom J. Clinical practice. Superior vena cava syndrome with malignant causes. *N Engl J Med.* 356(18):1862-1869.)

Pancoast Syndrome

Lung cancers arising in the superior sulcus cause Pancoast syndrome, manifested by pain (usually in the shoulder and less commonly in the forearm, scapula, and fingers); Horner syndrome (ptosis, miosis, and anhidrosis); bony destruction; and atrophy of hand muscles. It is more commonly seen in NSCLC (**Figure 11-3**).

Paraneoplastic Syndromes

Paraneoplastic effects of tumor are remote effects that are not related to direct invasion, obstruction, or metastasis. While paraneoplastic syndromes are most often diagnosed in the setting of a known malignancy, it is common for a paraneoplastic disorder to develop before a cancer is identified. Therefore, search for underlying malignancy is

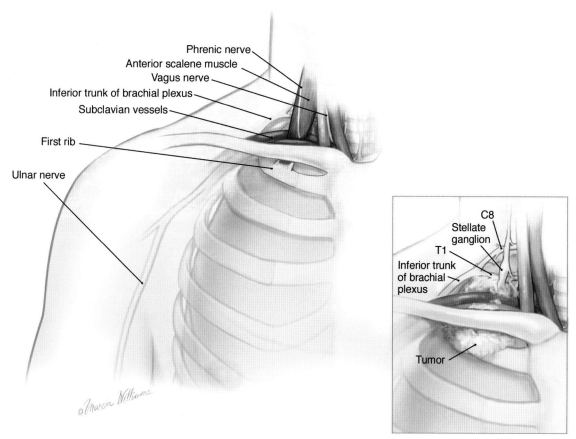

Phrenic nerve
Anterior scalene muscle
Vagus nerve
Inferior trunk of brachial plexus
Subclavian vessels
First rib
Ulnar nerve

C8
Stellate ganglion
T1
Inferior trunk of brachial plexus
Tumor

©Marcia Williams

Figure 11-3. Pancoast tumor in the superior sulcus. (Reproduced with permission from Sugarbaker DJ, Bueno R, Krasna MJ, Mentzer SJ, Zellos L. *Sugarbaker's Adult Chest Surgery.* 3rd ed. New York, NY: McGraw Hill; 2020: https://accesssurgery.mhmedical.com/content.aspx?bookid=2781&sectionid=239711663#239711671.)

important. In most instances, the tumor is revealed by computed tomography (CT) of the chest, abdomen, and pelvis.

Hypercalcemia: Most patients with hypercalcemia have advanced disease, which is associated with poor survival. It may arise from bony metastasis and less commonly due to tumor secretion of parathyroid hormone–related protein. It is more commonly associated with squamous cell lung cancer followed by adenocarcinoma and then SCLC.

> **CLINICAL PEARL:** Symptomatic patients with hypercalcemia of malignancy require immediate treatment with hydration and bisphosphonates.

Syndrome of inappropriate antidiuretic hormone secretion (SIADH) is frequently caused by SCLC.[11] Incidence is about 10%. Symptoms are related to severity of hyponatremia. Treatment focuses on treating the malignancy.

Hypertrophic pulmonary osteoarthropathy is defined by the presence of clubbing and periosteal proliferation of the tubular bones associated with lung cancer or lung disease causing symmetrical painful arthropathy. It is commonly caused by NSCLC. Incidence in lung cancer[12] varies between 4% and 17%.

Neurologic paraneoplastic syndromes are most commonly seen in lung cancer, especially SCLC. Incidence in SCLC is about 10%, most frequently Lambert-Eaton myasthenic syndrome (LEMS) (3.8%), sensory neuronopathy (1.9%), and limbic encephalitis (1.5%).[13] The following well-categorized paraneoplastic antibodies and associated paraneoplastic syndromes seen in lung cancer[14]:

- Anti-Hu (ANNA-1): Encephalomyelitis including cortical, limbic, and brainstem encephalitis; cerebellar degeneration; myelitis; sensory neuronopathy; and/or autonomic dysfunction
- Anti-Ri (ANNA-2): Cerebellar degeneration, brainstem encephalitis, opsoclonus-myoclonus
- Anti-CV2/CRMP5: Encephalomyelitis, cerebellar degeneration
- Anti-PCA-2 (MAP1B): Peripheral neuropathy, cerebellar ataxia, encephalopathy
- Anti-VGCC: cerebellar degeneration, LEMS

Lambert-Eaton myasthenic syndrome may be seen in about 3% of SCLC patients, but almost 60% of patients with LEMS have SCLC. It serves as a marker for early disease and precedes the diagnosis of SCLC in most cases. It usually presents as complaints of slowly progressive proximal muscle weakness. There is no significant muscle atrophy, and deep tendon reflexes are almost depressed or absent. The aggressive search for a primary underlying malignancy is central to the management of patients with LEMS.

Cushing syndrome secondary to ectopic production of corticotropin (ACTH) presents with muscle weakness, weight loss, hypertension, hirsutism, and osteoporosis. Also, it involves hypokalemic alkalosis and hyperglycemia. Incidence in SCLC is about 1%-5%, and patients with Cushing syndrome and SCLC together tend to have a worse prognosis.[15]

HISTORY AND PHYSICAL EXAMINATION

Every patient suspected of lung cancer should undergo thorough history and physical examination. Symptoms typically indicate advanced disease. Evaluation should be symptom directed, with particular attention to symptoms that might suggest metastasis.

- Medical history: Pay attention to other medical conditions like COPD, renal disease.
- Family history.
- Social history with attention to family/social support and smoking history.
- Performance status (Eastern Cooperative Oncology Group [ECOG] or Karnofsky performance scale).
- Elicit history about bone pain, back pain, neurologic symptoms (headache, focal weakness, blurry vision, confusion, slurred speech, etc.).
- Physical examination:
  - Evaluate for hypoxia.
  - Look for lymphadenopathy, finger clubbing.

- ○ Auscultate lung fields (evaluate for pleural effusion).
- ○ Every patient should undergo a brief neurologic examination; if neurologic symptoms are present, then perform a focused detailed neurologic examination to evaluate for brain metastasis and spinal cord compression.
- Symptom-directed evaluation prompts appropriate laboratory testing and imaging.

TESTING FOR LUNG CANCER

Laboratory

Consider performing the following laboratory studies if the history/physical examination or chest imaging are suspicious for lung cancer

- Complete blood count
- Creatinine
- Calcium
- Electrolytes
- Liver function test: alkaline phosphatase, alanine aminotransferase, aspartate aminotransferase, total bilirubin
- Albumin

No serum tumor markers have shown clinical utility in the diagnosis of lung cancer.

Imaging

If lung cancer is suspected based on signs/symptoms, the initial step is a CT of the chest and upper abdomen (including adrenal glands) with contrast.[16,17] A patient suspected of having lung cancer due to lung cancer screening or an incidental finding will already have initial chest imaging. Magnetic resonance imaging (MRI) of the brain with contrast should be performed for all patients with SCLC[16] and for stage IB, II, III, and IV cancer in patients with NSCLC.[17] An ^{18}F-fludeoxyglucose (FDG) positron emission tomographic (PET)/CT scan from the skull base to the midthigh should be considered in patients with suspected limited-stage SCLC[16] and in NSCLC patients during the initial evaluation.[17]

Patients with symptoms suspicious of metastasis should receive dedicated imaging.

- Back pain: MRI spine
- Headache, confusion, blurry vision: Brain MRI (preferred); if unable to obtain an MRI, then CT head with contrast
- Radicular back pain with focal weakness: MRI spine
- Abdominal pain: CT abdomen/pelvis with contrast
- Abnormal liver function test: CT abdomen/pelvis with contrast if liver not fully evaluated in CT chest

For patients who presented with CAP, a chest radiograph should be performed at 6 weeks following treatment of high-risk patients for malignancy[6,7]:

- Smokers
- >50 years of age

Biopsy

Tissue diagnosis is needed to diagnose lung cancer and differentiate between NSCLC (adenocarcinoma, squamous cell carcinoma) and SCLC. A biopsy that is the least invasive with the highest yield is preferred. Biopsy the site that would confer the highest stage, such as a biopsy of a suspected metastasis or mediastinal lymph node rather than the pulmonary lesion. Immunohistochemical (IHC) staining is used to classify NSCLC (adenocarcinoma, squamous cell carcinoma).

Patients with suspected nodal disease should receive a biopsy by endobronchial ultrasound (EBUS), endoscopic ultrasound (EUS), navigational bronchoscopy, or mediastinoscopy.[17]

- EBUS provides access to nodal stations 2R/2L, 4R/4L, 7, 10R/10L, and other hilar nodal stations if necessary.
- An EBUS transbronchial needle aspiration negative for malignancy in a clinically positive mediastinum should undergo subsequent mediastinoscopy prior to surgical resection.

Lung cancer patients with an associated pleural effusion should undergo thoracentesis and cytology. A negative cytology result on initial thoracentesis does not exclude pleural involvement, and an additional thoracentesis should be considered before starting therapy with a curative intent.

Molecular Testing

Multiple genetic alterations have been identified in NSCLC with approved targeted therapies. Molecular testing[17] is recommended in all metastatic lung cancer. The National Comprehensive Cancer Network (NCCN) guidelines recommend testing for the following gene mutations as a part of broader molecular profiling with the goal of identifying rare driver mutations:

- EGFR (epidermal growth factor receptor)
    - Exon 19 deletions or exon 21 L858R mutations are the most common mutations and are associated with responsiveness to EGFR tyrosine kinase inhibitor.
    - *EGFR* exon 20 insertions and p.T790M are less common and associated with lack of responsiveness to EGFR tyrosine kinase inhibitor.
- ALK (anaplastic lymphoma kinase)
- ROS1 (ROS proto-oncogene 1)
- *BRAF gene*
- PD-L1 (programmed death ligand 1)

Plasma cell-free/circulating tumor DNA (liquid biopsy) can be used in certain clinical situations for molecular testing:

- If a patient is clinically unfit to receive invasive tissue biopsy
- If a patient has no safe accessible site for invasive tissue biopsy
- In the setting of insufficient tissue after the initial diagnostic setting

Patients with suspected lung cancer, when possible, should be discussed in a multidisciplinary conference to move forward with the best approach for imaging and biopsy.

> **CLINICAL PEARL:** Tissue diagnosis is needed to diagnose lung cancer and differentiate between NSCLC (adenocarcinoma, squamous cell carcinoma) and SCLC. Biopsy the site that would confer the highest stage.

IMAGING OF LUNG CANCER

Chandler Park, MD, MSc, FACP, Samuel Reynolds, MD

A 68–year-old white male with a past medical history of malignant pleural mesothelioma is presented for discussion at a multidisciplinary lung tumor board meeting. The patient's CT chest scan with intravenous contrast only showed nodular lobular thickening in the left lower lobe, and no thoracic lymphadenopathy was seen. CT of the abdomen and pelvis with intravenous contrast showed no suspicious lesions. The cardiothoracic surgeon would like to consider the patient for surgery. What is the best imaging test to order next?

Learning Objectives:

1. What are the most common imaging modalities used in clinical practice?
2. What are the radiographic findings to suggest lung cancer in pulmonary nodules?
3. What are the characteristic radiographic features of SCLC?
4. For which lung cancer is a PET gallium scan the best to evaluate for metastatic cancer?
5. What is the lymphatic drainage pattern of left lower lobe lung cancer?

IMAGING MODALITIES

Radiographic imaging is essential in the evaluation of patients with suspected lung cancer. Imaging tests are very useful in distinguishing benign pulmonary nodules from metastatic lung lesions. Also, it is very useful in clinical practice to follow up patients with thoracic malignancy. Oncologists often use imaging tests such as CT of the chest and PET/CT tests to follow cancer patients after they complete treatments.

The main imaging modalities used in the initial diagnosis of lung cancers are chest x-ray and CT of the chest. A chest x-ray may show distinctive findings to suggest lung cancer. Chest CT is used to further characterize the chest x-ray findings. Once cancer is diagnosed by tissue biopsy, FDG PET/CT is often used for staging lung cancers. A bone scan with CT of the chest, abdomen, and pelvis may also be used for staging lung cancer. MRI is also used for patients who cannot tolerate iodinated contrast. Last, MRI is also used by cardiothoracic surgeons to evaluate patients for the possibility of surgical resection of localized malignant pleural mesothelioma.[18]

Chest Radiography

Patients who present with lung symptoms such as coughing and dyspnea are typically worked up starting with a chest x-ray (**Figure 11-4**). Chest x-rays allow an initial inspection of all lung structures, which often allows identification of radiographic

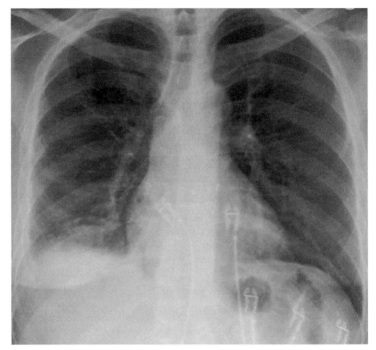

Figure 11-4. Chest x-ray.

abnormalities related to lung cancer. These include direct and indirect signs of cancer. Imaging findings of cancer include unexplained hilar lymphadenopathy, pleural effusions, atelectasis, infiltrates, and bone lesions.[19,20]

CT Chest

Chest CT is the most common imaging modality for the evaluation of lung cancers (**Figure 11-5**). CT images allow high spatial resolution for evaluation of pulmonary nodules, thoracic lymphadenopathy, pleural abnormalities, and locally invasive cancers. Metastatic bone lesions are also easily identified with this imaging modality.

Screening CT

In addition to diagnostic imaging, CT is valuable as a screening modality (**Figure 11-6**). Specifically, adult patients aged 55-80 with a 30 pack-year or more history of cigarette smoking who either actively smoke or have quit within 15 years are eligible for a low-dose CT (LDCT) of the chest for lung cancer screening. The difference between screening and standard non-contrast CT is in the radiation dose. The National Lung Screening Trial in 2011, for example, involved a LDCT dose of 2 millisievert (mSv), as compared to 8 mSv in standard CT scanning of the full chest.[21] The concept in utilizing LDCT is to provide a high-quality screening test for patients at risk for lung cancer while exposing them to as minimal a dose of radiation as possible. Identifying lung nodules long before symptoms arise will then, ideally, lead to earlier diagnosis and subsequent management.

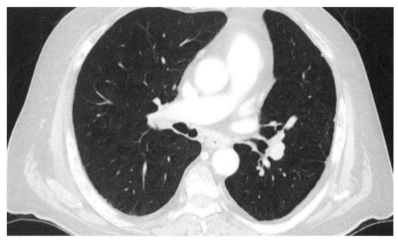

Figure 11-5. Chest CT with contrast visible in large vessels.

Positron Emission Tomography/Computed Tomography

Positron emission tomography with computed tomography is the current gold standard for staging of cancer (**Figure 11-7**). It is also used to evaluate undetermined pulmonary nodules for lung cancer. It is very important to remember that PET/CT does have limitations. Infectious and inflammatory diseases may lead to false-positive findings of high

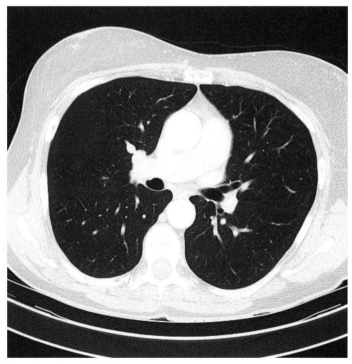

Figure 11-6. Screening chest CT without contrast.

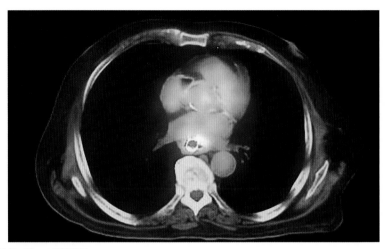

Figure 11-7. Chest PET/CT.

SUV. Also, slow-growing cancers with indolent features such as low-grade adenocarcinomas, bronchoalveolar carcinomas, and carcinoid cancers may exhibit a false-negative finding of low SUV.

Preoperative PET, Response Assessment, Surveillance

Currently, PET/CT is routine in preoperative staging in order to avoid unnecessary surgery. To highlight an example of its importance, a 2011 study published in the *New England Journal of Medicine* found that, of 189 total patients (98 randomized to the PET/CT group and 91 to conventional staging), 60 underwent thoracotomy in the PET/CT group (61%), compared to 73 (80%) in the conventional group. Approximately 41% of thoracotomies were then found to be futile in the conventional group, compared to only 21% in the PET/CT group. The authors concluded that PET/CT in preoperative NSCLC staging reduced both total and futile thoracotomies.[22] This study was followed by a study by Zelidat et al., who reported in 2014 on a cohort of 2,977 patients with NSCLC; there was a focus on 976 patient who underwent resection over an approximate 12-year period. Of patients who had surgery, 30.3% were later found to have distant metastases; however, the use of PET increased diagnosis of distant metastatic disease from 9% to 91% over this same period. By instrumental variable analyses, PET was associated with a reduction in unnecessary surgery (odds ratio 0.53, p = .004).[23]

Also, PET/CT may also be used in treatment response assessment, specifically when there is evidence or suspicion for either recurrence or metastatic spread of disease. The difficulty, however, is that PET/CT is often overused and may be misleading in some cases. Moreover, the efficacy of PET/CT in the context of formally assessing treatment response has not been established by clinical practice recommendations, making it difficult for physicians to justify its routine use.[24]

The role of PET/CT in lung cancer surveillance is also limited. A 2015 study published in the *Journal of Nuclear Medicine*, however, argued for its use when Antoniou et al. conducted a retrospective analysis of 261 patients from a single center with lung cancer, confirmed by biopsy. Within this population, 488 PET/CT scans were performed 6 months or longer from initial therapy completion; lung cancer recurrence was seen in 281 scans, while the other 207 demonstrated absence of disease. In a subpopulation of 245 patients in whom providers had no clinical suspicion of disease, PET/CT identified recurrence in 107 patients (43.7%). It was also found that overall survival was negatively correlated with a PET/CT study that demonstrated disease recurrence, as expected. Authors concluded that PET/CT could serve as a prognostic tool in following patients with lung cancer after primary treatment and could even assist in clinical judgment.[25] And while the latter of these conclusions is interesting, larger scale studies are needed to validate the authors' findings before PET/CT becomes a standardized component of lung cancer surveillance.

Magnetic Resonance Imaging

Magnetic resonance imaging is a very valuable imaging modality for oncologists and surgeons (**Figure 11-8**). For example, it is very useful to evaluate thymic lesions. MRI can be used to help distinguish benign thymic lesions from cancerous lesions. Also, MRI is the best modality for identification of soft tissue invasion. Therefore, when a surgeon is considering a resection of a malignant mesothelioma, the surgeon can order an MRI to see if the cancer has penetrated through the diaphragm, which would preclude surgery.[26]

Use of MRI for Brain Lesions, Pancoast Tumors, Spinal Metastases to Rule Out Cord Compression and/or Leptomeningeal Disease

Brain imaging is generally reserved for patients who demonstrate new neurologic symptoms, rather than as a routine screening modality (**Figure 11-9**). Given the propensity

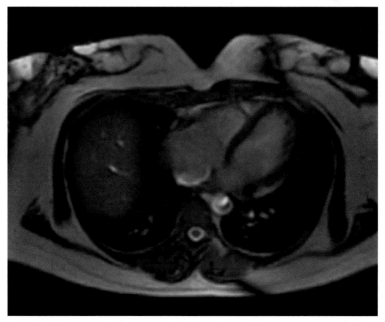

Figure 11-8. Chest MRI.

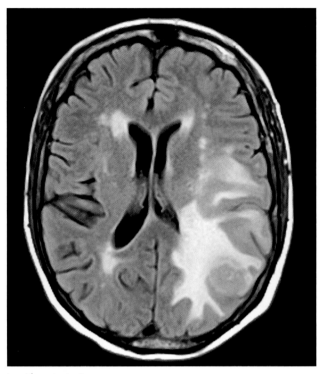

Figure 11-9. Brain with metastasis.

for intracranial extension of lung cancer, however, MRI of the brain can be a valuable tool for physicians. Most societal guidelines, including those put forth by the NCCN, European Society for Medical Oncology, and British Thoracic Society, recommend brain imaging in patients with stage III or greater NSCLC, but debate exists on how to screen in stages I-II. One group took a unique approach in a 2017 retrospective study that examined 585 patients who had undergone resection of diagnosed lung cancer, 471 of which had accessible radiographic records. Of the patients, 5.3% (25/471) had brain metastases on imaging, and 18/471 (3.8%) presented with metastases to the brain after surgical resection of lung cancer, 12 of which had adenocarcinoma. The authors concluded that preoperative brain MRI in patients with NSCLC, specifically those with adenocarcinoma histology, is indicated prior to surgery with curative intent. The idea here is that patients may be spared an invasive surgical procedure in favor of systemic therapy should intracranial metastases be discovered. Schoenmaekers et al. recently lauded the findings of this study in their own 2018 article published in the *Journal of Thoracic Disease*; the study recommended mandatory brain MRI in stage IIIA or higher NSLC or in those with stage II adenocarcinoma at a younger age.[27,28]

Magnetic resonance has other utilities in the context of both primary and metastatic lung cancer. It is useful, for example, in visualizing Pancoast tumors, as it provides detailed imagery of the regional extent of the tumor and involved surrounding soft tissue. Magnetic resonance angiography (MRA) is particularly useful in highlighting nervous and vascular structures of the superior sulcus. MRI is also critical in imaging the spinal cord and surrounding structures, specifically in the setting of suspected cord compression secondary to spinal metastases. Detecting such compression in a timely manner allows physicians to enact timely medical management and/or surgical intervention, if indicated. Last, MRI has utility in the radiographic diagnosis of leptomeningeal disease, which occurs most commonly when solid cancer, such as that of lung, breast, or skin, disseminates into the cerebrospinal fluid (CSF). The ideal image in suspected cases is a T1-weighted MRI with gadolinium contrast, which in the brain will demonstrate pial nodularity and enhancement overlying areas that include the basal cisterns, cerebral convexities, or ependymal surfaces of ventricles. In the spine, MRI with contrast will reveal patchy nerve root involvement and extramedullary nodules within the dura, specifically at the level of the cauda equina. And, as useful as these high-resolution images are, obtaining CSF to observe for malignant cytology remains the gold standard for diagnosis in leptomeningeal carcinomatosis.[29] This concept is best understood by recognizing that solid tumor, such as of the lung, may appear grossly on brain imaging, but hematogenous cancer (eg, acute lymphoblastic leukemia) will likely be radiographically negative but still very much involved in the CSF.

Bone Scan

A bone scan is also a very common radiographic test ordered by oncologists. It is a very sensitive nuclear medicine test to detect bone metastases. Metastatic bone cancers have increased radiotracer uptake. Lung cancers can be sclerotic or lytic. Squamous cell lung cancers can have mixed osteolytic and osteoblastic features. Lung adenocarcinomas typically are osteolytic.

RADIOGRAPHIC CLUES OF LUNG CANCER

In this section, we discuss radiographic clues of lung cancer. We focus on chest CT because this is the most common radiographic imaging test used to characterize lung cancers. On a chest CT examination, there are many radiographic findings that are identified by reviewing the images ourselves or by reading the radiology report interpreted by a radiologist. These radiographic findings of lung cancer include pulmonary nodules, pulmonary masses, cavitation, ground glass opacity (GGO), encasement, and lymphadenopathy.

Pulmonary Nodule

A pulmonary nodule is defined as a round lesion less than 3 cm in maximum diameter (**Figure 11-10**). Common pulmonary nodule characteristics help distinguish benign versus malignant lesions. For example, a spherical shape is more likely benign. On the other hand, spiculated margins imply cancer. There are also internal traits of pulmonary nodules, including solidity, GGO, fat inclusion, and calcifications. Fat-containing pulmonary nodules are commonly seen in benign hamartomas. Calcification of pulmonary nodules may be benign or cancerous. Pulmonary nodules with stippled or eccentric calcifications are suspicious for cancer. Central and laminar calcifications on pulmonary nodules are likely benign.

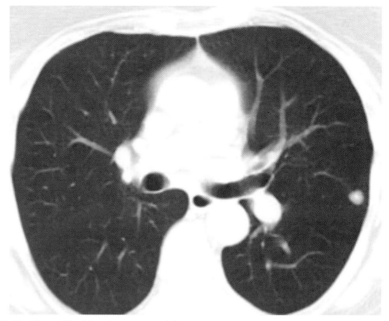

Figure 11-10. Chest CT with pulmonary nodule.

A pulmonary mass is defined as a lesion greater than 3 cm in maximum diameter. Differential diagnosis of pulmonary masses includes primary lung cancer, metastatic lung cancer, lymphoma, carcinoid tumor, infection, inflammation, and vasculitis. Image findings of cancer include borders that are spiculated, cavitations with thick walls (described in material that follows), and invasive lesions. Other clues to suggest malignancy include a mass with associated hilar or mediastinal lymphadenopathy and ipsilateral pleural effusion.[30,31]

Cavitation

Cavitation is defined as a lucency within a pulmonary nodule, mass, or consolidation (**Figure 11-11**). The gas-containing space is due to underlying lung necrosis. Differential diagnosis of cavitations includes necrotizing pneumonia, abscess, squamous cell lung cancer, metastatic cancer, and vasculitis. The wall thickness of the cavitation can be a clue to whether the underlying cause is an infection or cancer. Cavity wall thickness of less than 7 mm is most likely benign. On the other hand, cavity thickness more than 2 cm is most likely neoplastic.[30,31]

Ground-Glass Opacity

Ground glass opacity is defined as an increased density in an area in the lung that does not completely cover up the underlying structures (**Figure 11-12**). This is due to the fact that lung alveolus is filled with fluid, blood, or cancer cells. An alveolus can fill due to increased interstitial fluid, increased blood flow, or cancer cell invasion. Atypical infections, such as interstitial pneumonia caused by mycoplasma pneumonia, viral pneumonia, and pneumocystis jirovecii can also cause GGO. Interestingly, immunotherapies

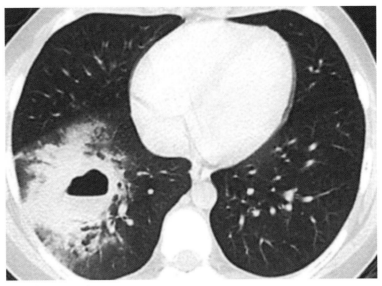

Figure 11-11. Chest CT with cavitation.

used in lung cancer can cause immunotherapy-associated pneumonitis that can be seen radiographically as GGO on CTs. Last, lung cancers can present as GGO. Lung adeno-carcinomas that are lepedic or minimally invasive appear as GGO. Therefore, clinical history is very important to fully analyze GGOs.[30,31]

Encasement

Encasement is due to surrounding a lung structure due to an underlying tissue (**Figure 11-13**). For example, aggressive cancers may encase and completely obstruct

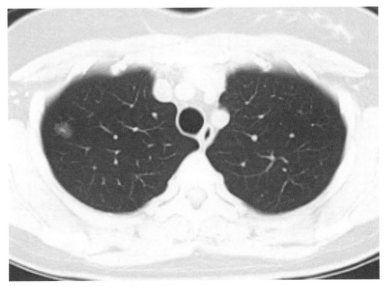

Figure 11-12. Chest CT with ground glass lesion.

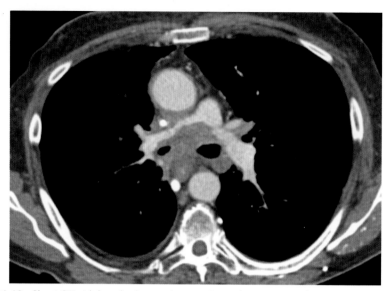

Figure 11-13. Chest CT with lymphadenopathy encasing pulmonary vessels.

the SVC, pulmonary artery, or main stem bronchus. If cancers encase the SVC, this is known as SVC syndrome. Lung cancers that are commonly centrally located in the thorax such as SCLC and squamous cell lung cancer can also encase and obliterate the main bronchus or nearby large great vessels.[32]

Lymphadenopathy is defined as abnormal enlargement of a lymph node. CT findings include intrathoracic lymph nodes that measure more than 1 cm on CT. There is an associated FDG uptake within the lymph node on PET/CT.

A good rule of thumb for abnormal lymph node size is location. For instance, a chest CT with a suspicious lung mass with an internal mammary lymph node, retrocrural lymph node, or extrapleural lymph node should always be considered abnormal and should be closely followed or biopsied.

On the other hand, the other lymph nodes have location-specific upper limit normal size criteria. For instance, lower paratracheal and subcarinal lymph nodes greater than 1.1 cm, high paratracheal and superior mediastinal lymph nodes greater than 7 mm, right hilar and paraesophageal lymph nodes greater than 1.0 cm, left hilar and paraesophageal lymph nodes greater than 7 mm, and peridiaphragmatic lymph nodes greater than 5 mm should be closely monitored.

Morphology of the lymph node may also be a clue to a cancerous lymph node. For example, abnormal lymph node features include rounded morphology, loss of fatty hilum, irregular borders, necrotic centers, and internal calcifications.[30,31]

LUNG CANCERS

Lung Adenocarcinoma

Lung adenocarcinomas are the most common histologic type of lung cancer (**Figure 11-14**). On imaging, there are many types of lung adenocarcinomas. Adenocarcinoma in situ (CIS) and minimally invasive adenocarcinomas have a GGO or

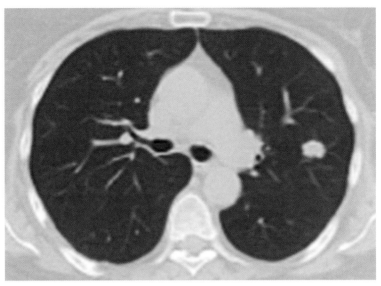

Figure 11-14. Chest CT and adenocarcinoma lung cancer.

part-solid nodule less than 3 cm. Lepidic-predominant adenocarcinomas are part solid or purely GGO. Acinar or papillary with mucin production nodules are usually solid and may include GGO. Last, invasive mucinous adenocarcinoma may be multilobar or bilateral lung cancers.

The most common radiographic findings of lung adenocarcinomas include peripheral or central mass, band-like features that look like fibrosis, postobstructive atelectasis or pneumonia, local invasion of mediastinum or chest wall, hilar or mediastinal lymphadenopathy, and ipsilateral pleural effusion. Also, interseptal thickening that is smooth or nodular can be present due to lymphangitic carcinomatosis.

There are also radiographic prognostic indictors for lung adenocarcinomas. For example, if a lung adenocarcinoma has an extensive ground glass component, that is considered a favorable prognostic indicator. On the other hand, if the lung adenocarcinoma is predominantly solid, that is a poor prognostic indicator. For mixed masses, if the mass is composed of mostly GGO, that is a favorable prognostic sign. Other predictors of poor outcomes include spiculated lesions, thick cavitations, and concave pull into the cancer. Last, the larger the adenocarcinoma is, the likelihood of central nervous systemic metastatic disease is increased. Therefore, any patient with a lung adenocarcinoma that is greater than 4 cm should receive a brain MRI for further evaluation.[33]

Squamous Cell Lung Cancer

Squamous cell lung cancer is thought to have developed from squamous metaplasia (**Figure 11-15**). Greater than 60% of these cancers arise in the main stem bronchus or lobar or main segmental branches. Apical lesions can also present as a Pancoast tumor. On radiographic x-rays, squamous cell lung cancer borders are commonly spiculated. Also, squamous cell lung cancers commonly exhibit internal cavitation or necrosis. Other common findings include a central airway mass with bronchial obstruction.

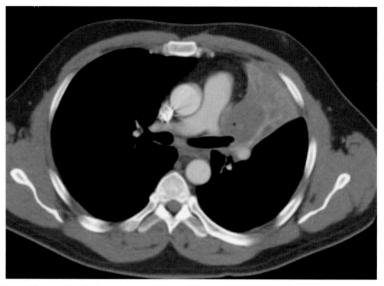

Figure 11-15. Chest CT with central squamous cell lung cancer and atelectasis.

This may manifest as postobstructive pneumonia in patients. On the other hand, the postobstructive pneumonia may also obscure an underlying cancer. Associated findings include wide mediastinum due to mediastinal lymphadenopathy.

Computed tomographic findings for squamous cell lung cancer include central necrosis and cavitations. Of squamous cell lung cancers, 15% have cavitation. Squamous cell lung cancers typically have an internal cavity wall thickness of greater than 1.5 cm. Other clues of squamous cell lung cancers on CT include assessment of local invasion. Squamous cell lung cancers can invade mediastinal structures such as great vessels, esophagus, pericardium, and myocardium. In terms of chest wall invasion, if the lung cancer and pleura are more than 3 cm in contact, there is a high likelihood of tumor invasion.

Lymphadenopathy is often a radiographic imaging clue to squamous cell lung cancer. Squamous cell lung cancers tend to have ipsilateral hilar lymph nodes greater than 1 cm on the short axis. Subcarinal lymph nodes greater than 1.2 cm, retrocrural lymph nodes greater than 0.8 cm, para-aortic lymph nodes greater than 0.8 cm, and pericardial lymph nodes greater than 0.8 cm are considered abnormal.[33]

Small Cell Lung Cancer

Small cell lung cancer is the most commonly diagnosed as a central pulmonary nodule or mass (**Figure 11-16**). Mediastinal and hilar encasement are also very common. This includes invasion of pericardium, myocardium, pulmonary arteries, SVC, and aorta. Unlike other lung cancers, SCLC can present with only mediastinal or hilar lymphadenopathy without a lung mass. A peripheral pulmonary nodule or mass is not as common in SCLC. Most common finding of SCLC is a central pulmonary mass, which may produce atelectasis and volume loss. Also malignant pleural effusion may occur. In terms of extrathoracic metastases, the most common areas of metastases are liver,

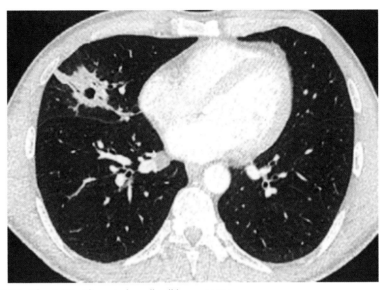

Figure 11-16. Chest CT with central small cell lung cancer.

bone, adrenal glands, and brain. On initial diagnosis, 15% of SCLC patients that are asymptomatic have metastatic brain lesions. Thus, all SCLC patients should receive an initial brain MRI.[33]

Large Cell Carcinoma

Large cell lung cancers are often considered a diagnosis of exclusion. Therefore, there are very few features of SCLC, adenocarcinoma, or squamous cell lung cancers on histological examination. This cancer occurs most commonly in the lung periphery. On CT, large cell lung cancers are not that different from lung adenocarcinomas. Spiculated pulmonary nodules or masses are seen. Also, the pulmonary nodules often have eccentric or punctate calcifications. On PET/CT, large cell carcinomas have increased FDG uptake. Large cell lung carcinomas are rarely centrally located on imaging.[33]

Carcinoid Tumors

Carcinoid tumors are low-grade malignant neuroendocrine cancers that typically do not metastasize to extrathoracic structures. These neuroendocrine cells arise from the bronchial epithelium. Most commonly, these cancers are found on imaging at the main stem, lobar, or segmental bronchi. They appear as a central hilar or perihilar well-defined mass. Metastases to liver or bone are very uncommon. Classic radiographic finding is seen with an expiratory air trapping that has a mosaic appearance on CT. Unlike other cancers, carcinoid tumors are not typically spiculated. These cancers typically have smooth pulmonary nodule borders. However, similar to other cancers, carcinoid tumors do spread to regional lymph nodes.

The best imaging modality for atypical carcinoid is PET with gallium 68–labeled somatostatin. This is because neuroendocrine tumors overexpress somatostatin receptors. PET with gallium 68–labeled somatostatin analogue binds to the somatostatin analogue. This is the best imaging modality to identify metastatic atypical carcinoid cancer.[33]

Malignant Pleural Mesothelioma

Malignant pleural mesothelioma has a circumferential nodular pleural thickening. There is also loss of volume on the affected hemithorax. Calcified plaques occur in 25% of the cases. MRI is most sensitive for local invasion. In terms of pleural thickening, it is more than 1 cm thick. Also, pleural effusion is typically unilateral. On PET/CT, there is avid pleural thickening the pleura.[34]

Thymoma and Thymic Carcinomas

Thymic carcinomas are malignant thymic epithelial cancers. It is difficult to distinguish thymic carcinoma from thymoma on CT imaging. On imaging, both cancers present as prevascular, circular soft tissue masses. These masses have smooth borders. There may be internal decreased density due to necrotic change. Invasive thymomas also commonly have pleural nodules. MRI is the best way to distinguish a benign thymic lesion from thymic carcinoma if tissue diagnosis cannot be obtained. Thymic carcinoma has a very characteristic MRI signal sequence that is not appreciated on benign thymic tissue.[26]

Teratoma

Teratomas are primary germ cell cancers that contain tissues derived from more than 1 germinal layer. Teratomas present as a well-defined circular anterior mediastinal mass with smooth borders. There is also a characteristic rim-like calcification in about 20% of the cases. The most characteristic finding is a fluid cyst that is thin walled (less than 7 mm thick) with septations. There may also be a fat-fluid level that is considered very diagnostic. Of note, teratomas rarely have lymphadenopathy. The best radiographic characteristics of a teratoma is a cystic mass that contains fat with a rim-like calcification.

Metastatic Cancer

Lung cancers commonly spread to intrathoracic and extrathoracic structures. On CT, there are usually multiple circular or ovoid pulmonary nodules in both lungs. Interestingly, EGFR-positive adenocarcinomas can present with a bilateral pulmonary miliary pattern metastatic cancer (**Figure 11-17**). Other findings include endoluminal lesions, pleural metastases, cardiac metastases, tumor emboli, chest wall metastases, and lymphangitic carcinomatosis. In terms of metastatic pleural effusion, there is typically a nodular thickening of the pleural effusion. Also, malignant pericardial effusion presents as a nodular thickening.[35]

Pancoast Tumor

Pancoast tumor presents as a lung mass in the pulmonary apex (**Figure 11-18**). Commonly there are rib destructions in the upper ribs. There are three main compartments in the lung apex: anterior, middle, and posterior.

The anterior compartment includes the subclavian vein. Therefore, if there is compression of the anterior compartment by a mass, this leads to SVC obstruction.

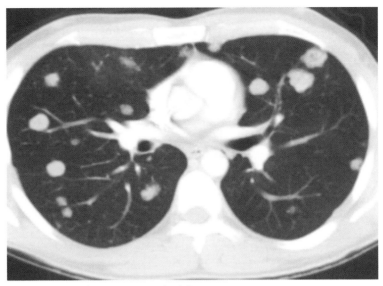

Figure 11-17. Chest CT with metastases to both lungs.

Associated findings of this condition commonly include dilated SVC, mediastinal widening, and intraluminal thrombus. Enlarged mediastinal widening is due to increased size of the mediastinal vessels, including the azygos vein, superior intercostal vein, and brachiocephalic vein.

Compression of the middle compartment leads to obstruction of the subclavian artery and portions of the brachial plexus. This leads to symptoms that include Horner syndrome.

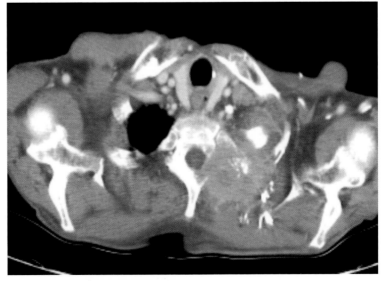

Figure 11-18. Chest CT with Pancoast tumor.

The posterior compartment has the brachial plexus roots. Compression of this compartment also leads to neurologic symptoms of the side of the body involved, which leads to smaller pupil, drooping eyelid, and decreased sweat production on the ipsilateral side.[36]

LYMPH NODE METASTATIC PATTERN IN LUNG CANCER
Lymph Node Map
A lymph node map helps us evaluate lymph node metastases. There are 7 lymph node zones and 14 lymph node stations that can be assessed on CT. The 7 lymph node zones are the supraclavicular zone, superior mediastinal zone, aortopulmonary zone, subcarinal zone, inferior mediastinal zone, hilar and interlobar zone, and peripheral zone.[37]

- The supraclavicular zone includes station 1R and station 1L. This zone includes right and left cervical, supraclavicular, and sternal notch lymph nodes.
- The superior mediastinal lymph zone (stations 2, 3, and 4) includes right and left upper paratracheal lymph nodes, prevascular lymph nodes, retrotracheal lymph nodes, right and left lower paratracheal lymph nodes.
- The aortopulmonary zone (stations 5 and 6) includes the subaortic and para-aortic lymph nodes.
- The subcarinal zone (station 7) includes the subcarinal lymph nodes.
- The inferior mediastinal zone (stations 8 and 9) includes paraesophageal lymph nodes and pulmonary ligament lymph nodes.
- The hilar and interlobar zone (station 10 and 11) includes hilar lymph nodes and interlobar lymph nodes.
- The peripheral zone (stations 12, 13, and 14) includes the lobar lymph nodes, segmental lymph nodes, and subsegmental lymph nodes.

LUNG CANCER LYMPHATIC DRAINAGE PATTERN
Lung cancer generally spreads from the intrapulmonary lymph nodes to the regional hilar lymph nodes then to mediastinal lymph nodes. Specific patterns also vary by the lobe involved, as discussed in the following material. And, while these patterns are useful for radiation and/or surgical planning, many variations in the lymphatic extension of lung cancer exist, and an individualized approach should be taken in guiding management.[37]

- Right upper lobe primary cancer cells drain to the right hilar lymph nodes, then into the paratracheal and anterior mediastinal lymph nodes.
- Left upper lobe primary cancer cells drain to the left hilar lymph nodes, then to the aorticopulmonary and para-aortic lymph nodes.
- Right middle lobe primary cancer cells drain from the right middle lobe pulmonary node to the right hilar lymph nodes, then to the subcarinal lymph nodes and afterward to the right paratracheal and anterior mediastinal lymph nodes.
- Right lower lobe primary cancer cells drain from right lower lobe pulmonary lymph node to right hilar lymph nodes, then to the subcarinal lymph nodes and afterward to the right paratracheal and anterior mediastinal lymph nodes.

- Left lower lobe primary cancer cells drain from the left lower lobe pulmonary lymph node to the left hilar lymph node, then to subcarinal and aorticopulmonary lymph nodes.[38]

BRONCHOSCOPY IN LUNG CANCER

Bilal Athar Jalil, MD, Umair Gauhar, MBBS

A 67-year-old ex-smoker with a 2-cm nodule in the right middle lobe is worked up for lung cancer. His CT shows hilar lymphadenopathy and a contralateral mediastinal adenopathy.

The adrenal gland has a 3-cm lesion that lights up on PET as well as the lesions in the chest.

What is the best way to obtain sufficient tissue to diagnose the nodule and help with treatment planning.

Learning Objectives:
1. What are the different types of bronchoscopy?
2. Can bronchoscopy treat lung cancer?
3. What are the complications of bronchoscopy?

Bronchoscopy is a minimally invasive procedure that allows access to the airways, mediastinum, and lung parenchyma. Bronchoscopy can be performed for both diagnostic and therapeutic purposes. While most bronchoscopy today is performed using a flexible fiber-optic bronchoscope (FOB), rigid bronchoscopy still plays an important role in the management of lung cancer–related complex airway problems. FOB can be performed with moderate sedation or general anesthesia and has a very good safety profile. In the last few decades, bronchoscopy has seen tremendous advances in both the therapeutic and the diagnostic arenas. The rigid bronchoscope was invented by Dr. Gustav Killian in 1898. Dr. Ikeda invented the flexible bronchoscope in 1967. In today's day and age, this minimally invasive tool has become an integral part of thoracic oncology, aiding in diagnosis and staging of lung cancer and minimizing the need for invasive procedures. In this chapter, we discuss the diagnostic and therapeutic applications of bronchoscopy in lung cancer.

FIBER-OPTIC BRONCHOSCOPY

Fiber-optic bronchoscopy is a very common procedure that involves intubation of the trachea with a flexible fiber-optic instrument. The FOB has a working channel that allows for instillation of topical anesthesia and suctioning of secretions and blood and facilitates the introduction of tissue sampling tools such as biopsy forceps, cytology brushes, needles for fine-needle aspirates or tissue cores, or therapeutic tools as mentioned further in the chapter.

Complications of bronchoscopy include hypoxemia, pneumonia, bronchitis, bleeding and trauma to vocal cords or the tracheobronchial tree, and pneumothorax.

The overall complication and mortality rates are extremely low, reported between less than 0.1% to 11% and 0% to 0.1%, respectively.[39]

Airway Inspection

The tracheobronchial tree is a 23-generation branching structure with the trachea being generation zero. A standard 5.9-mm bronchoscope with a 2-mm working channel only penetrates up to the fourth- to fifth-generation airways and allows visualization of the next 1-2 generations of airways.[40] Thus, the majority of the tracheobronchial tree is beyond the visual range of standard bronchoscopy.

Patients with known or suspected lung cancer with persistent atelectasis, unresolving pneumonia, or large pleural effusions should undergo bronchoscopy and airway inspection to evaluate for an obstructing endobronchial mass or stenosis/stricture of the central airways from radiation therapy. Similarly, hemoptysis in a patient with known or suspected lung cancer should be evaluated bronchoscopically to evaluate for endobronchial malignancy, radiation-induced tracheobronchitis, or tracheobronchial-vascular fistulas that may develop from the malignancy itself or radiation effects. Most standard bronchoscopy is performed using white light. White light bronchoscopy (WLB) can miss subtle endobronchial airway lesions, such as CIS. Narrow-band imaging (NBI) is a bronchoscopic modality that can improve detection of such lesions. The NBI technique involves decreasing the red wavelength and using the blue and green wavelengths of the light spectrum to enhance the superficial mucosal and deeper submucosal blood vessels, respectively. This depicts the angiogenesis associated with a malignant lesion. This technique has been used effectively in gastroenterology and now is being employed in bronchoscopy as well. In one study, NBI detected dysplasia or malignancy in 23% of the patients with normal WLB.[41] In another study, NBI performed after WLB led to a change in therapy in 10% of the patients.[42] The pattern of vascularization seen on NBI has been shown to correlate with the pathologic features of angiogenic squamous dysplasia.[43,44]

Endobronchial Tissue Sampling

In bronchology, the term *endobronchial* generally refers to a lesion that can be visualized during bronchoscopy. Endobronchial tissue sampling can be performed using biopsy forceps and various gauge needles for needle aspirates or tissue cores. Cytology brushes can be used for endobronchial tissue sampling but are only able to capture the superficial parts of such lesions, which are often necrotic, increasing the likelihood of a non-diagnostic sample. The sensitivity and specificity of bronchoscopically visible lesions is 88% to 100%.[45] Among different endobronchial tissue-sampling modalities, endobronchial biopsies have the highest sensitivity (74%), while cytology brushings and bronchial washings show poorer sensitivity at 59% and 48%, respectively.[46] The combination of all three modalities increases the sensitivity to 88%.[46] Thus, whenever feasible multiple sampling techniques should be utilized to obtain an adequate amount of diagnostic material, an issue that is even more important in the era of precision medicine.

Transbronchial Tissue Sampling Under Fluoroscopic Guidance

Fluoroscopy-guided transbronchial tissue sampling is used for lesions in the lung parenchyma and thus involves accessing pathologies that are "beyond visual range" of the bronchoscopist. These lesions can be pulmonary nodules, masses, or pulmonary infiltrates. The underlying etiology of these lesions is infectious, inflammatory, or neoplastic depending on the particular clinical context. The particular lobe of the lung and corresponding segment are identified during preprocedure review of chest imaging. During the procedure, the bronchoscope is advanced to the particular lobe and corresponding segment of concern. The tissue-sampling tool (biopsy forceps, cytology brushes, or aspiration needles) are then passed through the working channel of the bronchoscope and advanced under fluoroscopic guidance to access the parenchymal lesion. To maximize diagnostic yield and obtain abundant tissue for molecular analysis, a combination of sampling modalities is used, and multiple samples are usually obtained whenever feasible and safe. Transbronchial biopsies are generally safe, with a mortality rate of less than 0.04% and an overall complication rate of up to 6%.[47,48] Pneumothorax is the most common complication seen with transbronchial biopsies, with a rate of 5.8% in one study.[48]

Transbronchial tissue sampling involves operating beyond the visual range of the bronchoscopist using a 2-dimensional fluoroscopic view for guidance. As a result, the ability of a bronchoscopist to guide the sampling tool through the airways and the certainty of the relation of the tool to the parenchymal lesion as seen on the fluoroscopy view is decreased. While this factor is of limited concern in diffuse parenchymal processes such as pneumonia and pneumonitis, it can significantly compromise diagnostic yield in more focal lung lesions, such as pulmonary nodules and masses. Hence, the diagnostic yield of transbronchial sampling ranges widely, from 36% to 88%.[45] Various factors have been shown to affect the diagnostic yield, including the sampling method (forceps biopsy, cytology brushing, bronchoalveolar lavage [BAL]); number of samples taken; lesion size; and presence or absence of an airway leading to the lesion on chest CT scan.[45] Of these, the lesion size has the greatest impact on yield (63% for lesions greater than 2 cm and 34% with lesions less than 2 cm).

The diagnostic yield of CT-guided transthoracic needle aspirate (CT-TTNA) is higher at 90% compared to fluoroscopy-guided bronchoscopic biopsy.[45] However, CT-TTNA comes with a much higher complication rate of 15% for pneumothorax and 1% for hemorrhage (of these, 18% need a blood transfusion) based on cross-sectional analysis of 15,865 adults who had undergone CT-TTNA.[49] Over the last 2 decades, guided bronchoscopic techniques such as EBUS, electromagnetic navigation bronchoscopy, virtual bronchoscopy, and others have evolved to help bronchoscopists overcome the limitations of fluoroscopy-guided peripheral pulmonary tissue sampling and improve diagnostic yield. These techniques are discussed further in the chapter.

Bronchial Washings and Bronchoalveolar Lavage

Bronchial washings and BAL are performed by instilling fluid (usually normal saline) through the working channel of the bronchoscope and then aspirating to collect a specimen. The fluid can be instilled either on an endobronchial lesion (bronchial washing) or into the distal airways and alveolar tissue (BAL) after wedging the scope in a segment of the lung. Bronchial washing/BAL alone has a poor sensitivity for diagnosis of endobronchial lung cancer (48%) and even lower sensitivity (29%) for peripheral lung cancer.[45,50] In 1 study, only 1% of the lung cancer diagnoses would have been missed in the absence of BAL, and ground glass lesions were not associated with increased BAL yield.[50]

The main role of BAL in lung cancer is in the evaluation of patients who present with respiratory distress and pulmonary infiltrates on chest imaging in the setting of chemoimmunotherapy. In this situation, BAL can help diagnose an underlying infection or, by demonstrating negative cultures, favor a diagnosis of pneumonitis, whereby treatment with corticosteroids may be indicated.[51]

Curvilinear Endobronchial Ultrasound

Curvilinear EBUS (or convex probe EBUS) is a modification of the standard bronchoscope that includes an ultrasound transducer at the distal end of the bronchoscope (**Figure 11-19**). The ultrasound allows the visualization and sampling of structures outside the central airways. Malignant lymph nodes classically appear on ultrasound as round, heterogeneous structures with well-enhanced margins and loss of normal intranodal hilar structures (**Figure 11-20**). An aspiration needle is inserted through the working channel of the scope and exits at the distal end of the scope, making real-time sampling (called EBUS transbronchial needle aspirate or EBUS-TBNA) of central mediastinal masses and mediastinal and hilar lymph nodes possible (**Figure 11-21**). Since its introduction about 2 decades ago, curvilinear EBUS has radically changed the approach to mediastinal staging for lung cancer. Pooled analysis of 26 studies including 2,756 patients showed a sensitivity of 89%, specificity of 100%, positive predictive value of 100%, and negative predictive value of 91% for lung cancer.[52] These were significantly better than conventional unguided transbronchial needle aspiration.

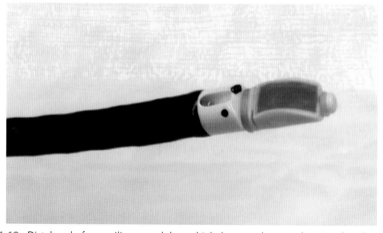

Figure 11-19. Distal end of a curvilinear endobronchial ultrasound scope showing the ultrasound transducer.

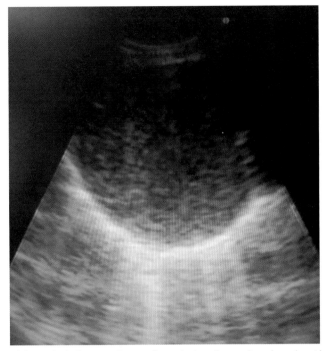

Figure 11-20. Endobronchial ultrasound view of a typical malignant lymph node with rounded shape, heterogeneous internal echotexture, loss of normal central hilar structure, and a distinct hyperechoic margin.

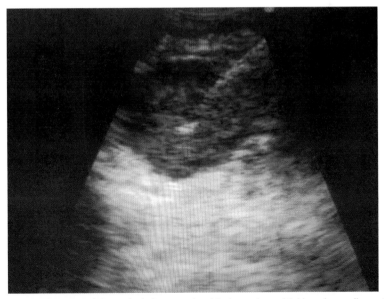

Figure 11-21. Real-time endobronchial ultrasound-guided transbronchial lymph needle aspiration of a malignant lymph node. The aspiration needle is seen entering diagonally into the lymph node.

Endobronchial ultrasound can provide access to the bilateral upper and lower paratracheal, subcarinal, and bilateral hilar lymph nodes. Combined EUS and fine-needle aspiration (EUS-FNA) and EBUS-TBNA ("medical mediastinoscopy") can provide access to inferior pulmonary ligament and esophageal lymph nodes, thus expanding the horizon of minimally invasive lung cancer staging. This medical mediastinoscopy can be performed in a single setting with a single scope using either moderate sedation or general anesthesia on an outpatient basis, thus saving time and cost.[53,54] Pooled analysis of 7 studies (811 patients) showed a sensitivity of 91%, specificity of 100%, positive predictive value of 100%, and negative predictive value of 96% for the combined approach, better than either approach alone.[52]

A multicenter randomized controlled trial of 241 patients compared mediastinoscopy alone for lung cancer staging to combined EBUS/EUS.[53] The patients underwent mediastinoscopy if the EUS/EBUS approach was negative. The sensitivities for mediastinoscopy, combined EBUS/EUS, and mediastinoscopy following a negative EBUS/EUS were 79%, 85%, and 94% respectively. The non-curative resection rate was reduced from 18% in the mediastinoscopy group to 7% ($p < .02$). The conclusions from this study were that patients should undergo EBUS/EUS staging first and if negative move on to mediastinoscopy.

Many studies have demonstrated cost savings with EBUS by reducing unnecessary mediastinocopies and other surgical procedures.[55-57] These savings persist even if EBUS is performed with general anesthesia.[55] Recent studies have shown that the EBUS scope can be used to sample the left adrenal gland and thus possibly allow evaluation of adrenal metastasis from lung cancer.[58,59]

The EBUS-TBNA samples have been found to be adequate for molecular analysis of non–small cell carcinoma. A systematic review and meta-analysis of 28 studies found a pooled probability of 94% for obtaining a sufficient sample for EGFR and ALK mutations.[60] EBUS samples have been found to be adequate for PD-L1 testing as well with an adequacy rate of 86%-90%.[61,62] EBUS needles are available as 21G, 22G, 25G cytology needles as well as a 19G histopathology needle. Multiple studies have been published to evaluate and compare the diagnostic yield and sample adequacy of these needles.[63] The studies showed good diagnostic yield with all available needles but were not conclusive enough to recommend one or another. Moreover, an EBUS microforceps needle has been introduced that can allow tissue biopsies. Multiple studies have shown feasibility and promising results with the miniforceps.[63]

Finally, EBUS has an excellent safety profile. Herth et al. studied the performance characteristics of EBUS in 124 patients with tissue-proven stage IIIA-N2 disease undergoing restaging after neoadjuvant chemotherapy.[64] The sensitivity, specificity, positive predictive value, negative predictive value, and diagnostic accuracy of EBUS in this patient population were 76%, 100%, 100%, 20%, and 77%, respectively. Of the 35 patients with no nodal metastases on EBUS-TBNA, 28 were found to have residual disease at thoracotomy. Because of a low negative predictive value in patients undergoing restaging after neoadjuvant chemotherapy, a negative result with EBUS should be confirmed surgically. In the ACCP (American College of Chest Physicians) Quality Improvement Registry, Evaluation, and Education (ACQuIRE) registry that includes 1,317 patients undergoing EBUS in 6 different hospitals, the overall complication rate was less than 1%, and the pneumothorax rate and major bleeding rate were 0.2% respectively.[65]

Guided Bronchoscopic Techniques for Peripheral Pulmonary Lesions

Guided bronchoscopic techniques for peripheral pulmonary lesions (PPLs) are technologies that allow the bronchoscopist to visualize and navigate the airways beyond the visual range of the standard bronchoscope, potentially increasing access to peripheral lung lesions and improving diagnostic yield. These technologies include radial probe endobronchial ultrasound (RP-EBUS), electromagnetic navigation bronchoscopy (ENB), and virtual bronchoscopy with ultrathin bronchoscopy (VB/UB).

Radial probe EBUS uses a thin, flexible ultrasound probe (**Figure 11-22**) that can be passed through the working channel of the bronchoscope and advanced to the peripheral lung tissue to provide a 360° ultrasonic view of the lung tissue. Normal lung tissue has a characteristic "snowstorm" appearance on lung ultrasound. PPLs appear heterogeneous with a bright hyperechoic margin if the RP-EBUS probe is within or near a lesion (**Figure 11-23**). RP-EBUS probe is usually used within a guide sheath as a single unit. Once the PPLs have been located, the RP-EBUS probe is removed, leaving the guide sheath in place. The guide sheath acts as an extended working channel (EWC) to allow sampling of PPLs with forceps, brushes, and needles. The biggest disadvantage of RP-EBUS is the inability of the bronchoscopist to maneuver the probe in the peripheral

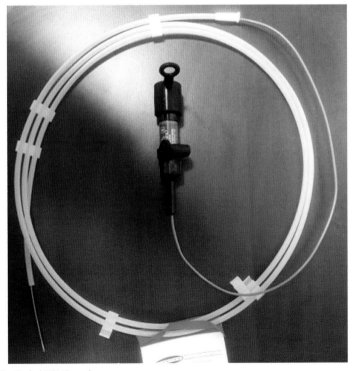

Figure 11-22. Radial EBUS probe.

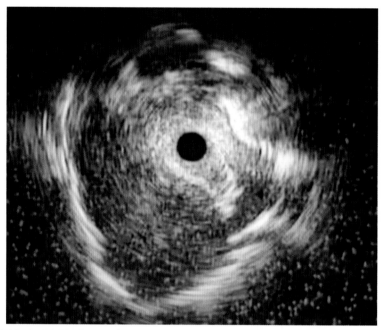

Figure 11-23. An RP-EBUS view of a malignant lung nodule. The dark central circle represents the RP-EBUS probe in a central position relative to the nodule. Notice the heterogeneous lesion and bright margin of the lesion around the probe.

smaller and tortuous airways. This is why this technique is often combined with ENB to provide better navigation and maneuverability.

While studies have shown a diagnostic yield of around 70% with RP-EBUS alone, real-world experience has been less impressive, with yields around 57% in the ACCP ACQuIRE bronchoscopy registry.[66,67] The biggest predictor of yield is the location of the RP-EBUS probe in relation to the lesion, with a more central location (as shown in Figure 11-23) associated with higher yields.[40] RP-EBUS probe can also be used to study tumor invasion of the tracheobronchial wall as in centrally located lung malignancies. This can help evaluate whether these central tumors are actually invading the trachea or simply abutting the central airways without actual tissue invasion. Herth et al. studied 131 consecutive such patients and found RP-EBUS had a sensitivity of 89%, specificity of 100%, and accuracy of 94% for assessing tumor invasion.[68] RP-EBUS performed better than CT in this study.

Electromagnetic navigation bronchoscopy involves uploading the patient's CT to planning software. The computer uses the information from the axial, coronal, and sagittal views of the CT to generate a virtual bronchoscopy view and a 3-dimensional tracheobronchial tree (**Figure 11-24**). The bronchoscopist selects the target of interest and locates any airway that may lead to the target on the CT. The planning software then generates a pathway from the central airways to the lesion. During bronchoscopy, an EWC that houses a steerable locatable guide (LG) is used to travel through the airways while the computer tracks the position of the LG in an electromagnetic field that surrounds the patient and provides instructions on where to make the turns. Once the

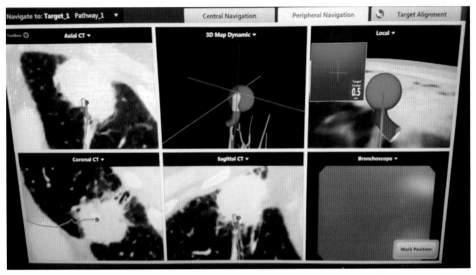

Figure 11-24. Electromagnetic bronchoscopy screen as seen during a procedure. The "green ball" represents the center of the lesion. Virtual view and triplanar CT views are depicted simultaneously.

LG is within a centimeter of the lesion, the LG can be removed, leaving the EWC in place. When combined technologies are utilized, an RP-EBUS probe can then be passed through the EWC at this point to obtain a real-time image of the lesion. The position of the probe is correlated with the patient's chest imaging and fluoroscopic view. RP-EBUS probe is then removed and samples obtained through the EWC using needles, brushes and biopsy forceps. The diagnostic yield of ENB with or without RP-EBUS has been very variable, ranging from 38.5% to 74%.[66,67,69] This wide variation in diagnostic yield can be due to a wide range of motion of pulmonary nodules during the respiration cycle, as shown in study by Chen et al.[70] In this study, the average motion of all nodules was 17.6 mm, with lower lobe nodules having greater motion than upper lobe nodules. Ongoing technologic advances in navigation bronchoscopy promise more accurate and real-time sampling of PPLs in the near future.

Virtual bronchoscopy with ultrathin bronchoscopy involves using planning software to reconstruct a virtual tracheobronchial tree. This can be combined with UB with a scope with an outer diameter of 2.8 mm that can be advanced under virtual guidance to visualize up to the ninth-generation airway. Diagnostic yields around 70% have been reported in the literature.[67] The small size of the tissue samples obtained with UB would be concerning when considering molecular analysis for lung cancer.[40]

Guided bronchoscopy has a good safety profile, with a pneumothorax rate of 1.5% in a meta-analysis of 39 studies including 3,052 patients.[67]

THERAPEUTIC BRONCHOSCOPY IN LUNG CANCER

The therapeutic role of bronchoscopy in lung cancer includes management of complications caused by the tumor or therapies. These problems can include hemoptysis, trachea-broncho-esophageal fistulas and airway stenosis from tumors or postradiation strictures (**Figures 11-25** through **11-31**). Bronchoscopy can also be used to assist in

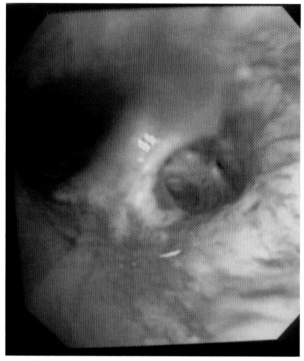

Figure 11-25. Postradiation scarring of left upper lobe anterior segment bronchus.

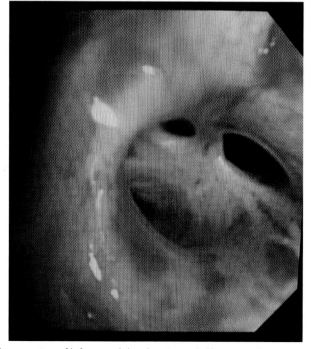

Figure 11-26. Close-up view of left upper lobe showing web-like postradiation scar.

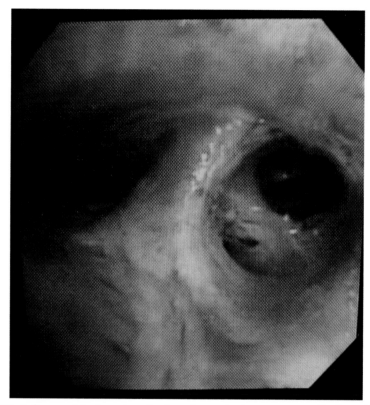

Figure 11-27. Left upper lobe bronchus after bronchoscopic electrocautery and balloon dilation showing normal-appearing bronchial orifice.

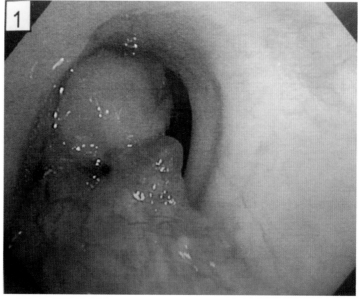

Figure 11-28. Large endobronchial malignant tumor in distal trachea causing near-complete obstruction of trachea and left main stem bronchus.

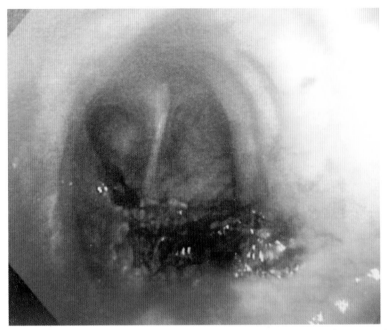

Figure 11-29. Distal trachea and bilateral main stem bronchi completely patent after tumor debulking with electrocautery.

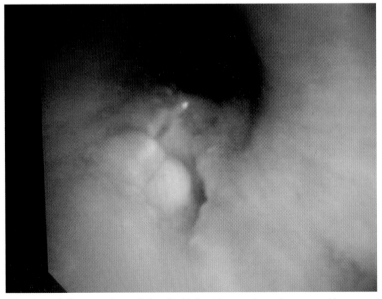

Figure 11-30. Large defect seen in medial wall of left main stem bronchus caused by tumor infiltration and radiation therapy.

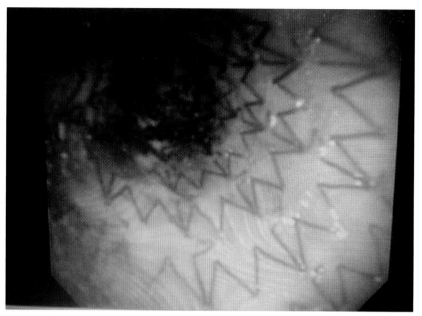

Figure 11-31. The same area after hybrid covered airway stent placement.

radiation therapy for lung cancer by placing fiducial markers and endobronchial brachytherapy catheters. Bronchoscopic intratumoral use of various antitumor agents has been tried in the past.[71] Bronchoscopic radio-frequency ablation (RFA) of lung cancer is also on the horizon.[71] A detailed discussion of the different bronchoscopic therapeutic modalities is beyond the scope of this book. **Table 11-1** highlights some of the common indications and available therapeutic interventions.

TABLE 11-1 Therapeutic Bronchoscopy and Indications in Lung Cancer	
Hemoptysis	Laser bronchoscopy, electrocautery, APC, airway stent placement
Complex airway stenosis (from tumor or postradiation fibrosis)	Laser bronchoscopy, electrocautery, APC, balloon dilation, PDT, cryodebridement, airway stent placement
Local endobronchial CIS	Laser bronchoscopy, electrocautery, APC, PDT
Airway perforation, fistulas	Airway stenting (metal, hybrid, silicone stents)
Assistance with radiation therapy	Fiducial marker placement, endobronchial brachytherapy catheter placement

APC, argon plasma coagulation; PDT, photodynamic therapy.

MOLECULAR MARKERS

Emily Jonczak, MD, Raja Mudad, MD, FACP

A 56-year-old male with a history of smoking presented to the clinic with complaints of cough and shortness of breath. He was found to have stage IV adenocarcinoma of the lung. Which molecular markers should be tested in this patient?

Learning Objectives:
1. Which molecular markers are found in lung cancer?
2. Which most common types of patients have molecular mutations?
3. Which patients should be tested for molecular mutations?
4. Which tests should be used?

The advent of molecular genetic testing has revolutionized the treatment of several different types of cancers, including NSCLC. Our ability to detect and understand how molecular genetic variations alter the pathogenesis and ultimately treatment of NSCLC has ushered in an era of practice-changing studies. In the past, treatment decisions have primarily been based on the clinicopathological staging and histology of the tumor, classically divided into two subgroups: SCLC and NSCLC.[72] In the last decade, it has become evident that NSCLC can be further divided into biologically heterogeneous subgroups based on molecular mutations to different cellular pathways. These discoveries have allowed for the development of specific genetic testing to become available and the advent of treatments that target these aberrant pathways, leading us away from the traditional platinum-based cytotoxic chemotherapy to targeted treatments.[73,74]

MOLECULAR MARKERS IN ADENOCARCINOMA NON–SMALL CELL LUNG CANCER

Multiple oncogenic driver mutations have been identified in NSCLC, particularly in adenocarcinoma, including, in order of prevalence, KRAS, EGFR, ALK, RET, BRAF, PI3K, MET, HER2, ROS1, MEK1, AKT1, FGFR1, VEGFR, and PDGFR. These so-called driver mutations induce the transformation from a benign cell to a malignant cell and result in constitutive activation of mutant signaling proteins sustaining tumorigenesis.[74-76] In development of targeted therapies, driver mutations are optimal candidates, as tumor cells are reliant on their activation for survival.[74]

MOLECULAR MARKERS

Molecular genetic testing has become the standard of care in the pathologic analysis of tissue samples for patients with advanced adenocarcinoma of the lung (**Figure 11-32**).[77,78] A limiting factor for this analysis has been appropriate tissue sampling and the amount available for review. Historically, the preferred method has been surgical resection or core needle biopsy due to the increased amount of tissue available with these modalities.[76] Several recent studies supported the use of minimally invasive techniques, including EBUS, to obtain cytologic specimens for testing.[74,76] A recent large multicenter study of 774 cytologic specimens obtained via EBUS reported that EGFR mutation analysis

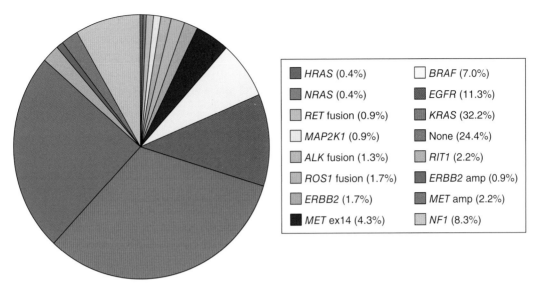

Figure 11-32. Adenocarcinoma markers. (Reproduced with permission from Cancer Genome Atlas Research Network: Comprehensive molecular profiling of lung adenocarcinoma. *Nature.* 2014;511(7511):543-50. Copyright © 2014, Springer Nature.)

was possible in 90% of the specimens for which it was requested.[79] Similar examples exist for testing ALK fusion genes and multiple-gene mutation analysis.[80,81] In addition to the use of cytology specimens, the use of liquid biopsies has become an acceptable alternative, especially in situations where adequate tissue is not available. A liquid biopsy is a blood draw in which the patient's blood sample undergoes centrifugation in order to collect plasma and isolate DNA shed by the tumor, known as cell-free DNA (cfDNA). The cfDNA undergoes analysis for multiple molecular mutations.[82] Finally, variations in testing exist across laboratories; therefore, only laboratories accredited by the Clinical Laboratory Improvement Amendments (CLIA) should be utilized for testing.[76]

Various methods of testing are used to assess for these multiple genomic alterations. Real-time polymerase chain reaction (PCR) and Sanger sequencing can be used to target specific mutations. Multiplex PCR systems can be used to detect multiple point mutations simultaneously (eg, Sequenom MassARRAY and SNapShot Multiplex system). In order to detect gene rearrangements, fluorescence in situ hybridization (FISH) is utilized. Increasingly, laboratories are using next-generation sequencing (NGS) to detect both point mutations and gene rearrangements, but this must be completed in a validated laboratory with CLIA accreditation.[76]

The NCCN recommends that all patients with adenocarcinoma histology, non-squamous NSCLC, and NSCLC not otherwise specified (NOS) be tested for EGFR mutations and have routine comprehensive testing for ALK gene rearrangements, ROS1 rearrangements, BRAF mutations, and programmed death (PD-1) receptor expression levels as all of these biomarkers have treatment options approved by the Food and Drug Administration (FDA).[78]

These various genetic mutations are typically mutually exclusive and do not occur together. A mutation in KRAS is a prognostic marker and may indicate patients who would not benefit from further molecular testing if present.[78] Additionally, although rare, ALK rearrangements mutations and EGFR mutations can be seen in patients with mixed squamous histology. Therefore, it is recommended that any patient with mixed histology, with squamous cell histology with a history of never smoking, and with small tissue samples used for testing be assessed for EGFR mutations and ALK gene rearrangements.[78]

Molecular Markers and Clinical Implications
KRAS Mutation

KRAS mutations are found in approximately 25% of patients with adenocarcinoma, making it the most common mutation found. KRAS proteins are a family of guanine nucleotide-binding proteins that have an important role in intracellular signaling pathways. Activating point mutations, typically occurring at codon 12, of this proto-oncogene lead to unregulated signaling through the MAP/ERK pathway.[83-85]

KRAS mutations are considered prognostic biomarkers as patients with mutations have poor survival when compared to those with wild-type KRAS. In addition, there is a clinical and therapeutic benefit to knowing if a patient has a KRAS mutation as these patients generally lack therapeutic benefit from treatment with targeted therapy, but the presence of a mutation does not appear to alter the efficacy of chemotherapy.[83-85]

> **CLINICAL PEARL:** Mutations in KRAS have been shown to be more prevalent among those patients who are older, with a smoking history, who are of the white race, and who have a lower frequency of bone metastasis.[5] These clinical features should not determine who is tested for the mutation.

Epidermal Growth Factor Receptor Mutation

The EGFR belongs to a family of growth factor receptor proteins, which consist of an extracellular ligand-binding domain, a transmembrane structure, and an intracellular tyrosine kinase domain normally found on the surface of epithelial cells. When binding of ligand to receptor occurs, there is activation of the receptor, resulting in dimerization and autophosphorylation of tyrosine kinase, leading to a cascade of cellular events.[86,87]

The two most common gene mutations on the EGFR are deletions on exon 19 and the L858R missense mutation on exon 21. Together, these mutations account for approximately 90% of EGFR mutations found in NSCLC and result in activation of the tyrosine kinase domain, constitutively activating cellular pathways and inhibiting cell death.[74] These are referred to as sensitizing EGFR mutations given their sensitivity to treatment with targeted therapy. There are additional, less common mutations, accounting for approximately 10%, which include exon 19 insertions, p.L861Q, p.G719X, and p.S768I. These mutations have also been found to be sensitive to targeted therapy.[74,88]

Resistance to targeted therapy has been shown in patients with EGFR exon 20 insertion mutations and p.T790M, which is typically found in relapsed disease. If a p.T790M mutation is noted prior to treatment with targeted therapies, the patient should be referred to genetic counseling as this is suggestive of a germline mutation and has significance in familial lung cancers.[89]

> **CLINICAL PEARL:** The EGFR mutations are typically mutually exclusive of KRAS and ALK rearrangements. They are more common among never-smokers, women, and those of Asian descent; however, they are not found exclusively among this cohort of patients.[74] A recent study examined 2,124 lung adenocarcinoma specimens with EGFR mutations and found that although mutations were common among never-smokers and women, there was a significant number found among smokers and men.[74,90,91] Therefore, these clinical features should not determine which patients undergoing testing.

As for testing, EGFR mutations should be assessed with DNA mutational analysis. IHC is not recommended. Test methods include: real-time PCR, Sanger sequencing, NGS, and mutation screening assays using multiplex PCR.[74,76]

Anaplastic Lymphoma Kinase Gene Rearrangement

Anaplastic lymphoma kinase is a receptor tyrosine kinase originally identified in a subset of anaplastic large cell lymphomas. In approximately 2%-7% of patients with NSCLC, an inversion of the short arm of chromosome 2 results in the fusion of a protein encoded by echinoderm microtubule-associated protein-like 4 (EML4) gene with ALK receptor tyrosine kinase, resulting in EML4-ALK translocation. This translocation results in activation of the ALK receptor tyrosine kinase, leading to inappropriate signaling through the ALK tyrosine kinase domain.[74,92] The presence of this rearrangement is associated with sensitivity to targeted treatment.

> **CLINICAL PEARL:** The EML4-ALK translocation is more commonly appreciated in patients younger than 55 years, men, and non-smokers; however, these clinical features should not be used when selecting patients who should be tested for ALK rearrangement.[3,19,20]

Regarding testing, a FISH break-apart probe was the first utilized method. IHC can be utilized as an effective screening modality, but if positive, then FISH analysis should be done. NGS can also be used to detect ALK fusions.[74,76,93]

ROS1 Rearrangements

Approximately 2% of patient with NSCLC have been found to have ROS1 gene rearrangement. ROS1 is a tyrosine kinase of the insulin receptor family located on chromosome 6. Gene rearrangements of ROS1 lead to inappropriate signaling through the ROS1 kinase domain.[94,95] The presence of this rearrangement is associated with sensitivity to targeted therapy.

> **CLINICAL PEARL:** ROS1 rearrangement is more commonly seen in younger women, never-smokers, those with adenocarcinoma histology, and those negative for EGFR mutation, KRAS mutation, and ALK rearrangement. These clinical features should not be used as the basis for patient selection for testing.

Regarding testing, a FISH break-apart probe similar to that used to detect ALK rearrangements is used to test. IHC can be utilized; however, this is only a screening modality, and confirmatory FISH testing is required. NGS can be used to assess if ROS1 rearrangements are present if appropriately designed and validated to detect ROS1 rearrangement.[94,95]

BRAF Mutation

BRAF (v-Raf murine sarcoma viral oncogene homolog 6) is a serine/threonine kinase part of the MAP/ERK signaling pathway, and mutations result in unregulated signaling through this pathway. BRAF mutations are found in approximately 1%-2% of patients with NSCLC.[96] About half of the mutations in NSCLC are BRAF V600E, for which targeted therapy has been studied. Other mutations in BRAF can be seen in NSCLC, but the clinical relevance of these mutations has yet to be determined with regard to treatment options.[96]

> **CLINICAL PEARL:** Mutations in BRAF V600E are more commonly found in patients with a history of smoking. Mutations in BRAF do not typically occur concurrently with EGFR mutations and ALK rearrangements.[96]

Testing uses real-time PCR, Sanger sequencing, and NGS.[6]

Other Mutations (HER, RET, MET)

Other, less common, driver mutations and gene rearrangements have been identified, including RET gene rearrangements, HER2 (also known as ERBB2), and MET. Targeted treatment is available for these mutations, but is approved for other indications; thus, the NCCN recommends broader molecular profiling to identify these rare mutations that may potentially benefit from targeted therapy.[78]

In addition, in all advanced-stage NSCLC regardless of histology, the PD-L1 expression should be measured. PD-1 is expressed on activated T cells in the tumor microenvironment. Tumors can express the ligand PD-L1 which binds to PD-1 and downregulates the immune response within the tumor. Monoclonal antibodies against PD-1 and PD-L1 have been developed and are currently approved in the treatment of NSCLC, improving antitumor immunity.[97]

MOLECULAR MARKERS IN SQUAMOUS CELL NON–SMALL CELL LUNG CARCINOMA

The discovery and understanding of molecular mutations and implementation of targeted therapies has disproportionally impacted adenocarcinoma when compared to squamous cell cancer. Many of the driver mutations found in adenocarcinoma are not found or found very rarely in squamous cell carcinoma. Despite this, efforts are being made to pursue potential targetable mutations, including FGFR1, EGFR, DDR2, PIK3CA, SOX2, IGF1R, EphA2, MET, PDGFRA, p53/MDM2, AKT, EGFR, LKB1, PTEN, and NRF2/KEAP1. The development of these potentially targetable mutations is actively under investigation on clinical trials.

Programmed Death Ligand 1

Program death ligand 1 is a transmembrane protein involved in immunosuppression. PD-L1 is the ligand for PD-1, and the binding of the two on activated T lymphocytes disrupts PD-1 signaling and effectively downregulates effector T-cell functions. In normal cells this maintains self-tolerance and helps prevent autoimmunity. In the setting of tumor cells, the binding of PD-L1 to PD-1 assists in protecting tumor cells from elimination by the immune system.[97] PD-L1 expression on tumor cells has been the focus of significant research and the development of checkpoint inhibitors. These monoclonal antibodies block either PD-L1 or PD-1 and improve antitumor immunity.[98,99]

> **CLINICAL PEARL:** All patients, regardless of histology, with NSCLC should have PD-L1 expression assessed by IHC, ideally prior to any first-line treatment. PD-L1 expression of greater than 1% can alter treatment decisions, and therapy should include a checkpoint inhibitor barring no contraindications.[99]

Regarding testing, IHC that focuses on the proportion of tumor cells expressing membranous staining at any level is used.

REFERENCES

1. Siegel RL, Miller KD, Jemal A. Cancer statistics, 2018. *CA Cancer J Clin.* 2018;68(1):7-30. Epub 2018/01/10. doi:10.3322/caac.21442.
2. U.S. Preventive Services Task Force Recommendation Statement. Screening for Lung Cancer, 2013.
3. Pham D, Bhandari S, Oechsli M, Pinkston C, Kloecker G. Lung cancer screening rates: data from the lung cancer screening registry. *J Clin Oncol.* 2018;36(15_suppl):6504.
4. Hyde L, Hyde CI. Clinical manifestations of lung cancer. *Chest.* 1974;65(3):299-306. Epub 1974/03/01.
5. Kocher F, Hilbe W, Seeber A, et al. Longitudinal analysis of 2293 NSCLC patients: a comprehensive study from the TYROL registry. *Lung Cancer.* 2015;87(2):193-200. Epub 2015/01/08. doi:10.1016/j.lungcan.2014.12.006.
6. Lim WS, Baudouin SV, George RC, et al. BTS guidelines for the management of community acquired pneumonia in adults: update 2009. *Thorax.* 2009;64(Suppl 3):iii1-iii55. doi:10.1136/thx.2009.121434.
7. Tang KL, Eurich DT, Minhas-Sandhu JK, Marrie TJ, Majumdar SR. Incidence, correlates, and chest radiographic yield of new lung cancer diagnosis in 3398 patients with pneumonia. *Arch Intern Med.* 2011;171(13):1193-1198. Epub 2011/04/27. doi:10.1001/archinternmed.2011.155.
8. Okoli GN, Kostopoulou O, Delaney BC. Is symptom-based diagnosis of lung cancer possible? A systematic review and meta-analysis of symptomatic lung cancer prior to diagnosis for comparison with real-time data from routine general practice. *PLoS One.* 2018;13(11):e0207686. Epub 2018/11/22. doi:10.1371/journal.pone.0207686.
9. Myers KA, Farquhar DR. The rational clinical examination. Does this patient have clubbing? *JAMA.* 2001;286(3):341-347. Epub 2001/07/24.
10. Yu JB, Wilson LD, Detterbeck FC. Superior vena cava syndrome—a proposed classification system and algorithm for management. *J Thorac Oncol.* 2008;3(8):811-814. Epub 2008/08/02. doi:10.1097/JTO.0b013e3181804791.
11. List AF, Hainsworth JD, Davis BW, Hande KR, Greco FA, Johnson DH. The syndrome of inappropriate secretion of antidiuretic hormone (SIADH) in small-cell lung cancer. *J Clin Oncol.* 1986;4(8):1191-1198. Epub 1986/08/01. doi:10.1200/jco.1986.4.8.1191.
12. Izumi M, Takayama K, Yabuuchi H, Abe K, Nakanishi Y. Incidence of hypertrophic pulmonary osteoarthropathy associated with primary lung cancer. *Respirology.* 2010;15(5):809-812. Epub 2010/05/26. doi:10.1111/j.1440-1843.2010.01769.x.
13. Gozzard P, Woodhall M, Chapman C, et al. Paraneoplastic neurologic disorders in small cell lung carcinoma: a prospective study. *Neurology.* 2015;85(3):235-239. Epub 2015/06/26. doi:10.1212/wnl.0000000000001721.
14. Graus F, Delattre JY, Antoine JC, et al. Recommended diagnostic criteria for paraneoplastic neurological syndromes. *J Neurol Neurosurg Psychiatry.* 2004;75(8):1135-1140. Epub 2004/07/20. doi:10.1136/jnnp.2003.034447.

15. Shepherd FA, Laskey J, Evans WK, Goss PE, Johansen E, Khamsi F. Cushing's syndrome associated with ectopic corticotropin production and small-cell lung cancer. *J Clin Oncol.* 1992;10(1):21-27. Epub 1992/01/01. doi:10.1200/jco.1992.10.1.21.

16. National Comprehensive Cancer Network. Small Cell Lung Cancer 2018. https://www.nccn.org/professionals/physician_gls/pdf/sclc.pdf. Accessed December 6, 2018; Version 1.2019.

17. National Comprehensive Cancer Network. Non-Small Cell Lung Cancer 2018. https://www.nccn.org/professionals/physician_gls/pdf/nscl.pdf. Accessed December 6, 2018; Version 2.2019.

18. Brant WE, Helms CA. *Fundamentals of Diagnostic Radiology.* Philadelphia, PA: Lippincott, Williams & Wilkins; 2007.

19. Ashizawa K, Hayashi K, Aso N, Minami K. Lobar atelectasis: diagnostic pitfalls on chest radiography. *Br J Radiol.* 2001;74(877):89-97. Epub 2001/03/03. doi:10.1259/bjr.74.877.740089.

20. Collins J SE. *Chest Radiology.* 2nd ed. Philadelphia, PA: Lippincott, Williams & Wilkins; 2008.

21. Mascalchi M, Sali L. Lung cancer screening with low dose CT and radiation harm-from prediction models to cancer incidence data. *Ann Transl Med.* 2017;5(17):360. Epub 2017/09/25. doi:10.21037/atm.2017.06.41.

22. Fischer BM, Lassen U, Hojgaard L. PET-CT in preoperative staging of lung cancer. *N Engl J Med.* 2011;364(10):980-981. Epub 2011/03/11. doi:10.1056/NEJMc1012974.

23. Zeliadt SB, Loggers ET, Slatore CG, et al. Preoperative PET and the reduction of unnecessary surgery among newly diagnosed lung cancer patients in a community setting. *J Nucl Med.* 2014;55(3):379-385. Epub 2014/01/23. doi:10.2967/jnumed.113.124230.

24. Sheikhbahaei S, Mena E, Yanamadala A, et al. The value of FDG PET/CT in treatment response assessment, follow-up, and surveillance of lung cancer. *AJR Am J Roentgenol.* 2017;208(2):420-433. Epub 2016/10/12. doi:10.2214/ajr.16.16532.

25. Antoniou AJ, Marcus C, Tahari AK, Wahl RL, Subramaniam RM. Follow-up or surveillance (18)F-FDG PET/CT and survival outcome in lung cancer patients. *J Nucl Med.* 2014;55(7):1062-1068. Epub 2014/04/30. doi:10.2967/jnumed.113.136770.

26. Engels EA. Epidemiology of thymoma and associated malignancies. *J Thorac Oncol.* 2010;5(10 Suppl 4): S260-S265. Epub 2010/10/05. doi:10.1097/JTO.0b013e3181f1f62d.

27. Schoenmaekers J, Dingemans AC, Hendriks LEL. Brain imaging in early stage non-small cell lung cancer: still a controversial topic? *J Thorac Dis.* 2018;10(Suppl 18):S2168-S2171. Epub 2018/08/21. doi:10.21037/jtd.2018.06.68.

28. Hudson Z, Internullo E, Edey A, Laurence I, Bianchi D, Addeo A. Brain imaging before primary lung cancer resection: a controversial topic. *Ecancermedicalscience.* 2017;11:749. Epub 2017/07/19. doi:10.3332/ecancer.2017.749.

29. Nayar G, Ejikeme T, Chongsathidkiet P, et al. Leptomeningeal disease: current diagnostic and therapeutic strategies. *Oncotarget.* 2017;8(42):73312-73328. Epub 2017/10/27. doi:10.18632/oncotarget.20272.

30. Parker MS, Chasen MH, Paul N. Radiologic signs in thoracic imaging: case-based review and self-assessment module. *AJR Am J Roentgenol.* 2009;192(3 Suppl):S34-S48. Epub 2009/03/03. doi:10.2214/ajr.07.7081.

31. Torigian D RP. *Radiology Secrets Plus.* 4th ed. Philadelphia, Pennsylvania: Elsevier; 2016.

32. Eren S, Karaman A, Okur A. The superior vena cava syndrome caused by malignant disease. Imaging with multi-detector row CT. *Eur J Radiol.* 2006;59(1):93-103. Epub 2006/02/16. doi:10.1016/j.ejrad.2006.01.003.

33. Yazawa T, Ishii H, Ito T, et al. Colliding primary lung cancers of adenosquamous carcinoma and large cell neuroendocrine carcinoma. *Pathol Int.* 2003;53(1):58-65. Epub 2003/02/01.

34. Truong MT, Viswanathan C, Godoy MB, Carter BW, Marom EM. Malignant pleural mesothelioma: role of CT, MRI, and PET/CT in staging evaluation and treatment considerations. *Semin Roentgenol.* 2013;48(4):323-334. Epub 2013/09/17. doi:10.1053/j.ro.2013.03.017.

35. Webb R BW, Major N. *Fundamentals of Body CT.* 4th ed. Philadelphia, PA: Saunders; 2014.

36. Heelan RT, Demas BE, Caravelli JF, et al. Superior sulcus tumors: CT and MR imaging. *Radiology.* 1989;170 (3 Pt 1):637-641. Epub 1989/03/01. doi:10.1148/radiology.170.3.2916014.

37. Shimada Y, Saji H, Kakihana M, et al. Retrospective analysis of nodal spread patterns according to tumor location in pathological N2 non-small cell lung cancer. *World J Surg.* 2012;36(12):2865-2871. Epub 2012/09/06. doi:10.1007/s00268-012-1743-5.

38. Kim AW. Lymph node drainage patterns and micrometastasis in lung cancer. *Semin Thorac Cardiovasc Surg.* 2009;21(4):298-308. Epub 2009/01/01. doi:10.1053/j.semtcvs.2009.11.001.

39. Lin CY, Chung FT. Central airway tumors: interventional bronchoscopy in diagnosis and management. *J Thorac Dis.* 2016;8(10):E1168-E1176. Epub 2016/11/22. doi:10.21037/jtd.2016.10.101.

40. Leong S, Shaipanich T, Lam S, Yasufuku K. Diagnostic bronchoscopy—current and future perspectives. *J Thorac Dis.* 2013;5(Suppl 5):S498-510. Epub 2013/10/29. doi:10.3978/j.issn.2072-1439.2013.09.08.

41. Vincent BD, Fraig M, Silvestri GA. A pilot study of narrow-band imaging compared to white light bronchoscopy for evaluation of normal airways and premalignant and malignant airways disease. *Chest.* 2007;131(6): 1794-1799. Epub 2007/05/17. doi:10.1378/chest.06-2794.

42. Zaric B, Becker HD, Perin B, et al. Narrow band imaging videobronchoscopy improves assessment of lung cancer extension and influences therapeutic strategy. *Jpn J Clin Oncol.* 2009;39(10):657-663. Epub 2009/08/04. doi:10.1093/jjco/hyp083.

43. Shibuya K, Hoshino H, Chiyo M, et al. High magnification bronchovideoscopy combined with narrow band imaging could detect capillary loops of angiogenic squamous dysplasia in heavy smokers at high risk for lung cancer. *Thorax.* 2003;58(11):989-995. Epub 2003/10/31.

44. Shibuya K, Nakajima T, Fujiwara T, et al. Narrow band imaging with high-resolution bronchovideoscopy: a new approach for visualizing angiogenesis in squamous cell carcinoma of the lung. *Lung Cancer.* 2010;69(2): 194-202. Epub 2010/06/15. doi:10.1016/j.lungcan.2010.04.023.

45. Rivera MP, Mehta AC, Wahidi MM. Establishing the diagnosis of lung cancer: diagnosis and management of lung cancer, 3rd ed: American College of Chest Physicians evidence-based clinical practice guidelines. *Chest.* 2013;143(5 Suppl):e142S-e165S. Epub 2013/05/10. doi:10.1378/chest.12-2353.

46. Schreiber G, McCrory DC. Performance characteristics of different modalities for diagnosis of suspected lung cancer: summary of published evidence. *Chest.* 2003;123(1 Suppl):115S-128S. Epub 2003/01/16.

47. Asano F, Aoe M, Ohsaki Y, et al. Deaths and complications associated with respiratory endoscopy: a survey by the Japan Society for Respiratory Endoscopy in 2010. *Respirology.* 2012;17(3):478-485. Epub 2012/01/10. doi:10.1111/j.1440-1843.2011.02123.x.

48. Milman N, Faurschou P, Munch EP, Grode G. Transbronchial lung biopsy through the fibre optic bronchoscope. Results and complications in 452 examinations. *Respir Med.* 1994;88(10):749-753. Epub 1994/11/01.

49. Wiener RS, Schwartz LM, Woloshin S, Welch HG. Population-based risk for complications after transthoracic needle lung biopsy of a pulmonary nodule: an analysis of discharge records. *Ann Intern Med.* 2011;155(3): 137-144. Epub 2011/08/04. doi:10.7326/0003-4819-155-3-201108020-00003.

50. Bezel P, Tischler V, Robinson C, et al. Diagnostic value of bronchoalveolar lavage for diagnosis of suspected peripheral lung cancer. *Clin Lung Cancer.* 2016;17(5):e151-e156. Epub 2016/02/03. doi:10.1016/j.cllc.2015.12.012.

51. Chuzi S, Tavora F, Cruz M, et al. Clinical features, diagnostic challenges, and management strategies in checkpoint inhibitor-related pneumonitis. *Cancer Manag Res.* 2017;9:207-213. Epub 2017/06/28. doi:10.2147/CMAR.S136818.

52. Silvestri GA, Gonzalez AV, Jantz MA, et al. Methods for staging non-small cell lung cancer: diagnosis and management of lung cancer, 3rd ed: American College of Chest Physicians evidence-based clinical practice guidelines. *Chest.* 2013;143(5 Suppl):e211S-e250S. Epub 2013/05/10. doi:10.1378/chest.12-2355.

53. Herth FJ, Krasnik M, Kahn N, Eberhardt R, Ernst A. Combined endoscopic-endobronchial ultrasound-guided fine-needle aspiration of mediastinal lymph nodes through a single bronchoscope in 150 patients with suspected lung cancer. *Chest.* 2010;138(4):790-794. Epub 2010/02/16. doi:10.1378/chest.09-2149.

54. Hwangbo B, Lee GK, Lee HS, et al. Transbronchial and transesophageal fine-needle aspiration using an ultrasound bronchoscope in mediastinal staging of potentially operable lung cancer. *Chest.* 2010;138(4):795-802. Epub 2010/03/30. doi:10.1378/chest.09-2100.

55. Chouaid C, Salaun M, Gounant V, et al. Clinical efficacy and cost-effectiveness of endobronchial ultrasound-guided transbronchial needle aspiration for preoperative staging of non-small-cell lung cancer: results of a French prospective multicenter trial (EVIEPEB). *PLoS One.* 2019;14(1):e0208992. Epub 2019/01/08. doi:10.1371/journal.pone.0208992.

56. Grove DA, Bechara RI, Josephs JS, Berkowitz DM. Comparative cost analysis of endobronchial ultrasound-guided and blind TBNA in the evaluation of hilar and mediastinal lymphadenopathy. *J Bronchology Interv Pulmonol.* 2012;19(3):182-187. Epub 2012/12/05. doi:10.1097/LBR.0b013e31825fdc52.

57. Sharples LD, Jackson C, Wheaton E, et al. Clinical effectiveness and cost-effectiveness of endobronchial and endoscopic ultrasound relative to surgical staging in potentially resectable lung cancer: results from the ASTER randomised controlled trial. *Health Technol Assess.* 2012;16(18):1-75, iii-iv. Epub 2012/04/05. doi:10.3310/hta16180.

58. Crombag L, Szlubowski A, Stigt JA, et al. EUS-B-FNA vs conventional EUS-FNA for left adrenal gland analysis in lung cancer patients. *Lung Cancer.* 2017;108:38-44. Epub 2017/06/20. doi:10.1016/j.lungcan.2017.02.011.

59. Meena N, Hulett C, Jeffus S, Bartter T. Left adrenal biopsy using the convex curvilinear ultrasound scope. *Respiration.* 2015;89(1):57-61. Epub 2014/12/17. doi:10.1159/000368370.

60. Labarca G, Folch E, Jantz M, Mehta HJ, Majid A, Fernandez-Bussy S. Adequacy of samples obtained by endobronchial ultrasound with transbronchial needle aspiration for molecular analysis in patients with non-small

cell lung cancer. Systematic review and meta-analysis. *Ann Am Thorac Soc.* 2018;15(10):1205-1216. Epub 2018/07/17. doi:10.1513/AnnalsATS.201801-045OC.

61. Biswas A, Leon ME, Drew P, et al. Clinical performance of endobronchial ultrasound-guided transbronchial needle aspiration for assessing programmed death ligand-1 expression in nonsmall cell lung cancer. *Diagn Cytopathol.* 2018;46(5):378-383. Epub 2018/02/25. doi:10.1002/dc.23900.

62. Smith A, Wang H, Zerbo A, et al. PD-L1 testing of EBUS-TBNA samples acquired for the diagnosis and staging of non-small cell lung cancer: feasibility and results. *Am J Respir Crit Care Med*; May 22 2018; San Diego, USA2018. p. A6158.

63. Colella S, Scarlata S, Bonifazi M, et al. Biopsy needles for mediastinal lymph node sampling by endosonography: current knowledge and future perspectives. *J Thorac Dis.* 2018;10(12):6960-6968. Epub 2019/02/13. doi:10.21037/jtd.2018.11.35.

64. Herth FJ, Annema JT, Eberhardt R, et al. Endobronchial ultrasound with transbronchial needle aspiration for restaging the mediastinum in lung cancer. *J Clin Oncol.* 2008;26(20):3346-3350. Epub 2008/06/04. doi:10.1200/JCO.2007.14.9229.

65. Eapen GA, Shah AM, Lei X, et al. Complications, consequences, and practice patterns of endobronchial ultrasound-guided transbronchial needle aspiration: results of the AQuIRE registry. *Chest.* 2013;143(4):1044-1053. Epub 2012/11/03. doi:10.1378/chest.12-0350.

66. Ost DE, Ernst A, Lei X, et al. Diagnostic yield and complications of bronchoscopy for peripheral lung lesions. Results of the AQuIRE registry. *Am J Respir Crit Care Med.* 2016;193(1):68-77. Epub 2015/09/15. doi:10.1164/rccm.201507-1332OC.

67. Wang Memoli JS, Nietert PJ, Silvestri GA. Meta-analysis of guided bronchoscopy for the evaluation of the pulmonary nodule. *Chest.* 2012;142(2):385-393. Epub 2011/10/08. doi:10.1378/chest.11-1764.

68. Herth F, Ernst A, Schulz M, Becker H. Endobronchial ultrasound reliably differentiates between airway infiltration and compression by tumor. *Chest.* 2003;123(2):458-462. Epub 2003/02/11.

69. Gex G, Pralong JA, Combescure C, Seijo L, Rochat T, Soccal PM. Diagnostic yield and safety of electromagnetic navigation bronchoscopy for lung nodules: a systematic review and meta-analysis. *Respiration.* 2014;87(2):165-176. Epub 2014/01/10. doi:10.1159/000355710.

70. Chen A, Pastis N, Furukawa B, Silvestri GA. The effect of respiratory motion on pulmonary nodule location during electromagnetic navigation bronchoscopy. *Chest.* 2015;147(5):1275-1281. Epub 2014/10/31. doi:10.1378/chest.14-1425.

71. Harris K, Puchalski J, Sterman D. Recent advances in bronchoscopic treatment of peripheral lung cancers. *Chest.* 2017;151(3):674-685. Epub 2016/06/14. doi:10.1016/j.chest.2016.05.025.

72. Alberts WM, American College of Chest P. Diagnosis and management of lung cancer executive summary: ACCP evidence-based clinical practice guidelines (2nd Edition). *Chest.* 2007;132(3 Suppl):1S-19S. Epub 2007/10/06. doi:10.1378/chest.07-1860.

73. Riess JW, Wakelee HA. Metastatic non-small cell lung cancer management: novel targets and recent clinical advances. *Clin Adv Hematol Oncol.* 2012;10(4):226-234. Epub 2012/06/19.

74. Lazarus DR, Ost DE. How and when to use genetic markers for nonsmall cell lung cancer. *Curr Opin Pulm Med.* 2013;19(4):331-339. Epub 2013/05/30. doi:10.1097/MCP.0b013e328362075c.

75. Lovly C, Horn L, Pao W. Molecular Profiling of Lung Cancer. My Cancer Genome 2018. https://www.mycancergenome.org/content/disease/lung-cancer/. Accessed March 16, 2018.

76. Sholl LM, Aisner DL, Varella-Garcia M, et al. Multi-institutional oncogenic driver mutation analysis in lung adenocarcinoma: the lung cancer mutation consortium experience. *J Thorac Oncol.* 2015;10(5):768-777. Epub 2015/03/05. doi:10.1097/JTO.0000000000000516.

77. Cancer Genome Atlas Research Network. Comprehensive molecular profiling of lung adenocarcinoma. *Nature.* 2014;511(7511):543-550. Epub 2014/08/01. doi:10.1038/nature13385.

78. Network NCC. NCCN Clinical Practice Guidelines in Oncology (NCCN Guidelines®): Non-Small Cell Lung Cancer 2018. https://www.nccn.org/professionals/physician_gls/default.aspx.

79. Navani N, Brown JM, Nankivell M, et al. Suitability of endobronchial ultrasound-guided transbronchial needle aspiration specimens for subtyping and genotyping of non-small cell lung cancer: a multicenter study of 774 patients. *Am J Respir Crit Care Med.* 2012;185(12):1316-1322. Epub 2012/04/17. doi:10.1164/rccm.201202-0294OC.

80. Sakairi Y, Nakajima T, Yasufuku K, et al. EML4-ALK fusion gene assessment using metastatic lymph node samples obtained by endobronchial ultrasound-guided transbronchial needle aspiration. *Clin Cancer Res.* 2010;16(20):4938-4945. Epub 2010/10/12. doi:10.1158/1078-0432.CCR-10-0099.

81. Nakajima T, Yasufuku K, Nakagawara A, Kimura H, Yoshino I. Multigene mutation analysis of metastatic lymph nodes in non-small cell lung cancer diagnosed by endobronchial ultrasound-guided transbronchial needle aspiration. *Chest.* 2011;140(5):1319-1324. Epub 2011/04/30. doi:10.1378/chest.10-3186.

82. Kwapisz D. The first liquid biopsy test approved. Is it a new era of mutation testing for non-small cell lung cancer? *Ann Transl Med*. 2017;5(3):46. Epub 2017/03/03. doi:10.21037/atm.2017.01.32.

83. Roberts PJ, Stinchcombe TE. KRAS mutation: should we test for it, and does it matter? *J Clin Oncol*. 2013;31(8):1112-1121. Epub 2013/02/13. doi:10.1200/JCO.2012.43.0454.

84. Tsao MS, Aviel-Ronen S, Ding K, et al. Prognostic and predictive importance of p53 and RAS for adjuvant chemotherapy in non small-cell lung cancer. *J Clin Oncol*. 2007;25(33):5240-5247. Epub 2007/11/21. doi:10.1200/JCO.2007.12.6953.

85. Eberhard DA, Johnson BE, Amler LC, et al. Mutations in the epidermal growth factor receptor and in KRAS are predictive and prognostic indicators in patients with non-small-cell lung cancer treated with chemotherapy alone and in combination with erlotinib. *J Clin Oncol*. 2005;23(25):5900-5909. Epub 2005/07/27. doi:10.1200/JCO.2005.02.857.

86. Jorissen RN, Walker F, Pouliot N, Garrett TP, Ward CW, Burgess AW. Epidermal growth factor receptor: mechanisms of activation and signalling. *Exp Cell Res*. 2003;284(1):31-53. Epub 2003/03/22.

87. Lynch TJ, Bell DW, Sordella R, et al. Activating mutations in the epidermal growth factor receptor underlying responsiveness of non-small-cell lung cancer to gefitinib. *N Engl J Med*. 2004;350(21):2129-2139. Epub 2004/05/01. doi:10.1056/NEJMoa040938.

88. Riely GJ, Politi KA, Miller VA, Pao W. Update on epidermal growth factor receptor mutations in non-small cell lung cancer. *Clin Cancer Res*. 2006;12(24):7232-7241. Epub 2006/12/26. doi:10.1158/1078-0432.CCR-06-0658.

89. Oxnard GR, Miller VA, Robson ME, et al. Screening for germline EGFR T790M mutations through lung cancer genotyping. *J Thorac Oncol*. 2012;7(6):1049-1052. Epub 2012/05/17. doi:10.1097/JTO.0b013e318250ed9d.

90. D'Angelo SP, Pietanza MC, Johnson ML, et al. Incidence of EGFR exon 19 deletions and L858R in tumor specimens from men and cigarette smokers with lung adenocarcinomas. *J Clin Oncol*. 2011;29(15):2066-2070. Epub 2011/04/13. doi:10.1200/JCO.2010.32.6181.

91. Lindeman NI, Cagle PT, Aisner DL, et al. Updated molecular testing guideline for the selection of lung cancer patients for treatment with targeted tyrosine kinase inhibitors: guideline from the College of American Pathologists, the International Association for the Study of Lung Cancer, and the Association for Molecular Pathology. *J Thorac Oncol*. 2018;13(3):323-358. Epub 2018/02/06. doi:10.1016/j.jtho.2017.12.001.

92. Pillai RN, Ramalingam SS. The biology and clinical features of non-small cell lung cancers with EML4-ALK translocation. *Curr Oncol Rep*. 2012;14(2):105-110. Epub 2012/02/09. doi:10.1007/s11912-012-0213-4.

93. Shaw AT, Solomon B, Kenudson MM. Crizotinib and testing for ALK. *J Natl Compr Can Netw*. 2011;9(12):1335-1341. Epub 2011/12/14.

94. Shaw A, Ou S, Bang Y, et al. Crizotinib in ROS1-rearranged non-small-cell lung cancer. *N Engl J Med*. 2014;371(21):1963-1971. doi:10.1056/NEJMoa1406766.

95. Lim SM, Kim HR, Lee JS, et al. Open-label, multicenter, phase II study of ceritinib in patients with non-small-cell lung cancer harboring ROS1 rearrangement. *J Clin Oncol*. 2017;35(23):2613-2618. Epub 2017/05/19. doi:10.1200/JCO.2016.71.3701.

96. Paik PK, Arcila ME, Fara M, et al. Clinical characteristics of patients with lung adenocarcinomas harboring BRAF mutations. *J Clin Oncol*. 2011;29(15):2046-2051. Epub 2011/04/13. doi:10.1200/JCO.2010.33.1280.

97. Ribas A. Releasing the brakes on cancer immunotherapy. *N Engl J Med*. 2015;373(16):1490-1492. Epub 2015/09/09. doi:10.1056/NEJMp1510079.

98. Duffy MJ, O'Byrne K. Tissue and blood biomarkers in lung cancer: a review. *Adv Clin Chem*. 2018;86:1-21.

99. Hui R, Millward M. *Treatment of Pulmonary Adenocarcinoma with Immune Checkpoint Inhibitors*. Pulmonary Adenocarcinoma: Approaches to Treatment: Elsevier; 2019:151-171.

12

STAGING OF LUNG CANCER

Susanne M. Arnold, MD

A 48-year-old female presents to her primary care physician with a 2-month history of shortness of breath. Chest radiographs reveal a large left upper lobe lung mass and a prominent mediastinum. A computed tomographic (CT) scan of the chest was performed and revealed enlarged aorticopulmonary window lymph nodes and pretracheal mediastinal adenopathy. She undergoes a bronchoscopy with biopsy of the lung mass and endobronchial ultrasound (EBUS)–guided biopsy of the mediastinal lymph nodes, both of which were positive for thyroid transcription factor-1 (TTF-1) adenocarcinoma consistent with lung cancer. What additional tests are needed for completion of staging?

Learning Objectives:
1. What are the current guidelines for staging of non–small cell lung cancer and small cell lung cancer by stage?
2. What are the diagnostic modalities of choice for staging non–small cell and small cell lung cancer?
3. How does the American Joint Committee on Cancer/International Association for the Study of Lung Cancer (AJCC/IASLC) eighth edition of its *Cancer Staging Manual* differ from prior versions of the staging system?

The standard nomenclature of the AJCC remains the tumor, node, metastasis (TNM) staging system, which is an internationally accepted mechanism to accurately describe the anatomic extent of cancer in the human at time of diagnosis. It not only allows communication across the world but also provides a framework for response assessment in clinical trials and the published record. On January 1, 2018, the eighth edition of the AJCC *Cancer Staging Manual* went into effect for all cancer types, including non–small cell and small cell lung cancer.[1,2] The IASLC revised the seventh edition of the AJCC manual, and both the IASCL and AJCC accepted the revision with the 2017 publication of the guidelines.[3,4] Concurrently, the National Comprehensive Cancer Network (NCCN) incorporated these changes into its guidelines.

While small cell carcinoma has traditionally been staged in a simplified nomenclature of "limited" versus "extensive" stage, the AJCC's TNM staging system has been adopted for small cell lung cancer to improve the specificity and reliability in reproducibility of small cell lung cancer staging across countries and in clinical trials.

DIAGNOSTIC EVALUATION

The AJCC and NCCN guidelines also confirm the appropriate evaluation of patients with lung cancer. This includes clinical staging: physical examination, non-invasive radiographic evaluations, and laboratory evaluations (complete blood count, electrolytes, calcium, alkaline phosphatase, alanine aminotransferase, aspartate aminotransferase, total bilirubin, creatinine, and albumin).[5] The staging guidelines also include pathologic staging, which requires invasive staging procedures, such as fine-needle aspiration, mediastinoscopy, and thoracotomy. The diagnostic workup should also include evaluation for paraneoplastic syndromes, performance status, and other comorbidities that might limit treatment options. To date, serum tumor markers have not been shown to have benefit in the assessment of small cell or non–small cell lung cancer. Together, these measures provide an important assessment of extent of disease, organ involvement, and organ function and ability to tolerate systemic treatment.

The foundation of radiographic assessment of lung cancer is CT scanning, as well as positron emission tomographic (PET) scans. There are non-invasive methods to assess tumor size, metabolic activity, and location. Contrast-enhanced magnetic resonance imaging (MRI) or contrast-enhanced CT scan of the brain is indicated in all subjects with documented lung cancer greater than 1 cm because of the high rate of dissemination to the brain in this disease. Clinical symptoms should guide further radiographic assessment, including the symptoms of bone pain, suspected disseminated disease in liver, or other suspicious symptoms of metastasis.

Tissue biopsy is required in all cases of lung cancer, and core needle biopsy is the minimum procedure that should be performed because of the need for adequate tissue for genomic testing in many stages of lung cancer. In general, the least invasive procedure required to provide adequate documentation of the highest possible stage is recommended. Adequately staging lung cancer is critical to appropriate decision-making for treatment. Mediastinal nodal staging is a critical component of adequate staging, and mediastinoscopy is still considered the gold standard of mediastinal staging. EBUS is a newer modality used to stage mediastinal lymph nodes in a less invasive manner (**Figure 12-1**).

While EBUS has become commonplace, one caveat to this procedure is that a negative EBUS biopsy of mediastinal lymph nodes that are suspected to be malignant (metabolically active on PET scan, enlarged greater than 2 cm, involvement of multiple nodes) require confirmatory surgical sampling to ensure adequate staging of the mediastinum.

> **CLINICAL PEARL:** *Clinical stage in the AJCC is based on all clinical investigations and assigned a prefix c. Pathological stage requires both clinical and histopathologic data to provide confirmation of stage. The surgical pathologic stage is assigned a prefix p.*

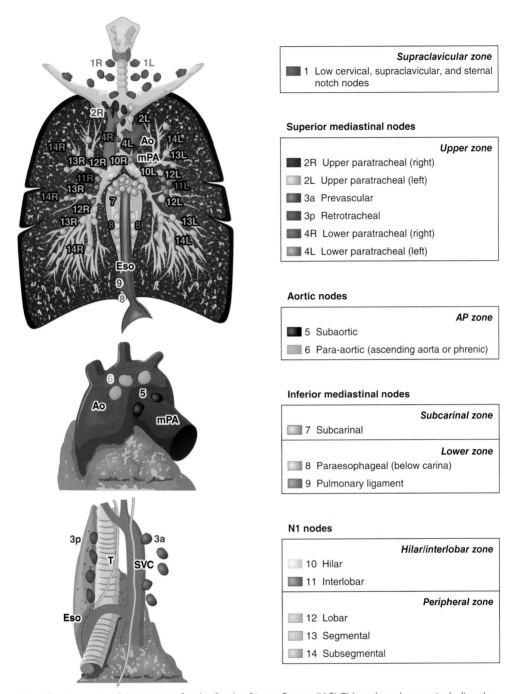

Supraclavicular zone
1 Low cervical, supraclavicular, and sternal notch nodes

Superior mediastinal nodes

Upper zone
2R Upper paratracheal (right)
2L Upper paratracheal (left)
3a Prevascular
3p Retrotracheal
4R Lower paratracheal (right)
4L Lower paratracheal (left)

Aortic nodes

AP zone
5 Subaortic
6 Para-aortic (ascending aorta or phrenic)

Inferior mediastinal nodes

Subcarinal zone
7 Subcarinal

Lower zone
8 Paraesophageal (below carina)
9 Pulmonary ligament

N1 nodes

Hilar/interlobar zone
10 Hilar
11 Interlobar

Peripheral zone
12 Lobar
13 Segmental
14 Subsegmental

Figure 12-1. The International Association for the Study of Lung Cancer (IASLC) lymph node map, including the proposed grouping of lymph node stations into "zones." (Reproduced with permission from Rusch VW, Asamura H, Watanabe H, Giroux DJ, Rami-Porta R, Goldstraw P. The IASLC lung cancer staging project: A proposal for a new international lymph node map in the forthcoming seventh edition of the TNM classification for lung cancer. *J Thorac Oncol.* 2009;4(5):568-577. doi:https://doi.org/10.1097/JTO.0b013e3181a0d82e. Copyright © 2009 International Association for the Study of Lung Cancer. Published by Elsevier Inc.)

NON–SMALL CELL LUNG CANCER STAGING

Standardized staging has been in practice for lung cancer for many years. The overall stage of a lung cancer (stages I-IV) is determined by all 3 descriptors: T, N, and M. The IASLC used a database of over 95,000 patients with lung cancer to update survival data according to staging and applied these clinical outcomes to suggested changes to the seventh edition of the AJCC lung cancer staging system.[6] The eighth edition staging system of the Union Internationale Contre le Cancer (UICC) and AJCC for lung cancer is listed in **Table 12-1**, and significant changes are presented in bold in the table.

Tumor Staging

Significant changes to the tumor staging in the eighth edition include the addition of a new T category "Tis," which includes carcinoma in situ, squamous cell carcinoma in situ (as CIS), and adenocarcinoma in situ (AIS), which is adenocarcinoma with pure lepidic pattern 3 cm or less in greatest dimension. "T1mi," which is minimally invasive adeno-carcinoma (≤3 cm in the greatest dimension) with a predominantly lepidic pattern and 5 mm or less invasion in the greatest dimension.

As seen in Table 12-1, the size of the tumor designation in each T stage differs in the eighth edition, with new stage groupings dividing T1 tumors into: T1a (≤1 cm or super-ficial spreading tumor in central airway); T1b (>1 to ≤2 cm); T1c (>2 to ≤3 cm); T2 (>3 to ≤5 cm or tumor involving visceral pleura main bronchus [not carina], atelectasis to the hilum); T3 (>5 to ≤7 cm or invading chest wall, pericardium, phrenic nerve, or separate tumor nodule in the same lobe); and T4 (>7 cm or tumor invading the medias-tinum, diaphragm, heart, great vessels, recurrent laryngeal nerve, carina, trachea, esophagus, spine, or tumor nodule in a different ipsilateral lobe) (**Table 12-2**).

> **CLINICAL PEARL:** In part-solid, nonmucinous adenocarcinoma, the clinical size is the size of the solid component, while the pathological size is the size of the invasive component. Additionally, the IASLC recommends measurement of tumor size using CT lung windows rather than soft tissue windows.

Special Categories for Cancers with Multiple Lesions

Patients with multiple primary tumors should receive one TNM stage for each tumor. Separate tumor nodules that are thought not to be synchronous tumors should be staged as T3, T4, or M1a depending on their position compared to the primary tumor. Multiple adenocarcinomas with lipidic growth features or ground glass opacities with at least one suspected or proven lesion to be cancer with or without biopsies require that the T stage is determined according to the highest T lesion, single N and M for all lesions collectively with the designation "#/m" indicating multiplicity.[7] For the dif-fuse pneumonic-type adenocarcinomas, these are staged as T3, T4, or M1a depending on their position compared to the primary tumor and designated as a single N and M for all.[8]

TABLE 12-1	Eighth Edition TNM Classification for Lung Cancer
colspan Proposed T, N, and M Descriptors for The Eight Edition of TNM Classification for Lung Cancer	
T: Primary Tumor	
Tx	Primary tumor cannot be assessed, or tumor proven by the presence of malignant cells in sputum or bronchial washings but not visualized by imaging or bronchoscopy
T0	No evidence of primary tumor
Tis	**Carcinoma in situ**
T1	Tumor ≤ 3 cm in greatest dimension surrounded by lung or visceral pleura without bronchoscopic evidence of invasion more proximal than the lobar bronchus (ie, not in the main bronchus)[a]
T1a(mi)	**Minimally invasive adenocarcinoma[b]**
T1a	Tumor ≤ 1 cm in greatest dimension[a]
T1b	Tumor > 1 cm but ≤ 2 cm in greatest dimension[a]
T1c	Tumor > 2 cm but ≤ 3 cm in greatest dimension[a]
T2	Tumor > 3 cm but ≤ 5 cm or tumor with any of the following features[c]: • Involves main bronchus regardless of distance from the carina but without involvement of the carina • Invades visceral pleura • Associated with atelectasis or obstructive pneumonitis that extends to the hilar region, involving part or all of the lung
T2a	Tumor > 3 cm but ≤ 4 cm in greatest dimension
T2b	Tumor > 4 cm but ≤ 5 cm in greatest dimension
T3	**Tumor > 5 cm but ≤ 7 cm** in greatest dimension or associated with separate tumor nodule(s) in the same lobe as the primary tumor or directly invades any of the following structures: chest wall (including the parietal pleura and superior suicus tumors), phrenic nerve, parietal pericardium
T4	**Tumor > 7 cm** in greatest dimension or associated with separate tumor nodule(s) in a different ipsilateral lobe than that of the primary tumor or invades any of the following structures: diaphragm, mediastinum, heart, great vessels, trachea, recurrent laryngeal nerve, esophagus, vertebral body, and carina
N: Regional lymph node involvement	
Nx	Regional lymph nodes cannot be assessed
N0	No regional lymph node metastasis
N1	Metastasis in ipsilateral peribronchial and/or ipsilateral hilar lymph nodes and intrapulmonary nodes, including involvement by direct extension
N2	Metastasis in ipsilateral mediastinal and/or subcarinal lymph node(s)
N3	Metastasis in contralateral mediastinal, contralateral hilar, ipsilateral or contralateral scalene, or supraclavicular lymph node(s)

(Continued)

TABLE 12-1	Eighth Edition TNM Classification for Lung Cancer (Continued)
Proposed T, N, and M Descriptors for The Eight Edition of TNM Classification for Lung Cancer	
M: Distant metastasis	
M0	No distant metastasis
M1	Distant metastasis present
M1a	Separate tumor nodule(s) in a contralateral lobe; tumor with pleural or pericardial nodule(s) or malignant pleural or pericardial effusion[d]
M1b	Single extrathoracic metastasis[e]
M1c	Multiple extrathoracic metastases in one or more organs

Reproduced with permission from Detterbeck FC, Boffa DJ, Kim AW, Tanoue LT. The Eighth Edition Lung Cancer Stage Classification. Chest. 2017;151(1):193-203. Epub 2016/10/27. doi:10.1016/j.chest.2016.10.010. Copyright © 2016 American College of Chest Physicians. Published by Elsevier Inc.

Note: Changes to the seventh edition are in bold.

[a]*The uncommon superficial spreading tumor of any size with its invasive component limited to the bronchial wall, which may extend proximal to the main bronchus, is also classified as T1a.*

[b]*Solitary adenocarcinoma ≤3 cm, with a predominantly lepidic pattern and ≤5 mm invasion in any one focus.*

[c]*T2 tumors with these features are classified T2a if ≤4 cm in greatest dimension or if size cannot be determined, and T2b if >4 cm but not ≤5 cm in greatest dimension.*

[d]*Most pleural (pericardial) effusions with lung cancer are due to tumor. In a few patients, however, multiple microscopic examinations of pleural (pericardial) fluid are negative for tumor and the fluid is nonbloody and is not an exudate. Where these elements and clinical judgement dictate that the effusion is not related to the tumor, the effusion should be excluded as a staging descriptor.*

[e]*This includes involvement of a single distant (nonregional) lymph node.*

Nodal Staging

Nodal staging in the eighth edition matches that of the seventh edition. No changes were made because the nodal staging consistently predicted the prognosis of these patients. N1 and N2 nodal stations are designated as follows:

1. N1: Involvement of ipsilateral intrapulmonary, peribronchial, or hilar lymph nodes.
   - pN1a: Single-station metastasis
   - pN1b: Multiple-station metastasis
2. N2: Involvement of ipsilateral mediastinal or subcarinal lymph nodes
   - pN2a1: Single N2 station without concurrent N1 station involvement (skip metastasis)
   - pN2a2: Single N2 station with concurrent N1 involvement
   - pN2b: Multiple N2 station metastasis
3. N3: Nodes represent contralateral mediastinal or contralateral hilar lymphadenopathy; ipsilateral/contralateral scalene or supraclavicular nodes

Metastasis Staging

As in previous versions, metastatic disease limited to the chest (contralateral lung, pericardial effusion, or pleural effusion, or pleural nodules) are considered M1a. However, a new distinction of cases where there is a single extrathoracic metastatic site was made in the eighth edition, with the designation M1b. The category M1c was created

TABLE 12-2	Lung Cancer Stage Grouping: Eighth Edition, AJCC/IASLC Staging System				
T/M	LABEL	N0	N1	N2	N3
T1	T1a ≤ 1 cm	IA1	IIB	IIIA	IIIB
	T1b > 1-2 cm	IA2	IIB	IIIA	IIIB
	T1c > 2-3 cm	IA3	IIB	IIIA	IIIB
T2	T2a Central (Cent) visceral pleura (VISC Pl)	IB	IIB	IIIA	IIIB
	T2a > 3-4 cm	IB	IIB	IIIA	IIIB
	T2b > 4-5 cm	IIA	IIB	IIIA	IIIB
T3	T3 > 5-7 cm	IIB	IIIA	IIIB	IIIC
	T3 Invasive (Inv)	IIB	IIIA	IIIB	IIIC
	T3 Satellite (Satell)	IIB	IIIA	IIIB	IIIC
T4	T4 > 7 cm	IIIA	IIIA	IIIB	IIIC
	T4 Invasive (Inv)	IIIA	IIIA	IIIB	IIIC
	T4 Ipsilateral Nodule (Ipsi Nod)	IIIA	IIIA	IIIB	IIIC
M1	M1a Contralateral Nodule (Contr Nod)	IVA	IVA	IVA	IVA
	M1a Pleural Dissimination (Pl Dissem)	IVA	IVA	IVA	IVA
	M1b single extrathoracic metastasis (Single)	IVA	IVA	IVA	IVA
	M1c Multiple (Multi)	IVB	IVB	IVB	IVB

T3 Inv, invades structures: chest wall (including the parietal pleura and superior sulcus tumors), phrenic nerve, parietal pericardium; T4 Inv, invades any of these structures: diaphragm, mediastinum, heart, great vessels, trachea, recurrent laryngeal nerve, esophagus, vertebral body, and carina; Ipsi Nod, ipsilateral nodule.

Reproduced with permission from Detterbeck FC, Boffa DJ, Kim AW, Tanoue LT. The Eighth Edition Lung Cancer Stage Classification. Chest. 2017;151(1):193-203. Epub 2016/10/27. doi:10.1016/j.chest.2016.10.010. Copyright © 2016 American College of Chest Physicians. Published by Elsevier Inc.

to designate multiple extrathoracic metastatic lesions in one or more organs. Stage IVa corresponds to disease limited to either intrathoracic or a single extrathoracic metastasis (M1a or M1b), which portends better prognosis (11.5- and 11.4-month median overall survival, respectively) compared to stage IVb with multiple extrathoracic metastases and a median overall survival of 6.3 months.[9]

Stage groupings are listed in Table 12-2 with a stage shift in T4 tumors invading the diaphragm, which moved from stage IIB to stage IIIA in the eighth edition; increase in tumor stage for T1N1 tumors, which moved from stage IIA to stage IIB; and a new stage IIIC category created for patients with N3 disease and T3 or T4 primary tumors. These changes better predict median survival by stage.

SMALL CELL LUNG CANCER

Staging for small cell lung cancer was developed as a simple, two-stage system in the mid-twentieth century, based on the lack of surgical options for most patients with small cell lung cancer. In the past 10 years, there has been movement to incorporate the AJCC TNM staging system into small cell lung cancer staging to further classify and clarify disease. Of note, many practitioners still use the Veterans Affairs Lung Study Group

(VALSG) staging system, which is a two-stage system developed in the 1950s for small cell lung cancer developed.[10] This has utility in treatment planning for those patients receiving multimodality radiation and concurrent chemotherapy. The system is as follows:

- Limited disease: Tumor confined to the ipsilateral hemithorax and regional nodes able to be included in a single tolerable radiotherapy port (corresponding to TNM stages I through IIIB).

- Extensive disease: Tumor beyond the boundaries of limited disease, including distant metastases, malignant pericardial or pleural effusions, and contralateral supraclavicular and contralateral hilar involvement.

The TNM system has been validated in small cell lung cancer beginning with the AJCC's sixth edition and in general is recommended for use for small cell lung cancer. Using the TNM staging system, limited-stage small cell lung cancer is defined as stages I-III (any T stage, any N stage, and M0 status). This implies that definitive radiation is possible in these earlier stages of the AJCC TNM categories (see Table 12-1). Extensive-stage disease therefore is any M1a, M1b, or M1c or any disease that is so extensive it renders radiation intolerable due to the size of a radiation port that would be required, such as in the case of multiple pulmonary nodules of T3 or T4 year for status.

REFERENCES

1. Detterbeck FC, Boffa DJ, Kim AW, Tanoue LT. The eighth edition lung cancer stage classification. *Chest.* 2017;151(1):193-203. Epub 2016/10/27. doi:10.1016/j.chest.2016.10.010.
2. Rami-Porta R, Asamura H, Travis WD, Rusch VW. Lung cancer—major changes in the American Joint Committee on Cancer eighth edition cancer staging manual. *CA Cancer J Clin.* 2017;67(2):138-155. Epub 2017/02/01. doi:10.3322/caac.21390.
3. Detterbeck FC, Chansky K, Groome P, et al. The IASLC lung cancer staging project: methodology and validation used in the development of proposals for revision of the stage classification of NSCLC in the forthcoming (eighth) edition of the TNM classification of lung cancer. *J Thorac Oncol.* 2016;11(9):1433-1446. Epub 2016/07/28. doi:10.1016/j.jtho.2016.06.028.
4. Goldstraw P, Chansky K, Crowley J, et al. The IASLC lung cancer staging project: proposals for revision of the TNM stage groupings in the forthcoming (eighth) edition of the TNM classification for lung cancer. *J Thorac Oncol.* 2016;11(1):39-51. Epub 2016/01/15. doi:10.1016/j.jtho.2015.09.009.
5. Ost DE, Jim Yeung SC, Tanoue LT, Gould MK. Clinical and organizational factors in the initial evaluation of patients with lung cancer: diagnosis and management of lung cancer, 3rd ed: American College of Chest Physicians evidence-based clinical practice guidelines. *Chest.* 2013;143(5 Suppl):e121S-e141S. Epub 2013/05/10. doi:10.1378/chest.12-2352.
6. Asamura H, Chansky K, Crowley J, et al. The International Association for the Study of Lung Cancer Lung Cancer Staging Project: proposals for the revision of the N descriptors in the forthcoming 8th edition of the TNM classification for lung cancer. *J Thorac Oncol.* 2015;10(12):1675-1684. Epub 2015/12/29. doi:10.1097/jto.0000000000000678.
7. Detterbeck FC, Marom EM, Arenberg DA, et al. The IASLC lung cancer staging project: background data and proposals for the application of TNM staging rules to lung cancer presenting as multiple nodules with ground glass or lepidic features or a pneumonic type of involvement in the forthcoming eighth edition of the TNM classification. *J Thorac Oncol.* 2016;11(5):666-680. doi:https://doi.org/10.1016/j.jtho.2015.12.113.
8. Detterbeck FC, Nicholson AG, Franklin WA, et al. The IASLC lung cancer staging project: summary of proposals for revisions of the classification of lung cancers with multiple pulmonary sites of involvement in the forthcoming eighth edition of the TNM classification. *J Thorac Oncol.* 2016;11(5):639-650. Epub 2016/03/05. doi:10.1016/j.jtho.2016.01.024.
9. Eberhardt WE, Mitchell A, Crowley J, et al. The IASLC lung cancer staging project: proposals for the revision of the M descriptors in the forthcoming eighth edition of the TNM classification of lung cancer. *J Thorac Oncol.* 2015;10(11):1515-1522. Epub 2015/11/05. doi:10.1097/jto.0000000000000673.
10. Kalemkerian GP, Gadgeel SM. Modern staging of small cell lung cancer. *J Natl Compr Canc Netw.* 2013;11(1):99-104. Epub 2013/01/12.

PART IV

Treatment: Non–Small Cell and Small Cell Lung Cancer

13

NON–SMALL CELL LUNG CANCER TREATMENT: EARLY STAGE

Victor van Berkel, MD, PhD • Michael J. Carr, MD, MS • Neal E. Dunlap, MD • Matthew Fox, MD
• Ignacio Gil-Bazo, MD, PhD • Rohit Kumar, MD • Katy Alyse Marino, MD • Mike May, MD • Phuong T. Ngo, MD
• Jose Pinto-Llerena, MD, FACP • Luis E. Raez, MD, FACP, FCCP • Jonathan Rice, MD, PhD

PREOPERATIVE WORKUP FOR EARLY STAGE NON–SMALL CELL LUNG CANCER

Michael J. Carr, MD, MS, Katy Alyse Marino, MD, Matthew Fox, MD

A 62-year-old African American male presents to his primary care physician for routine health maintenance. He has diabetes mellitus (DM) controlled on oral medications and hypertension (HTN), for which he takes hydrochlorothiazide and lisinopril. He has a 50 pack-year smoking history, so his physician orders low-dose chest computed tomography (CT), which shows a 2.1-cm mass in the left upper lobe area. His laboratory work is normal. He sees a pulmonology and undergoes endobronchial ultrasound (EBUS)–guided biopsy, which shows adenocarcinoma. The patient wonders if he will need surgery, radiation, chemotherapy, or all three.

Learning Objectives:
1. How do you determine the best modality for biopsy of a lung nodule?
2. Which lymph nodes are sampled with a mediastinoscopy?
3. Which tests should be done prior to lung cancer resection?

HISTORY AND PHYSICAL

Assessment of a newly found lung nodule should begin with a history and physical to determine the extent of the disease, focusing especially on areas that may imply presence of metastatic disease. Questioning should be directed toward possible symptoms within and outside of the pulmonary system, including pain within the long bones and vertebrae, new lesions of the skin, and focal neurological findings, such as headache, nausea, vomiting, or seizure. Other suggestions toward metastatic disease include constitutional symptoms such as anorexia, unintentional weight loss, and general malaise. Physical examination warrants attention to palpable lymph nodes, especially the cervical and supraclavicular basins; muscle wasting; and chest auscultation. Routine laboratory studies searching for paraneoplastic syndromes include complete blood count, basic metabolic panel, calcium, and the hepatic enzymes glutamic oxaloacetic transaminase and alkaline phosphatase.

ROLE OF CONTRASTED COMPUTED TOMOGRAPHY AND POSITRON EMISSION TOMOGRAPHY

Further assessment of a lung nodule should continue with non-invasive staging of disease using advanced imaging. The status of intrathoracic nodal disease will be the patient's major determining factor when discussing treatment options. If disease has not spread from the primary tumor to mediastinal or subcarinal lymph nodes, surgical resection would be the preferred choice.

If a patient does not already had a thin-cut chest CT, a scan with intravenous contrast should be performed for elucidation of the primary tumor size and characteristics as well as for mediastinal lymphadenopathy or other disease burden in relation to the major structures of the thorax. Extension of CT to the liver and adrenal glands can evaluate two common sites of metastasis at this initial scan. If there is an increase in the size of lymph nodes noted on CT, positron emission tomography (PET) is useful in distinguishing malignant tissue from benign forms of lymphadenopathy. PET provides benefit in the evaluation of regional disease as well as distant sites, with the exception of visualizing disease within the brain due to baseline metabolic activity. In the PLUS multicenter randomized controlled trial, addition of PET to the preoperative workup prevented futile thoracotomy in 20% of patients with suspected NSCLC.[1] Although an expensive imaging modality, the upfront cost of PET imaging has been proven to be worth it in the staging of newly diagnosed non–small cell lung cancer (NSCLC) and in the diagnosis of indeterminate solitary pulmonary nodules, as it is the most accurate non-invasive imaging modality to evaluate the mediastinum, offers additional evaluation of extrathoracic sites of possible disease, and can reduce the incidence of non-curative resections.[2,3]

Magnetic resonance imaging (MRI) of pulmonary or mediastinal nodules has little role to contribute at the staging period unless the patient has iodine contrast allergy. MRI is useful if the patient gives a reason for needing more detailed visualization of disease invading vascular structures, vertebral body, or the brain.

Computed tomographic scanning for identification of mediastinal lymph node metastasis was found to have sensitivity and specificity of approximately 55% and 81%, respectively.[3] Mediastinal lymph node staging by PET appears to have greater accuracy compared to CT, as proved in a meta-analysis with a pooled sensitivity of 84% (CI 78%-89%), specificity of 89% (CI 83%-93%), and overall prevalence of disease 32% (range 5%-56%). Combined CT and PET scan improved sensitivity to a range of 0.78-0.93 and specificity from 0.82 to 0.95, with a prevalence of mediastinal disease from 32% to 50%.[4]

A Cochrane review of 45 studies based on combined PET/CT positivity performed two main analyses based on PET uptake. In the first group where uptake was noted to be just greater than the background uptake, PET/CT correctly identified nodal disease metastasis beyond N1 nodes in 77.4% of patients (95% CI 65.3%-86.1%) and 90.1% (95% CI 85.3%-93.5%) of patients without disease metastasis beyond N1 nodes. In the second group where uptake was noted to have a SUVmax (maximum standard uptake value) of 2.5 or greater, PET/CT correctly identified nodal disease metastasis beyond N1 nodes in 81.3% of patients (95% CI 70.2%-88.9%) and 79.4% (95% CI 70%-86.5%) of patients without metastasis beyond the N1 nodes.[5]

Even with this high accuracy, it should be noted that PET analysis may lead to false negatives in disease that has low metabolic activity (eg, carcinoid and bronchioalveolar tumors). For peripherally located nodules less than 3 cm with no evidence of hilar, mediastinal, or other metastatic presentation on PET, it is indicated to forgo biopsy in favor of proceeding directly to wedge resection.[6] For centrally located tumors or for tumors greater than 3 cm, invasive staging of the mediastinum is recommended even if the PET is negative, as false-negative rates have been shown to approach 20%-25%.[3] Therefore, with high suspicion of malignancy, which can be aided through use of the Fleischner criteria, any imaging finding of mediastinal lymph node enlargement should be confirmed with tissue biopsy.[7] Confirmation of a histologic diagnosis via direct tissue sampling also makes available molecular testing. The differentiation of a cytologic specimen is tightly associated with chemotherapy treatment regimen, and as such early assessment of tissue is imperative. Tissue can be obtained through biopsy via CT-guided needle, EBUS, bronchoscopy, mediastinoscopy, or video-assisted thorascopic surgery (VATS).

ENDOSCOPIC BRONCHIAL ULTRASOUND

Endobronchial ultrasound represents a relatively new and alternative method for nodal staging of lung cancer. In a prospective controlled trial, Yasufuku et al. found no significant differences between EBUS transbronchial needle aspiration (TBNA) and mediastinoscopy in determining the true pathologic N stage in over 150 patients.[8] Further study has documented the ability to achieve high sensitivity and specificity using EBUS with rapid on-site evaluation by a cytopathologist. In a large report of 483 patients, Nakajima et al. found the sensitivity and specificity of EBUS TBNA samples to be 96.5% and 100%, respectively.[9] With the ability to diagnose not only tumor type, but also molecular genotype of cancers, EBUS TBNA may replace other more invasive staging methods in patients with advanced disease.[10]

> **CLINICAL PEARL:** In the most recent chest guidelines, all patients with either high or intermediate suspicion of N2,3 by avidity or increased size should undergo EBUS as a first-line staging strategy, over surgical staging.

Those with negative results, however, should still undergo surgical staging with mediastinoscopy when there is a high suspicion for N2,3 disease.[3]

MEDIASTINOSCOPY

Mediastinoscopy involves taking a patient to the operating room. Under general anesthesia, the surgeon will make a pretracheal incision just superior to the sternal notch, dissect inferiorly along the anterior trachea to the mediastinum, and insert a mediastinoscope. Through the scope, the surgeon performs biopsies of mediastinal lymph nodes. Risks of the procedure are minimal, with one study finding morbidity and mortality of 0% and 2.1%, respectively. Complications included hoarseness, which improved at follow-up, and wound infection.[11] Video mediastinoscopy uses an enhanced mediastinoscope with a camera at the distal tip of the scope blade. This technology outperforms conventional mediastinoscopy in that it yields more lymph nodes and more lymph node stations with higher accuracy, better negative predictive value, and increased sensitivity.[3,12]

Traditionally, the lymph nodes accessible for biopsy via mediastinoscopy are listed by station as follows: 1 (low cervical); 3a, 3p (prevascular, retrotracheal, respectively); 2R, 2L, 4R, 4L (paratracheal); and 7 (anterior subcarinal). The stations 2R, 2L, 4R, 4L, and 7 should be routinely sampled with all procedures. Video-assisted mediastinoscopic complete lymphadenectomy has been shown to have equal accuracy compared to open lymphadenectomy with the added benefit of easier access to the left paratracheal and tracheobronchial stations.[13] Video mediastinoscopy is also useful in surgical training, as both attending and resident can view a screen together, as opposed to taking turns visualizing a limited field. This leads to more rapid learning without added risk to patient safety.[14,15]

In comparison of techniques utilized to stage mediastinal disease involvement, it is important to note that often EBUS and PET are performed on patients with enlarged mediastinal lymph nodes, with mediastinoscopy is performed on patients to rule out disease even without mediastinal lymph node enlargement.[14,15]

DETERMINING OPERABILITY

Cardiopulmonary Testing

As staging of disease is confirmed, patients with stage I or II lung cancer should be considered for surgical resection. Prior to the operation, thorough history and physical examination of the patient's overall medical status and screening with chest plain films and electrocardiography should be performed. Additionally, pulmonary function testing (PFT) should be done routinely. Those patients with signs and symptoms of cardiopulmonary disease at this initial evaluation should undergo further testing of physiological fitness for ability to tolerate an operation and reduction in lung volume. If considering pneumonectomy and patients complain of chest pain or have signs of heart failure, then echocardiography and stress testing is recommended.

Pulmonary Function Tests

The pulmonary capability of patients needing treatment for lung cancer is often markedly hampered at the expense of a lifetime of abusing tobacco products. PFTs are the primary method to evaluate for operative risk, notably the forced expiratory volume in

1 second (FEV_1) measured in the forced vital capacity test and the diffusing capacity of the lungs for carbon monoxide (DLCO) measured by inhalation of a test gas.

> **CLINICAL PEARL:** There is a higher risk of postresection morbidity and mortality for both FEV_1 and DLCO if less than 60% of preoperative function remains, up to 48% and 5%, respectively.[16,17]

We can calculate the predicted postoperative lung function with the metric ppo-FEV_1 = FEV_1 [1 - (Number of segments resected × 0.0526)] (where ppo refers to predicted postoperative). This equation can substitute DLCO in the place of FEV_1. In the presence of significant obstruction, significant pleural disease, endobronchial obstruction, or history of prior resection, other modalities must be used to assess lung function. A variety of methods to predict postoperative functional status exists, including perfusion scans and quantitative CT. The correlations between pre- and postoperative functional status proved perfusion and CT scanning were useful predictors regardless of the extent of resection, with perfusion results being the most accurate. Predictions based on counting functional anatomic segments found on imaging were less accurate and could only be found useful for resections limited to one lobe.[18]

A quantitative or ventilation-perfusion lung scan is helpful in predicting the postoperative function in marginal cases where FEV_1 and DLCO are less than 60%-80%. If ppo-FEV_1 and ppo-DLVO are greater than 40% on this scan, there is an acceptable risk in attempting surgery.[19] If less than 60% but greater than 30% predicted, patients may be evaluated with a low-technology exercise test such as stair climb or shuttle walk test. If less than 30%, then a formal cardiopulmonary exercise test (CPET) with measurement of maximal oxygen consumption (VO_{2max}) is recommended.

Cardiac Evaluation

The Thoracic Revised Cardiac Risk Index (ThRCRI) is a branch of the Revised Cardiac Risk Index (RCRI) used to specifically evaluate patients for cardiac risk prior to lung resection. It can be used as a screening tool to separate those individuals who need further cardiac assessment from those who are fit for surgery. Of classes A (score 0-1), B (1.5-2.5), and C (>2.5), those within the class C category had a shorter 5-year overall survival (OS), shorter cancer-specific survival (CSS), and higher mortality from specifically cardiac events.[20,21] In patients with need of further cardiac assessment, exercise testing, echocardiography, or nuclear perfusion scans should be performed and any reversible pathology addressed prior to initiation of therapy for the cancer.

Exercise Tolerance (VO_{2max})

Cardiopulmonary exercise test is considered the gold standard for preoperative risk assessment. It includes recording electrocardiogram, heart rate, minute ventilation, and oxygen uptake per minute during exercise. The maximal oxygen consumption (VO_{2max}) is measured from this test. It has been studied extensively regarding consideration for preoperative risk stratification and found to be an independent predictor of postoperative pulmonary morbidity and mortality. Patients with VO_{2max} greater than 20 mL/kg/min can safely undergo resection up to pneumonectomy, as morbidity rates have been observed at 3.5% with no deaths. In patients with VO_{2max} less than 12 mL/kg/min, the morbidity and mortality rates were significantly higher at 33% and 13%, respectively.[22] If VO_{2max} is less than or equal to 10 mL/kg/min, surgery is contraindicated, and patients should be counseled on non-operative management of their lung cancer.

In general, regarding the fitness of a patient under consideration for surgical resection, there is acceptable risk if ppo-DLCO and ppo-FEV$_1$ are greater than 40% and VO_{2max} is greater than 15. High-risk patients are those with ppo-DLCO and ppo-FEV$_1$ within 20%-40% and VO_{2max} 10-15. With ppo-DLCO and ppo-FEV$_1$ less than 20% or VO_{2max} < 10, surgery is not indicated.[23]

OPERATIVE PREPARATION
Cessation of Smoking

Smoking is the foremost cause of preventable death.[24] While the proportion of adult daily smokers in the United States has declined in recent years, it continues to have a prevalence of 17.5% of men and 13.5% of women.[25,26] Recent reports have indicated that 66.7% of men and 69.4% of women expressed an interest in smoking cessation; however, less than half used counseling and/or medication in their efforts.[27]

Overall, cancer patients and cancer survivors who smoke have increased all-cause mortality, cancer-specific mortality, and risk for a second primary cancer.[24] In their study of lung cancer patients, Dobson Amato et al. found a median 9-month improvement in OS in patients who quit tobacco after diagnosis.[28] Specific to thoracic surgery, the association between smoking and adverse postoperative outcomes is well known.[29-31] Even as more minimally invasive procedures are utilized, smoking remains a risk factor for complications. In a prospective study of lung cancer patients undergoing VATS, multivariate analysis revealed current smoking as a significant independent risk factor for postoperative pulmonary complications.[32]

The American College of Chest Physicians recommends that all patients with lung cancer who are being considered for surgery and who are actively smoking be treated for tobacco dependence.[33] The 2013 guidelines recommend perioperative cessation with pharmacotherapy. If patients have contraindications to or refusal of pharmacotherapy, cessation counseling alone is recommended. Importantly, the authors of this chapter do not advocate for the delay of surgical procedures in favor of a longer period of abstinence, as the timing of cessation does not appear to increase the risk of postoperative complications.[34] The National Comprehensive Cancer Network has outlined concordant principles of smoking cessation, enforcing that surgical patients should be encouraged to quit smoking, emphasizing again that longer periods of abstinence should not delay the planned surgical procedure.[35] In light of this evidence, a recent survey of thoracic surgeons demonstrated significant variability in the management of smoking patients related to denying procedures to smokers, duration of preoperative abstinence from smoking, and nicotine testing prior to surgery.[36]

When instituting a smoking cessation regimen to a patient's care, multiple evidence-based methods are available. These included pharmacotherapy and behavioral therapy. Several randomized studies have shown the superiority of varenicline to both placebo and bupropion in patients who want to quit smoking.[37,38] Moreover, in patients not ready to quit smoking but willing to reduce, varenicline also demonstrated significantly better abstinence rates in a randomized study against a placebo.[39] The incorporation of the "five major steps to intervention" (ask, advise, assess, assist, arrange) allows the surgeon to document the smoking history, introduce smoking cessation and its benefits, evaluate the patient's readiness to quit, assist with pharmacotherapy initiation, and arrange follow-up to monitor progress toward smoking cessation.[1] This strategy can be assimilated into clinic workflow with the assistance of other personnel, making it possible for the physician to spend less than 60 s fulfilling this vital part of the preoperative visit.[35]

Preoperative Rehabilitation

The exercise capacity of patients undergoing lung resection, expressed as VO_{2max}, has been proven to be lower in those patients who develop pulmonary complications and inversely proportional to length of stay postoperatively. It has also been shown that preoperative pulmonary rehabilitation may lead to improvement in VO_{2max}.[40-42] One study testing pulmonary rehabilitation in patients with chronic obstructive pulmonary disease (COPD) noted a shorter hospital stay by 3 days, fewer prolonged chest tubes (defined as >7 days), and fewer days needing a chest tube compared to controls with 10 preoperative sessions involving inspiratory muscle training, endurance training, and practice of slow breathing.[43] The benefit of preoperative exercise training with the idea of improving a patient's postoperative recovery seems to fit logically but has proven difficult to quantify. Studies regarding preoperative physiotherapy effects on reduction of postoperative pulmonary complications thus far have been limited in power and statistical significance but do warrant further exploration with large, multicenter, randomized controlled trials.

SURGERY FOR EARLY STAGE NON–SMALL CELL LUNG CANCER

Jonathan D. Rice, MD, Katy A. Marino, MD, Victor H. van Berkel, MD, PhD

A 58-year-old gentleman presents to your office after a 1.1-cm right upper lobe nodule was found incidentally while undergoing CT examination workup after a car crash 1 month prior. He currently denies any shortness of breath, hematemesis, cough, or recent bought of pneumonia. He has a 20 pack-year history of cigarette smoking, yet he stopped smoking 18 years ago. He denies any past medical history or family history.

Learning Objectives:

1. What are the modalities for staging lung cancer?
2. What is the ideal treatment approach for resectable non-metastatic early stage lung cancer?
3. Which lymph nodes are sampled with a mediastinoscopy?
4. Should the patient have a robotic or video-assisted surgery?

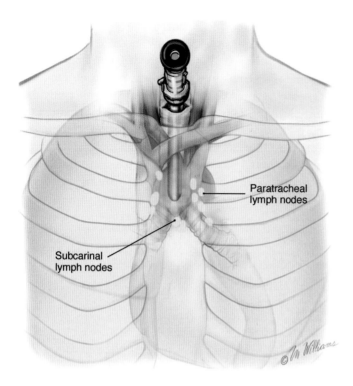

Paratracheal
lymph nodes

Subcarinal
lymph nodes

Figure 13-1. Standard mediastinal scope insertion technique used in a mediastinoscopy for
nodal staging. (Reproduced with permission
from E Hong, MJ Liptay. Techniques for staging
and restaging of lung cancer. In Sugarbaker DJ,
Bueno R, Colson YL, et al., eds. *Adult Chest
Surgery.* 2nd ed. McGraw Hill Medical; 2015:
Chap. 70. Available at https://accesssurgery
.mhmedical.com/content.aspx?bookid=
1317&sectionid=72431939. Accessed June 10,
2019.)

Treatment for patients with stage I and II cancer are reviewed in this chapter. Clinical
staging does not always correlate with pathological staging, leading to most patients being
restaged after surgical sampling of mediastinal nodes. For example, 28% of patients with
clinical stage I lung cancer were upstaged (14% stage II and 14% stage III) in a Cancer
and Leukemia Group B prospective clinical trial (CALGB 9761).[44] The mediastinum is
sampled either at the time of resection or prior to resection, depending on the suspicion
of the physician on the presentation of the patient (**Figure 13-1**).

Surgical resection presents the greatest opportunity for survival when patients present with early stage I or II NSCLC.[45,46] Although a mass may be amenable to surgical
resection, it does not mean that a patient is a surgical candidate for the operation at
hand. It is essential that all patients undergoing lung resection receive preoperative evaluation. Preoperative evaluation is discussed in detail in a separate chapter.

For patients who are considered surgical candidates, an R0 surgical resection is the
procedure of choice for patients who present with stage I and II disease. For patients
who undergo resection and are unable to obtain a negative margin, R1 resection, there
is a role for postoperative chemotherapy with radiation.

LOBECTOMY, BILOBECTOMY, PNEUMONECTOMY, AND SLEEVE RESECTIONS

Lobectomy continues to be the procedure of choice for resection in early stage NSCLC.[47]
Traditionally, lobectomy was performed with an open thoracotomy technique, yet as
technology has advanced, more studies continue to advocate for a minimally invasive

surgical approach.[48] The options for minimally invasive approaches include both the traditional VATS and newer robotic-assisted thoracic surgery (RATS), which is starting to gain favor among thoracic surgeons.

Bilobectomy is the removal of two lobes on the right side. Traditionally, it has been considered a high-risk procedure because it has the potential for significant morbidity and mortality with the addition of possible negative impact on OS.[49] Galetta et al. recently presented a retrospective review that had favorable survival rates based on stage when compared to lobectomy, with high morbidity but low mortality rates when performing bilobectomy.[49] Although not commonly performed and with high morbidity rates, bilobectomy appears to be an acceptable alternative operation when compared to lobectomy when criteria for bilobectomy are met but lobectomy would not be acceptable for oncologic reasons.

Although lobectomy might be considered the "gold standard" for peripheral tumors, as tumors become more proximal, a lobectomy may not be adequate for R0 resection. Such tumors can be approached with a pneumonectomy or a tracheobronchial sleeve resection. Pneumonectomy is an operative procedure in which the entirety of the lung is removed at the time of surgical resection. To undergo this operation, a patient has to have enough pulmonary reserve to tolerate the operation. Even with the significant advancements made in the field of thoracic surgery since the first reported successful 1-stage pneumonectomy performed in 1933 by Graham and Singer, pneumonectomy still has a high complication rate.[50] Due to the pulmonary insult a patient undergoes after pneumonectomy, this has led to the development and advancement of the tracheobronchial sleeve resection, commonly referred to in short as a sleeve resection. A sleeve resection is circumferential resection of the involved airway with primary end-to-end anastomosis.

Pneumonectomy is fraught with postpneumonectomy complications that not only involve the respiratory system of the patient but also can encompass cardiovascular and pleural space disease.[51] Due to the extent of morbidity that is associated with the postpneumonectomy state, a sleeve resection is generally favored.[52] Sleeve resections have been shown to have similar oncologic outcomes when compared to pneumonectomy. Furthermore, they allow for greater preservation of pulmonary function, have better outcomes with long-term survival, increase quality of life, and are overall more cost-effective.[52] With the advancement in surgical technique since its inception, tracheobronchial sleeve resection has established itself as the preferred resection for the majority of centrally located tumors.

SUBLOBAR RESECTION

Sublobar resection (SR) can be classified as either a non-anatomical wedge resection or an anatomical segmentectomy. Both of these resections allow patients who might not tolerate a formal lobectomy due to poor pulmonary status to undergo resection when the tumor is amenable to this type of resection.

The initial data reported by the Lung Cancer Study Group Trial 801 demonstrated an increased rate of local recurrence and lower survival rates when comparing limited resection to lobectomy.[47] This study's application to current practice, however, has its impediments, as it was reported over 20 years ago, without the use of PET imaging and included wedge resection with segmentectomy in 1 analysis.[47]

Another more recent series by Dai et al. investigated 15,760 patients with T1aN0M0 NSCLC tumors (≤2 cm, now T1a and T1b tumors) from the SEER (Surveillance, Epidemiology, and End Results) database. OS and lung cancer-specific survival (LCSS) were evaluated in patients comparing outcomes after lobectomy, anatomical segmentectomy, or non-anatomical wedge resection.[53] They showed that lobectomy had a greater survival advantage for patients with NSCLC ≤ 1 cm and 1 to 2 cm. OS and LCSS for tumors greater than 1 to 2 cm were lower after wedge resection compared to lobectomy. Yet, for patients who had a wedge resection for NSCLC tumors ≤ 1 cm, survival was similar.[53] Cardinale et al. reported another favorable database review comparing segmentectomy to lobectomy from 1998 to 2006 in the SEER database for early stage Ia NSCLC.[54] Their results favored segmentectomy with significant overall and LCSS when compared to wedge resection.[54]

As surgeons become more familiar with minimally invasive techniques and advancement in preoperative screening techniques detect smaller lung nodules, long-term outcomes can be evaluated on patients who receive SRs. Newer reports have had favorable results in favor of segmentectomy. Recently, a large retrospective study investigating the Poland National Lung Cancer Registry failed to show a statistical difference in 3-year and 5-year survival rates when comparing lobectomy to segmentectomy.[55] This survival advantage was not observed when comparing wedge resection to lobectomy, noting that 3- and 5-year survival was statistically less for patients who underwent wedge resection.[55]

Although more recent study results are starting to show segmentectomy as an oncologic equivalent in terms of survival to a lobectomy, the overall consensus appears to still be up for debate. It would be safe to say that a lobectomy can still be considered the gold standard for early stage NSCLC. Yet, for a patient who might not tolerate a complete lobe resection, a segmentectomy is a possible option for a patient with predicted borderline pulmonary function after a complete lobectomy.

Video-Assisted Thoracoscopic Surgery

The majority of lobectomies are still performed utilizing the open approach, despite an increasing amount of data that show the benefit of minimally invasive approach.[56] VATS offers a minimally invasive approach to the traditional open thoracotomy technique for early stage lung resections. Commonly accepted incision placements for VATS operative technique are shown in **Figure 13-2**. A typical operating room setup during VATS is pictured in **Figure 13-3**, with operating room bedside port placement shown in **Figure 13-4**.

In a prospective trial of 128 patients with peripheral lung nodules less than or equal to 3 cm, a standardized VATS technique was shown to have acceptable outcomes.[57]

CLINICAL PEARL: Further studies have shown VATS to be a safe alternative to open thoracotomy, with minimal morbidity and mortality.[58]

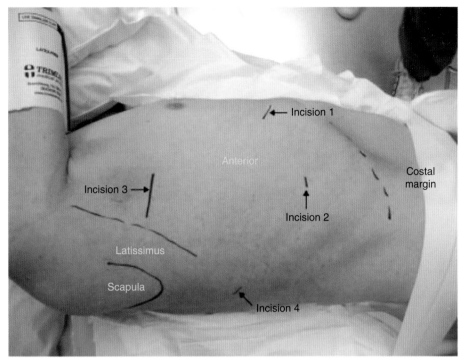

Figure 13-2. Commonly accepted incision proposal for port placement in a video-assisted thoracoscopic surgery. (Reproduced with permission from R. J. McKenna. *Atlas of Minimally Invasive Thoracic Surgery (VATS)*. Elsevier; January 1, 2011:3-14, Figure 1-2, Incisions for a video-assisted lobectomy. Copyright © 2011 by Saunders, an imprint of Elsevier Inc.)

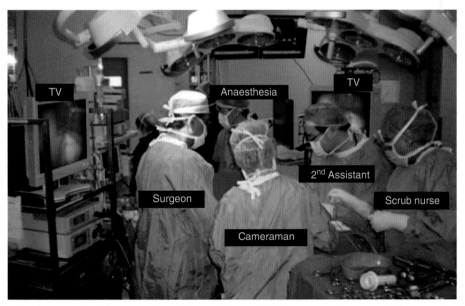

Figure 13-3. A common operating room setup during a video-assisted thoracoscopic surgery. (Reproduced with permission from Thirugnanam A. Video-assisted thoracoscopic surgery and open chest surgery in infectious lung diseases. *J Vis Surg.* 2017;3:3. Published 2017 Jan 6. doi:10.21037/jovs.2016.12.03.)

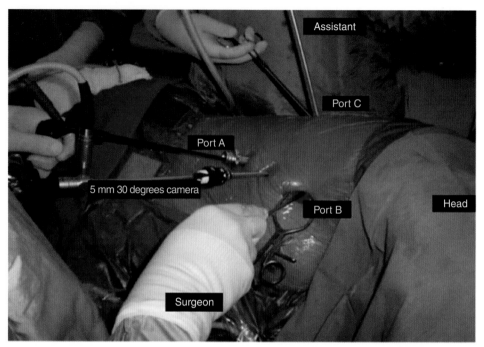

Figure 13-4. Picture of bedside placement of ports and trocars during a video-assisted thoracoscopic surgery. (Reproduced with permission from Thirugnanam A. Video-assisted thoracoscopic surgery and open chest surgery in infectious lung diseases. *J Vis Surg.* 2017;3:3. Published 2017 Jan 6. doi:10.21037/jovs.2016.12.03.)

VATS resection has been reported to reduce the length of stay without compromising oncologic outcomes when compared to an open technique.[48] Most recently, VATS lobectomy was shown to have overall lower 30-day morbidity when compared to the open approach.[59]

Robotic-Assisted Thoracoscopic Surgery

With the advancements of minimally invasive surgery and technology, RATS is starting to build steam as another acceptable alternative to open thoracotomy for early stage NSCLC. Port placement and a docked Xi robot are shown in **Figure 13-5**.

At the onset of RATS, early reports of RATS lobectomy appeared to have consistent and favorable outcomes when compared to the current standards of VATS lobectomy.[60] As this operation has developed over the years latter reports, including a large multi-institutional retrospective review of robotic lobectomy during an 8 year period showed low morbidity and mortality with acceptable long term survival that was similar to VATS and open resection.[61]

In addition, a more recent study retrospectively reviewed 10 years of robotic resection at their institution for stage I and II NSCLC and had favorable results.[62] They had excellent 30- and 90-day mortality, 0% and 0.3%, respectively.[62] In addition the oncologic survival at 3 and 5 years was similar to results seen from VATS and open technique, at 96.1% and 91.5%, respectively.[62]

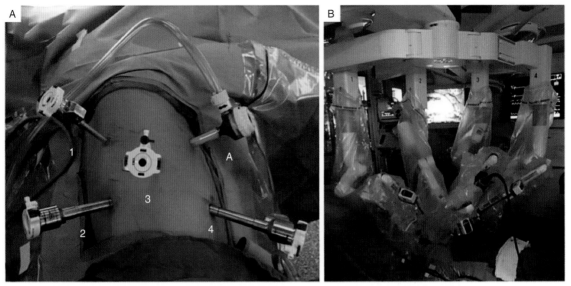

Figure 13-5. **A.** Trocar port placement for robotic-assisted thoracoscopy surgery right upper lobectomy. **B.** Xi robot docked in operative position. (Reproduced with permission from Kim MP, Chan EY. "Five on a dice" port placement for robot-assisted thoracoscopic right upper lobectomy using robotic stapler. *J Thorac Dis.* 2017;9(12):5355–5362. doi:10.21037/jtd.2017.11.0.)

Both of these studies are encouraging for the future of robotic-assisted resection in terms of oncologic outcomes and low morbidity and mortality from the operation itself. The technology continues to become more readily available for the thoracic surgeon to utilize in their practice. Since the majority of hospitals will not have a robot at their disposal, proficiency in open and VATS surgical approach is still necessary.

Postoperative Considerations

Although most early stage resections that undergo an open, VATS, or RATS approach will not need postoperative intensive care, its availability is imperative in case of intra-operative and postoperative complications.

Favorable data from advance recovery protocols seen from early implementation in elective colorectal surgery has led the field of thoracic surgery to investigate protocols for enhanced recovery protocols (ERPs) in thoracic resections.[63-65] Recent outcomes investigating results from implementation after ERP have been favorable but have not been widely adopted.[66]

As advances continue to occur in diagnostic and therapeutic interventions in NSCLC, the treatment algorithm will continue to evolve and improve. The surgical field continues to shift based on the data derived from prospective and retrospective studies. As data continue to support the use of the VATS and now RATS operative technique in terms of overall and oncologic survival outcomes, faster patient recovery, and overall patient satisfaction, these technologies are still not readily available to all surgeons but appear to be taking a strong hold on the future of operative intervention for early stage NSCLC.

RADIATION THERAPY FOR EARLY STAGE NON–SMALL LUNG CARCINOMA

Mike May, MD, Neal E. Dunlap, MD

A 60–year-old Asian female had a 4-cm lung mass biopsied by core needle biopsy. She never smoked and has no history of cancer or comorbidities. The pathology shows adenocarcinoma of the lung. PET and MRI are otherwise negative.

Learning Objectives:

1. Who would be a candidate for curative treatment of early stage lung cancer by radiation?
2. What are the risks of stereotactic radiation?
3. How long does the radiation treatment take?

PATIENT SELECTION FOR PRIMARY THERAPY

Patients with early stage NSCLC are managed with surgical resection or definitive radiation therapy (RT). Surgical considerations are discussed elsewhere, but, to briefly summarize, lobectomy is considered the standard of care for medically fit patients capable of tolerating the procedure.[67] Many patients in this population have long smoking histories, which carry associated pulmonary and cardiovascular medical comorbidities, increasing their operative risk. Patients deemed to be at a high operative risk are not candidates for lobectomy, at which point their options are less extensive surgery or non-operative management. While segmentectomy or wedge resection offers the ability to remove tumors with a smaller concomitant reduction of healthy lung parenchyma, these procedures are less ideal and not considered an oncologic surgery, as normal tissue sparing comes with the compromise of a greater incidence of local recurrence.[47] Determination of operability is guided by factors such as advanced age, cardiovascular or pulmonary impairment, and the burden of competing comorbidities. Objective quantification has mainly relied on PFT, specifically the FEV_1 and the DLCO. High operative risk and medically inoperable patients are candidates for definitive RT after multidisciplinary discussion has concluded the morbidity of surgical resection outweighs potential benefit.

PRIMARY SURGERY: POSTOPERATIVE RT

Surgical resection is recommended for patients deemed medically fit to undergo the procedure, with evidence-based guidelines available to aid this decision.[67] For these patients, RT is generally reserved for the postoperative setting when lymph node sampling demonstrates metastatic carcinoma, diagnosing the patient with locally advanced disease.[68] Multiple studies have sought to determine a role for postoperative radiation therapy (PORT) in early stage lung cancer, but results were mixed, with no clear improvement in survival. Ultimately, a meta-analysis of these trials demonstrated PORT to be detrimental in stage I-II patients.[69] A subsequent SEER database analysis further showed a negative impact on survival, with benefit seen only for locally advanced patients with N2 disease.[70] For patients with positive margins on resection (R2), PORT improves survival, and this effect is seen for all nodal stages.[71] For patients deemed high risk for lobectomy, SR provides a less morbid operation, but with a higher rate of local recurrence. In the American College of Surgeons Oncology Group (ACOSOG) Z4032 trial, investigators sought to improve local control (LC) with the addition of postoperative brachytherapy. Patients with stage I NSCLC meeting criteria warranting exclusion of lobectomy underwent SR and were randomized to observation or brachytherapy. The brachytherapy group underwent iodine 125 suture or mesh implant at the postresection staple line at time of SR. Unfortunately, final analysis demonstrated no statistical difference in local progression; however, on subset analysis there was a trend toward significance for a benefit with brachytherapy in patients with positive staple line cytology.[72]

PRIMARY RADIATION

Historically, primary RT was typically reserved for medically inoperable patients as the only available option for definitive treatment. While conventional RT increased survival compared to no treatment, the results were lackluster, with a survival benefit of 5-7 months and no change in 5-year OS.[73] Over the past few decades, as medical radiation technology improved, so did the treatments and results. Improved outcomes were seen when 3-dimensional RT was compared to older 2-dimensional techniques.[74] A retrospective series from Memorial Sloan Kettering Cancer Center (MSKCC) showed that for patients with stage I/II tumors, doses of 80 Gy or greater using 3-dimensional conformal RT with sequential chemotherapy yielded a median OS of 3.4 years.[75] An ability to better deliver a dose led to dose escalation studies demonstrating these treatments to be safe with acceptable toxicity, including when administered with chemotherapy.[76,77] To achieve these higher doses, conventional daily 2-Gy fractions required treatment periods of 6+ weeks, which can be very demanding on patients, especially those with significant comorbidities that have precluded surgery. Further work showed accelerating treatments with hypofractionated regimens to be feasible, reducing treatment time by up to 2-3 weeks with similar rates of control and low toxicity.[78]

Stereotactic Body Radiation Therapy

Stereotactic body radiation therapy (SBRT) has emerged as the standard of care for medically inoperable patients with early stage NSCLC. This technique utilizes patient immobilization, image guidance, and respiratory management to deliver very high doses of radiation in a much shorter course than previous conventional regimens. Early retrospective comparisons between SBRT and conventional RT demonstrated improved local control (LC) and OS in favor of SBRT, with a meta-analysis estimating an improvement in 5-year OS from 19% to 42% when comparing conventional RT to SBRT.[79,80] Since the mid-2000s, multiple fractionation schemes have been studied in single- and multiple-institution phase 2 studies with excellent results, reporting LC rates of more than 90% and 3-year OS rates of 55%-60% in stage I patients.[81,82] Of note, this treatment is also referred to as stereotactic ablative radiation therapy (SABR), but this nomenclature is not used in this chapter.

Treatment Technique

By increasing the dose of radiation delivered per treatment fraction, radiation oncologists are able to take advantage of radiobiological properties and achieve a higher biologically effective dose (BED). A higher dose delivered to a tumor necessarily results in a higher dose to surrounding normal tissue, and for these treatments to be feasible, the amount of normal tissue receiving a high dose must be minimized. The stereotactic approach involves creating a treatment setup and plan that maximally minimizes aspects of uncertainty in tumor location. The first step is creating reliable and reproducible patient positioning and may be accomplished with rigid immobilization techniques to ensure the same area of the body is targeted with each treatment with minimal change in the patient's body position in space (**Figure 13-6**).

Because of the movement of the chest and intrathoracic contents with respiration, the next step involves accounting for the position of the tumor in space and time. Multiple methods have been developed to accomplish this. Four-dimensional CT (4-D CT) simulations are performed for treatment planning, allowing tumor motion to be tracked through all phases of the breathing cycle. Qualitative and quantitative vector maps have been used to describe lung and tumor motion that must be accounted for during RT delivery. Lung tumors can move well over 2 cm depending on the tumor location within the lung (**Figure 13-7**).[83]

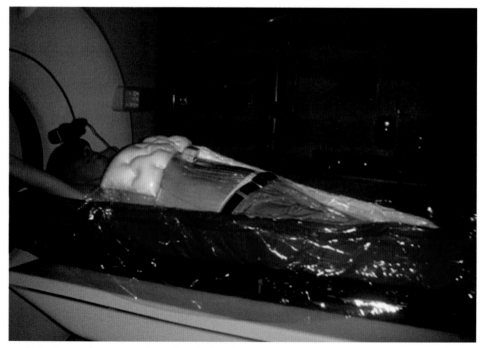

Figure 13-6. Patient setup for stereotactic body radiation therapy for treatment of a stage I lung cancer. A vacuum lock bag is used for rigid immobilization with plastic wrap over the top for further immobilization. Motion management is being used, with a block on the chest to measure surface position change with breathing, and a goggle screen gives the patient visual representation of this motion to help coordinate breathing actions.

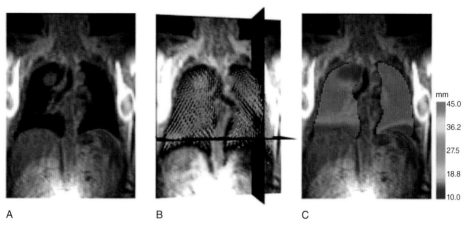

Figure 13-7. MRI depiction of parenchymal lung motion. **A.** Patient with solitary non–small cell lung cancer in upper right lung. **B.** Using simple vector field representation for a one-time frame of the breathing cycle, limited lung motion in right upper lung can hardly be seen. **C.** Using color map representation of the breathing cycle, from maximum expiration to maximum inspiration, limited asymmetric lung motion can clearly be seen. In this patient, overall lung motion was limited because of limited lung function. (Reproduced with permission from Plathow C, Schoebinger M, Herth F, Tuengerthal S, Meinzer HP, Kauczor HU. Estimation of pulmonary motion in healthy subjects and patients with intrathoracic tumors using 3D-dynamic MRI: initial results. *Korean J Radiol.* 2009;10(6):559-567.)

Using this information, the treating radiation oncologist can employ multiple techniques to ensure accurate targeting. For tumors that move minimally, a small extra margin can be applied to cover the target in all phases of the breathing cycle (**Figure 13-8**).[84] If there is substantial motion, radiation can be delivered in a gated fashion, with dose only being delivered at certain intervals of the breathing cycle as tracked by external monitoring or by having the patient hold his or her breath during the periods of radiation delivery to "fix" the tumor in space by eliminating intrathoracic respiratory motion (**Figure 13-9**).[85]

Pretreatment imaging is mandatory for SBRT to ensure accurate treatment localization prior to radiation delivery, but intratreatment radiographic imaging can also be

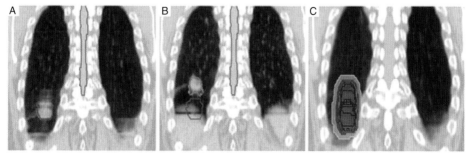

Figure 13-8. Example of internal target volume (ITV) creation. CT imaging is obtained for all phases of the breathing cycle, and the tumor is contoured in each phase to create a target volume that encompasses all areas it occupies. (Reproduced with permission from Glide-Hurst C, Chetty I. Improving radiotherapy planning, delivery accuracy, and normal tissue sparing using cutting edge technologies. *J Thorac Dis.* 2014;6(4):303-318. http://jtd.amegroups.com/article/view/2119.)

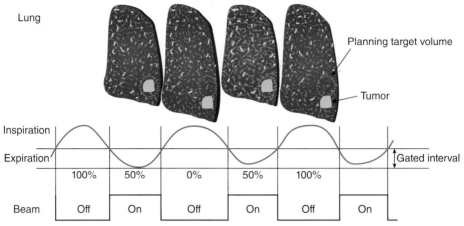

Figure 13-9. Principle of respiratory gating. The tumor is tracked during all stages of the respiratory cycle, and a particular phase is chosen for treatment. The radiation beam is turned on, and treatment is delivered during this pre-specified phase and is turned off at other times so that the beam targets the tumor at a particular point in time and space and avoids treatment of normal lung parenchyma when the tumor moves during the next phase of breathing. (Reproduced with permission from Kim JH. LINAC-based high-precision radiotherapy: radiosurgery, image-guided radiotherapy, and respiratory-gated radiotherapy. *J Korean Med Assoc.* 2008 Jul;51(7):612-618. https://doi.org/10.5124/jkma.2008.51.7.612.)

used to track the tumor, sometimes with the aid of fiducial markers or by confirmation of the positioning of adjacent bony structures (**Figure 13-10**). There is growing interest in using implanted fiducial markers with positional tracking radio transmission capabilities to track tumor motion, and this will be an area of active study in the coming years (**Figure 13-11**).

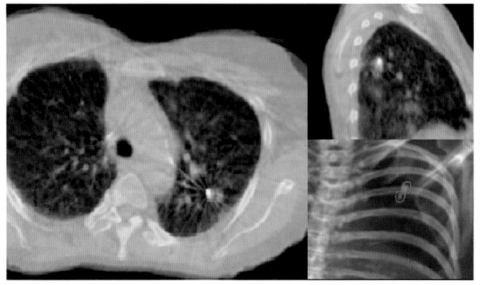

Figure 13-10. Fiducial markers. Metallic fiducial markers were bronchoscopically placed into a left upper lobe lung tumor and are utilized by the treatment delivery system to track the tumor throughout the breathing cycle to aid in targeting.

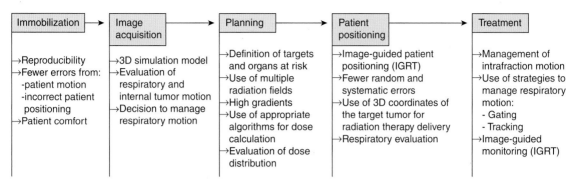

Figure 13-11. Workflow. This diagram details the steps for SBRT treatment of a lung tumor, from the initial planning stage to the delivery of treatment. (Reproduced with permission from Abreu CECV, Ferreira PPR, Moraes FY, Neves WFP Jr, Gadia R, Carvalho H A. Stereotactic body radiotherapy in lung cancer: an update. *J Bras Pneumol.* 2015;41(4):376-387. https://dx.doi.org/10.1590/S1806-37132015000000034.)

Medically Inoperable Patients

Stereotactic radiosurgery (SRS) is the use of high-dose RT, which is by definition delivered in a single fraction, to intracranial neoplasms, commonly in the form of brain metastases. As this technology gained widespread acceptance in the late twentieth century as an alternative to surgery, groups in Japan and the United States began exploring the feasibility of applying this technique to small lung tumors. First described as extracranial SRS, this technique then became known as SBRT to refer to RT delivered in a stereotactic manner to the body.

Uematsu et al. retrospectively analyzed a group of patients treated in the late 1990s undergoing RT to small primary lung tumors and lung metastases using motion evaluation, frame immobilization, and high dose per fraction (30-75 Gy delivered in 5-15 fractions). They found this technique was technically feasible, efficacious, and tolerable and yielded excellent LC.[86] This finding lead to implementation of SBRT for the treatment of stage I NSCLC in Japan; however, uncertainty remained regarding optimal dosing.

The Japanese Society of Radiation Oncology (JCOG) analyzed multiple fractionation regimens in both operable and inoperable patients receiving hypofractionated stereotactic radiation and found that doses with a BED of 100 Gy or greater provided better LC and OS.[87] Updated results demonstrated a persistent benefit at 5 years, with local failure of 43% versus 8% and 5-year OS of 31% versus 71% in tumors dosed to a BED less than 100 Gy versus BED greater than 100 Gy, respectively.[79]

While these previous findings were in a cohort receiving multiple fractionation regimens, Nagata et al. analyzed a population who had received 48 Gy in 4 fractions in a phase 1/2 study. In this retrospective study, no grade 3 toxicity was reported, and at 3-year disease-free survival (DFS) was greater than 70%, and OS was 83% and 72% for stage IA and IB (<4-cm tumor size) lung cancers, respectively.[88]

This led to a prospective clinical trial, JCOG 0403, evaluating this dose in both medically inoperable patients and patients who were operative candidates but had declined surgery. Grade 3 and 4 toxicity was observed in this study, likely owing to the more rigorous data collection inherent to a clinical trial, in 10 and 2 patients, respectively, out of a cohort of 169. Excellent LC and OS were once again demonstrated, with 3-year OS of 59.9% and 76.5% in the medically inoperable and operable groups, respectively, and due to the low incidence of severe toxicity, this regimen became the standard of care in Japan for medically inoperable patients with stage I NSCLC.[89]

Meanwhile, in the United States, a group at Indiana University led by Timmerman conducted a prospective phase 1 trial evaluating dose escalation in medically inoperable stage I NSCLC patients. Escalation was conducted separately between stage IA and IB patients, with both groups reaching a dose of 60 Gy in 3 fractions without reaching a maximum tolerated dose (MTD). Of note, 2 patients developed grade 3 toxicity; however, both received dose schedules less than the maximum of 20 Gy per fraction.[90] This was followed by a prospective phase 2 trial of medically inoperable patients. Patients were stratified by tumor size, with T1 patients receiving 60 Gy in 3 fractions and, as the MTD had not been reached on the phase 2 study, T2 patients receiving 66 Gy in 3 fractions. The 3-year LC was 88%, and CSS was 83%, with failures documented in the regional nodes in 9% and distantly in 13%.[91]

The success of this work led to the multi-institutional cooperative study Radiation Therapy Oncology Group (RTOG) 0236, a phase 2 trial delivering a dose of 54 Gy in 3 fractions to peripheral T1-2 tumors in non-operable patients, which further showed excellent disease response, with 98% primary tumor control and 91% LC (tumor and involved lobe) and a median OS of 4 years.[82] The recently issued final report demonstrated further recurrences as a consequence of longer follow-up, but outcomes were promising compared to historical data, with 5-year DFS and OS of 25.5% and 40%, respectively. At 5 years, primary tumor failure was 7.3%, with lobar, locoregional, and disseminated failures reported as 20%, 25.5%, and 23.6%, respectively. Disseminated disease was more common in T2 tumors, with 45.5% versus 18.2% incidence for T1 and non-squamous histologies, with 31.6% versus 5.9% incidence in those with squamous histology, following with our understanding of the course of larger and more biologically aggressive tumors.[92]

Medically Operable

Stereotactic body RT has provided major gains in survival and control in medically inoperable patients, and these results are also seen in the elderly population, for whom surgery, while feasible, comes with an increased risk of morbidity and mortality due to coexisting medical issues (**Table 13-1**).[93] With such promising results, the question has been posited regarding whether SBRT could be used as an alternative to surgical resection in the medically operable. This is a topic of multiple current clinical trials and is discussed further in the chapter. This section reviews the results of SBRT in the medically operable population.

In the JCOG 0403 trial, 39% ($n = 64$) of the study group were medically operable but had refused surgery and received 48 Gy in 4 fractions for their T1N0 lung tumor. The 3-year LC was 85.4%, with failure rates locally, locoregionally, and distantly of 9%, 25%, and 33%, respectively. The 3- and 5-year OS were 76.5% and 54%, respectively. Comparing the results to surgical patients in a national registry, the authors found their cohort tended to be older, and subgroup analysis of patients 80 years or older

TABLE 13-1	Radiation Dose Fractionation Schemes				
PROSPECTIVE TRIALS OF SBRT FOR STAGE I LUNG CANCER					
AUTHOR (yr)	TYPE/STAGE	NO. OF PATIENTS	DOSE	MEDIAN FOLLOW-UP (mo)	OUTCOMES
Timmerman et al. (2003) McGarry et al. (2005)	Phase I/Stage I NSCLC	47	8 Gy x 3 to 20 Gy x 3	19.1–27.4	1-yr LC: 64.7% 3-yr OS: 64%
Hoyer et al. (2006)	Prospective/ Stage I NSCLC	40	15 Gy x 3	28.8	2-yr LC: 85% 2-yr CSS: 62% 2-yr OS: 48%
Baumann et al. (2009)	Phase II/Stage I NSCLC	70	15 Gy x 3 to 67%	35	3-yr LC: 92% 3-yr CSS: 88% 3-yr OS: 60%
Timmerman et al. (2010)	RTOG Phase II/ T1-2N0M0 NSCLC (peripherally located)	55	18 Gy x 3	34.4	3-yr LC: 97.6% 3-yr DFS: 48.3% 3-yr OS: 55.8%
Ricardi et al. (2010)	Phase II/Stage I NSCLC	62	15 Gy x 3	28	3-yr LC: 87.8% 3-yr CSS: 72.5% 3-yr OS: 57.1%
Bral et al. (2011)	Phase II/ T1-3N0M0	40	20 Gy x 3 15 Gy x 4	16	2-yr LC: 84% 2-yr CSS: 64% 2-yr OS: 52%

A list of dose fractionation schemes from SBRT trials. CSS, cancer-specific survival; DFS, disease-free survival; LC, local control; NSCLC, non-small cell lung cancer; OS, overall survival; SBRT, stereotactic body radiotherapy; RTOG, Radiation Therapy Oncology Group.

Reproduced with permission from Ricardi U, Badellino S, Filippi AR. Stereotactic radiotherapy for early stage non-small cell lung cancer. Radiat Oncol J. 2015;33(2):57-65.

demonstrated similar 3- and 5-year OS, 73.8% and 62% for surgery and 80% and 54% for SBRT, respectively. These outcomes were deemed promising enough for the authors to posit that SBRT could be an acceptable alternative to surgical resection.[89]

RTOG 0618 evaluated 60 Gy in 3 fractions (54 Gy in 3 fractions with heterogeneity correction as per previous studies) for patients with tumors 5 cm or less in a peripheral location who all had PET/CT staging confirming disease extent. All patients had a Zubrod performance status of 0-1, and all were deemed fit for at least SR by a thoracic surgeon. Primary tumor and LC were 96%, locoregional control was 88%, and disseminated failure occurred in 12% of patients, with 4-year DFS and OS of 57% and 56%, respectively. Grade 3 toxicity was experienced by 15% of patients, with no grade 4-5 toxicity observed.[94]

Comparison to Surgery

For medically operable patients, while resection is the current standard of care, there is strong interest in determining whether SBRT provides equivalent or superior results. Comparable outcomes have been suggested in retrospective series, but to date no randomized trial has been completed to verify these data.[95,96] Two phase 3 studies were conducted in the United States and the Netherlands comparing SBRT to lobectomy in medically operable patients with stage I NSCLC (**Table 13-2**). The STARS trial was conducted in the United States, randomizing patients to robotic SBRT of 54 Gy in 3 fractions for peripheral lesions or 50 Gy in 4 fractions for central lesions, or surgical resection. The ROSEL trial, conducted in the Netherlands, randomized patients to

TABLE 13-2 Comparison of Studies of SBRT Versus Surgery					
STUDIES COMPARING SURGERY AND SBRT IN STAGE I NSCLC					
AUTHOR (yr)	STUDY DESIGN	NO. OF PATIENTS	SURGICAL PROCEDURE	OVERALL SURVIVAL	
				SURGERY	SBRT
Grills et al. (2010)	Retrospective	Surgery (69) SBRT (55)	Wedge resection	87% 30 mo	72% 30 mo
Crabtree et al. (2010)	Propensity-score matching	Unmatched: Surgery (458) SBRT (151) Matched: 112/group	(Bi)obectomy 78%; sublobar 19%; pneumonectomy 4%	78% 3 yr 68% 3 yr	47% 3 yr 52% 3 yr
Verstegen et al. (2013)	Propensity-score matching	Unmatched: Surgery (86) SBRT (527) Matched: 64/group	VATS lobectomy	77% 3 yr	80% 3 yr
Shirvani et al. (2014)	SEER population, propensity-score matching	Unmatched: Surgery (8,711) SABR (382) Matched: 251/group	Lobectomy 83% Sublobar 17%	Lobectomy vs. SBRT, HR 1.01 (SA: 1.16–1.28)	
Mokhles et al. (2015)	Propensity-score matching	Unmatched: Surgery (96) SBRT (481) Matched: 73/group	VATS lobectomy	95% 1 yr 80% 3 yr	94% 1 yr 53% 3 yr

This table lists details of recent studies comparing SBRT versus surgical resection of early stage NSCLC. HR, hazard ratio; NSCLC, non-small cell lung cancer; SA, sensitivity analyses; SBRT, stereotactic body radiotherapy; SEER Surveillance Epidemiology and End Results; VATS, video-assisted thoracoscopic surgery.

Reproduced with permission from Ricardi U, Badellino S, Filippi AR. Stereotactic radiotherapy for early stage non-small cell lung cancer. Radiat Oncol J. 2015;33(2):57-65.

surgery or SBRT of 54 Gy in 3 fractions, with only peripheral tumors treated. Due to low accrual, these were terminated early, but a pooled analysis of the results found better tolerability for SBRT and an estimated improved 3-year OS compared to surgical resection.[97] While these results were cautiously celebrated by proponents of SBRT, a pooled analysis does not deliver the same caliber of evidence as a completed phase 3 randomized controlled trial. Additionally, a meta-analysis of 12 cohort studies with over 13,000 patients showed worse OS with SBRT when compared to lobectomy and similar survival rates when compared to SR, raising further questions about the findings of the pooled analysis.[98]

High-level evidence in the form of fully accrued clinical trials is still needed to verify whether SBRT can be an equivalent alternative to lobectomy in the medically operable population. The failure to enroll a sufficient number of patients in these previous trials is likely multifactorial. Patients may balk at undergoing a surgical procedure requiring inpatient admission when the alternative consists of a few outpatient appointments in a radiation clinic. Likewise, due to the physiological stress and potential morbidity of a pulmonary resection, physicians may be biased in enrolling higher risk patients in a randomization that could result in allocation to surgery. The currently enrolling JoLT-CA STABLEMATES trial seeks to remedy these issues by prerandomizing eligible patients to SBRT or SR. If the patient consents to their allocated treatment, they will be treated per protocol and followed for OS, toxicity, and patterns of failure. Those who reject their allocated treatment and choose the other treatment arm will be consented to be followed in a registry for OS and patterns of failure.

The Veterans Affairs Lung Cancer or Stereotactic Radiotherapy (VALOR) trial is seeking to answer this question as well, with patients randomized to SBRT or anatomic surgical resection of their early stage lung cancer. The SABRTOOTH trial is another variation of this schema currently being investigated in the United Kingdom. While enrollment and follow-up are still underway, the results of these studies will have strong implications for the standard of care for early stage, medically operable patients going forward.

TOXICITY

As with conventional RT, toxicity from SBRT is related to the location of the lesion being treated, with adverse reactions ranging from radiographically detected, asymptomatic pulmonary fibrosis, to fatal complications such as exsanguination by hemoptysis. Radiation pneumonitis is the major dose-limiting factor in the treatment of lung cancers with RT (**Figure 13-12**). Symptoms can be as mild as a small cough to progressive dyspnea requiring steroid treatment or mechanical ventilation. Centrally located tumors present the greatest risk for morbidity and mortality due to the vital function of structures in the mediastinum. Damage to the great vessels, specifically the aorta, can lead to rupture, dissection, or fistula and can result in exsanguination events. Esophageal injury can manifest as mild esophagitis to serious complications like perforation and fistula. An excess dose to the vagus or recurrent laryngeal nerves has the potential to cause vocal cord paralysis, whereas superior sulcus tumors place patients at risk for brachial plexopathy. Peripheral tumors place the patient at risk of injury to the chest wall, which

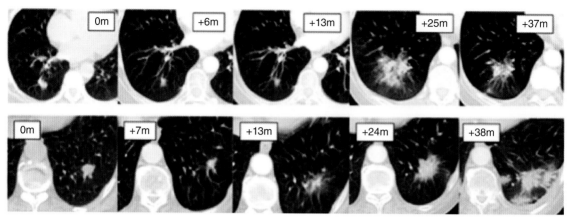

Figure 13-12. Radiation pneumonitis. Radiation pneumonitis is a common complication from radiation therapy to the lung and can manifest across a spectrum of symptoms, from mild to severe. This image demonstrates the progression of fibrotic change over 3 years after delivery of SBRT. (Reproduced with permission from Dahele M, Palma D, Lagerwaard F, Slotman B, Senan S. Radiological changes after stereotactic radiotherapy for stage I lung cancer. *J Thorac Oncol.* 2011; 6(7):1221-1228. https://doi.org/10.1097/JTO.0b013e318219aac5. http://www.sciencedirect.com/science/article/pii/ S1556086415310388. Copyright © 2011 by the International Association for the Study of Lung Cancer.)

may present as rib fracture or pain, as well as damage to the overlying skin.[99] Multiple resources are available with dosimetric constraints to help avoid these situations and guide treating physicians' choices in dose and fractionation to limit and avoid these toxicities (**Table 13-3**).

Role of Location in Toxicity

A noteworthy finding from the phase 2 Indiana study was grade 3-5 toxicity in 20% of patients at 2 years. Analysis showed a predilection for development of grade 3+ toxicity in those undergoing treatment for centrally located lesions in the proximal bronchial tree. Grade 3+ toxicity was 46% in these patients with tumors in the hilar/pericentral area, compared to 17% in those with peripheral tumors.[100] These initial findings prompted the study group to urge caution in using this regimen in patients with centrally located tumors. Final analysis of this study showed an increased rate of grade 3+ toxicity of 27% versus 10% in central versus peripheral lesions, but this did not reach statistical significance.[91]

> **CLINICAL PEARL:** Regardless, these findings led to the designation of a "no-fly zone" (**Figure 13-13**) in the area lying within 2 cm of the proximal bronchial tree, and this led to the exclusion of these patients in the RTOG 0236 study.

These findings led to the creation of the RTOG 0813 trial to study dose escalation for central tumors, with a starting dose of 10 Gy delivered in 5 fractions every other day, with a dose increase of 0.5 Gy per fraction up to a maximum dose of 60 Gy in 5 fractions. The rationale for increased fractionation relies on radiobiology. Sublethal damage is repaired between radiation fractions, and the combination of decreased daily dose over an increased time frame should allow for less damage and more repair of normal tissue, thus decreasing the incidence of greater toxicity. Preliminary results have been

TABLE 13-3   Treatment Planning Dose Constraints

SERIAL TISSUE	VOLUME	VOLUME MAX (Gy)	MAX POINT DOSE (Gy)	AVOIDANCE ENDPOINT
Spinal cord	<0.25 mL <0.5 mL	22.5 Gy (4.5 Gy/fx) 13.5 Gy (2.7 Gy/fx)	30 Gy (6 Gy/fx)	Myelitis
Ipsilateral brachial plexus	<3 mL	30 Gy (6 Gy/fx)	32 Gy (6.4 Gy/fx)	Neuropathy
Skin	<10 mL	30 Gy (6 Gy/fx)	32 Gy (6.4 Gy/fx)	Ulceration
PARALLEL TISSUE	CRITICAL COLUME	CRITICAL VOLUME DOSE MAX (Gy)		AVOIDANCE ENDPOINT
Lung (right & left)	1,500 mL	12.5 Gy (2.5 Gy/fx)		Basic lung function
Lung (right & left)	1,000 mL	13.5 Gy (2.7 Gy/fx)		Pneumonitis
Esophagus, non-adjacent wall	<5 mL	27.5 Gy (5.5 Gy/fx)	105% of PTV prescription	Stenosis/fistula
Heart/pericardium	<15 mL	32 Gy (6.4 Gy/fx)	105% of PTV prescription	Pericarditis
Great vessels, non-adjacent wall	<10 mL	47 Gy (9.4 Gy/fx)	105% of PTV prescription	Aneurysm
Trachea and ipsilateral bronchus, non-adjacent wall	<4 mL	18 Gy (3.6 Gy/fx)	105% of PTV prescription	Stenosis/fistula

This table details radiation dose constraints for normal tissues as per the RTOG 0813 protocol.

PTV: planning target volume.

Reproduced with permission from https://www.rtog.org/clinicaltrials/protocoltable/studydetails.aspx?action=openFile& FileID=9067.

reported in abstract form, and for patients receiving the 2 highest dose fractionation schemes, 11.5 and 12 Gy per fraction, 2-year grade 3+ toxicity was acceptable; there was excellent LC and 2-year OS of 70%, comparable to patients treated for peripheral tumors.[101] The currently active European Organization for Research and Treatment of Cancer (EORTC) 22113-08113 LungTech trial is investigating a slightly more fractionated scheme of 60 Gy in 8 fractions in medically inoperable patients with central lesions. Further delineation of central tumors into an ultracentral designation has been made, characterized as tumors where the planning treatment volume encompasses the central bronchial tree, esophagus, or pulmonary vasculature. The SUNSET study is currently underway in Canada and is investigating the safety of a regimen of 60 Gy delivered over 8 daily fractions for ultracentral tumors.[102]

Dose Fractionation Schedules

There are currently no standard dose fractionation schedules, and numerous trials are underway seeking to compare results between multiple accepted regimens. Schedules

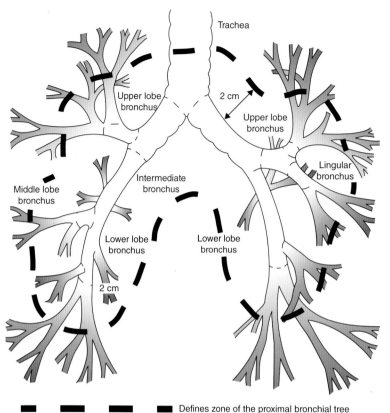

Trachea

Upper lobe bronchus

2 cm

Upper lobe bronchus

Lingular bronchus

Intermediate bronchus

Middle lobe bronchus

Lower lobe bronchus

Lower lobe bronchus

2 cm

2 cm

■ ■ ■ ■ Defines zone of the proximal bronchial tree

Figure 13-13. "No-fly zone" delineating locations of central versus peripheral tumors. This image from the RTOG 0236 protocol designates the areas within 2 cm of the proximal bronchial tree as a no-fly zone, which delineates central versus peripheral tumors given the additional toxicity seen when treating centrally located tumors. (Reproduced with permission from Timmerman R, McGarry R, Yiannoutsos C, et al. Excessive toxicity when treating central tumors in a phase II study of stereotactic body radiation therapy for medically inoperable early-stage lung cancer. *J Clin Oncol.* 2006;24(30):4833-4839. Copyright © 2006 American Society of Clinical Oncology.)

of 1-5 fractions have been reported with good success, with increased fractionation recommended for centrally located tumors due to the potential for increased toxicity with high doses to the proximal bronchial tree and mediastinal contents.[91] At this time, there are a number of dose fractionation schedules in use and various others under study, with many of these discussed previously in the chapter (**Table 13-4**).

The Japanese regimen of 48 Gy in 4 fractions has been used in both medically operable and inoperable patients for tumors in all locations. The Indiana series utilized doses of 60 Gy and 66 Gy in 3 fractions for T1 and T2 tumors, respectively, in a cohort of medically inoperable patients. The schedule of 60 Gy in 3 fractions was utilized in the RTOG 0236 trial, and when planning adjustments were made for tissue heterogeneity, the rationale of which is outside the scope of this text, the final prescribed dose was 54 Gy in 3 fractions. These patients were medically inoperable, and due to the findings of excessive toxicity for central tumors in the phase 2 Indiana study, the cohort was restricted to those patients with tumors outside of 2 cm from the proximal bronchial tree. The phase 2 RTOG 0915 trial further investigated fractionation schedules in medically inoperable patients with peripheral tumors, comparing treatments of 34 Gy in a single fraction to 48 Gy in 4 fractions, with the single-fraction arm meeting prespecified toxicity criteria, with a recommendation for further study of this regimen.[103] For central

TABLE 13-4   Common Dose Fractionation Schedules

COMMONLY EMPLOYED SBRT DOSE FRACTIONATION REGIMES FOR PERIPHERAL AND CENTRAL EARLY STAGE NON-SMALL CELL LUNG CANCER

LOCATION OF PRIMARY DISEASE	TOTAL DOSE (Gy)	NUMBER OF FRACTIONS	DOSE PER FRACTION (Gy)	BED_{10} (Gy)	EQD_2 TUMOR	BED_3 (Gy)	EQD_2 NORMAL TISSUE
Peripheral ES-NSCLC	34	1	34	150	125	420	252
	45	3	15	113	94	270	162
	54	3	18	151	126	378	227
	60	3	20	180	150	460	276
	48	4	12	106	88	240	144
Central ES-NSCLC	50	5	10	100	83	217	130
	55	5	11	116	96	257	154
	60	5	12	132	110	300	180
	60	8	7.5	105	88	210	126

This table lists common dose fractionation schedules used for SBRT treatment of lung tumors. BED_3, biological effective dose using alpha/beta 3; BED_{10}, biological effective dose using alpha/beta 10; EQD_2, normal tissue, equivalent dose in 2-Gy fractions using alpha/beta 3; EQD_2 tumor, equivalent dose in 2-Gy fractions using alpha/beta 10; ES-NSCLC, early stage non–small cell lung cancer; Gy, Gray.

Reproduced with permission from Dunne E, Fraser I, Liu M. Stereotactic body radiation therapy for lung, spine and oligometastatic disease: current evidence and future directions. Ann Transl Med. 2018;6(14):283. doi:10.21037/atm.2018.06.40.

tumors in medically inoperable patients, RTOG 0813 began with a dose of 50 Gy in 5 fractions and dose escalation to 60 Gy in 5 fractions, with the logic that fractionating the dose would improve normal tissue toxicity and put these patients at less risk for adverse events. In the Netherlands, 60 Gy was prescribed in 3, 5, and 8 fractions to an elderly, inoperable population with multiple medical comorbidities with acceptable toxicity. Yet another dose schedule of 45 Gy in 3 fractions is used in Scandinavian countries with good success.

Fewer studies have been conducted in medically operable patients; however, multiple trials are currently underway with dose fractionation schedules derived from previous work in the inoperable population and following on the same principles of fractionation for more centrally located lesions. The JCOG 0403 study utilized 48 Gy in 3 fractions for both medically operable and inoperable patients with T1 tumors. RTOG 0618 used 60 Gy in 3 fractions, with tumors greater than 5 cm or centrally located excluded from the trial. The STARS trial used robotic SBRT and fiducial tracking to deliver 54 Gy in 3 fractions to peripheral lesions and 50 Gy in 4 fractions to central lesions. The ROSEL protocol used fractionation schedules of 54 Gy in 3 fractions and 60 Gy in 5 fractions, with central tumors excluded from the study. In Europe, central lesions are being treated to 60 Gy in 8 fractions on the EORTC LungTech trial that is currently in progress. As mentioned, the current treatment planning goal is to deliver doses with a

BED of more than 100 Gy while optimally minimizing the risk of damage to adjacent normal tissues.

Significant progress has been made in the treatment of early stage NSCLC with definitive RT. As technology improved, so did the ability to deliver higher doses while respecting the tolerance of adjacent normal tissues. With the advent of SBRT, further improvement in control and survival has been appreciated in both the medically operable and inoperable populations. Further innovation will improve the accuracy and efficiency of SBRT treatments and it is hoped provide greater benefits to patients. The question about whether SBRT can be considered an alternative to surgical resection in the operable population has not been satisfactorily answered and is the current focus of multiple ongoing clinical trials. The results of these trials, as well as other studies evaluating optimal dose fractionation and site of tumor, are sure to impact clinical management of early stage NSCLC for the years to come.

CHEMOTHERAPY FOR EARLY NON–SMALL CELL LUNG CANCER
Phuong T. Ngo, MD

A 62-year-old Caucasian male with past medical history of tobacco abuse, hypertension, and COPD was found to have a 4-cm spiculated mass in the right lower lobe with no lymph node involvement. PET/CT and MRI brain showed no distant disease. He underwent right lobectomy without complications and now presents to discuss further management. What should be offered to this patient?

Learning Objectives:
1. What is the rationale for adjuvant chemotherapy?
2. Which patients should receive adjuvant chemotherapy?
3. What defines high-risk patients?
4. What are some common chemotherapy regimens for adjuvant treatment?

ADJUVANT CHEMOTHERAPY

Even with stage I disease, a portion of patients will relapse and die of distant disease within 5 years of curative surgical resection, hence the rationale of adjuvant chemotherapy. Its use in completely resected NSCLC began in the 1960s and 1970s through trials evaluating alkylating agents and certain immunotherapies (mainly levamisole and Bacillus Calmette-Guerin [BCG]), all of which failed to show any survival benefit. Following these were trials using cisplatin-based chemotherapy, but many of these had flaws, including sample size, incomplete mediastinal lymph node dissection, inadequate accrual, and inadequate dose and dose intensity. Thus, the majority of these trials failed to show benefit from adjuvant chemotherapy.

In 1995, however, an individual patient meta-analysis of 8 randomized clinical trials showed that patients who received cisplatin-based regimens had an improved survival rate of about 5% at 5 years, with borderline statistical significance, $p = .08$.[104] There was a 6% reduction in the risk of death in patients treated with postoperative radiation plus chemotherapy compared to radiation alone, but the results were also not significant, and adjuvant chemotherapy with long-term alkylating agents also appeared to have a detrimental effect. The applicability of this meta-analysis to clinical practice was limited by its imprecise results, the heterogeneity of surgical procedures, differences in staging modalities, and specific chemotherapy regimens. There was also no large prospective trial showing improved survival from adjuvant treatment. Subsequently, many large clinical trials emerged to definitively evaluate the role of adjuvant chemotherapy after resection in early stage NSCLC.

In the International Adjuvant Lung Trial (IALT), patients with stage I to IIIA disease were randomized to observation alone or chemotherapy with cisplatin plus vinorelbine, etoposide, vinblastine, or vindesine after resection. The study showed significant improvement in median survival, DFS, 5-year survival, and 5-year DFS with a hazard ratio (HR) of 0.86 for survival in favor of the chemotherapy arm.[105] The National Cancer Institute of Canada (NCI-C JBR.10) also conducted a trial in which 482 patients with resected stage IB or II disease were randomized to observation alone or to cisplatin and vinorelbine. They also found that OS was significantly prolonged for the chemotherapy arm, with OS of 94 versus 73 months (HR for death, 0.69; $p = .04$). Five-year survival rates were also significant at 69% versus 54% for the chemotherapy and observations groups, respectively ($p = .03$).[106]

ADJUVANT POPULATION

The benefits of adjuvant chemotherapy also appear to differ with disease stage. The Lung Adjuvant Cisplatin Evaluation (LACE) was an individual patient meta-analysis that pooled 5 large cisplatin-based adjuvant trials (ALPI, BLT, IALT, JBR.10, and ANITA [Adjuvant Navelbine International Trialist Association]) to show a 5.4% absolute 5-year survival benefit with chemotherapy (HR 0.89; 95% CI 0.82-0.96; $p = .005$).[107] Interestingly, adjuvant chemotherapy in stage IB patients had an HR for death of 0.93 (95% CI 0.78-1.10), while stage IA patients had an HR of 1.40 (95% CI 0.95-2.06), indicating additional systemic treatment actually had a detrimental effect in this latter group. The CALGB 9633 trial randomly assigned stage IB patients to surgery alone versus surgery followed by carboplatin/paclitaxel and found that in long-term follow up, only patients with tumors 4 cm or larger had a significant survival benefit with adjuvant chemotherapy.[108]

> **CLINICAL PEARL:** There are currently no data in favor of adjuvant chemotherapy for stage IA disease while "high-risk" stage IB patients, discussed next, can be considered for adjuvant chemotherapy.

HIGH-RISK PATIENTS

- Tumor 4 cm or greater
- Poorly differentiated tumors
- Presence of vascular invasion
- Wedge resection
- Visceral pleural involvement
- Unknown lymph node status (Nx)

The results of the CALGB 9633 trial were confounded by the use of carboplatin rather than cisplatin since cisplatin has been superior to carboplatin for stage IV NSCLC.

The role of adjuvant chemotherapy for stage II disease is more established compared to stage I. In the ANITAtrial, patients with stage IB to IIIA disease were randomized to surgery alone or surgery followed by cisplatin and vinorelbine for 4 cycles.[109] The median survival was 65.8 months for the chemotherapy arm compared to 43.7 months in the observation arm (HR 1.264; 95% CI 1.05-1.52; p = .013). Survival was measured at 2, 5, and 7 years, showing 68%, 51%, 45%, respectively, in the chemotherapy arm compared to 63%, 43%, and 37%, respectively. Overall 5-year survival was significantly improved in favor of chemotherapy, but the results were more evident with stage II and IIIA disease.

> **CLINICAL PEARL:** Adjuvant chemotherapy is recommended following resection of stage II and III NSCLC, though the optimal regimen remains unclear.

ADJUVANT AGENTS

Cisplatin plus vinorelbine was the most commonly used regimen in positive trials of adjuvant chemotherapy, but cisplatin can also be combined with etoposide, gemcitabine, or pemetrexed in non-squamous disease as well. Almost all studies have used cisplatin-containing doublets, with the exception of the CALGB 9633 trial, which used carboplatin. Cisplatin is recommended over carboplatin for the adjuvant setting with potential curative intent (**Table 13-5**).

Tyrosine Kinase Inhibitors

There is ongoing research regarding the incorporation of molecularly targeted agents into adjuvant treatment of early stage NSCLC, though the results of past trials have not been promising. The NCI-C JBR.19 trial looked at the administration of gefitinib, an epidermal growth factor receptor (EGFR) inhibitor, in stage I to III NSCLC patients after resection and found that OS did not improve. In fact, a subset of these patients who were found to have an EGFR mutation, a population expected to have more benefit from this regimen, potentially had a detrimental effect to gefitinib.[110] Stage IB to IIIA NSCLC patients were randomly assigned to erlotinib, another EGFR inhibitor, or placebo for 2 years in the RADIANT trial, but the results were not statistically significant.[111] The ALCHEMIST trial is currently ongoing in which stage IB to stage IIIA patients with EGFR or anaplastic lymphoma kinase (ALK) mutations are randomly assigned to adjuvant erlotinib or crizotinib versus placebo. *At this time, until more studies are available, the use of a molecularly targeted agent is not recommended as adjuvant therapy in early stage NSCLC outside of a clinical trial.*

ADJUVANT THERAPY IN ELDERLY PATIENTS

Elderly patients typically have a worse performance status, more comorbidities, and possibly organ failure, including declining renal function, which presents a challenge for chemotherapy administration. In addition, they also tend to have slower recovery

TABLE 13-5	Chemotherapy Table for Adjuvant Chemotherapy Following Surgical Resection in Early Stage Non–Small Cell Lung Cancer					
TRIAL	STAGES	PATIENTS	TREATMENT	5-YEAR SURVIVAL (%)	HAZARD RATIO	P-VALUE
ALPI	I-IIIA	603 606	Surgery alone vs. adjuvant mitomycin, vindesine, and cisplatin	51 43	0.96	0.589
IALT	IB-IIIA	405 361	Surgery alone vs. adjuvant cisplatin/etoposide or vinca alkaloids	40 44.5	0.86	0.03
CALGB	IB	172 172	Surgery alone vs. adjuvant carboplatin/paclitaxel	57 59	0.83	0.12
NCI-C	IB-II	241 241	Surgery alone vs. adjuvant cisplatin/vinorelbine	54 69	0.80	0.03
ANITA	IB-IIIA	433 407	Surgery alone vs. adjuvant cisplatin/vinorelbine	43 51	0.80	0.017

ANITA, Adjuvant Navelbine International Trialist Association; ALPI, Adjuvant Lung Project Italy; CALGB, Cancer and Leukemia Group B; IALT, International Adjuvant Lung Cancer Trial; NCI-C, National Cancer Institute of Canada.

from surgery and are at higher risk for treatment-related toxicities. However, they also make up a large percentage of lung cancer patients, with about 50% diagnosed after the age of 65 and about 30% diagnosed after the age of 70.[107] A retrospective analysis used the NCI-C JBR.10 trial to evaluate the effect of age on survival, chemotherapy compliance, and toxicity.[112] Of 482 patients, 155 were 65 years or older. These elderly patients received fewer doses of chemotherapy without significant differences in toxicities. Overall, their survival was also better with chemotherapy than without, though patients who were older than 75 years had a significantly shorter survival than those ages 66-75.

> **CLINICAL PEARL:** Adjuvant chemotherapy should therefore still be given to elderly patients fit enough to receive platinum-based chemotherapy.

NEOADJUVANT THERAPY

Chemotherapy given before surgery can downstage the disease to allow for complete resection and treat micrometastases earlier. Patients also tolerate preoperative chemotherapy better, with a greater percentage of patients completing it compared to postoperative chemotherapy. Two small randomized trials sought to establish its role in the treatment of stage IIIA patients; patients were assigned to surgery alone versus surgery plus neoadjuvant chemotherapy.[113,114] Both studies showed improved survival for the neoadjuvant arm, but each trial only had 60 patients, with imbalances between the two arms and poor survival of the control group. A larger study randomized patients to surgery alone versus neoadjuvant chemotherapy with mitomycin, ifosfamide, and cisplatin followed by surgery in patients with stage IB, II, and IIIA; the study did not show a survival benefit in the chemotherapy arm. Another large study randomly assigned 519 patients to surgery alone versus preoperative treatment with three cycles of platinum-based chemotherapy followed by surgery in which, again, there was no evidence of survival benefit (HR 1.02; 95% CI 0.80-1.31; $p = .86$).[115]

> **CLINICAL PEARL:** There is currently no evidence that neoadjuvant chemotherapy improves survival in early stage NSCLC patients.

IMMUNOTHERAPY FOR EARLY STAGE NON–SMALL CELL LUNG CANCER

Joseph A. Pinto-Llerena, MD, Luis E. Raez, MD, FACP, FCCP, Ignacio Gil-Bazo, MD, PhD

A 60-year-old patient had a stage II adenocarcinoma of the lung resected. She received adjuvant chemotherapy but is aware of the ongoing risk of having a recurrence. She asks if immunotherapy could prevent a relapse and improve her chances of cure.

Learning Objectives:
1. What kind immunotherapies for lung cancer have been tested?
2. Would you advise the patient to participate in a clinical trial with this modality?

Although early stage lung cancers are treated surgically with curative intent, recurrence rates after complete anatomic resection remain unacceptably high, ranging from 30% to 70%, with a peak of recurrence at the 10th month after surgery.[107,116] Thus, very few NSCLC patients achieve cure even with surgery; in fact, tumor recurrence is the primary obstacle to long-term survival (OS) with no further curative options after relapse. Only 36% to 73% of patients with stage IA-IIB lung cancer are alive at 5 years; for those with stage III disease, the 2-year survival is less than 50% despite definitive therapy. We have learned that adjuvant cisplatin-based doublet chemotherapy can marginally improve survival by eradicating occult micrometastases. The LACE trial, a pooled analysis of 5 large clinical trials accounting for 4,584 patients, demonstrated a 5-year OS benefit of 5.4% with adjuvant chemotherapy. This is a fairly modest gain considering the toxicity associated with cisplatin-based chemotherapy. Moreover, no predictive biomarkers have ever been developed in order to select patients in which a greater benefit from adjuvant chemotherapy may be estimated. This caveat leaves us in dire need of novel adjuvant approaches to improve cure rates.

> **CLINICAL PEARL:** Currently, the indication for adjuvant treatment with platinum-based doublets is only limited to stages II (A and B) and IIIA and selected patients with stage IB (>4 cm in longest diameter) with weaker evidence.[117,118]

After several trials failing to prove clinical benefit in terms of OS for patients harboring EGFR-positive NSCLC,[110,111] more recently a benefit of the adjuvant gefitinib has been shown (over vinorelbine plus cisplatin),[119] but there have been controversies with the study, and validation trials are warranted to see if this is real or not and finally we can move forward with adjuvant therapy for lung cancer other than chemotherapy.

The manipulation of patients' immune system offers new therapeutic opportunities where several approaches are being developed with great potential for becoming the new standard of care. There is an increasing amount of data regarding the role of immunotherapy in metastatic NSCLC as well in other malignant tumors. Activation or restoration of immune surveillance could treat and eradicate cancers; this is something well known now that we have several agents approved for stage III and IV NSCLC. Despite the efforts and promising results in the advanced and metastatic setting, many immunotherapies, especially vaccines, have failed to move forward to localized disease, revealing also that there are many immunological phenomena influencing these treatments that remain in the darkness.

We cover in this section vaccines, antiangiogenic antibodies, and checkpoint inhibitors that are the most common types of immunotherapy interventions that have been studied in NSCLC. Some promissory types of immunotherapy in development for other malignancies but not clinically tested in lung cancer yet (like chimeric antigen receptor [CAR] T cells in hematology malignancies) are not covered here, but we have to keep them in mind if they find a role in NSLC in the near future.

ACTIVE IMMUNOTHERAPY

In NSCLC, several strategies of active immunotherapy have been evaluated with contrasting results. Active immunotherapy using tumor-associated antigens is the oldest approach to immunotherapy in NSCLC. Hollinshead et al.[120] aimed to study the role of vaccines (active immunotherapy) for NSCLC after surgery, observing significant differences in 5-year OS in favor of the immunized group compared to the control group (69% vs. 49%; p = .0002) in stage II and III NSCLC patients. However, after the communication of this and other promising phase 2 trials, there were several randomized multinational phase 3 studies that also tried to address this question. Nevertheless, none of those trials resulted in success. The most relevant studies are as follows:

The melanoma-associated antigen 3 (MAGE-A3), a protein involved in embryonal development and tumor transformation and progression, is expressed in 30%-50% of NSCLC tumor samples depending on the stage, and it is associated with poor outcome.[121-123] MAGE-A3 is associated with the immune adjuvant AS15 in the vaccine GSK1572932A and has been evaluated in NSCLC.[124] In a randomized, placebo-controlled phase 2 trial, after a median follow-up of 44 months after surgery, recurrence rates were 35% in patients treated with MAGE-A3 and 43% in patients with placebo, although differences were not statistically significant. Even though no significant differences were observed in terms of disease-free interval, DFS, or OS, the promising results justified a phase 3 study.[125]

The phase 3 MAGRIT trial screened more than 13,000 patients for MAGE-A3 expression and enrolled 2,312 patients randomly assigned to a 2:1 ratio to receive vaccine or placebo (13 doses over 27 months). Three co-primary study endpoints were established: DFS in the overall population, DFS in patients not receiving chemotherapy treatment, and DFS in patients with a potentially favorable gene signature. This study failed to show an improvement in the three primary endpoints when patients received MAGE-A3 vaccination. In fact, the results showed, for the general population, HR = 1.02 (95% CI 0.89–1.18) and HR = 1.04 (95% CI 0.86–1.24) for DFS and OS, respectively. In the no-chemotherapy cohort, the authors found HR = 0.97 (95% CI 0.80–1·18) and HR = 1.00 (95% CI 0.78–1.29) for DFS and OS, respectively.[126]

Other vaccines were evaluated in phase 3 trials in NSCLC patients, with unsuccessful results after several promising phase 2 studies were published.[127-130] A more recent meta-analysis of adjuvant immunotherapy studies for NSCLC (excluding checkpoint inhibitors) in patients treated with surgery or radiotherapy with curative intent showed no benefit from this type of intervention yet.[131]

MONOCLONAL ANTIBODIES TARGETING ANGIOGENESIS

Angiogenesis is an essential cancer hallmark for oncogenesis, disease progression, and metastases.[132] The interaction between the vascular endothelial growth factor (VEGF) and its receptor is a key player of angiogenesis in malignant tumors, where targeting angiogenesis has been an attractive therapeutic strategy for a long time.[133] Bevacizumab is a humanized monoclonal antibody targeting VEGF that is widely used in several malignant tumors, including lung cancer.[134]

The phase 3 study ECOG 4599 comparing paclitaxel and carboplatin alone versus paclitaxel and carboplatin plus bevacizumab evaluated 878 NSCLC patients with recurrent or advanced disease. A significant improvement in the OS and DFS of patients treated with bevacizumab plus chemotherapy compared with those treated with chemotherapy alone was demonstrated (HR = 0.79, 95% CI 0.67-0.92, p = .003 and HR = 0.66, 95% CI 0.57-0.77, p < .001).[135] Thanks to this trial, the study of bevacizumab gained Food and Drug Administration approval in the United States as first-line therapy for NSCLC combined with carboplatin and paclitaxel and became a new standard of care.

This promising result led to the development of the ECOG 1505 study, in which a potential survival advantage gained by the addition of bevacizumab to chemotherapy (platinum based) in the adjuvant setting after surgery for early stage NSCLC was investigated. In total 1,501 patients with stage IB to IIIA with surgically resected disease were randomly assigned to either treatment arm. Despite the advantage seen in adding bevacizumab to chemotherapy in the advanced setting, the ECOG 1505 study showed no significant differences between the treatment arms (HR = 0.99, 95% CI 0.82–1.19, p = .90 and HR = 0.99, 95% CI 0.86–1.15, p = .95 for OS and DFS, respectively, in the primary analysis population). Moreover, the addition of bevacizumab produced more cases of grade 3-5 toxicity in the bevacizumab arm compared to the standard of care (83% vs. 67%).[136] For this reason, bevacizumab was not added to the standard adjuvant therapy for NSCLC, which still comprises platinum-based chemotherapy alone. There are other antiangiogenic agents approved for NSCLC, such as ramucirumab, but no data regarding its use in the adjuvant setting have been produced yet.

IMMUNE CHECKPOINT INHIBITORS

One of the most important steps in cancer evolution occurs when tumor cells are able to evade immune system surveillance; in fact, the tumor manipulates the immune system to promote a tumor-friendly microenvironment.[137] One of the most relevant mechanisms allowing tumor evasion is the creation of immune tolerance by activating inhibitory checkpoints on T cells.[138] The receptors CTLA-4, PD-1, and its ligand PD-L1 are the better characterized immune checkpoints, and several antibodies have been developed to target these molecules with the aim of activating the antitumor immune response against several malignancies, including NSCLC. These drugs include ipilimumab, targeting CTLA-4; nivolumab and pembrolizumab, targeting PD-1; atezolizumab, avelumab, and durvalumab, directed against PD-L1.[139]

Phase 2/3 trials evaluating combinations of ipilimumab with carboplatin/paclitaxel in the treatment of advanced NSCLC have not demonstrated an improvement in overall survival (OS) or progression free survival (PFS) when compared with carboplatin/paclitaxel alone.[140,141] Novel strategies looking for the abscopal effect by combining ablation radiotherapy with ipilimumab are showing promising results.[142] In addition, combinations of ipilimumab with an anti-PD-1 antibody are being evaluated. The trial CheckMate 816 (NCT02998528) is evaluating ipilimumab plus nivolumab in combination with platinum doublet chemotherapy in the adjuvant setting of early stage NSCLC.

Approved immune checkpoint inhibitor monoclonal antibodies for NSCLC include nivolumab (anti-PD-1, for metastatic tumors with progression during or after platinum chemotherapy); pembrolizumab (anti-PD-1, for metastatic tumors expressing PD-L1 with progression during or after platinum chemotherapy or as first-line treatment in PD-L1 expression > 50%); atezolizumab (anti-PD-L1, for metastatic setting progressed during or following platinum-containing chemotherapy); and more recently, durvalumab (anti-PD-L1, in unresectable stage III tumors without progression following concurrent platinum-based chemotherapy and radiotherapy).

There is great interest to move these drugs forward to the adjuvant and neoadjuvant setting in NSCLC, and efforts are focused on a combination of two immune checkpoint inhibitors (an anti-CTLA-4 agent and anti-PD-1/PD-L1) or combinations with radiotherapy. The ALCHEMIST master protocol (NCT02194738) is an ongoing clinical trial platform evaluating several targeted therapies in the adjuvant setting in NSCLC, including nivolumab. The ANVIL study (NCT02595944) included in the ALCHEMIST camp are nivolumab versus placebo in patients with tumors without EGFR mutations or ALK translocations. The idea is to offer this to patients with stage IB-III targeted therapy or immunotherapy after they have received the standard of care: surgery followed by chemotherapy. Patients with actionable genes EGFR or ALK will be administered targeted therapy (substudies E45412 and A081105), and the rest of the patients with no actionable genes will be randomized, in the substudy E5142, to either fixed-dose 240 mg nivolumab or placebo for 1 year.

The Canadian Cancer Trials Group (CCTG) has launched a study, BR.31, aiming to accrue 1,100 patients with stages IB-IIIA who will be randomized to durvalumab versus placebo after surgery, looking for DFS in PD-L1 high as the main endpoint. This study will include EGFR-/ALK-positive patients. Also, KEYNOTE-091 study is testing pembrolizumab for 1 year (vs. placebo) in stage IB/II-IIIA NSCLC patients who have undergone complete surgical resection followed by standard adjuvant chemotherapy.[143]

New approaches changing the tumor immunity by tumor exposition to chemoradiation prior to immune checkpoint inhibitors show dramatic changes in the efficacy of these drugs.

The initial results of the PACIFIC trial with durvalumab has increased PFS in patients with unresectable stage III disease who have completed chemotherapy and radiation (16.8 months with durvalumab vs. 5.6 months with placebo; stratified HR for disease progression or death = 0.52; 95% CI 0.42-0.65, $p < .001$); the updated analysis of this study (with a median of 25.2 months of follow-up) showed a meaningful increase of the 2-year OS rates in patients treated with durvalumab in contrast to patients treated with placebo (66.3% vs. 55.6%, respectively; $p = .005$).[144,145]

> **CLINICAL PEARL:** Adjuvant Durvalumab improved PFS and OS in unresectable Stage 3 NSCLC after chemoradiation.

Technically, we call this "consolidation" immunotherapy, but probably we could also conceive that this benefit from durvalumab might be derived from local or distant microscopic disease in some patients in whom the recurrence may be delayed. With that perspective, this agent might also be useful in the adjuvant setting if there is microscopic disease after surgery.

Finally, the other great opportunity is the combination of immunotherapy and chemotherapy; in patients with metastatic disease, we have learned from the studies KEYNOTE 024, 189 and IMPOWER 150 that the addition of immunotherapy to combination chemotherapy increases not only DFS but also sometimes OS[146-148]; maybe the adjuvant immunotherapy of the future will include a combination of agents with chemotherapy and not immunotherapy agents alone.

In summary, after close to 15 years since the approval of adjuvant chemotherapy for NSCLC, we are finally getting closer to find better and less toxic alternatives that can prolong PFS and OS. Targeted therapy is very promissory in this context, with the results already presented using tyrosine kinase inhibitors (TKIs) in the adjuvant setting for NSCLC. Immunotherapy has several studies that have showed success with a strong HR in the metastatic setting and recently in stage III NSCLC after chemotherapy and radiation (PACIFIC trial). We hope that it is only a matter of time before this benefit translates to the early stage setting, where we know definitely that there is microscopic disease that needs to be eradicated to prolong PFS and OS (**Table 13-6**). The low-toxicity profile of immunotherapy also provides desirable options where the benefits probably outweigh the risks.

TABLE 13-6		Phase 3 Trials Evaluating Immune Checkpoint Inhibitors in Early Stage NSCLC			
PACIFIC (NCT02125461)	3	NSCLC patients with 2 cycles of platinum-based chemotherapy with radiation therapy	Durvalumab vs. placebo	PFS; OS	PFS medians: 16.8 vs. 5.6; 2-year OS rates: 66.3% vs. 55.6%
CheckMate 816 (NCT02998528)	3	Early stage IB-IIIA, operable NSCLC	Nivolumab plus chemotherapy vs. chemotherapy alone	Event-free survival, PCR	Recruiting
ANVIL (NCT02595944)	3	Stage IB, stage II, stage IIA, stage IIB, and stage IIIA NSCLC	Nivolumab vs. observation	DFS, OS	Recruiting
BR.31 (NCT02273375)	3	Stage IB, II, III, and IIIA NSCLC	Durvalumab vs. placebo	DFS in PD-L1+ and in all patients	Recruiting
KEYNOTE-091 (NCT02504372)	3	Stage IB NSCLC, II-IIIA NSCLC after complete surgical resection and carcinoma in situ at the bronchial margin	Pembrolizumab vs. placebo	DFS	Recruiting

REFERENCES

1. van Tinteren H, Hoekstra OS, Smit EF, et al. Effectiveness of positron emission tomography in the preoperative assessment of patients with suspected non-small-cell lung cancer: the PLUS multicentre randomised trial. *Lancet*. 2002;359(9315):1388-1393.

2. Cao JQ, Rodrigues GB, Louie AV, Zaric GS. Systematic review of the cost-effectiveness of positron-emission tomography in staging of non--small-cell lung cancer and management of solitary pulmonary nodules. *Clin Lung Cancer*. 2012;13(3):161-170.

3. Silvestri GA, Gonzalez AV, Jantz MA, et al. Methods for staging non-small cell lung cancer: diagnosis and management of lung cancer, 3rd ed: American College of Chest Physicians evidence-based clinical practice guidelines. *Chest*. 2013;143(5 Suppl):e211S-e250S.

4. Toloza EM, Harpole L, McCrory DC. Noninvasive staging of non-small cell lung cancer: a review of the current evidence. *Chest*. 2003;123(1 Suppl):137S-146S.

5. Schmidt-Hansen M, Baldwin DR, Hasler E, Zamora J, Abraira V, Figuls MRI. PET-CT for assessing mediastinal lymph node involvement in patients with suspected resectable non-small cell lung cancer. *Cochrane Database Syst Rev*. 2014(11):CD009519.

6. De Leyn P, Dooms C, Kuzdzal J, et al. Revised ESTS guidelines for preoperative mediastinal lymph node staging for non-small-cell lung cancer. *Eur J Cardiothorac Surg*. 2014;45(5):787-798.

7. MacMahon H, Naidich DP, Goo JM, et al. Guidelines for management of incidental pulmonary nodules detected on CT images: from the Fleischner Society 2017. *Radiology*. 2017;284(1):228-243.

8. Yasufuku K, Pierre A, Darling G, et al. A prospective controlled trial of endobronchial ultrasound-guided transbronchial needle aspiration compared with mediastinoscopy for mediastinal lymph node staging of lung cancer. *J Thorac Cardiovasc Surg*. 2011;142(6):1393-1400 e1.

9. Nakajima T, Yasufuku K, Saegusa F, et al. Rapid on-site cytologic evaluation during endobronchial ultrasound-guided transbronchial needle aspiration for nodal staging in patients with lung cancer. *Ann Thorac Surg*. 2013;95(5):1695-1699.

10. Ghigna MR, Crutu A, Florea V, et al. Endobronchial ultrasound-guided fine-needle aspiration for pulmonary carcinomas genotyping: experience with 398 cases including rapid EGFR/KRAS analysis in 43 cases. *J Thorac Dis*. 2018;10(7):4653-4658.

11. Choi YS, Shim YM, Kim J, Kim K. Mediastinoscopy in patients with clinical stage I non-small cell lung cancer. *Ann Thorac Surg*. 2003;75(2):364-366.

12. Leschber G, Sperling D, Klemm W, Merk J. Does video-mediastinoscopy improve the results of conventional mediastinoscopy? *Eur J Cardiothorac Surg*. 2008;33(2):289-293.

13. Witte B, Wolf M, Huertgen M, Toomes H. Video-assisted mediastinoscopic surgery: clinical feasibility and accuracy of mediastinal lymph node staging. *Ann Thorac Surg*. 2006;82(5):1821-1827.

14. Martin-Ucar AE, Chetty GK, Vaughan R, Waller DA. A prospective audit evaluating the role of video-assisted cervical mediastinoscopy (VAM) as a training tool. *Eur J Cardiothorac Surg*. 2004;26(2):393-395.

15. Anraku M, Miyata R, Compeau C, Shargall Y. Video-assisted mediastinoscopy compared with conventional mediastinoscopy: are we doing better? *Ann Thorac Surg*. 2010;89(5):1577-1581.

16. Berry MF, Villamizar-Ortiz NR, Tong BC, et al. Pulmonary function tests do not predict pulmonary complications after thoracoscopic lobectomy. *Ann Thorac Surg*. 2010;89(4):1044-1051; discussion 1051-1052.

17. Licker MJ, Widikker I, Robert J, et al. Operative mortality and respiratory complications after lung resection for cancer: impact of chronic obstructive pulmonary disease and time trends. *Ann Thorac Surg*. 2006;81(5):1830-1837.

18. Bolliger CT, Gückel C, Engel H, et al. Prediction of functional reserves after lung resection: comparison between quantitative computed tomography, scintigraphy, and anatomy. *Respiration*. 2002;69(6):482-489.

19. Datta D, Lahiri B. Preoperative evaluation of patients undergoing lung resection surgery. *Chest*. 2003;123(6):2096-2103.

20. Brunelli A, Varela G, Salati M, et al. Recalibration of the revised cardiac risk index in lung resection candidates. *Ann Thorac Surg*. 2010;90(1):199-203.

21. Brunelli A, Ferguson MK, Salati M, Vigneswaran WT, Jimenez MF, Varela G. Thoracic revised cardiac risk index is associated with prognosis after resection for stage I lung cancer. *Ann Thorac Surg*. 2015;100(1):195-200.

22. Brunelli A, Belardinelli R, Refai M. et al. Peak oxygen consumption during cardiopulmonary exercise test improves risk stratification in candidates to major lung resection. *Chest*. 2009;135(5):1260-1267.

23. Blackmon S, Vapociyan A. Thoracic malignancies. In: Feig B, Ching D, eds. *The MD Anderson Surgical Oncology Handbook*. 5th ed. Philadelphia, PA: Lippincott, Williams, & Wilkins; 2012.

24. Warren GW, Alberg AJ, Kraft AS, Cummings KM. The 2014 Surgeon General's report: "The health consequences of smoking—50 years of progress": a paradigm shift in cancer care. *Cancer*. 2014;120(13):1914-1916.

25. Jamal A, King BA, Neff LJ, Whitmill J, Babb SD, Graffunder CM. Current cigarette smoking among adults—United States, 2005-2015. *MMWR Morb Mortal Wkly Rep*. 2016;65(44):1205-1211.

26. Jamal A, Phillips E, Gentzke AS, et al. Current cigarette smoking among adults—United States, 2016. *MMWR Morb Mortal Wkly Rep*. 2018;67(2):53-59.

27. Babb S, Malarcher A, Schauer G, Asman K, Jamal A. Quitting smoking among adults—United States, 2000-2015. *MMWR Morb Mortal Wkly Rep*. 2017;65(52):1457-1464.

28. Barrera R, Shi W, Amar D, et al. Smoking and timing of cessation: impact on pulmonary complications after thoracotomy. *Chest*. 2005;127(6):1977-1983.

29. Mason DP, Subramanian S, Nowicki ER, et al. Impact of smoking cessation before resection of lung cancer: a Society of Thoracic Surgeons General Thoracic Surgery Database study. *Ann Thorac Surg*. 2009;88(2):362-370; discussion 370-371.

30. Nakagawa M, Tanaka H, Tsukuma H, Kishi Y. Relationship between the duration of the preoperative smoke-free period and the incidence of postoperative pulmonary complications after pulmonary surgery. *Chest*. 2001;120(3):705-710.

31. Agostini PJ, Lugg ST, Adams K, et al. Risk factors and short-term outcomes of postoperative pulmonary complications after VATS lobectomy. *J Cardiothorac Surg*. 2018;13(1):28.

32. Marino KA, Little MA, Bursac Z, Sullivan JL, Klesges R, Weksler B. Operating on patients who smoke: a survey of thoracic surgeons in the United States. *Ann Thorac Surg*. 2016;102(3):911-916.

33. Leone FT, Evers-Casey S, Toll BA, Vachani A. Treatment of tobacco use in lung cancer: diagnosis and management of lung cancer, 3rd ed: American College of Chest Physicians evidence-based clinical practice guidelines. *Chest*. 2013;143(5 Suppl):e61S-e677S.

34. Shields PG, Herbst RS, Arenberg D, et al. Smoking Cessation, Version 1.2016, NCCN Clinical Practice Guidelines in Oncology. *J Natl Compr Canc Netw*. 2016;14(11):1430-1468.

35. Steliga MA. Smoking cessation in clinical practice: how to get patients to stop. *Semin Thorac Cardiovasc Surg*. 2018;30(1):87-91.

36. Brunelli A, Kim AW, Berger KI, Addrizzo-Harris DJ. Physiologic evaluation of the patient with lung cancer being considered for resectional surgery: diagnosis and management of lung cancer, 3rd ed: American College of Chest Physicians evidence-based clinical practice guidelines. *Chest*. 2013;143(5 Suppl):e166S-e190S.

37. Gonzales D, Rennard SI, Nides M, et al. Varenicline, an alpha4beta2 nicotinic acetylcholine receptor partial agonist, vs sustained-release bupropion and placebo for smoking cessation: a randomized controlled trial. *JAMA*. 2006;296(1):47-55.

38. Jorenby DE, Hays JT, Rigotti NA, et al. Efficacy of varenicline, an alpha4beta2 nicotinic acetylcholine receptor partial agonist, vs placebo or sustained-release bupropion for smoking cessation: a randomized controlled trial. *JAMA*. 2006;296(1):56-63.

39. Ebbert JO, Hughes JR, West RJ, et al. Effect of varenicline on smoking cessation through smoking reduction: a randomized clinical trial. *JAMA*. 2015;313(7):687-694.

40. Weinstein H, Bates AT, Spaltro BE, Thaler HT, Steingart RM. Influence of preoperative exercise capacity on length of stay after thoracic cancer surgery. *Ann Thorac Surg*. 2007;84(1):197-202.

41. Nagarajan K, Bennett A, Agostini P, Naidu B. Is preoperative physiotherapy/pulmonary rehabilitation beneficial in lung resection patients? *Interact Cardiovasc Thorac Surg*. 2011;13(3):300-302.

42. Benzo R, Kelley GA, Recchi L, Hofman A, Sciurba F. Complications of lung resection and exercise capacity: a meta-analysis. *Respir Med*. 2007;101(8):1790-1797.

43. Benzo R, Wigle D, Novotny P, et al. Preoperative pulmonary rehabilitation before lung cancer resection: results from two randomized studies. *Lung Cancer*. 2011;74(3):441-445.

44. D'Cunha J, Herndon JE 2nd, Herzan DL, et al. Poor correspondence between clinical and pathologic staging in stage 1 non-small cell lung cancer: results from CALGB 9761, a prospective trial. *Lung Cancer*. 2005;48(2):241-246.

45. Uzel EK, Abacioglu U. Treatment of early stage non-small cell lung cancer: surgery or stereotactic ablative radiotherapy? *Balkan Med J*. 2015;32(1):8-16.

46. Scott WJ, Howington J, Feigenberg S, Movsas B, Pisters K, American College of Chest Physicians. Treatment of non-small cell lung cancer stage I and stage II: ACCP evidence-based clinical practice guidelines (2nd edition). *Chest*. 2007;132(3 Suppl):234S-242S.

47. Ginsberg RJ, Rubinstein LV. Randomized trial of lobectomy versus limited resection for T1 N0 non-small cell lung cancer. Lung Cancer Study Group. *Ann Thorac Surg*. 1995;60(3):615-622; discussion 622-623.

48. Flores RM, Park BJ, Dycoco J, et al. Lobectomy by video-assisted thoracic surgery (VATS) versus thoracotomy for lung cancer. *J Thorac Cardiovasc Surg*. 2009;138(1):11-18.

49. Galetta D, Solli P, Borri A, et al. Bilobectomy for lung cancer: analysis of indications, postoperative results, and long-term outcomes. *Ann Thorac Surg*. 2012;93(1):251-257; discussion 257-258.

50. Fuentes PA. Pneumonectomy: historical perspective and prospective insight. *Eur J Cardiothorac Surg*. 2003;23(4):439-445.

51. Kopec SE, Irwin RS, Umali-Torres CB, Balikian JP, Conlan AA. The postpneumonectomy state. *Chest*. 1998;114(4):1158-1184.

52. Ferguson MK, Lehman AG. Sleeve lobectomy or pneumonectomy: optimal management strategy using decision analysis techniques. *Ann Thorac Surg*. 2003;76(6):1782-1788.

53. Dai C, Shen J, Ren Y, et al. Choice of surgical procedure for patients with non-small-cell lung cancer ≤ 1 cm or > 1 to 2 cm among lobectomy, segmentectomy, and wedge resection: a population-based study. *J Clin Oncol*. 2016;34(26):3175-3182.

54. Smith CB, Swanson SJ, Mhango G, Wisnivesky JP, et al. Survival after segmentectomy and wedge resection in stage I non-small-cell lung cancer. *J Thorac Oncol*. 2013;8(1):73-78.

55. Dziedzic R, Zurek W, Marjanski T, et al. Stage I non-small-cell lung cancer: long-term results of lobectomy versus sublobar resection from the Polish National Lung Cancer Registry. *Eur J Cardiothorac Surg*. 2017;52(2):363-369.

56. Abdelsattar ZM, Allen MS, Shen KR, et al. Variation in hospital adoption rates of video-assisted thoracoscopic lobectomy for lung cancer and the effect on outcomes. *Ann Thorac Surg*. 2017;103(2):454-460.

57. Swanson SJ, Herndon JE 2nd, D'Amico TA, et al. Video-assisted thoracic surgery lobectomy: report of CALGB 39802—a prospective, multi-institution feasibility study. *J Clin Oncol*. 2007;25(31):4993-4997.

58. McKenna RJ, Jr., Houck W, Fuller CB. Video-assisted thoracic surgery lobectomy: experience with 1,100 cases. *Ann Thorac Surg*. 2006;81(2):421-425; discussion 425-426.

59. Laursen LO, Petersen RH, Hansen HJ, Jensen TK, Ravn J, Konge L. Video-assisted thoracoscopic surgery lobectomy for lung cancer is associated with a lower 30-day morbidity compared with lobectomy by thoracotomy. *Eur J Cardiothorac Surg*. 2016;49(3):870-875.

60. Park BJ, Flores RM, Rusch VW. Robotic assistance for video-assisted thoracic surgical lobectomy: technique and initial results. *J Thorac Cardiovasc Surg*. 2006;131(1):54-59.

61. Park BJ, Melfi F, Mussi A, et al. Robotic lobectomy for non-small cell lung cancer (NSCLC): long-term oncologic results. *J Thorac Cardiovasc Surg*. 2012;143(2):383-389.

62. Casiraghi M, Galetta D, Borri A, et al. Ten years' experience in robotic-assisted thoracic surgery for early stage lung cancer. *Thorac Cardiovasc Surg.* 2019;67(7):564-572.

63. Kehlet H. Multimodal approach to control postoperative pathophysiology and rehabilitation. *Br J Anaesth.* 1997;78(5):606-617.

64. Kehlet H. Fast-track colorectal surgery. *Lancet.* 2008;371(9615):791-793.

65. Ljungqvist O, Scott M, Fearon KC. Enhanced recovery after surgery: a review. *JAMA Surg.* 2017;152(3):292-298.

66. Rogers LJ, Bleetman D, Messenger DE, et al. The impact of enhanced recovery after surgery (ERAS) protocol compliance on morbidity from resection for primary lung cancer. *J Thorac Cardiovasc Surg.* 2018;155(4):1843-1852.

67. Howington JA, Blum MG, Chang AC, Balekian AA, Murthy SC. Treatment of stage I and II non-small cell lung cancer: diagnosis and management of lung cancer, 3rd ed: American College of Chest Physicians evidence-based clinical practice guidelines. *Chest.* 2013;143(5 Suppl):e278S-e313S.

68. Rodrigues G, Choy H, Bradley J, et al. Adjuvant radiation therapy in locally advanced non-small cell lung cancer: executive summary of an American Society for Radiation Oncology (ASTRO) evidence-based clinical practice guideline. *Pract Radiat Oncol.* 2015;5(3):149-155.

69. Burdett S, Stewart L. Postoperative radiotherapy in non-small-cell lung cancer: update of an individual patient data meta-analysis. *Lung Cancer.* 2005;47(1):81-83.

70. Lally BE, Zelterman D, Colasanto JM, Haffty BG, Detterbeck FC, Wilson LD. Postoperative radiotherapy for stage II or III non-small-cell lung cancer using the surveillance, epidemiology, and end results database. *J Clin Oncol.* 2006;24(19):2998-3006.

71. Wang EH, Corso CD, Rutter CE, et al. Postoperative radiation therapy is associated with improved overall survival in incompletely resected stage II and III non–small-cell lung cancer. *J Clin Oncol.* 2015;33(25):2727-2734.

72. Fernando HC, Landreneau RJ, Mandrekar SJ, et al. Impact of brachytherapy on local recurrence rates after sublobar resection: results from ACOSOG Z4032 (Alliance), a phase III randomized trial for high-risk operable non-small-cell lung cancer. *J Clin Oncol.* 2014;32(23):2456-2462.

73. Wisnivesky JP, Bonomi M, Henschke C, Iannuzzi M, McGinn T. Radiation therapy for the treatment of unresected stage I-II non-small cell lung cancer. *Chest.* 2005;128(3):1461-1467.

74. Fang LC, Komaki R, Allen P, Guerrero T, Mohan R, Cox JD. Comparison of outcomes for patients with medically inoperable stage I non-small-cell lung cancer treated with two-dimensional vs. three-dimensional radiotherapy. *Int J Radiat Oncol Biol Phys.* 2006;66(1):108-116.

75. Sura S, Yorke E, Jackson A, Rosenzweig KE. High-dose radiotherapy for the treatment of inoperable non-small cell lung cancer. *Cancer J.* 2007;13(4):238-242.

76. Bradley J, Graham MV, Winter K, et al. Toxicity and outcome results of RTOG 9311: a phase I-II dose-escalation study using three-dimensional conformal radiotherapy in patients with inoperable non-small-cell lung carcinoma. *Int J Radiat Oncol Biol Phys.* 2005;61(2):318-328.

77. Bradley JD, Moughan J, Graham MV, et al. A phase I/II radiation dose escalation study with concurrent chemotherapy for patients with inoperable stages I to III non-small-cell lung cancer: phase I results of RTOG 0117. *Int J Radiat Oncol Biol Phys.* 2010;77(2):367-372.

78. Bogart JA, Hodgson L, Seagren SL, et al. Phase I study of accelerated conformal radiotherapy for stage I non-small-cell lung cancer in patients with pulmonary dysfunction: CALGB 39904. *J Clin Oncol.* 2010;28(2):202-206.

79. Onishi H, Shirato H, Nagata Y, et al. Hypofractionated stereotactic radiotherapy (HypoFXSRT) for stage I non-small cell lung cancer: updated results of 257 patients in a Japanese multi-institutional study. *J Thorac Oncol.* 2007;2(7 Suppl 3):S94-S100.

80. Grutters JP, Kessels AGH, Pijls-Johannesma M, De Ruysscher D, Joore MA, Lambin P. Comparison of the effectiveness of radiotherapy with photons, protons and carbon-ions for non-small cell lung cancer: a meta-analysis. *Radiother Oncol.* 2010;95(1):32-40.

81. Baumann P, Nyman J, Hoyer M, et al. Outcome in a prospective phase II trial of medically inoperable stage I non-small-cell lung cancer patients treated with stereotactic body radiotherapy. *J Clin Oncol.* 2009;27(20):3290-3296.

82. Timmerman R, Paulus R, Galvin J, et al. Stereotactic body radiation therapy for inoperable early stage lung cancer. *JAMA.* 2010;303(11):1070-1076.

83. Plathow C, Schoebinger M, Herth F, Tuengerthal S, Meinzer H-P, Kauczor H-U. Estimation of pulmonary motion in healthy subjects and patients with intrathoracic tumors using 3D-dynamic MRI: initial results. *Korean J Radiol.* 2009;10(6):559-567.

84. Glide-Hurst CK, Chetty IJ. Improving radiotherapy planning, delivery accuracy, and normal tissue sparing using cutting edge technologies. *J Thorac Dis.* 2014;6(4):303-318.

85. Kim JH. LINAC-based high-precision radiotherapy: radiosurgery, image-guided radiotherapy, and respiratory-gated radiotherapy. *J Korean Med Assoc.* 2008;51(7):612-618.

86. Uematsu M, Shioda A, Tahara K, et al. Focal, high dose, and fractionated modified stereotactic radiation therapy for lung carcinoma patients: a preliminary experience. *Cancer.* 1998;82(6):1062-1070.

87. Onishi H, Araki T, Shirato H, et al. Stereotactic hypofractionated high-dose irradiation for stage I nonsmall cell lung carcinoma: clinical outcomes in 245 subjects in a Japanese multiinstitutional study. *Cancer.* 2004;101(7):1623-1631.

88. Nagata Y, Takayama K, Matsuo Y, et al. Clinical outcomes of a phase I/II study of 48 Gy of stereotactic body radiotherapy in 4 fractions for primary lung cancer using a stereotactic body frame. *Int J Radiat Oncol Biol Phys.* 2005;63(5):1427-1431.

89. Nagata Y, Hiraoka M, Shibata T, et al. Prospective trial of stereotactic body radiation therapy for both operable and inoperable T1N0M0 non-small cell lung cancer: Japan Clinical Oncology Group Study JCOG0403. *Int J Radiat Oncol Biol Phys.* 2015;93(5):989-996.

90. Timmerman R, Papiez L, McGarry R, et al. Extracranial stereotactic radioablation: results of a phase I study in medically inoperable stage I non-small cell lung cancer. *Chest.* 2003;124(5):1946-1955.

91. Fakiris AJ, McGarry RC, Yiannoutsos CT, et al. Stereotactic body radiation therapy for early-stage non-small-cell lung carcinoma: four-year results of a prospective phase II study. *Int J Radiat Oncol Biol Phys.* 2009;75(3):677-682.

92. Timmerman RD, Hu C, Michalski JM, et al. Long-term results of stereotactic body radiation therapy in medically inoperable stage I non-small cell lung cancer. *JAMA Oncol.* 2018;4(9):1287-1288.

93. Haasbeek CJ, Lagerwaard FJ, Antonisse ME, Slotman BJ, Senan S. Stage I nonsmall cell lung cancer in patients aged > or =75 years: outcomes after stereotactic radiotherapy. *Cancer.* 2010;116(2):406-414.

94. Timmerman RD, Paulus R, Pass HI, et al. Stereotactic body radiation therapy for operable early-stage lung cancer: findings from the nrg oncology rtog 0618 trial. *JAMA Oncology.* 2018;4(9):1263-1266.

95. Grills IS, Mangona VS, Welsh R, et al. Outcomes after stereotactic lung radiotherapy or wedge resection for stage I non-small-cell lung cancer. *J Clin Oncol.* 2010;28(6):928-935.

96. Crabtree TD, Denlinger CE, Meyers BF, et al. Stereotactic body radiation therapy versus surgical resection for stage I non-small cell lung cancer. *J Thorac Cardiovasc Surg.* 2010;140(2):377-386.

97. Chang JY, Senan S, Paul MA, et al. Stereotactic ablative radiotherapy versus lobectomy for operable stage I non-small-cell lung cancer: a pooled analysis of two randomised trials. *Lancet Oncol.* 2015;16(6):630-637.

98. Deng HY, Wang YC, Ni PZ, et al., Radiotherapy, lobectomy or sublobar resection? A meta-analysis of the choices for treating stage I non-small-cell lung cancer. *Eur J Cardiothorac Surg.* 2017;51(2):203-210.

99. Kang KH, Okoye CC, Patel RB, et al. Complications from stereotactic body radiotherapy for lung cancer. *Cancers (Basel).* 2015;7(2):981-1004.

100. Timmerman R, McGarry R, Yiannoutsos C, et al. Excessive toxicity when treating central tumors in a phase II study of stereotactic body radiation therapy for medically inoperable early-stage lung cancer. *J Clin Oncol.* 2006;24(30):4833-4839.

101. Bezjak A, et al. Efficacy and Toxicity Analysis of NRG Oncology/RTOG 0813 Trial of Stereotactic Body Radiation Therapy (SBRT) for Centrally Located Non-Small Cell Lung Cancer (NSCLC). *Int J Radiat Oncol Biol Phys.* 2016;96(2):S8.

102. Giuliani M, Mathew AS, Bahig H, et al. SUNSET: stereotactic radiation for ultracentral non-small-cell lung cancer—a safety and efficacy trial. *Clin Lung Cancer.* 2018;19(4):e529-e532.

103. Videtic GM, Hu C, Singh AK, et al. A randomized phase 2 study comparing 2 stereotactic body radiation therapy schedules for medically noperable patients with stage I peripheral non-small cell lung cancer: NRG oncology RTOG 0915 (NCCTG N0927). *Int J Radiat Oncol Biol Phys.* 2015;93(4):757-764.

104. NCLCCG, Chemotherapy in non-small cell lung cancer: a meta-analysis using updated data on individual patients from 52 randomised clinical trials. Non-small Cell Lung Cancer Collaborative Group. *BMJ.* 1995;311(7010):899-909.

105. Arriagada R, Bergman B, Dunant A, et al. Cisplatin-based adjuvant chemotherapy in patients with completely resected non-small-cell lung cancer. *N Engl J Med.* 2004;350(4):351-360.

106. Winton T, Livingston R, Johnson D, et al. Vinorelbine plus cisplatin vs. observation in resected non-small-cell lung cancer. *N Engl J Med.* 2005;352(25):2589-2597.

107. Pignon JP, Tribodet H, Scagliotti GV, et al. Lung adjuvant cisplatin evaluation: a pooled analysis by the LACE Collaborative Group. *J Clin Oncol.* 2008;26(21):3552-3559.

108. Strauss GM, Herndon JE 2nd, Maddaus MA, et al. Adjuvant paclitaxel plus carboplatin compared with observation in stage IB non-small-cell lung cancer: CALGB 9633 with the Cancer and Leukemia Group B, Radiation Therapy Oncology Group, and North Central Cancer Treatment Group Study Groups. *J Clin Oncol.* 2008;26(31):5043-5051.

109. Douillard JY, Rosell R, De Lena M, et al. Adjuvant vinorelbine plus cisplatin versus observation in patients with completely resected stage IB-IIIA non-small-cell lung cancer (Adjuvant Navelbine International Trialist Association [ANITA]): a randomised controlled trial. *Lancet Oncol*. 2006;7(9):719-727.

110. Goss GD, O'Callaghan C, Lorimer I, et al. Gefitinib versus placebo in completely resected non-small-cell lung cancer: results of the NCIC CTG BR19 study. *J Clin Oncol*. 2013;31(27):3320-3326.

111. Kelly K, Altorki NK, Eberhardt WEE, et al. Adjuvant erlotinib versus placebo in patients with stage IB-IIIA non-small-cell lung cancer (RADIANT): a randomized, double-blind, phase III trial. *J Clin Oncol*. 2015;33(34):4007-4014.

112. Pepe C, Hasan B, Winton TL, et al. Adjuvant vinorelbine and cisplatin in elderly patients: National Cancer Institute of Canada and Intergroup Study JBR.10. *J Clin Oncol*. 2007;25(12):1553-1561.

113. Rosell R, Gómez-Codina J, Camps C, et al. A randomized trial comparing preoperative chemotherapy plus surgery with surgery alone in patients with non-small-cell lung cancer. *N Engl J Med*. 1994;330(3):153-158.

114. Roth JA, Fossella F, Komaki R, et al. A randomized trial comparing perioperative chemotherapy and surgery with surgery alone in resectable stage IIIA non-small-cell lung cancer. *J Natl Cancer Inst*. 1994;86(9):673-680.

115. Gilligan D, Nicolson M, Smith I, et al. Preoperative chemotherapy in patients with resectable non-small cell lung cancer: results of the MRC LU22/NVALT 2/EORTC 08012 multicentre randomised trial and update of systematic review. *Lancet*. 2007;369(9577):1929-1937.

116. Yamauchi Y, Muley T, Safi S, et al. The dynamic pattern of recurrence in curatively resected non-small cell lung cancer patients: experiences at a single institution. *Lung Cancer*. 2015;90(2):224-229.

117. Kris MG, Gaspar LE, Chaft JE, et al. Adjuvant systemic therapy and adjuvant radiation Therapy for stage I to IIIA completely resected non-small-cell lung cancers: American Society of Clinical Oncology/Cancer Care Ontario Clinical Practice Guideline Update. *J Clin Oncol*. 2017;35(25):2960-2974.

118. Thomas A, Liu SV, Subramaniam DS, Giaccone G. Refining the treatment of NSCLC according to histological and molecular subtypes. *Nat Rev Clin Oncol*. 2015;12(9):511-526.

119. Zhong W-Z, Wang Q, Mao W-M, et al. Gefitinib versus vinorelbine plus cisplatin as adjuvant treatment for stage II-IIIA (N1-N2) EGFR-mutant NSCLC (ADJUVANT/CTONG1104): a randomised, open-label, phase 3 study. *Lancet Oncol*. 2018;19(1):139-148.

120. Hollinshead A, Stewart TH, Takita H, Dalbow M, Concannon J. Adjuvant specific active lung cancer immunotherapy trials. Tumor-associated antigens. *Cancer*. 1987;60(6):1249-1262.

121. Sienel W, Varwerk C, Linder A, et al. Melanoma associated antigen (MAGE)-A3 expression in stages I and II non-small cell lung cancer: results of a multi-center study. *Eur J Cardiothorac Surg*. 2004;25(1):131-134.

122. Gure AO, Chua R, Williamson B, et al. Cancer-testis genes are coordinately expressed and are markers of poor outcome in non-small cell lung cancer. *Clin Cancer Res*. 2005;11(22):8055-8062.

123. Kim SH, Lee S, Lee CH, et al. Expression of cancer-testis antigens MAGE-A3/6 and NY-ESO-1 in non-small-cell lung carcinomas and their relationship with immune cell infiltration. *Lung*. 2009;187(6):401-411.

124. Melero I, Gaudernack G, Gerritsen W, et al. Therapeutic vaccines for cancer: an overview of clinical trials. *Nat Rev Clin Oncol*. 2014;11(9):509-524.

125. Vansteenkiste J, Zielinski M, Linder A, et al. Adjuvant MAGE-A3 immunotherapy in resected non-small-cell lung cancer: phase II randomized study results. *J Clin Oncol*. 2013;31(19):2396-2403.

126. Vansteenkiste JF, Cho BC, Vanakesa T, et al. Efficacy of the MAGE-A3 cancer immunotherapeutic as adjuvant therapy in patients with resected MAGE-A3-positive non-small-cell lung cancer (MAGRIT): a randomised, double-blind, placebo-controlled, phase 3 trial. *Lancet Oncol*. 2016;17(6):822-835.

127. Butts C, Socinski MA, Mitchell PL, et al. Tecemotide (L-BLP25) versus placebo after chemoradiotherapy for stage III non-small-cell lung cancer (START): a randomised, double-blind, phase 3 trial. *Lancet Oncol*. 2014;15(1):59-68.

128. Giaccone G, Bazhenova L A, Nemunaitis J, et al. A phase III study of belagenpumatucel-L, an allogeneic tumour cell vaccine, as maintenance therapy for non-small cell lung cancer. *Eur J Cancer*. 2015;51(16):2321-2329.

129. Quoix E, Lena H, Losonczy G, et al. TG4010 immunotherapy and first-line chemotherapy for advanced non-small-cell lung cancer (TIME): results from the phase 2b part of a randomised, double-blind, placebo-controlled, phase 2b/3 trial. *Lancet Oncol*. 2016;17(2):212-223.

130. Kotsakis A, Papadimitraki E, Vetsika EK, et al. A phase II trial evaluating the clinical and immunologic response of HLA-A2(+) non-small cell lung cancer patients vaccinated with an hTERT cryptic peptide. *Lung Cancer*. 2014;86(1):59-66.

131. Zhu J, Li R, Tiselius E, et al. Immunotherapy (excluding checkpoint inhibitors) for stage I to III non-small cell lung cancer treated with surgery or radiotherapy with curative intent. *Cochrane Database Syst Rev*. 2017;12:CD011300.

132. Hanahan D, Weinberg RA. Hallmarks of cancer: the next generation. *Cell*. 2011;144(5):646-674.

133. Bergers G, Benjamin LE. Tumorigenesis and the angiogenic switch. *Nat Rev Cancer.* 2003;3(6):401-410.

134. Ferrara N, Hillan KJ, Gerber HP, Novotny W. Discovery and development of bevacizumab, an anti-VEGF antibody for treating cancer. *Nat Rev Drug Discov.* 2004;3(5):391-400.

135. Sandler A, Gray R, Perry MC, et al. Paclitaxel-carboplatin alone or with bevacizumab for non-small-cell lung cancer. *N Engl J Med.* 2006;355(24):2542-2550.

136. Wakelee HA, Dahlberg SE, Keller SM, et al. Adjuvant chemotherapy with or without bevacizumab in patients with resected non-small-cell lung cancer (E1505): an open-label, multicentre, randomised, phase 3 trial. *Lancet Oncol.* 2017;18(12):1610-1623.

137. Turley SJ, Cremasco V, Astarita JL. Immunological hallmarks of stromal cells in the tumour microenvironment. *Nat Rev Immunol.* 2015;15(11):669-682.

138. Topalian SL, Drake CG, Pardoll DM. Immune checkpoint blockade: a common denominator approach to cancer therapy. *Cancer Cell.* 2015;27(4):450-461.

139. Pardoll DM. The blockade of immune checkpoints in cancer immunotherapy. *Nat Rev Cancer.* 2012; 12(4):252-264.

140. Lynch TJ, Bondarenko I, Luft A, et al. Ipilimumab in combination with paclitaxel and carboplatin as first-line treatment in stage IIIB/IV non-small-cell lung cancer: results from a randomized, double-blind, multicenter phase II study. *J Clin Oncol.* 2012;30(17):2046-2054.

141. Govindan R, Szczesna A, Ahn M-J, et al. Phase III trial of ipilimumab combined with paclitaxel and carboplatin in advanced squamous non-small-cell lung cancer. *J Clin Oncol.* 2017;35(30):3449-3457.

142. Tang C, Welsh JW, de Groot P, et al. Ipilimumab with stereotactic ablative radiation therapy: phase I results and immunologic correlates from peripheral T cells. *Clin Cancer Res.* 2017;23(6):1388-1396.

143. O'Brien MER, et al. EORTC-ETOP randomized, phase 3 trial with anti-PD-1 monoclonal antibody pembrolizumab versus placebo for patients with early stage non-small cell lung cancer (NSCLC) after resection and standard adjuvant chemotherapy: PEARLS (NCT02504372). *J Clin Oncol.* 2016;34(15_suppl):TPS8571-TPS8571.

144. Antonia SJ, Villegas A, Daniel D, et al. Durvalumab after chemoradiotherapy in stage III non-small-cell lung cancer. *N Engl J Med.* 2017;377(20):1919-1929.

145. Antonia SJ, Villegas A, Daniel D, et al. Overall survival with durvalumab after chemoradiotherapy in stage III NSCLC. *N Engl J Med.* 2018;379(24):2342-2350.

146. Reck M, Rodríguez-Abreu D, Robinson AG, et al. Pembrolizumab versus chemotherapy for PD-L1-positive non-small-cell lung cancer. *N Engl J Med.* 2016;375(19):1823-1833.

147. Gandhi L, Rodríguez-Abreu D, Gadgeel S, et al. Pembrolizumab plus Chemotherapy in Metastatic Non-Small-Cell Lung Cancer. *N Engl J Med.* 2018;378(22):2078-2092.

148. Socinski MA, Jotte RM, Cappuzzo F, et al. Atezolizumab for first-line treatment of metastatic nonsquamous NSCLC. *N Engl J Med.* 2018;378(24):2288-2301.

14

NON–SMALL CELL LUNG CANCER TREATMENT: LOCALLY ADVANCED

Andrea Anampa-Guzmán, MD • Neal E. Dunlap, MD • Matthew Fox, MD • Ignacio Gil-Bazo, MD, PhD
• Rohit Kumar, MD • Michael May, MD • Cesar A. Perez, MD • Luis E. Raez, MD, FACP, FCCP
• Susan Ansley Smith, MD

SURGERY FOR LOCALLY ADVANCED NON–SMALL CELL LUNG CANCER

Susan Ansley Smith, MD, Matthew Fox, MD

A 60-year-old male has a 6-cm right apical lung mass that invades the chest wall. He has chronic obstructive pulmonary disease (COPD) and smokes 1 pack of cigarettes per day.

The mass is biopsied by computed tomographic (CT)–guided core needle and is positive for adenocarcinoma of the lung. The pathology shows non–small cell lung cancer (NSCLC) of the lung.

Positron emission tomography (PET) shows one ipsilateral PET-positive, non-bulky medastinal lymph node that is pathologically positive on mediastinoscopy. Magnetic resonance images (MRI) of the brain and neck are negative for metastases or extension into the plexus.

Learning Objectives:

1. What is the role of surgery in stage III NSCLC?
2. What surgical techniques are available to resect lung cancer invading adjacent organs?
3. How are Pancoast tumors of the lung treated?

Locally advanced NSCLC includes tumors that invade the surrounding structures, including the chest wall, vertebrae, great vessels, diaphragm, and structures of the superior sulcus. Treatment typically involves multimodal therapy, with surgical resection providing the best chance at improving 5-year survival. In this chapter, the surgical management of locally advanced NSCLC is discussed.

PANCOAST TUMORS

Pancoast tumors were originally described by Henry Pancoast, the first president of the American Board of Radiology.[1] Also known as superior sulcus tumors, these tumors invade the apical chest wall and surrounding structures, including the brachial plexus, sympathetic chain, subclavian artery and vein, vertebrae, spinal cord, clavicle, and ribs.[2] Approximately 90% of all Pancoast tumors are NSCLCs[2] and are classified according to the tumor, node, metastasis (TNM) staging system as T3 or T4 lesions depending on the extent of invasion. The National Comprehensive Cancer Network (NCCN) guidelines can be used to determine treatment strategies. Treatment options are multimodal and include a combination of chemotherapy, radiation therapy, and surgical excision.[3] However, because less than 5% of all NSCLCs are Pancoast tumors, no prospective head-to-head randomized controlled trials comparing treatment strategies have been conducted.[2]

PREOPERATIVE CHEMORADIATION

The NCCN guidelines recommend neoadjuvant concurrent chemoradiation for T3N0-1 and possibly resectable T4N0-1 Pancoast tumors. Standard regimens include platinum-based chemotherapy along with 45- to 54-Gray (Gy) radiation given in 1.8- to 2-Gy fractions.[3] Induction chemoradiotherapy is associated with an improved 5-year survival rate, complete pathologic response, and R0 resection rate compared to the historical treatment regimen of preoperative radiotherapy followed by surgery. Furthermore, trimodal therapy has been shown to downstage tumors.[2]

OVERVIEW OF SURGERY

Surgical resection is the mainstay of treatment of Pancoast tumors, with the goal of R0 resection, including the upper lobe with one rib with attached intercostal muscles below the inferior margin of the tumor and all invaded structures en bloc.[4] Absolute contraindications to surgical resection include extrathoracic metastases, N2 disease, and invasion of the trachea, esophagus, spinal canal, or brachial plexus above the T1 nerve root because of the functional loss that occurs with resection of the lower trunk.[5,6] Resection can be approached anteriorly or posteriorly depending on structures involved. Most Pancoast tumors are found in the posterior compartment of the thoracic inlet[5] where neural structures are located[6] and are accessed through a posterolateral approach.[5] Anterior lesions extending into the subclavian vessels[5] or first rib[6] are approached anteriorly.[5,6] Several anterior approaches exist, including anterior transcervical-transthoracic, hemiclamshell, modified hemiclamshell, and Masoaka incision.[4-9] Pancoast tumors can also be resected using minimally invasive techniques.[10,11]

ANTERIOR APPROACH

Anterior Transcervical-Transthoracic

Lesions involving the anterior sulcus can be resected using a transcervical incision, which was first described by Dartevelle.[12] The patient is placed supine, and a large L-shaped cervicotomy is made along the sternocleidomastoid muscle and extended laterally to the deltopectoral groove just inferior to the clavicle.[8,12] Full exposure of the thoracic inlet is obtained by dividing the sternal head of the sternocleidomastoid muscle and the clavicular attachment of pectoralis major and resecting the medial clavicle.[7,8] The subclavian vein is exposed and resected if invaded by tumor.[8] The phrenic nerve is then identified along the anterior scalene muscle and preserved if uninvolved by tumor. The anterior scalene is divided at its insertion on the first rib. The phrenic nerve is resected as well as the anterior scalene at its attachment on the transverse processes of the third through sixth cervical vertebrae if either is grossly involved.[6,8] The subclavian artery is then exposed and dissected away from the tumor if possible. Resection and revascularization with end-to-end anastomosis or with polytetrafluoroethylene (PTFE) graft is required if the tumor invades the wall of the subclavian artery.[7,8] At its insertion on the first rib, the middle scalene is divided to expose the brachial plexus. If tumor involvement extends beyond the first rib, it is also divided at its attachment on the transverse processes of the second through seventh cervical vertebrae. Divide prevertebral muscles and sympathetic chain and ganglia from the seventh cervical and first thoracic vertebral bodies and then transect the first thoracic nerve root lateral to the intervertebral foramen.[8] Finally, the first rib is disarticulated, and ribs two and three are resected.[7,8] Upper lobectomy is then performed and removed en bloc.[12]

Hemiclamshell/Trapdoor Incision

The hemiclamshell or trapdoor incision extends a partial upper sternotomy into an anterior thoracotomy.[8,11] An *oblique* incision along the anterior border of the sternocleidomastoid just superior to the midsternal notch is extended into an upper median sternotomy down to the third or fourth intercostal space and then extended laterally along that intercostal space to the anterior axillary line.[8] After the sternum and internal mammary artery are transected, the chest wall is retracted, thereby exposing the superior sulcus and mediastinum.[8] The superior vena cava (SVC) is dissected superiorly to the subclavian vein. The ribs are resected posterolaterally and at the costochondral junctions. The subclavian vein, artery, and brachial plexus are then resected if involved by tumor in the same fashion as in the transcervical approach,[9] and lobectomy is performed. If optimal exposure of the thoracic inlet structures is not achieved with chest wall retraction alone, then the clavicle can also be resected.[8]

Modified Hemiclamshell

The hemiclamshell approach can be modified to include resection of the costoclavicular ligament and first costal cartilage, creating a larger sternocostal flap and better exposure of the hilar structures as well as the thoracic inlet and posterior chest wall.[4]

Masoaka Incision

This is an anterior trans-sternal approach described by Masoaka to provide extended exposure of the anterior part of the superior sulcus.[11] A transverse incision is made at the base of the neck just superior to the clavicle, followed by an upper median sternotomy to the fourth intercostal space.[8,11]

POSTERIOR APPROACH
Posterolateral

The posterolateral approach was first described by Shaw and Paulson to allow sufficient exposure of the vertebral bodies, transverse processes, and brachial plexus.[6,11] However, it may be difficult to achieve R0 resection with this approach if local invasion of the tumor extends to the vasculature above these structures.[6] A posterolateral thoracotomy is made with the patient in the lateral decubitus position and extended posteriorly just medial to the scapula to the level of the seventh cervical vertebra.[8] The trapezius, levator scapulae, rhomboid major, and rhomboid minor muscles are divided posteriorly while the latissimus dorsi is retracted anteriorly, and the serratus anterior and posterior muscles are divided to allow for retraction of the scapula.[8] Chest wall resection is then carried out with a 4-cm anterior margin and an inferior margin extending 1 rib and intercostal muscle beneath the gross inferior margin of the tumor.[8] Scalene muscles are divided, and the involved ribs are transected. The first rib is disarticulated from the costovertebral joint to expose the brachial plexus, and the first thoracic nerve root is subsequently transected lateral to the intervertebral foramen. The subclavian artery and vein are then resected if necessary in the same fashion as described. The sympathetic chain and ganglia are transected along with up to one-fourth of the corresponding vertebral bodies if involved by tumor. With the specimen attached, upper lobectomy is completed. Chest wall reconstruction is not needed as the scapula and clavicle close off the defect.[8]

MINIMALLY INVASIVE APPROACH

The thoracoscopic approach to both pulmonary resection and chest wall resection for Pancoast tumors is also used. The thoracoscope allows for optimal views of the apical chest wall and superior sulcus and for a more accurate evaluation of the correct level of chest wall resection. Furthermore, the minimally invasive approach requires only a small incision for en bloc resection and permits the preservation of the musculature overlying the area of resection, resulting in less postoperative pain.[10,11]

LOWER CHEST WALL RESECTION

Tumors that invade the chest wall are at least T3 by definition and account for roughly 5% of all lung cancers.[13] Chest wall invasion generally arises from the local spread of peripheral tumors.[13] Surgical resection is the mainstay of *initial* therapy for all T3 tumors with chest wall invasion.[3] NCCN guidelines recommend neoadjuvant chemotherapy or concurrent chemoradiation for all T4N0-1 (stage IIIA) tumors invading the chest wall.[3]

RECONSTRUCTION OPTIONS

As in the resection of Pancoast tumors, lateral margins of tumors invading the chest wall should be 4 cm, and superior and inferior margins should include 1 intact rib with intercostal muscles.[13] Similarly, reconstruction is not necessary for defects deep to the scapula. However, reconstruction is needed to cover large defects to preserve the structure and function of the chest wall. The chest wall can be reconstructed using a variety of prosthetic materials, including polypropylene mesh, PTFE mesh, soft tissue xenografts, and titanium plates.[13]

Vertebral Body Resection

Tumors that invade the vertebra are also classified as T4. Surgical resection involves the removal of at least three hemivertebrae, one above and one below tumor invasion, followed by spinal fixation.[7] Vertebrae can be resected first or after the resection of other involved structures and lobectomy. In the latter, the previously described transcervical approach is first completed. Prior to closure, the trachea and esophagus are retracted, and the anterior longitudinal ligament is dissected to *expose* the lower cervical and upper thoracic vertebrae. The transcervical incision is closed, and the patient is then placed prone; a vertical midline incision from C7 to T4 is made followed by unilateral laminectomies. Involved nerve roots are divided, and the corresponding vertebral bodies are transected in the midline, which allows for en bloc removal of the specimen. The spine is then fixed with hooks and screws.[7] Alternatively, spinal resection with fixation can be done prior to chest wall resection and lobectomy without exposure of the tumor itself.[14]

Resection of Great Vessel

The NCCN guidelines recommend initial en bloc surgical resection of tumors invading the great vessels and the heart without mediastinal lymph node involvement or metastatic disease.[3]

Aorta

Resection of NSCLC invading the aorta can be performed with or without cardiopulmonary bypass.[15,16] Depending on the size of the defect, it can be closed primarily, with a prosthetic patch graft, or replaced with a prosthetic interposition graft.[17] When cardiopulmonary bypass is used, resection and reconstruction of the invaded segment is performed after aortic cross-clamping.[15] Shunting from the ascending aorta and the descending aorta distal to the lesion can also be used, which preserves blood flow to the spinal cord, abdominal viscera, and lower extremities.[17] Alternatively, the placement of non-fenestrated endovascular stents is also used to avoid bypass and shunting altogether. The stent can be placed at the same time as surgical resection or several days prior.[15,18] The stent forms a framework that maintains flow both during the resection and after, does not require defect coverage, and should be placed at least 3 cm from the expected aortic defect.[15,18] After endograft placement, a hemiclamshell or thoracotomy incision can be used for the lobectomy or pneumonectomy, with en bloc resection of the tumor and all invaded structures.[17,18]

Superior Vena Cava

Non–small cell lung cancer invasion into the SVC is exceedingly rare.[19] An endovascular stent can be placed in patients with unresectable disease and/or SVC syndrome to provide relief of symptoms caused by obstruction.[19] Surgical resection is indicated in patients without N2 or metastatic disease. If the brachiocephalic vein is involved, then a sternotomy incision is made; otherwise, a thoracotomy incision provides adequate exposure to the SVC.[20,21] Extent of invasion cannot be assessed without opening the pericardium.[20] If less than one-fourth of the circumference of the SVC is involved, a side clamp can be used to resect and primarily repair the defect.[21,22] A prosthetic patch or autologous pericardial patch is used to repair defects up to 50% of the diameter.[21,22] For defects greater than 50%, a ringed prosthetic graft or autologous spiral saphenous vein graft is placed after circumferential resection of the involved segment.[20-22] Cross-clamping of the SVC is avoided if the graft is placed between the brachiocephalic vein and the right atrial appendage rather than a brachiocephalic vein and the SVC.[21] Lobectomy or pneumonectomy is then performed and en bloc resection is complete.

Atrium

Despite a poor prognosis for localized NSCLCs invading the left atrium, surgical resection remains the gold standard.[23] Because the right pulmonary veins are shorter, invasion of the left atrium is more commonly seen with right-sided tumors.[24] A thoracotomy incision is made, and the pericardium is opened. The involved atrial wall is clamped and resected. The stump can be repaired primarily or with a patch graft if the reduction in atrial volume affects hemodynamics.[25] Lobectomy or pneumonectomy is then performed to complete en bloc resection.

Diaphragm

Tumors with diaphragmatic involvement are now classified as T4 (previously T3) in the latest TNM staging classification because of their poorer prognosis.[26] These tumors should be considered potentially curable by resection; however, literature regarding these outcomes is limited and often single center.[27-32] Within the English literature, Weksler et al. first reported on the postsurgical outcomes of NSLC invading the diaphragm. In their series of 8 patients, all surgical specimens showed invasion of the diaphragmatic musculature, and all 4 patients with N2 disease died of recurrent disease, highlighting the importance of mediastinal staging and chemotherapy in this patient population.[28] In a more recent series, Galetta et al. reported a series of 19 patients in which depth of invasion to the muscular diaphragm and again, nodal involvement, were associated with a worse prognosis for survival. In this study, patients with pathologically confirmed N2 disease received induction chemotherapy and were only offered surgery if the tumor showed a response or no progression.[27] After resection of the diaphragm, closure of the defect can usually be done primarily, with bridging prosthetic rarely required.[27,28,30] In one series, prosthetic replacement of the diaphragmatic defect was associated with improved survival, supporting a hypothesis of interrupting the drainage of the diaphragmatic lymphatics to the abdomen; therefore, the authors advocated for a larger margin of resection.[30] Because of the difficulty in preoperatively diagnosing diaphragmatic involvement, thoracoscopic investigation and MRI have both been advocated prior to determination of therapy in cases where diaphragmatic involvement is suspected.[27,28,31] The NSCLC tumor invading the diaphragm is a prime example of the importance of a multidisciplinary team approach to cancer staging and treatment where input from surgery, pathology, oncology and radiology are used to optimize patient outcomes.

SURGERY AS PART OF MULTIDISCIPLINARY CARE

The surgical management of locally-advanced NSCLC is complex due to extrapulmonary invasion by the tumor. Because of the aggressive nature of the disease, large randomized controlled trials have not been conducted comparing the various treatment strategies. Nevertheless, it is becoming more widely accepted that surgical resection, in the absence of mediastinal node involvement or other contraindications described previously, in conjunction with other treatment modalities can provide better outcomes.

RADIATION THERAPY FOR LOCALLY ADVANCED NON–SMALL CELL LUNG CANCER
Neal Dunlap, MD, Michael May, MD

A 72-year-old male has a 4-cm lung mass biopsied by core needle biopsy. He has COPD and smokes 1 pack of cigarettes per day.

The biopsy pathology shows NSCLC of the lung. PET shows bulky mediastinal lymph nodes that are pathologically positive on mediastinoscopy. Brain MRI brain is negative.

Learning Objectives:
1. What is the role of radiation therapy in locally advanced NSCLC?
2. How do you combine it with other treatment modalities?

Radiation therapy is an essential modality in treatment of locally advanced NSCLC. It can be used in a variety of sequences with surgery and chemotherapy depending on the cancer stage, individual patient characteristics, and institutional preference. It is estimated that 84% of stage II and 66% of stage III lung cancer cases require radiotherapy.[33] This area of lung cancer treatment is rapidly evolving as new technologies and combinations with systemic agents are being developed.

LOCALLY ADVANCED RESECTABLE NSCLC

Tumor resectability must be determined in a multidisciplinary discussion prior to starting treatment.[34] An experienced thoracic surgeon is needed as there are no definite rules that determine resectability, and the patients need to be approached on a case-by-case basis. This is particularly so given that the staging system does not completely correlate with surgical resectability, and that newer surgical techniques may enable resection of previously unresectable disease. In general, counterindications to resection include significant mediastinal fat invasion; invasion of vital mediastinal structures such as heart, great vessels, aorta, esophagus, vertebrae, or trachea; malignant pleural or pericardial effusion; N2 disease that is bulky or with extracapsular spread; N3 disease; and distant metastases.[35]

Surgical resection offers superior staging ability as nodal metastases are not always detectable with certainty despite CT scanning, especially when evaluating subcarinal lymph nodes.[36] After surgery alone as definitive treatment, survival is poor. A 3-year survival was found to be 9%.[36] For stage IIIB disease, the 5-year survival was only 5%.[37] Because of this, combined modality trials were designed in order to improve distant and local failures and thus improve survival.

PREOPERATIVE RADIOTHERAPY FOLLOWED BY SURGERY

To improve the outcomes of locally advanced NSCLC patients treated with surgery, neoadjuvant therapy was explored. The goal was to lead to tumor downstaging, increasing the chance of a complete resection and to improve local control and survival. A randomized controlled trial published in 1972 demonstrated inferior survival in patients with lung adenocarcinoma treated with preoperative radiotherapy. Radiation doses were between 30 and 60 Gy, with most patients receiving 40 to 50 Gy, followed by surgery; this was compared to surgery alone.[38] In the first 12 months, the difference was statistically significant, but even at longer follow-up, while not reaching statistical significance, the survival in the radiotherapy group was 12.5% compared to 21% in a surgery-only one. Notably, older radiotherapy techniques were used in the study, which pre-dated CT-guided radiation therapy. Therefore, the outcomes with modern radiotherapy techniques would be expected to be superior due to more accurate radiation delivery, as illustrated in **Figure 14-1.**

PREOPERATIVE CHEMORADIOTHERAPY FOLLOWED BY SURGERY

Given the lack of clinical improvement with neoadjuvant radiation therapy alone, neoadjuvant radiation therapy combined with chemotherapy was investigated. In a prospective trial, Southwest Oncology Group (SWOG) 8805, concurrent cisplatin-etoposide with 45 Gy in 25 fractions of radiotherapy followed by surgery resulted in an encouraging 3-year survival rate of 27% and 24% for stage IIIA and stage IIIB NSCLC, respectively.[39] The toxicity was acceptable as well. Another prospective multicenter trial confirmed these findings in stage IIIB disease using cisplatin and docetaxel with 44 Gy in 22 fractions followed by definitive surgery.[40] A higher dose of radiotherapy to 61.2 Gy concurrently with chemotherapy was subsequently evaluated in a prospective phase 2 study, RTOG 0229, in N2-3 stage III NSCLC patients to sterilize the mediastinal lymph nodes.[41] The results were promising, showing 63% of patients achieved mediastinal nodal clearance and 2-year overall survival of 54% and 2-year progression-free survival of 33%. The toxicity was acceptable with grade 3 or 4 hematologic, pulmonary, and gastrointestinal toxicity occurring in 35%, 23% and 14% of patients, respectively.

INDUCTION CHEMOTHERAPY FOLLOWED BY SURGERY COMPARED TO CHEMORADIOTHERAPY OR RADIOTHERAPY ALONE

With the success of chemoradiation given prior to surgery, the question becomes whether surgery is necessary in every case of an operable locally advanced lung cancer. In patients with stage IIIA NSCLC, EORTC 08941 showed that overall survival did not differ between surgery and radiotherapy after induction chemotherapy with cisplatin, carboplatin, and one other chemotherapy drug as illustrated in **Figure 14-2.**[42] More distant recurrences occurred after surgery and more local failures after radiation therapy.

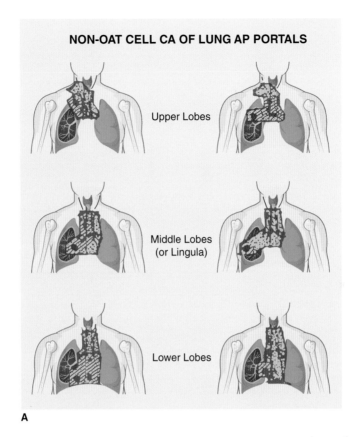

A

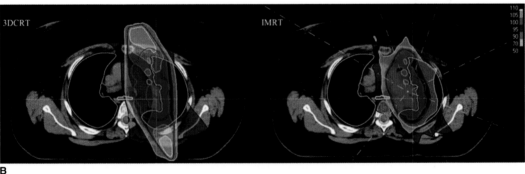

B

Figure 14-1. **A.** Technique used prior to CT-guided radiotherapy from a 1980s publication of RTOG 7301.[65] Treatment fields are illustrated for different tumor locations. Without using CT guidance, it was difficult to clearly visualize the tumor and avoid normal structures. Moreover, the use of posterior spinal cord blocks likely resulted in missing some of mediastinal lymph nodes affected by cancer. (Reproduced with permission from Perez CA, Stanley K, Rubin P, et al. A prospective randomized study of various irradiation doses and fractionation schedules in the treatment of inoperable non-oat-cell carcinoma of the lung. *Cancer.* 1980;45:2744-2753. © American Cancer Society.) **B.** CT-guided radiotherapy results in improved accuracy of treatment. With IMRT, there is additional improvement in conformity of the high-dose region to the target volume and normal organ sparing compared to 3-dimentional conformation radiation therapy. The colored regions in the pictures show the areas of radiation dose deposition. The legend in the upper right indicates the percentage of the prescribed dose delivered to each colored area. (Reproduced with permission from Reference 118 by Diwanji TP, Mohindra P, Vyfhuis M, et al. Advances in radiotherapy techniques and delivery for non-small cell lung cancer: benefits of intensity-modulated radiation therapy, proton therapy, and stereotactic body radiation therapy. *Transl Lung Cancer Res.* 2017;6(2):131-147.)

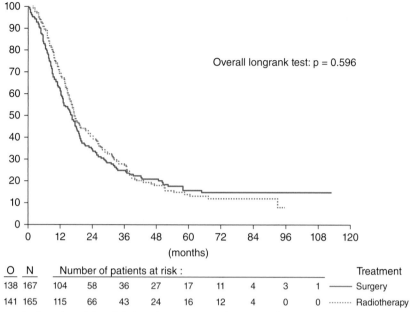

Figure 14-2. Data from EORTC 08941 showing equivalent survival in stage IIIA-N2 NSCLC patients who received induction chemotherapy followed by either surgery or radiotherapy. (Reproduced with permission by van Meerbeeck JP, Kramer GWPM, Van Schil PE, et al. Randomized controlled trial of resection versus radiotherapy after induction chemotherapy in stage IIIA-N2 non-small-cell lung cancer. *J Natl Cancer Inst.* 2007;99(6):442-450.)

The radiotherapy group had less than 1% of esophageal and 4% of pulmonary toxicity and 7% late esophageal or pulmonary toxicities with 1 death. Postoperative mortality ranged from 9% for left-sided pneumonectomy to 0% after lobectomy. Therefore, radiation therapy after chemotherapy is the preferred locoregional treatment to surgery after chemotherapy due to its low morbidity and mortality. The phase III study of surgery versus definitive concurrent chemoradiotherapy boost in patients with resectable stage IIIA(N2) and selected IIIB non-small-cell lung cancer after induction chemotherapy and concurrent chemoradiotherapy (ESPATUE) trial of stage III NSCLC patients evaluated induction chemotherapy with cisplatin-paclitaxel followed by concurrent chemoradiotherapy with cisplatin-vinorelbine with radiation therapy to 45 Gy in 1.5-Gy fractions given twice a day followed by either a radiotherapy boost to 65-71 Gy or surgical resection.[43] There was no difference in overall survival or progression-free survival between the two arms. Therefore, both treatment modalities are acceptable in stage III disease.

INDUCTION CHEMORADIOTHERAPY FOLLOWED BY SURGERY COMPARED TO DEFINITIVE CHEMORADIOTHERAPY

Another prospective randomized controlled trial, INT-0139, compared radiotherapy to 45 Gy plus cisplatin-etoposide chemotherapy with surgery to a group that did not receive surgery but underwent continued radiotherapy to 61 Gy.[44] In the surgery group, there was a better progression-free survival (12.8 vs. 10.5 months) and disease-free survival at 5 years (22% vs. 11%). While there was no difference in overall survival, the surgery group had more treatment-related deaths (8% vs. 2%). The toxicity was comparable. This study helped establish that chemotherapy with radiotherapy with or without resection is an acceptable option for stage T1-3pN2M0 NSCLC.

Superior sulcus tumors are a special consideration in NSCLC due to their unique location, making surgery more challenging. Neoadjuvant chemoradiation in attempt to downstage the tumor prior to resection is therefore an attractive option for superior sulcus tumors. A prospective phase 2 study, JCOG 9806, showed that a trimodality approach with mitomycin, vindesine, cisplatin, 45 Gy of radiotherapy followed by surgical resection is safe and effective in superior sulcus tumors.[45] The disease-free and overall survival rates at 5 years were 45% and 56%, respectively. Another prospective trial INT 0160 using cisplatin-etoposide followed by 45 Gy of radiotherapy followed by surgery and two more cycles of additional adjuvant chemotherapy resulted in an encouraging 55% 2-year survival and 70% rate of complete response.[46]

POSTOPERATIVE RADIATION THERAPY

Postoperative radiation therapy (PORT) is a well-studied area of locally advanced lung cancer treatment but continues to be a clinical challenge. A PORT meta-analysis trialists group in 1998, using older radiation techniques, evaluated all stages of NSCLC from 9 studies including 2,128 patients.[47] It showed that PORT was detrimental to overall and progression-free survival in patients with early stage completely resected NSCLC and should not be used, as illustrated in **Figure 14-3A**.

The role of PORT in stage III was not clear. The Surveillance, Epidemiology, and End Results (SEER) database retrospective review of 7,495 patients with NSCLC stage II and III disease demonstrated that PORT increased overall survival in patients with N2 disease but decreased the survival of N0 and N1 patients.[48] A 2008 retrospective analysis of the Adjuvant Navelbine International Trialist Association (ANITA) trial of 840 NSCLC patients with stage IB to IIIA disease compared outcomes of patients treated with and without PORT.[49] Of note, patients were originally randomized to either observation or adjuvant vinorelbine-cisplatin. The data were retrospectively analyzed to compare the outcomes of PORT and no radiotherapy. The patients who received PORT had improved median survival in both observation and chemotherapy arms in pN2 disease (23.8 vs. 47.4 in chemotherapy and 12.7 vs. 22.7 in observation) and in the observation arm alone in pN1 disease, 25.9 versus 50.2 months (while it was detrimental in the chemotherapy arm, 23.8 vs. 47.4 months).

A National Cancer Database analysis of 4,483 patients with N2 NSCLC revealed that there was a 5-year overall survival advantage to PORT compared to no PORT—39.3% compared to 34.8%[50]—as shown in **Figure 14-3B**. While there is a lack of consensus, patients whose tumors have not been completely resected (R1/R2 resection) and probably individuals with N2 disease may benefit from PORT.[34]

LOCALLY ADVANCED UNRESECTABLE NSCLC
Definitive Radiotherapy

As surgical resection is not possible in these patients, the question was whether radiation therapy alone would provide adequate outcomes in locally advanced disease. Cancer

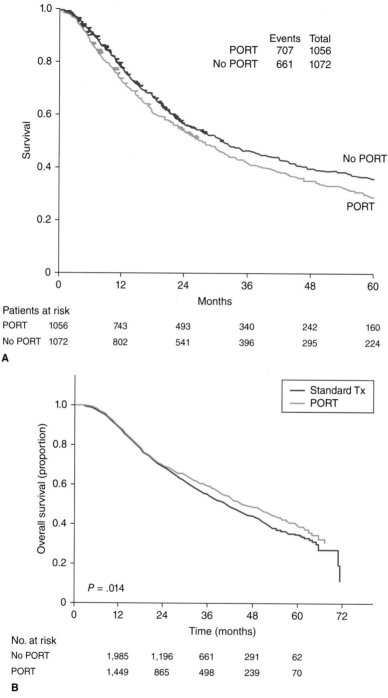

Figure 14-3. A. PORT Meta-analysis Trialists Group data showing worsening survival in patients of all stages receiving postoperative radiotherapy. **B.** Patients with pathologic N2 NSCLC who underwent complete resection and adjuvant chemotherapy had a statistically significant improvement in overall survival with PORT in an National Cancer Database (NCDB) analysis. (Reproduced with permission by Robinson CG, Patel AP, Bradley JD, et al. Postoperative radiotherapy for pathologic N2 non-small-cell lung cancer treated with adjuvant chemotherapy: a review of the National Cancer Data Base. *J Clin Oncol.* 2015;33(8):870-876. Copyright © 2015 American Society of Clinical Oncology.)

and Leukemia Group B (CALGB 8433) investigated whether sequential chemoradiation therapy performed better than radiation therapy alone in stage III lung cancer.[51] The combination of cisplatin-vinblastine chemotherapy with 60-Gy radiation in 30 fractions of radiation therapy resulted in median survival improvement of 4.1 months compared to radiation therapy to 60 Gy in 30 fractions alone. While the addition of chemotherapy did not appear to affect local recurrence, there was a significant improvement in distant failure-free survival. Based on this, chemotherapy should not be omitted. However, for patients who are too frail to tolerate both chemotherapy and radiotherapy, one or the other modality may be used.

Sequential Compared to Concurrent Chemoradiotherapy

For unresectable disease, various sequences of chemotherapy and radiation therapy have been investigated. In RTOG 9410, stage III NSCLC patients underwent either definitive concurrent or sequential chemoradiotherapy.[52] In both cases, radiation therapy was delivered to 63-Gy radiation, and chemotherapy consisted of cisplatin and vinblastine. A concurrent arm showed an improved 5-year survival from 10% to 16%, as illustrated in **Figure 14-4**. There was greater acute grade 3 or higher toxicity with the concurrent regimen, but there was no difference in late toxicity.

Another 3-arm prospective trial, LAMP (Locally Advanced Multimodality Protocol), evaluated induction chemotherapy followed by radiotherapy, induction chemotherapy followed by concurrent chemoradiation, and concurrent chemoradiation followed by additional chemotherapy in stage III disease.[53] The paclitaxel-carboplatin combination was used for chemotherapy, and radiation therapy was administered to 63 Gy.

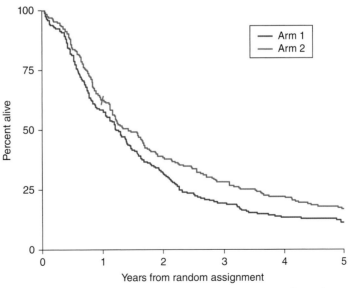

Figure 14-4. Results of RTOG 9410 showing improved survival in patients who underwent concurrent chemoradiotherapy (Arm 2) compared to sequential delivery of chemotherapy and radiation therapy (Arm 1). (Reproduced with permission by Curran WJ Jr, Paulus R, Langer CJ, et al. Sequential vs. concurrent chemoradiation for stage III non-small cell lung cancer: randomized phase III trial RTOG 9410. *J Natl Cancer Inst.* 2011;103(19):1452-1460.)

The concurrent chemoradiation followed by chemotherapy arm resulted in the best overall survival (16.3 compared to 13 and 12.7 months) at the expense of a higher rate of esophagitis with radiotherapy. Because of this, concurrent chemoradiation therapy is recommended for patients with inoperable stage III NSCLC. However, patients who are frail and are unable to tolerate concurrent therapy may be treated with the sequential approach.

PROPHYLACTIC CRANIAL IRRADIATION

Prophylactic cranial irradiation (PCI) has been investigated as NSCLC commonly metastases to the brain. In a prospective study (RTOG 0214), patients previously treated definitively with no evidence of disease progression were assigned to either PCI to 30 Gy in 15 fractions or observation.[54] While patients treated with PCI were 2.5 times more likely to develop brain metastases, the 1-year overall survival and disease-free survival did not differ.

A more recent prospective study, NVALT-11/DLCRG-02 evaluated the quality of life and compared the development of symptomatic brain metastases between PCI and observation in stage III patients treated with chemoradiotherapy with or without surgery. While PCI decreased the proportion of patients with symptomatic brain metastases from 27% to 7%, the quality of life was decreased 3 months post-PCI, memory impairment was worse (30% compared to 8%), and cognitive disturbances were present more often (19% compared to 3%) when PCI was not used. Because of this, PCI is not used in NSCLC due to its toxicity and lack of sufficient clinical benefit.

RADIATION TOXICITY

Both acute and late toxicity are a major concern with radiation therapy. To minimize the risk of developing these, normal organ dose constraints have been developed. Studies, including QUANTEC[55,56] and RTOG studies such as RTOG 0617,[57] are used to determine which radiation doses are safe for certain organs at risk. These include spinal cord, esophagus, brachial plexus, heart/pericardium, great vessels, tracheal and proximal bronchi, ribs, skin, and stomach depending on the exact location of the tumor. The toxicities depend on the exact location of the tumor, patient's comorbidities, prior radiation therapy, and individual genetic susceptibility. Radiation-induced adverse events include acute skin reaction, fatigue, dysphagia, odynophagia, cough, and myelosuppression. Late toxicities include radiation pneumonitis, lung fibrosis, brachial plexopathy, Lhermitte syndrome, radiation myelitis, esophageal fibrosis and strictures, pericarditis, and secondary malignancies.[58] Advanced radiation treatment techniques such as intensity-modulated radiation therapy (IMRT) have been shown to reduce the chance of developing these problems.[59]

RADIATION TECHNIQUES
Radiation Treatment Planning
General principles of radiation therapy include determining the tumor location, finding how much tissue to include in the radiation field, avoiding delivery of radiation to the normal structures, and maximizing the precision of radiation treatment delivery.

The gross tumor volume (GTV) is determined from the CT scan in treatment planning combined with the information obtained from a PET scan. Biopsy-proven lymph nodes or any nodes larger than 15 mm on CT are included in the radiation field. GTV is expanded to an internal target volume (ITV) to provide a margin for target motion. Planning target volume (PTV) is subsequently re-created, which has a 1- to 1.5-cm margin to account for setup uncertainties and patient movement. The margin can be decreased by immobilization, motion management, and image-guided radiation therapy (IGRT).[60,61] Radiation therapy interruptions and dose reductions should be avoided if possible.

Radiation Treatment Volume

Omitting irradiation of elective nodes in NSCLC stage I-IIIB was investigated in a retrospective study.[62] Only the involved lymph nodes by the tumor were included in the radiation treatment field. Elective nodal control was 92.4%, and local control was 51% at 2 years. As nodal failure was rare and only treating the involved field resulted in a reduced radiation dose to the normal tissues, involved-field radiation therapy without treating the elective nodes is the standard of care.

A prospective study of 200 patients with inoperable stage III NSCLC involved randomization of patients to cisplatin concurrently with radiotherapy to either 68-74 Gy for involved-field irradiation only compared to 60-64 Gy for elective nodal irradiation as well as involved-field irradiation.[63] Two-year overall survival was higher in the involved-field irradiation group, 39.4% compared to 25.6%. A 5-year local control was also better with involved-field irradiation, 51% compared to 36%. Moreover, omission of elective nodal irradiation resulted in less toxicity, manifested as radiation pneumonitis in 17% of involved-field irradiation compared to 29% in the other group. However, it is unknown whether the decrease in local control and survival could be mainly because a lower radiation dose was used in the elective nodal irradiation group. However, there are circumstances under which irradiation of elective lymph node regions may be considered. This depends on various variables related to the tumor, patient, staging, and treatment-related issues and should be evaluated on a case-by-case basis.[64]

Radiation Dose

The total radiation dose must be chosen such that the tumor or the remaining microscopic disease is adequately addressed without causing excessive toxicity. In a definitive chemoradiation or radiation-alone setting, the dose of 60 to 70 Gy in 30-35 fractions is the most commonly used.[34] The dose of 60 Gy in 30 fractions was shown to be superior to 40 or 50 Gy in the RTOG 7301 study.[65] The 3-year overall survival was improved from 6% in patients treated to 40 Gy, 10% in those treated to 50 Gy, to 15% in patients who received 60 Gy, as shown in **Figure 14-5A**. Dose escalation to 74 Gy appears to be detrimental compared to 60 Gy in patients treated with concurrent and consolidation carboplatin plus paclitaxel with or without cetuximab in a prospective trial (RTOG 0617), as shown in **Figure 14-5B**.[57] The higher radiation dose resulted in lower mean and overall survival (29 vs. 20 months and 67 vs. 54%). Surprisingly, fewer local regional failures and better quality of life were noted in the 60-Gy arm.

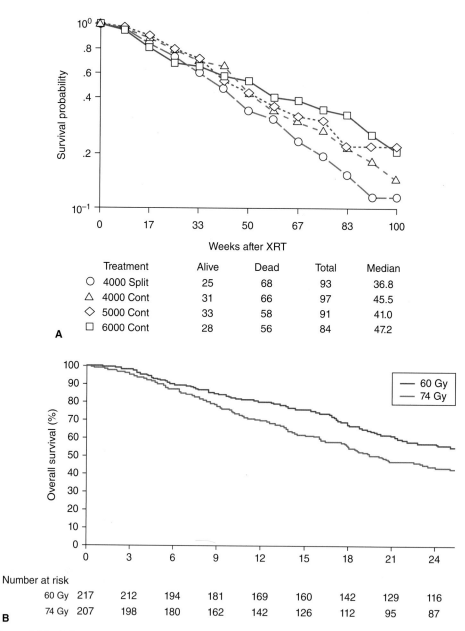

Treatment	Alive	Dead	Total	Median
○ 4000 Split	25	68	93	36.8
△ 4000 Cont	31	66	97	45.5
◇ 5000 Cont	33	58	91	41.0
□ 6000 Cont	28	56	84	47.2

Number at risk

60 Gy	217	212	194	181	169	160	142	129	116
74 Gy	207	198	180	162	142	126	112	95	87

Figure 14-5. A. Improvement in survival was achieved with doses up to 60 Gy in a classic study, RTOG 7031.[65] **B.** Worsening of overall survival was shown when the radiation dose was escalated to 74 Gy from 60 Gy. (Reproduced with permission by Bradley JD, Paulus R, Komaki R, et al. Standard-dose versus high-dose conformal radiotherapy with concurrent and consolidation carboplatin plus paclitaxel with or without cetuximab for patients with stage IIIA or IIIB non-small-cell lung cancer (RTOG 0617): a randomised, two-by-two factorial phase 3 study. *Lancet Oncol.* 2015;16:187-199. Copyright © 2015 Elsevier.)

For postoperative cases, 60-70 Gy are typically given for gross residual tumor, 54-60 Gy to extracapsular nodal extension and positive margin, and 50-54 Gy to negative margin.

The preoperative radiotherapy dose usually ranges from 45 to 54 in 25-27 fractions. It is important to note that institutional protocols and experience vary, and that the patients treated in high-volume centers have superior outcomes with radiotherapy.[34,61]

Radiation Fractionation

Radiation fractionation is important as different tumor types benefit from various treatment schemes depending on the biology of a specific cancer. In NSCLC, using modified fractionation of radiation therapy such as 54 Gy total given 3 times a day instead of daily radiation treatments to a total of 60 Gy was explored. A CHART (continuous, hyperfractionated, accelerated radiotherapy) randomized trial demonstrated a 9% absolute improvement in overall survival at 2 years.[66] This was postulated to be due to accelerated delivery of therapy preventing cancer cellular repopulation from a more protracted regimen. A meta-analysis looking at 10 trials with a total of 2,000 patients revealed that while there was a significant overall survival benefit at 5 years with modified fractionation compared to conventional fractionation (10.8% compared to 8.3%, respectively), this came at the expense of greater acute esophageal toxicity (odds ratio of 2.44) but not the other types of toxicity.[67] Overall, further research is needed to identify whether modified fractionation has benefits over a once-a-day schedule.

Intensity-Modulated Radiation Therapy

Intensity-modulated radiation therapy is an advanced mode of high-precision radiotherapy that uses computer-controlled linear accelerators to deliver radiation to a tumor.[58] The technique uses the accuracy of CT scanning to define the 3-dimensional target volume and normal structures and delivers treatments in a non-uniform intensity of the radiation beams using computerized inverse planning. Because variable radiation intensity is generated across each beam, in contrast to the uniform intensity used in other radiotherapy techniques, very complex plans can be constructed. Using this technology, tumors can be targeted precisely while avoiding normal structures. A secondary analysis of a prospective randomized study (RTOG 0617) of definitive chemoradiation for stage III NSCLC compared outcomes of patients treated with IMRT to 3-dimensional conventional radiation therapy (3D-CRT).[59] IMRT resulted in decreased incidence of high-grade radiation pneumonitis, 3.5% compared to 7.9%. The cardiac radiation dose was also significantly lower with IMRT compared to 3D-CRT. The tumor control and overall survival were similar.

Other Radiation Techniques

Other advanced technologies, such as 4-dimensional CT (4D-CT) scan, PET/CT simulation, respiratory motion management, and proton therapy may be appropriate to deliver curative radiation therapy safely. No randomized trials showed their superiority over older techniques, but non-randomized comparisons showed promising toxicity and survival outcomes. For instance, a phase 2 study of carboplatin-paclitaxel chemotherapy with proton beam radiation therapy to 74-Gy relative biological effectiveness resulted in medial overall survival of 26.5 months, with toxicity outcomes that compared favorably with prior conventional radiation therapy.[68] Further trials prospectively comparing modalities and evaluating cost-effectiveness are needed.

ONGOING STUDIES

Radiotherapy to NSCLC is a rapidly changing field. Various clinical trials are currently open to accrual. One emerging technology is adaptive radiation therapy. This technique allows for adjustment in the radiation treatment plan as the patient is undergoing radiation therapy as the tumor shrinks and lungs may undergo changes.[69] RTOG 1106 is prospective trial using ^{18}F-fludeoxyglucose (FDG)–PET/CT to modify the radiotherapy treatment plan.[70] Modern treatment regimens that maximize radiation dose delivery to areas that are the most likely to bear tumor and minimize radiation dose to normal tissues are currently being evaluated prospectively. One example of this is the ongoing phase 3 randomized trial Lung ART (Adjuvant Radiation Therapy) that uses information from the thoracic CT and PET scan obtained prior to surgery as well as the description of the mediastinal exploration and histopathological results for treatment planning.[71]

There is of course great interest in using immunotherapy for every cancer type. This is clearly the case with NSCLC, especially after durvalumab has been shown to improved progression-free survival after chemoradiation therapy of stage III patients.[72] Radiotherapy and immunotherapy combinations are currently being investigated in multiple studies, such as the PARIS trial, which is a phase 1 study of pembrolizumab in combination with radiotherapy in locally advanced NSCLC.[73] Another area of interest is hypofractionation. University of Texas Southwestern is conducting a trial comparing 60 Gy in 15 fractions compared to the standard 60-66 Gy in 30-33 fractions in patients with poor functional status.[74] Using fewer radiation fractions decreases the number of times the patients need to come to the clinic and may result in better outcomes. Proton therapy for lung cancer has been evaluated in retrospective studies showing promising results. PRONTOX is a prospective trial comparing proton to photon radiation therapy given to 66 Gy (or Gray radiological equivalent in the case of proton therapy).[75] The primary aim of this study is to show a decrease of radiation pneumonitis and esophagitis by proton therapy.

CENTRAL NERVOUS SYSTEM RADIATION

Asymptomatic brain metastases have been described for patients with locally advanced NSCLC with guidelines from the US NCCN recommending contrasted brain MRI as part of pretreatment staging for patients with stage II-IV NSCLC.[3] Patients with locally advanced NSCLC have a high risk for developing brain metastases during the course of their disease.[76] Subsequently, the development of new neurologic symptoms warrants central nervous system (CNS) imaging. Given this proclivity for intracranial failure, the RTOG attempted to perform a phase 3 study investigating if PCI was associated with improved survival in patients with locally advanced NSCLC.[54] Though this study demonstrated PCI significantly reduced the rate of brain metastasis development at 1 year (p = .004; 7.7% vs. 18.0% for PCI vs. observation), no significant difference in overall survival was found, and PCI is not currently standard of care for patients with locally advanced NSCLC.

CHEMOTHERAPY FOR LOCALLY ADVANCED NON–SMALL CELL LUNG CANCER

Rohit Kumar, MD

A 65-year-old white male with a past medical history of COPD presents with persistent cough and weight loss. He has a 60 pack-year smoking history. Chest CT reveals a 5-cm right lower lobe mass with 3-cm, single-station mediastinal lymphadenopathy. Endobronchial ultrasound–guided fine-needle aspiration biopsy confirms adenocarcinoma. No other metastatic site is identified.

Learning Objectives:
1. What is the best approach to the management of stage III NSCLC?
2. What is the benefit of chemotherapy in stage III NSCLC?
3. What is the role of immunotherapy in stage III NSCLC?

Stage III NSCLC is a heterogeneous group of diseases, and the optimal management of these patients remains challenging. An individualized treatment strategy should be sought from a multidisciplinary assessment for the best outcome in these patients. As a general rule, T4N0-3 or T1-4N3 tumors are unresectable, and definitive concurrent chemoradiation is the standard of care. In resectable tumors, adjuvant chemotherapy has shown a survival benefit. A subset of patients with N2 disease can benefit from induction chemotherapy with or without radiation therapy followed by surgery.

RESECTABLE STAGE III NSCLC

Adjuvant Chemotherapy

Several phase 3 randomized studies and meta-analyses have established the survival benefit of adjuvant chemotherapy in resected stage III NSCLC. The Lung Adjuvant Cisplatin Evaluation (LACE) meta-analysis of 4,584 patients from 5 large randomized trials evaluated the benefit of postoperative cisplatin-based chemotherapy in stage I-III NSCLC. At the median follow up period of 5.2 years, there was 5.4% absolute survival benefit favoring adjuvant chemotherapy in the overall study population (hazard ratio [HR] 0.89, 95% CI 0.82-0.96, $p = .005$). In this pooled analysis, approximately 1,200 patients had stage III disease and derived the most survival benefit from adjuvant chemotherapy. The HR for stage III was 0.83 (95% CI 0.72-0.94). The benefit of chemotherapy increased with better performance status (PS) and may be detrimental for PS of 2.[77]

The largest study included in the LACE meta-analysis was the International Adjuvant Lung Cancer Trial. A total of 1,867 patients underwent randomization, with enrollment of 39% pathologically confirmed stage III disease. Patients were randomly assigned to either 3 or 4 cycles of cisplatin-based chemotherapy or observation. The subset of patients with stage III NSCLC had a significantly higher 5-year overall survival rate (37.4% vs. 29.9%, $p < .05$).[78]

> **CLINICAL PEARL:** There is a 7.5% absolute 5-year survival benefit of adjuvant chemotherapy in stage III NSCLC.

TABLE 14-1	Chemotherapy Regimens (Neoadjuvant or Adjuvant)[a]

1. Cisplatin 50 mg/m² days 1 and 8; vinorelbine 25 mg/m² days 1, 8, 15, 22, every 28 days for 4 cycles
2. Cisplatin 100 mg/m² day 1; vinorelbine 30 mg/m² days 1, 8, 15, 22, every 28 days for 4 cycles
3. Cisplatin 75–80 mg/m² day 1; vinorelbine 25–30 mg/m² days 1 + 8, every 21 days for 4 cycles
4. Cisplatin 100 mg/m² day 1; etoposide 100 mg/m² days 1-3, every 28 days for 4 cycles
5. Cisplatin 75 mg/m² day 1; gemcitabine 1,250 mg/m² days 1, 8, every 21 days for 4 cycles
6. Cisplatin 75 mg/m² day 1; docetaxel 75 mg/m² day 1 every 21 days for 4 cycles

Non-squamous–only regimens
7. Cisplatin 75 mg/m² day 1; pemetrexed 500 mg/m² day 1 every 21 days for 4 cycles

Patients with significant comorbidities or not candidates for cisplatin:
1. Carboplatin AUC 6 day 1, paclitaxel 200 mg/m² day 1, every 21 days for 4 cycles
2. Carboplatin AUC 5 day 1, gemcitabine 1,000 mg/m² days 1, 8, every 21 days for 4 cycles

Non-squamous–only regimens
3. Carboplatin AUC 5 day 1, pemetrexed 500 mg/m² day 1 every 21 days for 4 cycles

[a]Available from https://www.nccn.org/professionals/physician_gls/default.aspx#nscl.[94]

Choice of Chemotherapy

All chemotherapy regimens mentioned in **Table 14-1** are equally efficacious. The treating physician may choose any of the chemotherapy regimens based on clinical judgment and patient preference. This recommendation is supported by the open-label randomized phase 3 trial (E1505) that assigned 1,501 patients to either chemotherapy alone or chemotherapy plus bevacizumab. Four cisplatin-based chemotherapy regimens were used: 25% of patients received vinorelbine, 23% received docetaxel, 19% received gemcitabine, and 33% received pemetrexed. At a median follow-up of 50.3 months, there was no survival benefit of adding bevacizumab to chemotherapy. In the pooled analysis across both arms and subdivided based on histology (non-squamous and squamous to account for use of pemetrexed only for the former)m there was no significant difference in overall survival or disease-free survival between the four chemotherapy regimens, suggesting use of either of the regimens in the adjuvant setting as a viable option.[79]

Preoperative Chemotherapy

Besides N2 disease, the data supporting neoadjuvant chemotherapy is not robust compared to adjuvant therapy, but benefits appear to be comparable. In a meta-analysis of 15 randomized trials that enrolled 2,385 patients (including 529 with stage III disease), there was a 13% relative risk reduction in mortality (HR 0.87, 95% CI 0·78-0.96, $p = .007$). There was a 5% absolute survival benefit at 5 years (45% vs. 40%), similar to the LACE meta-analysis. Whether additional postoperative chemotherapy would improve the survival outcomes remains unanswered.[80]

> **CLINICAL PEARL:** Neoadjuvant therapy can downstage a patient and improve resectability, and chemotherapy is more likely to be better tolerated before a major surgery.

TABLE 14-2 Neoadjuvant Chemotherapy Trials in Stage III/N2 Disease			
STUDY	SIZE (n)	ARMS	OUTCOMES
Rosell et al. (1994)[81]	60	1. Surgery with adjuvant mediastinal radiation Three cycles mitomycin, ifosfamide, and cisplatin followed by surgery with adjuvant mediastinal radiation	3-year overall survival: 0% vs. 23%
Roth et al. (1994)[82]	60	1. Surgery alone 2. Six cycles of cyclophosphamide, etoposide, and cisplatin followed by surgery	3-year overall survival: 15% vs. 56%

The role of preoperative chemotherapy specifically in patients who have N2 disease was evaluated in 2 small studies in the 1990s (**Table 14-2**). Both of these studies enrolled approximately 60 patients each. The study by Rosell et al. randomized patients to surgery followed by mediastinal radiation therapy with or without preoperative chemotherapy. The 3-year survival rate was 23% versus 0% in favor of preoperative chemotherapy.[81] Similarly, the study by Roth et al. randomized patients to surgery alone or preoperative chemotherapy followed by surgery. The 3-year survival was significantly improved with preoperative chemotherapy (56% vs. 15%).[82] The optimal neoadjuvant therapy for N2 disease remains unknown. A randomized phase 3 trial evaluated induction docetaxel and cisplatin versus docetaxel plus cisplatin followed by radiotherapy. There was no difference in the event-free survival between the arms, suggesting chemotherapy alone may be sufficient.[83] No overall survival data were reported by the study, which had several limitations due to the small sample size and slow accrual process. Current guidelines support use of chemotherapy alone or chemoradiotherapy as the induction regimen.

Postoperative radiation may be considered for patients who did not receive radiation in the neoadjuvant setting for N2 disease but is not recommended for pathological N0-1 because it has been associated with increased mortality, especially when older radiotherapy techniques are used. In a meta-analysis of 9 randomized controlled trials that mostly used older radiotherapy techniques, PORT was found to be detrimental in completely resectable NSCLC. The survival HR was 1.21 (95% CI 1.08–1.3) for PORT versus no PORT. In the subset analysis by nodal status, worse survival was noted in N0-1 and no survival impact in N2 disease.[84] A retrospective study from the National Cancer Database analyzed the impact of modern radiotherapy techniques. There was a detriment in 5-year overall survival with PORT for pathologically N0 (48% vs. 37.7%, $p < .001$) and N1 patients (39.4% vs. 34.8%, $p < .001$), although 5-year overall survival improved with PORT in N2 patients (27.8% vs. 34.1%, $p < .001$).[85]

Postoperative radiation therapy is recommended for all stages with positive resection margins. A randomized phase 3 trial (Lung Adjuvant Radiotherapy Trial NCT00410683) that is currently recruiting participants should be able to address the controversy around the impact of PORT.

> **CLINICAL PEARL:** Although mediastinal involvement (N2/N3 disease) precludes surgery in general, data suggest that a select subset of patients with N2 disease can benefit from surgery after induction chemotherapy or chemoradiotherapy: medically fit patients, single-station N2 disease less than 3 cm, and plan for lobectomy. If pneumonectomy is a possibility, evidence supports giving definitive chemoradiotherapy alone.

In the North America Intergroup trial (INT0139), over 400 patients with stage T1-3pN2M0 disease were randomized to either induction chemotherapy (two cycles of cisplatin and etoposide) plus radiotherapy (45 Gy) followed by surgery or definitive chemoradiotherapy (61 Gy). The median overall survival was not statistically different between the groups. On subgroup analysis, patients who underwent lobectomy had significantly better overall survival versus the no surgery group (5-year survival rate of 36% vs. 18%). Patients who had a nodal status of N0 after induction chemoradiotherapy had a higher median overall survival (34.4 months) compared to N1-3 or unknown status (**Table 14-3**). A repeat pathologic evaluation should be considered in these patients after induction treatment, and lobectomy can be opted for patients who clear their mediastinum (N0).[44]

UNRESECTABLE STAGE III NSCLC

Concurrent chemoradiation is the standard of care for unresectable stage III NSCLC or patients who are unfit for the surgery. Multiple randomized controlled trials have established that concurrent chemoradiation significantly improves overall survival, but as expected has more toxicity compared to sequential chemoradiation. In the United States, the most commonly used regimens are cisplatin and etoposide and dose-reduced weekly carboplatin and paclitaxel during radiation followed by 2 cycles of the same agents at systemic doses. Pemetrexed is a relatively newer agent that has been adopted widely as the chemotherapeutic agent of choice for non-squamous histology (**Table 14-4**).

In the absence of clear evidence supporting one particular regimen, a shared decision between the clinicians and patients should be made, keeping various factors into

TABLE 14-3	Phase 3 Trials Evaluating Survival Based on Nodal Response to Induction Therapy in Stage III/N2 Disease		
STUDY	SIZE (n)	NODAL STATUS	5-YEAR OS RATE
Van Meerbeeck et al. (2007)[42]	64	ypN0-1	29%
	86	ypN2	7%
Albain et al. (2009)[44]	76	ypN0	41%
	85	ypN1-3	24%

TABLE 14-4	Concurrent Chemoradiation Regimens[a]

1. Cisplatin 50 mg/m^2 on days 1, 8, 29, and 36 plus etoposide 50 mg/m^2 days 1-5, 29-33
2. Paclitaxel 45-50 mg/m^2 weekly, carboplatin AUC 2, concurrent radiotherapy with/without additional 2 cycles of paclitaxel 200 mg/m^2 and carboplatin AUC 6
3. Cisplatin 100 mg/m^2 days 1 and 29 plus vinablastine 5 mg/m^2/weekly for 5 weeks

Non-squamous–only regimens:

4. Cisplatin 75 mg/m^2 on day 1, pemetrexed 500 mg/m^2 on day 1 every 21 days times 3, concurrent radiotherapy with/without additional pemetrexed 500 mg/m^2 times 4
5. Carboplatin AUC 5 on day 1, pemetrexed 500 mg/m^2 on day 1 every 21 days times 4

Consolidation therapy:

1. Durvalumab 10 mg/kg IV every 2 weeks for up to 12 months

[a]Available from https://www.nccn.org/professionals/physician_gls/default.aspx#nscl.[94]

consideration: histology (pemetrexed is effective only in non-squamous histology); adverse effects (eg, renal dysfunction for cisplatin, neuropathy for paclitaxel); treatment duration (cisplatin/paclitaxel and pemetrexed-containing regimens are usually given with consolidation chemotherapy, whereas its role in etoposide/cisplatin and vinblastine-containing regimens is controversial); and cost (pemetrexed is significantly more expensive).

Concurrent Chemoradiation

During the 1990s, several studies showed the benefit of adding chemotherapy to the radiation. A meta-analysis that pooled data for 1,887 patients compared combined radiotherapy plus chemotherapy versus radiotherapy alone. For the cisplatin-based group, the estimated pooled odds ratio of death at 2 years was 0.70 (95% CI 0.5-0.9) and 0.82 (95% CI 0.5-1.3) for the non–cisplatin-based group. With the knowledge of the radio-sensitization effects of the chemotherapy, several studies followed to demonstrate the benefits of concurrent chemoradiation.

The landmark trial that established the advantage of concurrent chemoradiation was RTOG 9410. In this randomized phase 3 trial, 610 patients with stage III disease were assigned to 2 concurrent and 1 sequential chemoradiation arms. The sequential arm (arm 1) included cisplatin-vinblastine with 60-Gy TRT (thoracic radiation therapy) beginning on day 50. Arm 2 used the same chemotherapy regimen as arm 1 with 60-Gy TRT once daily beginning on day 1. Arm 3 used cisplatin with oral etoposide with 69.6 Gy delivered as 1.2-Gy twice-daily fractions beginning on day 1. The overall 5-year survival rates were 10% for arm 1, 16% for arm 2, and 13% for arm 3. The response rate was 70% in arm 2, 61% in arm 1, and 65% in arm 3. The response rate in arm 2 was statistically significantly higher ($p < .05$) compared with arm 1, but arms 2 and 3 were not statistically significantly different in response rate. There were statistically significantly higher rates of acute esophagitis in both concurrent arms than in the sequential arm.[52]

The concurrent chemoradiation with the cisplatin and etoposide combination was evaluated in SWOG 9019. The treatment regimen was 2 cycles of cisplatin plus etoposide concurrent with daily radiation (45 Gy). In patients with no disease progression, radiotherapy was completed to 61 Gy, and 2 additional cycles of cisplatin plus etoposide were given. The overall median survival was 15 months, with a 5-year survival rate of 15%.[86]

The efficacy of concurrent radiation with cisplatin-etoposide or carboplatin-paclitaxel was compared in a phase 3 multicenter trial. Patients in the etoposide/platinum (EP) arm received etoposide 50 mg/m^2 on days 1–5 and cisplatin 50 mg/m^2 on days 1 and 8 every 4 weeks for 2 cycles; patients in the paclitaxel/carboplatin (PC) arm received 45 mg/m^2 paclitaxel and carboplatin (area under the curve [AUC] 2) on day 1 once a week. A dose of 60-66 Gy (2 Gy per fraction) started on the first day of chemotherapy. TRT was given as per the treatment protocol in 96.9% in both arms. The overall response rate (ORR) was 73.7% versus 64.5% in the EP and PC arms, respectively (p = .21). The 5-year overall survival rate was 28% in the EP arm versus 19.7% in the PC arm. The incidence of grade 3 esophagitis was significantly higher in the EP arm than in the PC arm (20% vs. 6.3%).[87]

The phase 3 PROCLAIM study randomized patients with stage IIIA/B unresectable non-squamous NSCLC to either pemetrexed and cisplatin intravenously every 3 weeks for 3 cycles plus concurrent radiation followed by pemetrexed consolidation every 3 weeks for 4 cycles or etoposide and cisplatin every 4 weeks for 2 cycles plus concurrent radiation followed by 2 cycles of consolidation platinum-based doublet chemotherapy. Approximately 75% of patients had adenocarcinoma histology. There was no statistically significant difference in overall survival or objective response between the 2 chemotherapy regimens, but the incidence of grade 3 or above adverse events was significantly lower in the pemetrexed arm (64.0% vs. 76.8%, p = .001).[88] These data supported the use of platinum and pemetrexed in non-squamous histology with fewer toxicities.

There is no direct comparison of cisplatin-pemetrexed to carboplatin-paclitaxel or cisplatin-vinblastine, which are less toxic to cisplatin-etoposide. In an individual patient data meta-analysis of 9 trials, cisplatin- versus carboplatin-based chemotherapy were compared. The objective response rate was significantly higher with cisplatin (30% vs. 24%, p < .001) compared to carboplatin, but the latter had a non-significant higher mortality (HR 1.07, 95% CI 0.99-1.15). Cisplatin was associated with more severe nausea, vomiting, and nephrotoxicity.[89]

The best chemotherapy regimen for the concurrent chemoradiation is not well defined. In the United States, cisplatin-etoposide, carboplatin-paclitaxel, and cisplatin-pemetrexed (non-squamous) are the most commonly used chemotherapy regimens. The general consensus based on the available data is to give a cisplatin-based regimen to eligible patients, but a less toxic regimen like carboplatin-paclitaxel is a reasonable alternative for patients who cannot tolerate cisplatin.

Induction Chemotherapy

The role of induction chemotherapy in stage III unresectable NSCLC was studied in the CALGB 39801 trial. The patients were randomized to concurrent chemoradiotherapy with carboplatin (AUC 2) and paclitaxel (50 mg/m^2) weekly or 2 cycles of induction chemotherapy with carboplatin (AUC 6) and paclitaxel (200 mg/m^2) followed by identical concurrent chemoradiotherapy. Survival differences were not statistically significant, with 2-year survival of 31% and 29% in patients with or without induction chemotherapy, respectively. Additionally, the induction chemotherapy arm had significantly more toxicity; therefore, routine use of this approach is not recommended.[90]

> **CLINICAL PEARL:** Induction chemotherapy in stage III unresectable NSCLC has no survival benefit and may add to toxicities. In certain settings, such as limited access to radiotherapy in a timely fashion or with the goal of reducing the size of a radiation port in large tumors to minimize radiation toxicities, some centers may give induction chemotherapy.

Consolidation Chemotherapy

In a phase 3 randomized trial by the Hoosier Oncology Group and US Oncology, patients received cisplatin 50 mg/m^2 intravenously (IV) on days 1, 8, 29, and 36 and etoposide 50 mg/m^2 IV on days 1-5 and 29-33 with concurrent thoracic radiotherapy to 59.40 Gy. Patients who did not have progression were randomized to docetaxel 75 mg/m^2 IV every 21 days for 3 cycles versus observation. The median survival time was 21.2 months for the docetaxel arm versus 23.2 months for the observation arm ($p = .883$). In the docetaxel arm, 10.9% of patients had febrile neutropenia, 9.6% had grade 3 or above pneumonitis, and 5.5% of deaths were attributed to docetaxel. In the observation arm, only 1.4% of patients had grade 3 or higher pneumonitis after randomization. Hospitalization was higher in the docetaxel arm (28.8%) compared to the observation arm (8.1%) during the follow-up period after random assignment.[91]

> **CLINICAL PEARL:** Consolidation chemotherapy after chemoradiation is too toxic due to pneumonitis.

In a pooled analysis of 41 studies (7 phase 3 and 34 phase 2 studies), there was no statistically significant difference in median overall survival between the consolidation chemotherapy group (19.0 months) and the no consolidation group (17.9 months) (HR 0.94, 95% CI 0.81-1.09, $p = .40$). There were no differences between the two groups with regard to grade 3-5 toxicities in pneumonitis, esophagitis, and neutropenia.[92]

The benefit of consolidation chemotherapy has also been evaluated in several trials, but these have failed to demonstrate any survival advantage. However, there has been a trend to give 2 cycles of consolidation chemotherapy after concurrent chemoradiation with cisplatin and paclitaxel. The rationale behind this practice is that the doses of these chemotherapeutic agents given during the concurrent phase are not effective to treat systemic disease. Therefore, 2 cycles of higher doses of the same agents are given during the consolidation phase. Although consolidation chemotherapy may be given with other regimens at some centers, there are no good data to support this practice. With advent of consolidation immunotherapy, this has become less of an issue.

Consolidation Immunotherapy

In the era of immunotherapy, the prognosis has significantly improved with addition of a PD-L1 (programmed death ligand 1) inhibitor, durvalumab, as a consolidation therapy for patients with unresectable stage III NSCLC who did not progress on platinum-based chemotherapy. Durvalumab is a selective, high-affinity, engineered, human immunoglobulin (Ig) G1 monoclonal antibody that blocks PD-L1 binding to PD-1 (programmed cell death protein 1) and CD80, allowing T cells to recognize and kill tumor cells.

The data from the PACIFIC trial represent an important advancement in treatment of unresectable stage III NSCLC. In the trial, 709 patients were randomized in a 2:1 ratio to receive durvalumab (10 mg/kg IV) or placebo every 2 weeks for up to 12 months. The study included both squamous (46%) and non-squamous histology (54%). Patients were enrolled regardless of PD-L1 expression status. The median progression-free survival from randomization was 16.8 months with durvalumab versus 5.6 months with placebo (HR 0.52, 95% CI 0.42-0.65, $p < .001$). The response rate was higher with durvalumab than with placebo (28.4% vs. 16.0%, respectively; $p < .001$).[72] In updated overall survival data, at the median follow-up of 25.2 months, the 2-year overall survival rate was 66.3% in the durvalumab group versus 55.6% in the placebo group (two-sided $p = .005$).[93] Adjuvant Durvalumab has become a standard of care in this setting following the NCCN guidelines.[94] This benefit appears to be present regardless of PD-L1 immunohistochemistry (IHC) expression, with a notable trend for even further benefit for PD-L1-high patients (HR = 0.59 for PD-L1 IHC < 25%, while HR = 0.41 for PD-L1 IHC > 25%). Additionally, a 12% reduction in distant metastases (20% vs. 32%) and 50% reduction in CNS metastases (5.5% vs. 11%) were also significant highlights of the study. A total of 30.5% of the patients in the durvalumab group and 26.1% of those in the placebo group had any grade 3 or 4 adverse events.[72]

> **CLINICAL PEARL:** Durvalumab consolidation has become the standard of care following chemoradiation for patients with unresectable stage III NSCLC. The question remains whether some patients may have differential benefit.

IMMUNOTHERAPY FOR LOCALLY ADVANCED NON–SMALL CELL LUNG CANCER

Andrea Anampa-Guzmán, MD, Luis E. Raez, MD, Ignacio Gil-Bazo, MD

A 59-year-old female with a history of smoking is diagnosed with stage IIIB squamous cell carcinoma of the lung. She is treated with concurrent chemoradiotherapy with weekly carboplatin and paclitaxel. What is the role of maintenance immunotherapy for her disease and stage?

Learning Objectives:

1. Describe the data for adjuvant cancer vaccines for patients with locally advanced NSCLC.
2. Understand the role of checkpoint inhibitors as maintenance therapy after chemoradiotherapy for patients with stage III NSCLC.

The treatment of patients with stage III NSCLC is multidisciplinary, and historically included surgery, radiation, and systemic chemotherapy.[94] However, the prognosis for unresectable tumors, IIIA or IIB, remains poor.[95] Definitive chemoradiotherapy was the standard of care for many years for scenario IIIB and IIIA patients who are not candidates for surgery.[96] The selection of chemoradiotherapy agents that control the disease and increase survival is complex.

There have been efforts before to improve the chemoradiation standard of care: The SWOG has published several phase II and III trials in this topic. The phase 2 clinical trial SWOG S9504 analyzed the effect of consolidation chemotherapy, 3 cycles of docetaxel, after concurrent chemoradiation with cisplatin and etoposide in patients with stage 3B NSCLC.[97,98] The vast majority of patients in SWOG S9504 had a functional status of 0-1 at the start of treatment, and the trial rigorously excluded patients with stage IV disease or with inadequate staging to document the NSCLC IIIB or rule out stage IV of the disease. Three toxic deaths occurred during consolidation treatment with docetaxel, 2 due to pneumonitis and 1 due to aspiration pneumonia. This trial did not confirm the benefit of the addition of docetaxel but had the highest overall survival results reported at that time. The median survival with this regimen was 27 months, and the 1-year, 2-year, and 3-year survival rates were 76%, 54%, and 40%, respectively. The confirmatory phase 3 trial done by Nasser Hanna and the HOG (Hoosier Oncology Group) group showed that there was no benefit in adding consolidation chemotherapy with docetaxel after chemotherapy and radiation, and the standard of care remained again in chemotherapy with cisplatin and etoposide and concomitant radiation.[91]

Gefitinib was the first selective inhibitor of epidermal growth factor receptor (EGFR) to be approved.[99] SWOG S0023[100] was a phase 3 trial that compared the effectiveness of combination chemotherapy plus radiation therapy with or without gefitinib in treating unresectable stage III NSCLC. The trial was closed early following an unplanned interim analysis that showed that the median overall survival with gefitinib was non-significantly lower compared with placebo (19 months and 29 months, respectively). The survival rate of SWOG 0023 was not as high as in SWOG 9504, even though both arms were treated with the same scheme of the SWOG 9504. This led to suspicion of a negative interaction between EGFR tyrosine kinase inhibitors (TKIs) and radical radiation. After a median 27-month follow-up, the results were updated.[101] Overall survival was 23 months with gefitinib and 35 months with placebo (HR 0.63, $p = .01$), with 2-year survival of 46% and 59%, respectively.

The first immunotherapy attempt to be used after concurrent chemotherapy and radiation was tecemotide (L-BLP25), which was a synthetic peptide used in a cancer vaccine called stivumax. It targeted the aberrantly glycosylated mucin 1 (MUC1) glycoprotein overexpressed in NSCLC, especially in the non-squamous types. The cellular immune response may lead then to a rejection of tumor tissue expressing the MUC1 antigen. After a successful randomized phase 2 study,[102] the START[103] trial was initiated; it was a phase 3 trial that investigated tecemotide versus placebo as maintenance therapy after completion of chemoradiation in 1,239 patients with unresectable stage III NSCLC. Even though the endpoint of overall survival was met without significant difference, preplanned subgroup analyses showed statistically significant improvement in overall survival of the subgroup of patients who received concurrent chemoradiotherapy (30.8 vs. 20.6 months; adjusted HR 0.78, $p = .016$), the standard of care.[104] No difference in survival between treatment groups was observed in patients who received sequential chemoradiotherapy. Due to these findings, the study was unable to change the standard of care.

The START2 trial[105] intended to confirm the results observed in the predefined subset of 806 patients treated with concurrent chemoradiotherapy who experienced improved overall survival in the START trial. The START2 study was a global, randomized, double-blind, placebo-controlled, phase 3 trial investigating tecemotide in patients with unresectable stage III NSCLC who did not progress after completing first-line concurrent chemoradiotherapy 4–12 weeks before randomization. At the same time, there was another study on the works, INSPIRE,[106] a phase 3 clinical trial of tecemotide in Asian subjects with stage III, unresectable, NSCLC who had demonstrated either stable disease or objective response following primary chemoradiation.

Both studies were discontinued due to the analysis of a smaller trial, EMR 63325-009, conducted in Japanese patients, the majority of whom received concurrent chemoradiation.[107] EMR 63325-009 was a randomized, double-blind, placebo-controlled, phase 1/2 study in Japanese patients with stage III unresectable, locally advanced NSCLC who had received concurrent or sequential chemoradiotherapy, with a minimum of 2 cycles of platinum-based chemotherapy and radiotherapy. The results indicated that no effect was been observed for either the primary endpoint, overall survival, or for any of the secondary endpoints (progression-free survival, time to progression, and time to treatment failure). Although the trial did not aim to demonstrate a statistically significant difference in benefit between the two arms, the company decided to stop START2 and PROCLAIM after EMR 63325-009 showed no benefit from the addition of tecemotide to chemoradiation.

Another disappointment was MAGE-A3 (melanoma antigen A3) peptide vaccine. MAGE-A3 is a protein that is not expressed in normal tissue but appears in 55% of advanced stages of NSCLC. The MAGE-A3 vaccine can potentially stimulate the immune system against tumor cells expressing MAGE-A3, resulting in tumor cell lysis.[108] The MAGRIT trial was a phase 3 randomized, double-blind, placebo-controlled trial. In this trial, 12,820 MAGE-A3–positive patients with completely resected stage IB, II, or IIIA NSCLC were randomized to receive MAGE-A3 vaccine or placebo after they also had received adjuvant chemotherapy. MAGE-A3 did not significantly increase disease-free survival compared with placebo in patients, 58 months versus 57.9 months, respectively.[109]

After many disappointments trying to develop immunotherapy as "adjuvant" or "consolidation" for stage III NSCLC patients (**Table 14-5**), durvalumab was the first checkpoint inhibitor to successfully complete a clinical trial for these patients. Durvalumab is an IgG1 monoclonal antibody that specifically targets PD-L1.[110] The PACIFIC trial[93,111] was a randomized trial that recruited 709 adults (median age 64 years, 70% men) with unresectable stage III NSCLC who had concurrent chemoradiation and were randomized to consolidation therapy with durvalumab 10 mg/kg IV every 2 weeks

TABLE 14-5	Ongoing Trials Using Immunotherapy in Stage III NSCLC		
NCT#	PHASE	IT	TREATMENT SEQUENCE
NCT02434081	II	Nivolumab	CRT + concurrent IT
NCT03102242	II	Atezolizumab	Induction IT → CRT
NCT03379441	II	Pembrolizumab	CRT (concomitant or sequential) → IT; CRT (concomitant or sequential) → observation
NCT02343952	II	Pembrolizumab	Concurrent CRT → IT
NCT03053856	II	Pembrolizumab	Neoadjuvant concurrent CRT → curative resection → IT
NCT02428764	II	Nimotuzumab	Neodjuvant IT + chemotherapy → S
NCT03519971	II	Durvalumab	Concurrent IT + CRT
NCT02987998	II	Pembrolizumab	Neoadjuvant concurrent CRT + IT → consolidation IT

CRT, chemoradiotherapy; IT, immunotherapy; NSCLC, non–small cell lung cancer; S, surgery; SBRT, stereotactic body radiation therapy.

Current approaches include consolidation trials as well as other opportunities as the use of neoadjuvant immunotherapy or the concomitant use of immunotherapy with chemotherapy and/or radiation therapy and to try to bring to the front lines for stage III disease other checkpoint inhibitors like nivolumab and pembrolizumab.

versus placebo for 12 months or less and followed for a median of 14.5 months. Durvalumab was associated with significant improvement in progression-free survival: median progression-free survival 16.8 months versus 5.6 months ($p < .001$); 12-month progression-free survival 55.9% versus 35.3% ($p < .001$) and 18-month progression-free survival 44.2% versus 27% ($p < .001$). Moreover, durvalumab was associated with increased progression-free survival regardless of PD-L1 expression levels before chemoradiation. Patients treated with durvalumab had a significantly higher time to death or distant metastases, 23.2 months versus 14.6 months ($p < .001$). The most common adverse events reported included pneumonia, pneumonitis, anemia, and dyspnea. It was concluded that consolidation durvalumab improves progression-free survival in patients with unresectable stage III NSCLC who had received chemoradiation.

Currently, patients with unresectable disease who have not progressed after concurrent platinum-based chemotherapy and radiotherapy and who are candidates for immunotherapy are offered durvalumab as the new standard of care. It is important to mention that patients who are not candidates for a combined modality treatment approach can be considered for radiotherapy alone or sequential chemoradiotherapy.

> **CLINICAL PEARL:** Based on the results of the PACIFIC trial, adjuvant durvalumab is now considered a category 1 recommendation for maintenance therapy after concurrent chemoradiotherapy in patients with stage III NSCLC.

ONCOGENE INHIBITION FOR EARLY AND LOCALLY ADVANCED NON–SMALL CELL LUNG CANCER

Cesar A. Perez, MD

A never-smoker 45-year-old male is found to have a lung mass and is diagnosed with a Stage IIB adenocarcinoma of the lung. He undergoes complete resection of his tumor, which was found to have a EGFR exon 19 deletion. Should he start treatment with EGFR tyrosine kinase inhibitors?

Learning Objectives:
1. What is the role of EGFR mutation in the adjuvant setting?
2. What other mutations are important in this setting?

Patients with stage I, III, and III NSCLC have an overall survival of 63%, 52%, and 42%, respectively.[112] Since molecular testing and next-generation sequencing has been reserved for patients with metastatic disease, it is unclear if patients with early NSCLC with oncogene drivers have a lower rate of relapse and disease-related mortality compared to patients without molecular drivers. However, since patients with genomic abnormalities as EGFR mutations can have better prognosis in the metastatic setting because of a less aggressive disease and higher response to systemic chemotherapy, it has been hypothesized that these populations might have a better prognosis in the early stages compared to their wild-type counterparts. Nevertheless, adjuvant therapy with oncogene kinase inhibitors has been logically proposed as a mechanism to increase cure rates and prolong survival for patients with NSCLC with oncogene targets.

Most of the data currently available concerning using oncogene inhibition in the adjuvant setting is with EGFR inhibitors, which are the first targeted therapy developed for the disease. Since EGFR is overexpressed in NSCLC, initial trials of EGFR inhibitors in both the locally advanced and metastatic setting included all comers and not only EGFR mutation positive patients.

EGFR INHIBITION IN THE ADJUVANT SETTING

The first-generation EGFR inhibitor gefitinib was initially evaluated in addition to standard therapy for patients with stage III disease. The SOG S0023 was a randomized phase 3 trial that compared the efficacy of combined chemotherapy plus radiation therapy with or without gefitinib in treating unresectable stage 3 NSCLC (PMID 18378568). An interim analysis showed that the median overall survival with gefitinib was nonsignificantly lower compared with placebo (19 months and 29 months, respectively), leading to the early closure of the trial. The SWOG 9404, a trial with a similar treatment backbone, had a median survival of 26 months.[98] This led to a hypothesis that using EGFR inhibitors during concurrent chemoradiotherapy might actually decrease tumor control since the lower overall survival of SWOG 0023 was not related to gefitinib toxicity but to disease progression. Updated results revealed that after a median 27-month follow-up, overall survival was 23 months with gefitinib and 35 months with placebo (HR 0.63, $p = .01$), with a 2-year survival of 46% and 59%, respectively.[101]

The RADIANT trial was a randomized, placebo-controlled trial for completely resected stage IB to IIIA NSCLC patients whose tumor expressed EGFR protein by IHC or by EGFR amplification.[113] The trial randomized 973 patients into a 2:1 randomization of erlotinib 150 mg orally daily versus placebo. Results showed no statistically significant difference in disease-free survival, the primary outcome. For the small population with EGFR-mutant tumors (161 patients), there was a non-significant improvement in disease-free survival (median 46.4 vs. 28.5 months, HR 0.61, 95% CI 0.38-0.98, $p = .039$). The negative results have been attributed to the inclusion of patients who had mostly wild-type EGFR mutants, a population for which the activity of EGFR inhibitors is now known to be poor (despite having overexpression of the EGFR protein).

After data from the IPASS and EURTAC trials confirmed that the activity of EGFR inhibitors was driven by patients with an EGFR mutation, attention focused on the development of these agents in this population.[114,115] The SELECT trial was an open-label phase 2 trial that included patients with stage IA to IIIA resected, EGFR-mutant–positive NSCLC.[116] A total of 100 patients received erlotinib for 2 years after their surgery and adjuvant standard chemotherapy or radiotherapy. The 5-year disease-free survival was 56% (95% CI 45% to 66%), and 5-year overall survival was 86% (95% CI 77% to 92%). Disease recurred in 40 patients, and most of these recurrences were after the patient had stopped erlotinib. These individuals were re-treated with the agent, with a median duration of re-treatment of 13 months. A total of 56% of the patients in the erlotinib arm required a dose reduction, with the intended 2-year course achieved in 69%.[116] The trial was therefore considered a positive trial compared with historic genotype controls.

The Chinese thoracic oncology group (CTONG) 1104 was a randomized phase 3 trial that included 222 patients with resected EGFR-mutation–positive stage II-IIIA NSCLC treated in 27 institutions in China.[117] The trial randomized the patients in a 1:1 ratio to adjuvant treatment with vinorelbine plus cisplatin versus gefitinib. The trial demonstrated an improvement of the median disease-free survival for the patients treated with gefitinib compared to the group treated with chemotherapy (28.7 vs. 18.0 months, HR 0.60, 95% CI 0.42-0.87, $p = .0054$). The study mainly included patients with a high risk of recurrence (N1-N2 disease), but demonstrated the superiority of gefitinib over adjuvant chemotherapy for this high-risk population. The international ADAURA trial (NCT02511106) has now finished accrual of patients with EGFR mutations to receive treatment with the third-generation EGFR inhibitor osimertinib versus placebo; the trial has met its primary endpoint of disease-free survival (DFS), although the overall survival benefit is not yet known.

OTHER ONCOGENE INHIBITION IN THE ADJUVANT SETTING

Several other trials are currently recruiting patients with other genomic alterations after curative therapy to receive treatment with an appropriate specific inhibitor. Alectinib, a second-generation anaplastic lymphoma kinase (ALK) inhibitor, is currently being evaluated in a randomized phase 3 trial for patients with resected ALK-positive NSCLC (NCT03456076) comparing adjuvant alectinib versus adjuvant platinum-based chemotherapy. The ALCHEMIST trial also included patients with ALK-rearranged NSCLC to treatment with crizotinib versus placebo for 2 years.

Adjuvant oncogene inhibition has therefore the potential of improving the disease-free survival for patients with NSCLC and oncogene drivers. However, since patients might derive similar benefit after progression, it is possible that the early toxicity experienced by giving the treatment in the adjuvant setting might not translate into prolonging overall survival. The use of these agents in the adjuvant setting requires further studies, and their benefits will certainly be for the specific targeted population, with a high risk of recurrence and using the agent with the best tolerability.

REFERENCES

1. Miller WT. Certificate issued by the ABR to Henry Pancoast in June 1934. *Radiology*. 1986;161(2):412.
2. Peedell C, Dunning J, Bapusamy A. Is there a standard of care for the radical management of non-small cell lung cancer involving the apical chest wall (Pancoast tumours)? *Clin Oncol (R Coll Radiol)*. 2010;22(5):334-346.
3. Ettinger DS, Aisner DL, Wood DE, et al. NCCN Guidelines Insights: Non-Small Cell Lung Cancer, Version 5.2018. *J Natl Compr Canc Netw*. 2018;16(7):807-821.
4. Rusca M, Carbognani P, Bobbio P. The modified "hemi-clamshell" approach for tumors of the cervicothoracic junction. *Ann Thorac Surg*. 2000;69(6):1961-1963.
5. Solli P, Casiraghi M, Brambilla D, Maisonneuve P, Spaggiari L. Surgical treatment of superior sulcus tumors: a 15-year single-center experience. *Semin Thorac Cardiovasc Surg*. 2017;29(1):79-88.
6. Parissis H, Young V. Treatment of pancoast tumors from the surgeons prospective: re-appraisal of the anterior-manubrial sternal approach. *J Cardiothorac Surg*. 2010;5:102.
7. Fadel E, Missenard G, Chapelier A, et al. En bloc resection of non-small cell lung cancer invading the thoracic inlet and intervertebral foramina. *J Thorac Cardiovasc Surg*. 2002;123(4):676-685.
8. Dartevelle P, Macchiarini P. Surgical management of superior sulcus tumors. *Oncologist*. 1999;4(5):398-407.
9. Grunenwald D, Spaggiari L. Transmanubrial osteomuscular sparing approach for apical chest tumors. *Ann Thorac Surg*. 1997;63(2):563-566.
10. Giaccone A, Solli P, Pardolesi A, Brandolini J, Bertolaccini L. Video-assisted thoracoscopic surgery en bloc chest wall resection. *J Vis Surg*. 2017;3:73.
11. Marulli G, Battistella L, Mammana M, Calabrese F, Rea F. Superior sulcus tumors (Pancoast tumors). *Ann Transl Med*. 2016;4(12):239.
12. Dartevelle PG, Chapelier AR, Macchiarini P, et al. Anterior transcervical-thoracic approach for radical resection of lung tumors invading the thoracic inlet. *J Thorac Cardiovasc Surg*. 1993;105(6):1025-1034.
13. Filosso PL, Sandri A, Guerrera F, et al. Primary lung tumors invading the chest wall. *J Thorac Dis*. 2016;8(Suppl 11):S855-S862.
14. Anraku M, Waddell TK, de Perrot M, et al. Induction chemoradiotherapy facilitates radical resection of T4 non-small cell lung cancer invading the spine. *J Thorac Cardiovasc Surg*. 2009;137(2):441-447 e1.
15. Honguero-Martinez AF, García-Jiménez MD, León-Atance P, Landaluce-Chaves M. Non-small cell lung cancer invading the descending thoracic aorta: surgical resection without using cardiopulmonary bypass and without cross-clamping the aorta: long-term follow-up of 2 cases. *Vasc Endovascular Surg*. 2018;52(5):357-360.
16. Park B, Cho JH, Kim HK, et al. Long-term survival in locally advanced non-small cell lung cancer invading the great vessels and heart. *Thorac Cancer*. 2018;9(5):598-605.
17. Ohta M, Hirabayasi H, Shiono H, et al. Surgical resection for lung cancer with infiltration of the thoracic aorta. *J Thorac Cardiovasc Surg*. 2005;129(4):804-808.
18. Santana-Rodriguez N, Martel E, Clavo B, et al. Oncological resection of lung cancer invading the aortic arch in full thickness using a non-fenestrated endograft. *J Surg Oncol*. 2016;114(4):412-415.
19. Sobrinho G, Aguiar P. Stent placement for the treatment of malignant superior vena cava syndrome—a single-center series of 56 patients. *Arch Bronconeumol*. 2014;50(4):135-140.
20. Picquet J, Blin V, Dussaussoy C, Jousset Y, Papon X, Enon B. Surgical reconstruction of the superior vena cava system: indications and results. *Surgery*, 2009;145(1):93-99.
21. Leo F, Bellini R, Conti B, Delledonne V, Tavecchio L, Pastorino U. Superior vena cava resection in thoracic malignancies: does prosthetic replacement pose a higher risk? *Eur J Cardiothorac Surg*. 2010;37(4):764-769.
22. Sato H, Soh J, Hotta K, et al. Is surgery after chemoradiotherapy feasible in lung cancer patients with superior vena cava invasion? *Ann Thorac Cardiovasc Surg*. 2018;24(3):131-138.
23. Lee P, Kishan AU. Radiotherapy is effective for a primary lung cancer invading the left atrium. *BMJ Case Rep*. 2012;2012.
24. Galvaing G, Chadeyras JB, Merle P, et al. Extended resection of non-small cell lung cancer invading the left atrium, is it worth the risk? *Chin Clin Oncol*. 2015;4(4):43.

25. Stella F, Dell'Amore A, Caroli G, et al. Surgical results and long-term follow-up of T(4)-non-small cell lung cancer invading the left atrium or the intrapericardial base of the pulmonary veins. *Interact Cardiovasc Thorac Surg.* 2012;14(4):415-419.

26. Rami-Porta R, Bolejack V, Crowley J, et al. The IASLC lung cancer staging project: proposals for the revisions of the T descriptors in the forthcoming eighth edition of the TNM classification for lung cancer. *J Thorac Oncol.* 2015;10(7):990-1003.

27. Galetta D, Borri A, Casiraghi M, et al. Outcome and prognostic factors of resected non-small-cell lung cancer invading the diaphragm. *Interact Cardiovasc Thorac Surg.* 2014;19(4):632-636; discussion 636.

28. Weksler B, Bains M, Burt M, et al. Resection of lung cancer invading the diaphragm. *J Thorac Cardiovasc Surg.* 1997;114(3):500-501.

29. Inoue K, Sato M, Fujimura S, et al. Prognostic assessment of 1310 patients with non-small-cell lung cancer who underwent complete resection from 1980 to 1993. *J Thorac Cardiovasc Surg.* 1998;116(3):407-411.

30. Rocco G, Rendina EA, Meroni A, et al. Prognostic factors after surgical treatment of lung cancer invading the diaphragm. *Ann Thorac Surg.* 1999;68(6):2065-2068.

31. Riquet M, Porte H, Chapelier A, et al. Resection of lung cancer invading the diaphragm. *J Thorac Cardiovasc Surg.* 2000;120(2):417-418.

32. Yokoi K, Tsuchiya R, Mori T, et al. Results of surgical treatment of lung cancer involving the diaphragm. *J Thorac Cardiovasc Surg.* 2000;120(4):799-805.

33. Tyldesley S, Boyd C, Schulze K, Walker H, Mackillop WJ. Estimating the need for radiotherapy for lung cancer: an evidence-based, epidemiologic approach. *Int J Radiat Oncol Biol Phys.* 2001;49(4):973-985.

34. Ettinger DS, Aisner DL, Wood DE., et al, NCCN Guidelines Version 5.2018 Non-Small Cell Lung Cancer. nccn.org.

35. LE Q. Lung cancer: assessing resectability. *Cancer Imaging.* 2004;4(1):15-18.

36. Martini N, Flehinger BJ. The role of surgery in N2 lung cancer. *Surg Clin North Am.* 1987;67(5):1037-1049.

37. Mountain CF. The new international staging system for lung cancer. *Surg Clin North Am.* 1987;67(5):925-935.

38. Shield TW. Preoperative radiation therapy in the treatment of bronchial carcinoma. *Cancer.* 1972; 30(5):1388-1394.

39. Albain KS, Rusch VW, Crowley JJ, et al. Concurrent cisplatin/etoposide plus chest radiotherapy followed by surgery for stages IIIA (N2) and IIIB non-small-cell lung cancer: mature results of Southwest Oncology Group phase II study 8805. *J Clin Oncol.* 1995;13(8):1880-1892.

40. Stupp R, Mayer M, Kann R, et al, Neoadjuvant chemotherapy and radiotherapy followed by surgery in selected patients with stage IIIB non-small-cell lung cancer: a multicentre phase II trial. *Lancet Oncol.* 2009;10(8):785-793.

41. Suntharalingam M, Paulus R, Edelman MJ, et al. Radiation therapy oncology group protocol 02-29: a phase II trial of neoadjuvant therapy with concurrent chemotherapy and full-dose radiation therapy followed by surgical resection and consolidative therapy for locally advanced non-small cell carcinoma of. *Int J Radiat Oncol Biol Phys.* 2012;84(2):456-463.

42. van Meerbeeck JP, Kramer GW, Van Schil PE, et al. Randomized controlled trial of resection versus radiotherapy after induction chemotherapy in stage IIIA-N2 non-small-cell lung cancer. *J Natl Cancer Inst.* 2007;99(6):442-450.

43. Ebernhardt WEE, Pöttgen C, Gauler TC, et al. Phase III study of surgery versus definitive concurrent chemoradiotherapy boost in patients with resectable stage IIIA(N2) and selected IIIB non–small-cell lung cancer after induction chemotherapy and concurrent chemoradiotherapy (ESPATUE). *J Clin Oncol.* 2015;33(35):4194-4201.

44. Albain KS, Swann R, Rusch VW, et al. Radiotherapy plus chemotherapy with or without surgical resection for stage III non-small-cell lung cancer: a phase III randomised controlled trial. *Lancet.* 2009;374:379-386.

45. Kunitoh H, Kato H, Tsuboi M, et al. Phase II trial of preoperative chemoradiotherapy followed by surgical resection in patients with superior sulcus non-small-cell lung cancers: report of Japan Clinical Oncology Group trial 9806. *J Clin Oncol.* 2008;26(4):644-649.

46. Rusch VW, Giroux DJ, Kraut MJ, et al. Induction chemoradiation and surgical resection for non-small cell lung carcinomas of the superior sulcus: Initial results of Southwest Oncology Group Trial 9416 (Intergroup Trial 0160). *J Thorac Cardiovasc Surg.* 2001;121(3):472-483.

47. PORT Meta-analysis Trialist Group. Postoperative radiotherapy in non-small-cell lung cancer: systematic review and meta-analysis of individual patient data from nine randomised controlled trials. *Lancet.* 1998;352(9124):257-263.

48. Lally BE, Zelterman D, Colasanto JM, et al. Postoperative radiotherapy for stage II or III non-small-cell lung cancer using the surveillance, epidemiology, and end results database. *J Clin Oncol.* 2006;24(19):2998-3006.

49. Douillard JY, Rosell R, De Lena M, et al, Impact of postoperative radiation therapy on survival in patients with complete resection and stage I, II, or IIIA non-small-cell lung cancer treated with adjuvant chemotherapy: the adjuvant Navelbine International Trialist Association (ANITA) Randomized Trial. *Int J Radiat Oncol Biol Phys.* 2008;72(3):695-701.

50. Robinson CG, Patel A, Bradley JD, et al. Postoperative radiotherapy for pathologic N2 non-small-cell lung cancer treated with adjuvant chemotherapy: a review of the National Cancer Data Base. *J Clin Oncol.* 2015;33(8):870-876.

51. Dillman RO, Herndon J, Seagren SL, et al. Improved survival in stage III non-small-cell lung cancer: seven-year follow-up of cancer and leukemia group B (CALGB) 8433 trial. *J Natl Cancer Inst.* 1996;88(17):1210-1215.

52. Curran WJ, Jr., Paulus R, Langer CJ, et al. Sequential vs. concurrent chemoradiation for stage III non-small cell lung cancer: randomized phase III trial RTOG 9410. *J Natl Cancer Inst.* 2011;103(19):1452-1460.

53. Belani CP, Choy H, Bonomi P, et al. Combined chemoradiotherapy regimens of paclitaxel and carboplatin for locally advanced non-small-cell lung cancer: a randomized phase II locally advanced multi-modality protocol. *J Clin Oncol.* 2005;23(25):5883-5891.

54. Gore EM, Bae K, Wong SJ, et al. Phase III comparison of prophylactic cranial irradiation versus observation in patients with locally advanced non-small-cell lung cancer: primary analysis of radiation therapy oncology group study RTOG 0214. *J Clin Oncol.* 2011;29(3):272-278.

55. Emami B, Lyman J, Brown A, et al. Tolerance of normal tissue to therapeutic irradiation. *Int J Radiat Oncol Biol Phys.* 1991;21(1):109-122.

56. Marks LB, Yorke ED, Jackson A, et al. Use of normal tissue complication probability models in the clinic. *Int J Radiat Oncol Biol Phys.* 2010;76(3 Suppl):S10-S19.

57. Bradley JD, Paulus R, Komaki R, et al. Standard-dose versus high-dose conformal radiotherapy with concurrent and consolidation carboplatin plus paclitaxel with or without cetuximab for patients with stage IIIA or IIIB non-small-cell lung cancer (RTOG 0617): a randomised, two-by-two factorial p. *Lancet Oncol.* 2015;16:187-199.

58. Gunderson L, Tepper J. *Clinical Radiation Oncology.* 3rd ed. Philadelphia, PA: Elsevier Saunders; 2011.

59. Chun SG, Hu C, Choy H, et al. Impact of intensity-modulated radiation therapy technique for locally advanced non-small-cell lung cancer: a secondary analysis of the NRG oncology RTOG 0617 randomized clinical trial. *J Clin Oncol.* 2017;35(1):56-62.

60. Landberg T, Chavaudra J, Dobbs J, et al. ICRU Report 62: prescribing, recording and reporting photon beam therapy (supplement to ICRU report 50). *Journal of the International Commission on Radiation Units and Measurements.* 1999;32,1,1.

61. Lee NY, Riaz N, Lu JJ, et al. *Target Volume Delineation for Conformal and Intensity-Modulated Radiation Therapy.* New York, NY: Springer; 2015.

62. Rosenzweig KE, Sura S, Jackson A, et al. Involved-field radiation therapy for inoperable non small-cell lung cancer. *J Clin Oncol.* 2007;25(35):5557-5561.

63. Yuan S, Sun X, Li M, et al. A randomized study of involved-field irradiation versus elective nodal irradiation in combination with concurrent chemotherapy for inoperable stage III nonsmall cell lung cancer. *Am J Clin Oncol.* 2007;30(3):239-244.

64. Belderbos JS, Kepka L, Spring Kong FM, et al. Report from the International Atomic Energy Agency (IAEA) consultants' meeting on elective nodal irradiation in lung cancer: non-small-Cell lung cancer (NSCLC). *Int J Radiat Oncol Biol Phys.* 2008;72(2):335-342.

65. Perez CA, Pajak TF, Rubin P, et al. Long-term observations of the patterns of failure in patients with unresectable non-oat cell carcinoma of the lung treated with definitive radiotherapy. Report by the Radiation Therapy Oncology Group. *Cancer.* 1987;59(11):1874-1881.

66. Saunders M, Dische S, Barrett A, Harvey A, Griffiths G, Palmar M. Continuous, hyperfractionated, accelerated radiotherapy (CHART) versus conventional radiotherapy in non-small cell lung cancer: mature data from the randomised multicentre trial. CHART Steering committee. *Radiother Oncol.* 1999;52(2):137-148.

67. Mauguen A, Le Pechoux C, Saunders MI, et al. Hyperfractionated or accelerated radiotherapy in lung cancer: an individual patient data meta-analysis. *J Clin Oncol.* 2012;30(22):2788-2797.

68. Chang JY, Verma V, Li M, et al. Proton beam radiotherapy and concurrent chemotherapy for unresectable stage III non-small cell lung cancer: final results of a phase 2 study. *JAMA Oncol.* 2017;3(8):e172032.

69. Guy CL, Weiss E, Jan N, et al. Effect of atelectasis changes on tissue mass and dose during lung radiotherapy. *Med Phys.* 2016;43(11):6109.

70. Kong F, Miller MS, Bradley J, et al. Randomized phase II trial of individualized adaptive radiotherapy using during-treatment FDG-PET/CT and modern technology in locally advanced non-small cell lung cancer (NSCLC). NRG Oncology ECOG-ACRIN 6697, 2016.

71. Le Péchoux C. Role of postoperative radiotherapy in resected non-small cell lung cancer: a reassessment based on new data. *Oncologist.* 2011;16(5):672-681.

72. Antonia SJ, Villegas A, Daniel D, et al. Durvalumab after chemoradiotherapy in stage III non-small-cell lung cancer. *N Engl J Med.* 2017;377(20):1919-1929.

73. Kordbacheh T, Chan C, Bossons A, et al. PARIS: a phase 1 study of pembrolizumab anti-PD-1 monoclonal antibody in combination with radiotherapy (RT) in locally advanced non-small cell lung cancer (NSCLC). *Lung Cancer.* 2017;S1-S81.

74. Iyengar P, et al. Hypofractionated Image-Guided Radiation Therapy (IGRT) in Patients With Stage II-III Non-Small Cell Lung Cancer. https://clinicaltrials.gov/ct2/show/NCT01459497, 2018.

75. Troost E, Proton Therapy to Reduce Acute Normal Tissue Toxicity in Locally Advanced Non-small-cell Lung Cancer (PRONTOX). clinicaltrials.gov NCT02731001, 2017.

76. Jensen GL, Tang C, Hess KR, Liao Z, Gomez DR. Patterns of metastatic progression after definitive radiation therapy for early-stage and locally advanced non-small cell lung cancer. *Clin Exp Metastasis.* 2017;34(5):315-322.

77. Pignon JP, Tribodet H, Scagliotti GV, et al. Lung adjuvant cisplatin evaluation: a pooled analysis by the LACE Collaborative Group. *J Clin Oncol.* 2008;26(21):3552-3559.

78. Arriagada R, Bergman B, Dunant A, et al. Cisplatin-based adjuvant chemotherapy in patients with completely resected non-small-cell lung cancer. *N Engl J Med.* 2004;350(4):351-360.

79. Wakelee HA, Dahlberg SE, Keller SM, et al. Adjuvant chemotherapy with or without bevacizumab in patients with resected non-small-cell lung cancer (E1505): an open-label, multicentre, randomised, phase 3 trial. *Lancet Oncol.* 2017;18(12):1610-1623.

80. NSCLC Meta-analysis Collaborative Group. Preoperative chemotherapy for non-small-cell lung cancer: a systematic review and meta-analysis of individual participant data. *Lancet.* 2014;383(9928):1561-1571.

81. Rosell R, Gómez-Codina J, Camps C, et al. A randomized trial comparing preoperative chemotherapy plus surgery with surgery alone in patients with non-small-cell lung cancer. *N Engl J Med.* 1994;330(3):153-158.

82. Roth JA, Fossella F, Komaki R, et al. A randomized trial comparing perioperative chemotherapy and surgery with surgery alone in resectable stage IIIA non-small-cell lung cancer. *J Natl Cancer Inst.* 1994;86(9):673-680.

83. Pless M, Stupp R, Ris H-B, et al. Induction chemoradiation in stage IIIA/N2 non-small-cell lung cancer: a phase 3 randomised trial. *Lancet.* 2015;386(9998):1049-1056.

84. Postoperative radiotherapy in non-small-cell lung cancer: systematic review and meta-analysis of individual patient data from nine randomised controlled trials. PORT Meta-analysis Trialists Group. *Lancet.* 1998;352(9124):257-263.

85. Corso CD, Rutter CE, Wilson LD, Kim AW, Decker RH, Husain ZA. Re-evaluation of the role of postoperative radiotherapy and the impact of radiation dose for non-small-cell lung cancer using the National Cancer Database. *J Thorac Oncol.* 2015;10(1):148-155.

86. Albain KS, Crowley JJ, Turrisi AT 3rd, et al. Concurrent cisplatin, etoposide, and chest radiotherapy in pathologic stage IIIB non-small-cell lung cancer: a Southwest Oncology Group phase II study, SWOG 9019. *J Clin Oncol.* 2002;20(16):3454-3460.

87. Liang J, Bi N, Wu S, et al. Etoposide and cisplatin versus paclitaxel and carboplatin with concurrent thoracic radiotherapy in unresectable stage III non-small cell lung cancer: a multicenter randomized phase III trial. *Ann Oncol.* 2017;28(4):777-783.

88. Senan S, Brade A, Wang LH, et al. PROCLAIM: Randomized Phase III Trial of pemetrexed-cisplatin or etoposide-cisplatin plus thoracic radiation therapy followed by consolidation chemotherapy in locally advanced nonsquamous non-small-cell lung cancer. *J Clin Oncol.* 2016;34(9):953-962.

89. Ardizzoni A, Boni L, Tiseo M, et al. Cisplatin-versus carboplatin-based chemotherapy in first-line treatment of advanced non-small-cell lung cancer: an individual patient data meta-analysis. *J Natl Cancer Inst.* 2007;99(11):847-857.

90. Vokes EE, Herndon JE 2nd, Kelley MJ, et al. Induction chemotherapy followed by chemoradiotherapy compared with chemoradiotherapy alone for regionally advanced unresectable stage III non-small-cell lung cancer: Cancer and Leukemia Group B. *J Clin Oncol.* 2007;25(13):1698-1704.

91. Hanna N, Neubauer M, Yiannoutsos C, et al. Phase III study of cisplatin, etoposide, and concurrent chest radiation with or without consolidation docetaxel in patients with inoperable stage III non-small-cell lung cancer: the Hoosier Oncology Group and U.S. Oncology. *J Clin Oncol.* 2008;26(35):5755-5760.

92. Tsujino K, Kurata T, Yamamoto S, et al. Is consolidation chemotherapy after concurrent chemo-radiotherapy beneficial for patients with locally advanced non-small-cell lung cancer? A pooled analysis of the literature. *J Thorac Oncol.* 2013;8(9):1181-1189.

93. Antonia SJ, Villegas A, Daniel D, et al., Overall survival with durvalumab after chemoradiotherapy in stage III NSCLC. *N Engl J Med*. 2018;79(24):2342-2350.

94. Available from: https://www.nccn.org/professionals/physician_gls/default.aspx#nscl.

95. Auperin A, Le Péchoux C, Rolland E, et al. Meta-analysis of concomitant versus sequential radiochemotherapy in locally advanced non-small-cell lung cancer. *J Clin Oncol*. 2010;28(13):2181-2190.

96. Pritchard RS, Anthony SP. Chemotherapy plus radiotherapy compared with radiotherapy alone in the treatment of locally advanced, unresectable, non-small-cell lung cancer. A meta-analysis. *Ann Intern Med*. 1996;125(9):723-729.

97. Gandara DR, Chansky K, Albain KS, et al. Long term survival in stage IIIb non-small cell lung cancer (NSCLC) treated with consolidation docetaxel following concurrent chemoradiotherapy (SWOG S9504). *J Clin Oncol*. 2005;23(16_suppl):7059-7059.

98. Gandara DR, Chansky K, Albain KS, et al. Consolidation docetaxel after concurrent chemoradiotherapy in stage IIIB non-small-cell lung cancer: phase II Southwest Oncology Group Study S9504. *J Clin Oncol*. 2003;21(10):2004-2010.

99. Singh M, Jadhav HR. Targeting non-small cell lung cancer with small-molecule EGFR tyrosine kinase inhibitors. *Drug Discov Today*. 2018;23(3):745-753.

100. Thatcher N, Chang A, Parikh P, et al. Gefitinib plus best supportive care in previously treated patients with refractory advanced non-small-cell lung cancer: results from a randomised, placebo-controlled, multicentre study (Iressa Survival Evaluation in Lung Cancer). *Lancet*. 2005;366(9496):1527-1537.

101. Kelly K, Chansky K, Gaspar LE, et al. Phase III trial of maintenance gefitinib or placebo after concurrent chemoradiotherapy and docetaxel consolidation in inoperable stage III non-small-cell lung cancer: SWOG S0023. *J Clin Oncol*. 2008;26(15):2450-2456.

102. Butts C, Murray N, Maksymiuk A, et al. Randomized phase IIB trial of BLP25 liposome vaccine in stage IIIB and IV non-small-cell lung cancer. *J Clin Oncol*. 2005;23(27):6674-6681.

103. Butts C, Socinski MA, Mitchell PL, et al. Tecemotide (L-BLP25) versus placebo after chemoradiotherapy for stage III non-small-cell lung cancer (START): a randomised, double-blind, phase 3 trial. *Lancet Oncol*. 2014;15(1):59-68.

104. Bradley JD, Paulus R, Komaki R, et al. Standard-dose versus high-dose conformal radiotherapy with concurrent and consolidation carboplatin plus paclitaxel with or without cetuximab for patients with stage IIIA or IIIB non-small-cell lung cancer (RTOG 0617): a randomised, two-by-two factorial phase 3 study. *Lancet Oncol*. 2015;16(2):187-199.

105. Ramalingam SS, et al. START2: Tecemotide in unresectable stage III NSCLC after first-line concurrent chemoradiotherapy. *J Clin Oncol*. 2014;32(15_suppl):TPS7608-TPS7608.

106. Wu YL, Park K, Soo RA, et al. INSPIRE: a phase III study of the BLP25 liposome vaccine (L-BLP25) in Asian patients with unresectable stage III non-small cell lung cancer. *BMC Cancer*. 2011;11:430.

107. Daly ME, Monjazeb AM, Kelly K. Clinical trials integrating immunotherapy and radiation for non-small-cell lung cancer. *J Thorac Oncol*. 2015;10(12):1685-1693.

108. Sienel W, Varwerk C, Linder A, et al. Melanoma associated antigen (MAGE)-A3 expression in Stages I and II non-small cell lung cancer: results of a multi-center study. *Eur J Cardiothorac Surg*. 2004;25(1):131-134.

109. Vansteenkiste JF, Cho BC, Vanakesa T, et al. Efficacy of the MAGE-A3 cancer immunotherapeutic as adjuvant therapy in patients with resected MAGE-A3-positive non-small-cell lung cancer (MAGRIT): a randomised, double-blind, placebo-controlled, phase 3 trial. *Lancet Oncol*. 2016;17(6):822-835.

110. Copur MD, Gauchan D, Ramaekers R. Durvalumab in stage III non-small-cell lung cancer. *N Engl J Med*. 2018;378(9):868.

111. Uemura T, Hida T. Durvalumab showed long and durable effects after chemoradiotherapy in stage III non-small cell lung cancer: results of the PACIFIC study. *J Thorac Dis*. 2018;10(Suppl 9):S1108-S1112.

112. Douillard JY, Rosell R, De Lena M, et al. Adjuvant vinorelbine plus cisplatin versus observation in patients with completely resected stage IB-IIIA non-small-cell lung cancer (Adjuvant Navelbine International Trialist Association [ANITA]): a randomised controlled trial. *Lancet Oncol*. 2006;7(9):719-727.

113. Kelly K, Altorki NK, Eberhardt WEE, et al. Adjuvant erlotinib versus placebo in patients with stage IB-IIIA non-small-cell lung cancer (RADIANT): a randomized, double-blind, phase III trial. *J Clin Oncol*. 2015;33(34):4007-4014.

114. Mok TS, Wu YL, Thongprasert S, et al. Gefitinib or carboplatin-paclitaxel in pulmonary adenocarcinoma. *N Engl J Med*. 2009;361(10):947-957.

115. Rosell R, Carcereny E, Gervais R, et al. Erlotinib versus standard chemotherapy as first-line treatment for European patients with advanced EGFR mutation-positive non-small-cell lung cancer (EURTAC): a multicentre, open-label, randomised phase 3 trial. *Lancet Oncol*. 2012;13(3):239-246.

116. Pennell NA, Neal JW, Chaft JE, et al. SELECT: a phase II trial of adjuvant erlotinib in patients with resected epidermal growth factor receptor-mutant non-small-cell lung cancer. *J Clin Oncol.* 2019;37(2):97-104.
117. Zhong WZ, Wang Q, Mao W-M, et al. Gefitinib versus vinorelbine plus cisplatin as adjuvant treatment for stage II-IIIA (N1-N2) EGFR-mutant NSCLC (ADJUVANT/CTONG1104): a randomised, open-label, phase 3 study. *Lancet Oncol.* 2018;19(1):139-148.
118. Diwanji TP, Mohindra P, Vyfhuis M, et al. Advances in radiotherapy techniques and delivery for non-small cell lung cancer: benefits of intensity-modulated radiation therapy, proton therapy, and stereotactic body radiation therapy. *Transl Lung Cancer Res.* 2017;6(2):131-147.

15

NON–SMALL CELL LUNG CANCER TREATMENT: METASTATIC

Victor van Berkel, MD, PhD • Jennifer Cudris, MD • Neal E. Dunlap, MD • Ignacio Gil-Bazo, MD, PhD • Steven Mandish, MD • Katy Alyse Marino, MD • Phuong T. Ngo, MD • Cesar A. Perez, MD • Jose Pinto Llerena, MD • Edgardo S. Santos, MD, FACP • Andrew Tumen, MD, MS • Moises Harari Turquie, MD

SURGERY FOR OLIGOMETASTATIC DISEASE NON–SMALL CELL LUNG CANCER

Andrew Tumen, MD, MS, Katy Alyse Marino, MD, Victor van Berkel, MD, PhD

Learning Objectives:

1. What is oligometastatic non–small cell lung cancer (NSCLC)?
2. What clinicopathological features are suggestive of oligometastatic disease?
3. How does the eighth edition of the TNM (tumor, node, metastasis) staging system account for this concept?
4. How can the clinician determine whether 2 foci of lung cancer represent metastatic disease or independent primary tumors?
5. What is the ideal treatment approach and extent of resection in this subgroup of patients?

DEFINITION OF OLIGOMETASTATIC DISEASE

Most patients with advanced NSCLC receive systemic therapies as primary treatment, with therapeutic goals focused on palliation. However, it is becoming increasingly evident that patients with stage III-IV NSCLC are a heterogeneous group in regard to disease burden and prognosis. In its eighth edition, the TNM staging system was updated to reflect the diversity in this patient population, increasing our capacity to refine prognosis. Radiologic and therapeutic advances such as positron emission tomography (PET) and immunotherapy have improved survival for many patients with advanced lung cancer and led some to reconsider surgical intervention with curative intent for select patients with advanced NSCLC.[1,2] In this chapter, we define oligometastatic disease, summarize the current literature regarding the role of surgical resection, and discuss key considerations in the surgical management of patients with suspected oligometastatic NSCLC.

The term *oligometastatic disease* was first introduced by Hellman and Weichselbaum in 1995 to describe patients with a more indolent tumor biology and limited number of metastases that could be amenable to cure by means of local surgical therapies.[3] "In these cases the slow progression of the malignancy raises the opportunity for an aggressive local approach to control the disease" (page 9). While no clear consensus on the criteria defining oligometastatic disease has been reached, the patients most often included in this category are those with 1-5 metastases, locally advanced stage III, and metachronous second primary lung cancer (SPLC). There is growing evidence to suggest that oligometastatic lung cancer is a biologically and clinically distinct entity, which may redefine the prognosis and treatment approaches for many patients with historically incurable disease. Several studies have demonstrated long-term survival in certain patients with stage III and IV NSCLC following definitive surgical resection of both locoregional and distant metastases. Early evidence is, however, based almost exclusively on retrospective series, limiting conclusions on which patients benefit most from surgery and the most effective treatment approaches. As our understanding of oligometastatic NSCLC improves, characterization of predictable and reliable prognostic factors may facilitate proper patient selection.

DIAGNOSIS OF OLIGOMETASTATIC DISEASE

Identifying patients with oligometastatic disease is clinically challenging. Many patients presenting with apparent oligometastatic lung cancer progress to overtly metastatic disease. Objective predictors of the rate of metastatic progression are necessary to improve selection of patients who may achieve long-term disease control with aggressive oligometastasis-directed surgical therapy. Ashworth et al. conducted a meta-analysis characterizing outcomes and prognostic factors associated with oligometastatic stage IV NSCLC. The meta-analysis involved 757 patients with 1-5 metastases undergoing surgical resection of all lesions with curative intent. Median and 5-year overall survival (OS) were 26 months and 29.4%, respectively, while 8-year OS was 23.4%.[4] Low-risk patients, defined as those with metachronous metastases and any N stage, exhibited 47.8% 5-year OS, compared to 36.2% and 13.8% for intermediate-risk (synchronous metastases, N0) and high-risk (synchronous, N1-2) patients, respectively.[4] Here and for the purpose of this chapter, *metachronous* disease is diagnosed at least 2 months after the primary tumor, while *synchronous* disease is of course discovered concurrently. Significant factors portending long-term survival include R0 resection of the primary tumor, a long disease-free interval with metachronous rather than synchronous presentation, negative mediastinal nodal status, adenocarcinoma histology, and metastases limited in number and organ sites.[1,4,5]

Lussier et al. compared microRNA expression of lung metastasis specimens resected with curative intent between patients with high and low rates of recurrence. Several prioritized microRNAs were identified that consistently distinguished a high from a low rate of metastatic progression and OS.[6,7] Interestingly, this pattern of microRNA expression was not found in primary tumor specimens, which may be attributed to high genetic heterogeneity within the primary tumor and clonal selection within metastatic sites.[6] Further investigation of a molecular basis for tumor phenotype in NSCLC may aid in identification of patients most likely to experience long-term disease-free survival following surgical resection.

The most common sites of metastasis in NSCLC are lung, brain, adrenal glands, and bone. Intracranial lesions are found in 25%-35% of patients at the time of NSCLC diagnosis.[8] Retrospective studies have reported long-term survival in patients with solitary brain metastases following surgical treatment of both locoregional and intracranial disease.[9-11] A recent Surveillance Epidemiology and End Results (SEER) Program database study of the survival impact of combined surgical resection of the primary tumor and oligometastatic disease in 220 patients with brain-only M1 disease demonstrated combined surgery was associated with improved OS ($p < .0001$).[11] A Mayo Clinic study published in 2001 showed that surgical resection of synchronous brain metastases and primary NSCLC resulted in significantly superior 5-year survival in patients with N0 disease compared to those with N1/2 disease, with median OS of 44 months versus 10 months, respectively.[12] In their latest edition of clinical practice guidelines, the American College of Chest Physicians (ACCP) recommended resection or radiosurgical ablation in patients with metachronous single brain metastasis as well as those presenting with synchronous brain metastasis and resectable N0-1 primary NSCLC.[13] In most instances, the preferred strategy is surgical or ablative therapy of brain metastases prior to lung resection given the clinical levity of neurological symptoms due to mass effect (**Figure 15-1**).

The adrenal glands are the second most common extrathoracic site of NSCLC metastasis. A systematic review of isolated adrenal metastasis published in 2008 again showed patients with synchronous disease had a shorter median OS compared to those with metachronous disease, yet had equivalent 5-year survival estimates of 26% and 25%, respectively.[14] A study by Barone et al. found that median OS time of patients who underwent adrenalectomy was 31 months, likened to 13 months for patients who only underwent medical treatment. It is of no surprise that OS was significantly worse for bilateral than ipsilateral or contralateral metastasis (11 months vs. 27 months vs. 29 months, respectively).[15] The ACCP recommends resection of isolated metachronous and N0,1 synchronous adrenal metastases along with the primary tumor given negative invasive mediastinal staging (Figure 15-1).[13] Recent anatomical evidence of direct lymphatic channels between the chest and adrenal glands suggests that metastatic disease in the adrenal glands may represent locoregional lymphatic spread rather than hematogenous metastasis.[16]

Bone metastases carry a dismal prognosis associated with substantial morbidity and mortality. Poor outcomes are repeatedly reported despite surgical resection and radiotherapy, with median OS ranging from 0 to 13 months.[10,17,18] As a result, it may be argued

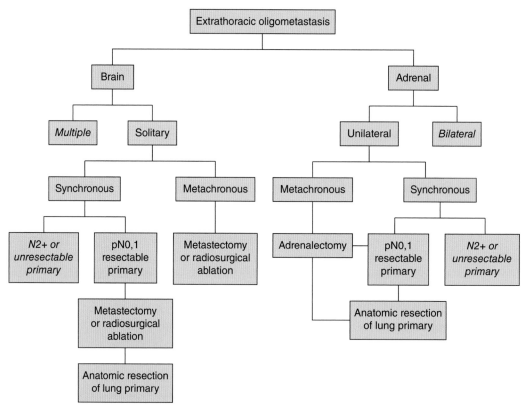

Figure 15-1. Suggested algorithm for surgical management of NSCLC with extrathoracic oligometastasis. Only the most common organ sites are included. Chemotherapy and radiation have been omitted, as has the management of frankly metastatic states indicated in italics.

that bony metastasis can seldom, if ever, be considered oligometastatic disease in the setting of an NSCLC primary.

MULTIPLE PULMONARY LESIONS

The incidence of metachronous and synchronous lung cancer is increasing due to advances in early detection and treatment in recent years. The management of patients with multiple pulmonary lesions suspicious for lung cancer is clinically challenging and raises many unique issues to consider. Take, for instance, the patient with potentially operable lung cancer found to have an additional small lesion on imaging. A great majority of additional pulmonary nodules with typical computed tomographic (CT) appearance are benign and should be surveilled according to published guidelines irrespective of accompanying malignancy.[19,20] The diagnostic dilemma is determining whether 2 foci of lung cancer represent metastatic disease or independent primary tumors.

Clinicians traditionally have relied on criteria proposed by Martini and Melamed in 1975 to help make this distinction.[21] SPLCs may be identified histologically if a different cell type than the primary tumor is found; however, two thirds of SPLCs reported in the literature have been the same cell type as the primary cancer.[13] Some authors suggested primary NSCLCs may be distinguished on the basis of the most dominant histological subtype (papillary, acinar, etc.) and a variety of cytologic and stromal features.[22]

There has been recent interest in utilizing genetic and molecular characterization to differentiate SPLCs and pulmonary metastases on the basis of tumor clonality.[23,24] Liu et al. examined the clonal relationship between lung tumors in several patients with multiple synchronous pulmonary lesions meeting 2007 ACCP criteria for hematogenous or intrapulmonary metastases using whole-genome and exome sequencing. The authors found that despite their clinicopathological classification, tumors harboring shared mutations in the same patient were extraordinarily rare. Such genetic heterogeneity suggests multiple primary tumors may be widely underdiagnosed.[24] While whole-genome sequencing and whole-exome sequencing of every lung tumor is not clinically practical, several studies have reported limited molecular analysis of cancer-related genes such as EGFR (epidermal growth factor receptor), P53, and ERBB2, with mixed results.[23,25] Tumor histology and genetic characterization have been challenged on theoretical grounds based on the tendency of malignant neoplasms to acquire mutations, intratumoral genetic heterogeneity, and even the ability to transform from adenocarcinoma to small cell lung cancer.[26,27] While not to be regarded as empirically definitive alone, these features should be taken into account and considered alongside the spatial and temporal relationship of the 2 foci of cancer, as well as the mediastinal nodal status.

Furthermore, concordance of nodal status, histology, anatomy, and timing may be most indicative of a diagnosis. For instance, pulmonary lesions of identical histology in a patient with multiple systemic metastases may suggest pulmonary metastases, as do histologically identical tumors in different lobes with N2-3 involvement.[13,28] An interval less than 2 years between occurrences of lung cancer suggests pulmonary metastasis, while a metachronous interval greater than 4 years between occurrences favors multiple primary lung cancers.[13,29] Tumors of the same histology in different lobes may be considered independent primary cancers in the absence of N2,3 nodal involvement and systemic/extrathoracic metastases. A second lesion of different histology arising from a nearby focus of carcinoma in situ is suggestive of multiple primary lung cancers.[13,29] Given the number of factors at play, it is critical that cases be discussed in a multidisciplinary setting involving an experienced radiologist, pathologist, oncologist, and thoracic surgeon, as this distinction will influence the prognosis and management of these patients.

Multiple primary lung cancers should be staged independently and managed as distinct tumors. Surgery is the treatment modality of choice for patients with multiple NSCLCs, if feasible. Pooled 5-year OS after resection of metachronous second primary NSCLC ranges from 41% to 46% in meta-analyses[13,30] and is as high as 54.5%-77% in recent series; however, a majority of patients included in the latter studies had stage I disease.[31-35] Anatomic resection of the second tumor is preferred in most studies, with the remaining 30%-40% of patients undergoing segmentectomy or wedge resection.[13,30] A handful of series have reported survival in regard to extent of resection, with mixed results.[31,32,34]

Despite the association of limited resection with locoregional recurrence, OS rates are not significantly different after wedge resection or segmentectomy compared to lobectomy in most studies, and sublobar resection is an acceptable alternative for patients with limited pulmonary reserve unable to tolerate more extensive resection.[31,35,36] It may be argued that segmentectomy or wedge resection is the most appropriate approach for early stage metachronous primary tumors in such patients. There is some recent evidence to suggest that segmentectomy is associated with lower recurrence as well as better progression-free and OS than wedge resection for early stage NSCLC, but this has not been evaluated in patients with oligometastatic disease.[37,38]

The eighth edition of the AJCC staging system subclassified stage IV disease into M1a, M1b (single extrathoracic metastasis in solitary organ), and M1c (multiple metastases in a single organ or in multiple organs), with median OS of 22.5, 17.8, and 13.6 months, respectively ($p < .001$).[39] Patients with pulmonary metastases typically undergo multimodal treatment, with more favorable outcomes compared to those with extrathoracic metastases. Patients with contralateral pulmonary metastases exhibited superior OS compared to patients with pleural/pericardial M1a disease or extrathoracic metastasis, but inferior OS compared to those with multiple primary lung cancers.[18,39,40]

In a SEER database study, Morris et al. examined the survival impact of a contralateral tumor nodule with that of regionally advanced contralateral N3 involvement. Compared to N3M0 disease, N0-1M1a patients with contralateral pulmonary metastasis experienced superior OS for primary tumors 2 cm or less (T1b), equivalent survival for primary tumors 2-7 cm (T1c-T3), and inferior survival for those 7 cm or greater (T4). This suggests that T stage of the primary tumor may carry greater prognostic significance in patients with intrapulmonary metastases than those with advanced locoregional disease, as the former are subject to multiple pulmonary resections. Survival outcomes of intrapulmonary M1a patients in this study were not significantly different from patients of comparable T and N stages with a second early stage primary lung cancer. This may reflect difficulty differentiating multiple primary lung cancers from metastatic disease from pooled retrospective data.[40]

MEDIASTINAL STAGING OF OLIGOMETASTATIC DISEASE

Few studies have investigated the survival impact of surgery for stage IV NSCLC with isolated pulmonary metastasis. The 5-year OS following definitive surgery is 22.5%-48.5%.[18,41] Patients with N0-1 and metachronous pulmonary metastases who underwent complete R0 resection of the primary tumor had the most favorable long-term outcomes.[4,18] Invasive mediastinal staging with video-assisted mediastinoscopy is essential prior to surgical intervention, even with negative CT/PET imaging.[42] A staged approach, including lobectomy of the primary tumor with systematic lymph node dissection followed by limited resection of contralateral metastases, may be appropriate for patients with multiple pulmonary lesions.[18,43] Systematic mediastinal lymph node dissection (MLND) has been shown in several randomized clinical trials to be far superior to selective lymph node sampling and no different from complete MLND in identifying positive N2 nodal stations.[44] The goals of surgery should be curative, with emphasis on complete resection of the primary tumor, as well as adequate mediastinal lymph node harvesting (**Figure 15-2**).

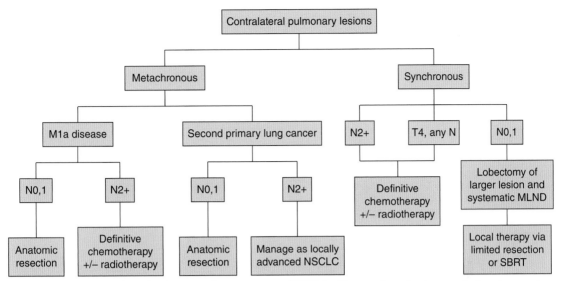

Figure 15-2. Suggested algorithm for surgical management of NSCLC with contralateral pulmonary lesion. A second primary lung cancer may less frequently present in a synchronous manner. SBRT, stereotactic body radiation therapy.

Low-Burden N2 Disease

The management of stage IIIA-IIIB-N2 NSCLC is one of the most controversial topics in thoracic oncology despite results from a handful of phase 3 randomized trials having been available for years. Although N2 nodal disease typically has negative prognostic implications in terms of long-term survival, a subset of patients with stage IIIA-N2 lung cancer may benefit from surgery as part of multimodal therapy. The eighth edition of the AJCC staging system subclassifies N2 disease into N2a$_1$ (single ipsilateral mediastinal or subcarinal nodal station without pN1 involvement, ie, skip N2); N2a$_2$ (single pN2 nodal station with pN1 involvement); and N2b (multiple pN2 nodal stations involved). Corresponding 5-year survival rates following definitive surgery are 52%, 41%, and 36%, respectively ($p < .01$).[45] Survival outcomes of N2a$_1$ patients are not significantly different from those with only N1b disease.[45]

Two recent studies indicated that the number of metastatic N2 lymph nodes and total metastatic lymph node ratio are independent predictive factors of disease-free survival.[46,47] Utilization of validated invasive mediastinal staging techniques is essential to provide patients every opportunity for long-term survival. There is roughly a 20% chance of N2 nodal station involvement in the setting of negative CT or PET imaging of the mediastinum.[44] Complete restaging after induction therapy is crucial in guiding subsequent treatment and has been shown to improve OS independently. This should include invasive mediastinal staging, head CT magnetic resonance imaging (MRI), plus either whole-body PET or abdominal CT and a bone scan.[13]

One of the dilemmas in management of patients with oligometastatic N2 disease is the timing of surgery and systemic therapy, as one modality of treatment may affect the patient's tolerance of the other. Advantages of upfront surgery include the procurement

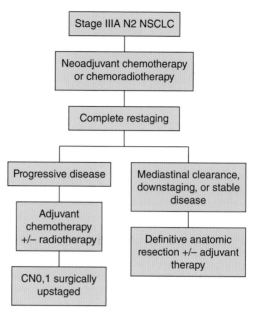

Figure 15-3. Suggested algorithm for surgical management of locally advanced NSCLC.

of tissue to guide systemic therapy and timely control of the primary tumor. Treatment-naïve patients have preserved functional status and tend to tolerate surgery better in general. Benefits of neoadjuvant therapy followed by surgery include early initiation and superior compliance with systemic therapy. Some advocate a period of neoadjuvant therapy in the setting of N2 disease to gauge tumors' metastatic potential, reserving surgery for patients with more favorable tumor biology who demonstrate some degree of mediastinal clearance (**Figure 15-3**).[48,49] Furthermore, patients who do not constitutionally tolerate chemotherapy may be less likely to tolerate an aggressive operation.[50]

Three relevant phase 3 randomized clinical trials have been conducted in patients with stage IIIA-N2 lung cancer; however, they did not provide definitive evidence regarding the optimal treatment approach.[51-53] In the Intergroup and ESPATUE trials, patients underwent induction chemoradiotherapy before being randomized to either surgery or further radiotherapy; patients in the ESPATUE trial also received platinum-based chemotherapy concurrently with chemoradiation prior to randomization. In the European Organization for Research and Treatment of Cancer (EORTC) trial, patients received induction platinum-based chemotherapy alone; those who responded were randomized to surgery or radiotherapy. OS was not significantly different between arms in any trial, although progression-free survival (PFS) in the Intergroup trial was superior in the surgery arm. Of note, 44% of patients in this study underwent pneumonectomy, with unacceptable perioperative mortality. A matched subgroup analysis excluding pneumonectomy found a significant survival difference favoring neoadjuvant chemo-radiation therapy (CRT) plus lobectomy over chemoradiation alone, with median and 5-year survival of 33.6 versus 21.7 months and 36.1% versus 17.8%, respectively ($p < .002$).[52] The best long-term results may be obtained with proven mediastinal clearance or downstaging, when a lobectomy is feasible to achieve R0 resection

(Figure 15-3).[52,54] The evidence of survival benefit associated with surgery is much stronger in studies of trimodal therapy than bimodal therapy, reflecting the synergistic effects of metastasis source control, ablation of locoregional micrometastatic lymph node disease, and systemic chemotherapy.[55]

Another subset of patients is found to have pN2 disease at the time of surgery for cN1 or clinically node-negative cancer (cN0). Patients typically undergo adjuvant chemotherapy with or without radiation therapy, with 5-year survival rates ranging from 30% to 47%.[56,57] This has been described as incidental, unsuspected, ignored, or underappreciated pN2 disease, depending on the clinical circumstances and extent of preoperative staging.[58] This is essentially the only group of patients with stage III-N2 lung cancer commonly treated with upfront surgery in the current era of systemic therapies. Most evidence suggests a clear survival benefit of mediastinal downstaging prior to surgery for N2 disease (Figure 15-3). However, recent studies of patients upstaged to pN2 at the time of surgery and given adjuvant therapy have failed to show a difference in survival compared to patients receiving neoadjuvant therapy prior to surgery.[57,58] Similarly, a recent comparison of neoadjuvant and adjuvant chemotherapy alone in combination with surgery for stage III-N2 disease demonstrated no survival difference.[56] Again, a wide range of survival outcomes and conflicting findings reflect a high degree of heterogeneity among N2 patients and further necessitates ongoing randomized prospective trials with standardized chemo- and radiation therapy regimens.

FUTURE PERSPECTIVE

As diagnostic and therapeutic advances improve survival of patients with NSCLC, we can expect to encounter more patients with oligometastatic disease. Large randomized trials with standardized systemic therapy regimens and patient selection criteria are needed to further investigate surgical management of oligometastatic NSCLC. Thorough staging and restaging prior to intervention and judicious patient selection based on validation of clinical and biological prognostic indicators will enhance delivery of appropriate treatment to this complex group of patients. While controversial, a definitive surgical approach appears to be associated with favorable long-term outcomes in select patients with advanced NSCLC undergoing multimodal therapy.

RADIATION FOR METASTATIC NON–SMALL CELL LUNG CANCER

Neal Dunlap, MD, Steven Mandish, MD

A 69-year-old female presents to the emergency room with complaint of lower back pain. She has a 45 pack-year smoking history, but no other significant past medical history and no trauma.

Lumbar spine CT shows a 1.4-cm lytic lesion in the L4 vertebral body. Chest, abdomen, and pelvis CT show a 3.6-cm left upper lobe lesion with associated mediastinal adenopathy. The brain MRI shows a 1.2-cm left frontal lobe lesion concerning for metastasis. The spine biopsy is positive for adenocarcinoma and is TTF-1 positive.

Learning Objectives:

1. The incidence of bone metastases in NSCLC is discussed.
2. Risks, benefits, and rationale of radiotherapy in the palliative setting are examined.
3. Understanding the emerging indications for local therapy, including stereotactic body radiation therapy (SBRT), in the oligometastatic patient is delineated.
4. The incidence of brain metastases in NSCLC is discussed.
5. Elucidation of information for understanding the risk, benefit, and rationale of radiotherapy, both stereotactic radiosurgery (SRS) and whole-brain radiotherapy (WBRT), for central nervous system (CNS) metastases is given.

BONE METASTASES

Bone metastases are a common sequela of NSCLC and can become very debilitating secondary to pain, pathologic fracture, and spinal cord compression. Bone metastases are becoming more common as patients live longer with cancer and imaging becomes more sensitive and aggressively used. Studies have shown bone metastases in 5%-30% of patients with lung cancer.[59] There is high-level evidence that external beam radiotherapy (EBRT) can be effective and safe in treating bone metastases.

PAIN CONTROL

Multiple studies have shown a significant improvement in pain with both fractionated and single-fraction EBRT. Studies suggested that 53%-88% of patients can expect at least partial response for pain, while 17%-24% can expect complete resolution of symptoms.[60-63] A meta-analysis by Chow et al. analyzed 25 randomized trials including 5,617 patients and reported a 60%-61% response rate.[61] Of patients with some response, 70% noticed pain relief within 2 weeks and 90% noticed within 2 months.[61]

FRACTIONATION

Traditional palliative radiotherapy courses for bone metastases include 8 Gy in 1 fraction, 20 Gy in 5 fractions, 24 Gy in 6 fractions, and 30 Gy in 10 fractions, among others. These have been compared in multiple studies. Chow et al. showed that single-fraction and multifraction treatments did not show a difference in any response (60% vs. 61%) or complete response (23% vs. 24%).[61] Also, 8 Gy in 1 fraction was found to be equivalent to 24 Gy in 6 fractions (response rate 53% vs. 56%).[63]

Re-treatment rates were increased for patients receiving single-fraction treatment versus a multifraction approach (20% vs. 8%[61]; 13.3% vs. 8.8%[60]; 15% vs. 5%[62]).

TOXICITY

Treatment for bone metastases is minimally toxic but can present issues depending on the location of treatment. Specifically, when considering if fractionation affects toxicity, Majumder et al. showed equivalent toxicity rates in patients receiving 30 Gy in 10 fractions versus 8 Gy in 1 fraction to vertebral body metastases.[64] Chow et al. also showed equivalent rates of pathologic fracture and spinal cord compression between the 2 groups.[61]

A well-recognized side effect of palliative radiotherapy for bone metastases is the pain flare, or a temporary worsening in pain at the treatment site shortly after radiotherapy. It is theorized that cytokine release is responsible and can be seen in 30%-40% of patients.[65] A phase 3 study randomizing patients to prophylactic dexamethasone (8 mg 1 hour before treatment and the following 4 days) versus placebo showed a reduced frequency of pain flare with prophylactic steroids (26% vs. 35%, $p = .05$). In the dexamethasone arm, 3/148 patients had a hyperglycemic event. The duration of pain flare was 3 days with dexamethasone and 2 days with placebo.[66] While this study supported prophylactic dexamethasone, the adoption of this as a standard of care is debated secondary to dexamethasone toxicities and the relatively limited clinical improvement.[67]

RE-TREATMENT

According to the most recent American Society for Radiation Oncology (ASTRO) bone metastases guidelines, patients with persistent or recurrent pain 1 month after palliative treatment are eligible for re-treatment.[68] A meta-analysis showed that 58% of patients who received retreatment will have a response to radiotherapy. The majority of these patients received single-fraction therapy, both primarily and in the re-treatment setting. Of these patients, 23% had lung primary cancer.[69]

There is high-level evidence that radiotherapy is safe and effective for bone metastases. Patients can be treated with single-fraction or multifraction regimens with similar responses and toxicity. Toxicity is limited and corresponds to treatment area. Pain flares are common and can be treated with dexamethasone. Re-treatment is possible and effective.

VERTEBRAL BODY METASTASES

The treatment algorithm for vertebral body metastases has become increasingly complicated with more advanced surgical and radiotherapy techniques. Memorial Sloan Kettering developed a systematic framework for decision-making: neurologic, oncologic, mechanical instability, and systemic disease, or NOMS.[70] The following discussion provides details about each. It is important to note that neurologic and oncologic effects are considered together to determine the appropriate treatment option (**Figure 15-4**).

Neurologic Consideration

The neurologic consideration is determining the amount of epidural spinal cord compression (ESCC) present. The Spine Oncology Study Group developed a 6-point, MRI-based grading system for ESCC (**Figure 15-5**).[71] Using axial T2-weighted images at the level of greatest compression, a score is given. Scores 0-1b are considered for radiation, scores of 2-3 are considered for surgery unless the tumor is of a radiosensitive histology (see oncologic consideration next). Score 1c treatment is not fully defined but may be amenable to SRS or separation surgery followed by radiation.[70]

Oncologic Consideration

The oncologic consideration is essentially deciding the radiosensitivity of the tumor, which is based on the response to conventional EBRT. Traditionally, NSCLC has been considered an unfavorable, radioresistant histology along with melanoma and renal cell

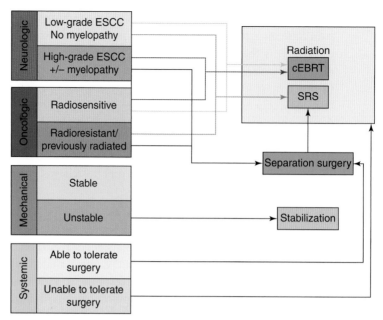

Figure 15-4. Treatment algorithm for the management of vertebral body metastases. CEBRT, conventional external-beam radiation. (Reproduced with permission from Laufer I, Rubin DG, Lis E, et al. The NOMS framework: approach to the treatment of spinal metastatic tumors. *Oncologist.* 2013;18(6):744-751. © 2013 AlphaMed Press.)

carcinoma. Lymphoma, seminoma, and myeloma are radiosensitive. Radiosensitive tumors can be treated with radiotherapy regardless of the ESCC score. Radioresistant tumors should follow the treatment algorithm based on the point score presented previously in this section.[70]

Mechanical Instability

The Spine Oncology Study Group published an evidence-based system to determine the Spinal Instability in Neoplastic Disease, or SINS, score (**Table 15-1**). SINS is a point-based, objective measurement system using the spinal location, presence of pain, bone lesion appearance (blastic/mixed/lytic), radiographic alignment of the vertebral body, amount of vertebral body collapse, and amount of posterior involvement. Patients whose metastasis scores a 7-13 represent those patients with a potentially unstable

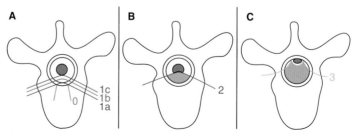

Figure 15-5. Spine Oncology Study Group MRI-based grading system for ESCC. (Reproduced with permission from Bilsky MH, et al. Reliability analysis of the epidural spinal cord compression scale. *J Neurosurg Spine.* 2010;13(3):324-328.)

TABLE 15-1	Spinal Instability in Neoplastic Disease
	SCORE
Location	
Junctional (occiput-C2, C7-T2, T11-L1, L5-S1)	3
Mobile spine (C3-C6, L2-L4)	2
Semirigid (T3-T10)	1
Rigid (S2-S5)	0
Pain	
Yes	3
Occasional pain but not mechanical	1
Pain-free lesion	0
Bone lesion	
Lytic	2
Mixed (lytic/blastic)	1
Blastic	0
Radiographic spinal alignment	
Subluxation/translation present	4
De novo deformity (kyphosis/scoliosis)	2
Normal alignment	0
Vertebral body collapse	
>50% collapse	3
<50% collapse	2
No collapse with >50% body involved	1
None of the above	0
Posterolateral involvement of spinal elements	
Bilateral	3
Unilateral	1
None of the above	0
Total score	
Stable	0-6
Indeterminate	7-12
Unstable	13-18

Reproduced with permission from Fisher CG, DiPaola CP, Ryken TC, et al. Spine. 2010 Oct 15;35(22): E1221-E1229.

lesion, and scores of 13 or greater represent an unstable lesion.[72] All patients scoring 7 or greater warrant neurosurgical assessment. A 2014 study of the SINS score showed nearly identical intraobserver and interobserver agreement, confirming that it was reliable and reproducible.[73]

Systemic Assessment

Systemic assessment is determining the patient's ability to tolerate intervention, particularly paying attention to tumor burden, aggressiveness of disease, medical comorbidities, and the like. There are no hard-and-fast rules in this scenario, and a multidisciplinary discussion as well as the patient's own goals should be considered.[70]

SBRT VERSUS CONVENTIONAL RADIATION THERAPY

Spine metastases had been treated like other bone metastases, but it had been questioned if an increasing dose would lead to better, more durable pain control and fewer re-treatments. Conventional EBRT has limitations with dose escalation secondary to the sensitive structures near the vertebral bodies (ie, the spinal cord and esophagus). Stereotactic body radiation is highly conformal, allowing for safe dose escalation. Multiple phase 2 studies have shown that this is both safe and effective. Radiation Therapy Oncology Group (RTOG) 0631 is a phase 2/3 study where patients with a numerical rating pain scale of 5 or greater were treated with 16 Gy in 1 fraction. This showed that SBRT for spine lesions is feasible in terms of tumor coverage, normal tissue constraints, and toxicity.[74] Phase 3 data, comparing 16-18 Gy in 1 fraction to 8 Gy in 1 fraction, are pending.

Tseng et al. analyzed 279 de novo metastases in 145 patients receiving 24 Gy in 2 fractions. The 1- and 2-year local failure rates were 9.7% and 17.6%, respectively. No grade 3 toxicity was noted.[75] Sprave et al. randomized patients to 24 Gy in 1 fraction versus 30 Gy in 10 fractions. There was no difference in pain relief at 3 months, although pain scores decreased faster with SBRT. SBRT also had greater pain relief at 6 months. No patients experienced grade 3 or higher toxicity.[76]

Contouring guidelines for SBRT alone[77] and postoperative SBRT[78] are available.

RADIONUCLIDES

Radionuclides or radiopharmaceuticals are radioactive, bone-seeking medications that can be used in patients with bone metastases. Through different mechanisms, these medications are selectively absorbed into metabolically active bone, thus delivering high doses of radiation to the diseased sites. Sumarium 153 is the most commonly used today, but other examples include strontium 89 and phosphorus 32. These are primarily used in breast and prostate cancers, but could be considered in the case of multifocal, painful bone metastases. Contraindications include severe marrow suppression and renal dysfunction.

OLIGOMETASTASES

Oligometastatic disease is generally defined as a maximum of 5 metastatic lesions. Distinct categories include the following:

1. Synchronous: diagnosed within months of the primary tumor
2. Metachronous: appear after primary treatment

Oligometastatic disease was previously considered incurable, but this treatment paradigm is now under question. Limited data on the benefit of local therapy are available, but studies have shown promising results.

A propensity-matched analysis studying patients with synchronous metastases at the time of diagnosis showed a benefit to comprehensive local therapy. Inclusion criteria were pathologic confirmation of NSCLC; 1-3 metastases at time of diagnosis; radical treatment to metastases, including radiation or surgery; and completion of 2 cycles of induction chemotherapy or concurrent chemoradiation without disease progression. Exceptions were made for patients who had early intracranial treatment.

There were 90 patients who met inclusion criteria. The majority had metastases that had non-squamous histology (89%) and had 1 metastasis (72%). Of the patients, 44/90 (49%) had metastases confined to the brain and 59% had brain metastases and metastases to other organs. Chemotherapy included a carboplatin-based doublet in 78% and a cisplatin-based doublet in 14%. Median number of chemotherapy cycles was 6. Out of 90 patients 69 received comprehensive local therapy (CLT). Median follow-up was 46.6 months.

Cox proportional hazards regression analysis showed that patients who received CLT had a significant improvement in OS versus patients who did not (27.1 vs. 13.1 months). Univariate analysis showed that comprehensive local therapy, non-squamous histology ($p = .03$), T stage ($p = .05$), and favorable Eastern Cooperative Oncology Group (ECOG) performance status predicted for improved OS ($p \leq .01$), although favorable ECOG was the only measure that remained significant in adjusted analysis. Non-brain/adrenal, single-organ metastases predicted increased PFS ($p = .05$) compared to brain/adrenal metastases. Eventually, 46/90 developed a new metastatic lesion, with 20 of those being in the brain. This study suggests that there is a subset of patients who would benefit from local therapy in the setting of oligometastatic NSCLC at diagnosis, particularly in patients with at least stable disease after primary therapy, limited metastases, and favorable performance status.[79]

Gomez et al. conducted a multicenter, randomized, phase 2 study in an attempt to define any benefit from aggressive local therapy in oligometastatic patients. Inclusion criteria were pathologically confirmed NSCLC stage IV disease according to the seventh edition of the AJCC guidelines, 3 or fewer metastases after first-line systemic therapy, ECOG less than 2, and standard chemotherapy (defined as 4 or more cycles of platinum doublet therapy, erlotinib/other first-line EGFR tyrosine kinase inhibitor [TKI] for 3 or more months if a patient had an EGFR mutation, or crizotinib for 3 or more months if the patient harbored an anaplastic lymphoma kinase [ALK] rearrangement). Patients with N1-N3 nodal involvement were considered to have 1 metastasis such that 2 additional extranodal metastases would qualify. Again, patients needing immediate treatment for CNS involvement were included in this study.

Randomization included local therapy (surgery and/or radiation) and maintenance therapy versus maintenance therapy alone (which could be observation) in patients with 3 or fewer metastatic sites with stable/responsive disease after first-line systemic therapy. After systemic therapy, 74 patients were eligible for the study, of which 49 entered randomization. Twenty-five patients received consolidative local therapy, with

24 undergoing maintenance. Patient characteristics were comparable between the 2 groups.

Most patients had adenocarcinoma histology and N0-N1 disease. A quarter of the patients had brain metastases. Of patients receiving local therapy, 48% were treated with radiation alone, 24% had surgery and radiation, 20% received chemoradiation, and 4% received surgery alone. In the maintenance group, 67% (16) received pemetrexed, 8% (2) erlotinib, 4% (1) afatinib, 4% (1) bevacizumab, and observation in 17% (4; 3 with squamous cell carcinoma [SCC] and 1 with sarcomatoid features). Median PFS in the local therapy arm was 11.93 months versus 3.9 months with maintenance therapy alone ($p = .0054$).[80]

Another potential benefit of radiotherapy in the setting of oligometastasis is the "abscopal effect," or the ability of radiation to induce tumor regression in non-irradiated, distant tumor sites. This was first theorized in 1953.[81]

WIDELY METASTATIC DISEASE

Patients with widely metastatic disease should have their cases discussed in a multidisciplinary setting. Radiotherapy is an important treatment option in this palliative setting.

CNS METASTASES

Brain metastases are diagnosed at presentation for 10% of patients with NSCLC,[82] with the prevalence of intracranial disease as high as 26% for stage IV disease at presentation. The incidence of brain metastases varies with the molecular mutational profile of the primary tumor, with the rates of brain metastases higher in patients with EGFR mutations.[83,84] Additionally, mutation status is prognostic for survival in NSCLC, with a median OS of almost 4 years for patients with adenocarcinoma and a graded pogostic assessment (GPA) of 3.5-4.0.[85] Steroids should be promptly initiated for symptomatic patients with 4-32 mg of dexamethasone administered twice daily with a taper after maximal neurologic improvement.[86] Surgical resection can be considered for patients with limited (1-3) brain metastases, lesions 3 cm or greater, controlled or absent systemic disease, and good performance status. Postoperative radiation should be delivered after surgical resection given high local recurrence rates with surgery alone.[87] Definitive SRS is an effective and increasingly used treatment for patients with brain metastases, with local control rates greater than 80%. WBRT can be used to palliate patients with poor performance status or extensive intracranial disease. Best supportive care (BSC) may be considered for selected patients with poor performance status.[88]

Additionally, the development of targeted therapy for select patients with EGFR and ALK mutations has led to interest in deferring upfront radiation for limited, asymptomatic brain metastases. Pending level I evidence, caution may be warranted, with a multiinstitutional retrospective suggesting upfront treatment with a first-generation EGFR TKI such as erlotinib with deferral of radiation therapy was associated with worsened survival.[89] Multidisciplinary evaluation by providers, including thoracic surgeons, medical oncologists, and radiation oncologists, to determine optimal management for these patients is critical pending the results of prospective trials (NCT03497767).

CHEMOTHERAPY FOR METASTATIC NON–SMALL CELL LUNG CANCER

Phuong Ngo, MD

A 59-year-old Caucasian male with a past medical history of tobacco abuse, hypertension, chronic obstructive pulmonary disease (COPD), and multiple sclerosis currently on treatment presents with persistent abdominal pain and weight loss for 3 months. Chest CT shows a right lower lobe mass and hilar adenopathy. Abdomen/pelvis CT shows 2 liver lesions, one of which is biopsied and returns with a finding of squamous cell carcinoma. Brain MRI is negative for metastatic disease. He has no driver mutations, and the programmed death ligand 1 (PD-L1) value is 3%.

Learning Objectives:
1. What basic molecular testing should be done for all metastatic NSCLC patients?
2. Which treatments should be avoided in squamous cell histology?
3. What are first-line treatment options for metastatic non-squamous NSCLC?
4. What are the first treatment options for metastatic squamous NSCLC?
5. Which agents are approved for continuation maintenance?
6. Which options are used for subsequent therapy?

SELECTING TREATMENT REGIMENS

Driver Mutations

All patients with metastatic disease require systemic therapy, though cases of limited metastatic disease may have a multimodality approach, including radiation and surgery. Tissue biopsies should be sent for predictive biomarkers, such as EGFR, ALK, ROS1 (ROS proto-oncogene 1), BRAF, and PD-L1, all of which will help tailor treatment regimens. Of note, actionable mutations are more likely to be found in non-squamous and not otherwise specified (NOS) NSCLC than squamous histology. Though rare, ALK and EGFR mutations can be found in some squamous cell patients, especially those with no smoking history, small tissue sample, and mixed histology.

> **CLINICAL PEARL:** All metastatic non-squamous NSCLC should be checked for EGFR, ALK, ROS1, BRAF, and PD-L1 at a minimum.

More recently, additional predictive markers have emerged, namely, neurotrophic receptor tyrosine kinase (NTRK) gene fusions, ERBB2 (HER2), RET (REarranged during Transfection) gene rearrangements, MET amplifications, and tumor mutational burden (TMB), although there is still no consensus on the best way to measure some of these markers. The National Comprehensive Cancer Network (NCCN) panel suggested broad molecular testing in order to ensure identification of any driver mutations that may help guide therapies. Differing from these predictive markers is KRAS, which is a poor prognostic marker for survival and also indicates lack of response to EGFR TKIs.

Histology: Squamous Versus Non-squamous

Histology is not a significant prognostic indicator, but it does affect treatment sensitivities and possible adverse effects. NSCLC mainly comprises adenocarcinoma, squamous cell carcinoma, and large cell carcinoma. Each of these is discussed in more detail in the pathology section, but for purposes of treatment, histology for NSCLC is generally divided into squamous and non-squamous histology since certain chemotherapies are less efficacious or contraindicated in the squamous subtype.

Pemetrexed

Pemetrexed is a thymidylate synthase inhibitor often used as part of a platinum doublet and is considered a chemotherapy backbone in the treatment of NSCLC. However, it appears to be less effective in squamous cell histology.

A large trial consisting of 1.700 treatment-naïve patients with advanced NSCLC compared cisplatin/pemetrexed to cisplatin/gemcitabine in the first-line setting. Investigators found that the OS was similar in both arms (median survival, 10.3 vs. 10.3 months, respectively; hazard ratio [HR] = 0.94; 95% CI 0.84-1.05), but that the pemetrexed arm had fewer toxicities. However, subset analysis showed OS was significant for the cisplatin/pemetrexed arm compared to the cisplatin/gemcitabine arm mainly in patients with adenocarcinoma (12.6 vs. 10.9 months, respectively) and large cell carcinoma histology (10.4 vs. 6.7 months, respectively). Meanwhile, those with squamous cell histology had significant improvement in survival with the cisplatin/gemcitabine arm over the cisplatin/pemetrexed arm (10.8 vs. 9.4 months, respectively).[90] This difference in response may be due to higher expression of thymidylate synthase in the squamous subtype.[91] Many other studies have confirmed this result, leading to the approval of pemetrexed for non-squamous NSCLC.

> **CLINICAL PEARL:** Pemetrexed is only used in non-squamous NSCLC; it does not appear to be as effective in squamous histology.

Bevacizumab

Another agent not approved for treatment in squamous cell histology is bevacizumab, which is a recombinant monoclonal antibody that inhibits vascular endothelial growth factor (VEGF) and blocks angiogenesis. Its use was evaluated in the ECOG 4599 study, which assigned patients to either carboplatin/paclitaxel or carboplatin/paclitaxel and bevacizumab every 3 weeks. Median survival and median duration of PFS for the chemotherapy plus bevacizumab arm were superior to the chemotherapy-alone arm. However, this study was restricted to non-squamous cell carcinoma due to increased bleeding seen in the preceding phase 2 study.[92] Since bleeding is a major complication of bevacizumab, the study patients also did not have brain metastases, hemoptysis, bleeding disorders, or anticoagulation requirements, though other studies have questioned some of these restrictions.

The dangers of bevacizumab in squamous cell histology were thought to be due to the central location of these tumors and their proximities to vascular structures, but these do not appear to be definite, independent risk factors. In the Avastin in Lung (AVAiL) trial in which patients were assigned to cisplatin/gemcitabine with placebo, cisplatin/gemcitabine with 7.5 mg/kg of bevacizumab every 3 weeks, or cisplatin/ gemcitabine with 15 mg/kg of bevacizumab every 3 weeks, central lesions were present in 38% of patients and did not appear to increase the rate of pulmonary hemorrhage.[93] The trial also had 86 patients who developed venous thromboembolism requiring therapeutic anticoagulation and found that despite a higher bleeding rate in these patients, the risk appeared to be independent of whether the patient was receiving bevacizumab.[94] Last, the PASSPORT trial used chemotherapy plus bevacizumab in 115 patients with brain metastases and had no cases of CNS hemorrhage.[95]

Still, the risk of bleeding is present. Despite the restrictions in ECOG 4599, patients receiving bevacizumab still had more bleeding compared to those who did not receive bevacizumab (4.4% vs. 0.9%; $p = .001$). Of the 15 treatment-related deaths in the bevacizumab group, 5 were from pulmonary hemorrhage. Thus, bevacizumab is contraindicated in those with squamous cell histology, and its serious side effects should be properly discussed with all other patients.

> **CLINICAL PEARL:** Bevacizumab is contraindicated in squamous cell NSCLC.

FIRST-LINE TREATMENT

Treatment in metastatic NSCLC is highly dependent on histology and whether the cancer has driver mutations, the PD-L1 status, and performance status.

Targeted Therapies

Specific TKIs are available for each driver mutation and are discussed separately in the TKI section. It is important to note, however, that when specific driver mutations such as EGFR, ALK, and ROS1 are present, treatment should be with the corresponding TKI regardless of PD-L1 status.

Chemotherapy Versus Immunotherapy

With the rapid success and subsequent approval of many immunotherapies, chemotherapy has moved away from being the first-line treatment in metastatic NSCLC. Instead, immunotherapy is now preferred alone or in combination with chemotherapy, depending on the PD-L1 status of treatment-naïve patients without targetable mutations.

Immune checkpoint inhibitor antibodies inhibit PD-1 (programmed cell death protein 1) receptors expressed on activated cytotoxic T cells or PD-L1 to improve immunity against tumors. For this reason, immunotherapy is contraindicated in those with autoimmune disorders and those who are on high doses of immunosuppressive agents. The immune checkpoint inhibitors currently available are pembrolizumab, nivolumab, durvalumab, and atezolizumab.

Single-Agent Immunotherapy

KEYNOTE-024 was a landmark trial involving previously untreated advanced squamous or non-squamous NSCLC patients who had PD-L1 expression of at least 50%

with no other targetable mutations. They were randomized to either pembrolizumab 200 mg every 3 weeks or the investigator's choice of platinum-based chemotherapy. The respective median PFS (10.3 vs. 6.0 months) and OS (80.2% vs. 72.4% at 6 months) were both statistically significant in favor of pembrolizumab. The response rate was also higher (44.8% vs. 27.8%), the median duration of response (DOR) longer (not reached vs. 6.3 months), and the treatment-related adverse events (TRAEs) fewer (73.4% vs. 90.0%) compared to the chemotherapy arm. Thus, pembrolizumab was approved as first-line monotherapy in those with PD-L1 greater than or equal to 50%.[96]

> **CLINICAL PEARL:** All patients with metastatic NSCLC should have PD-L1 status checked.

> **CLINICAL PEARL:** Single-agent pembrolizumab is approved as first-line treatment in patients with PD-L1 of 50% or greater.

Given these significant outcomes in patients with high PD-L1 expression, there was understandable curiosity regarding those who had less than 50% PD-L1. Another trial, KEYNOTE-042, followed again with treatment-naïve patients randomized to pembrolizumab versus platinum-based chemotherapy as first-line therapy but now included patients with PD-L1 of 1% or greater. These patients also had no actionable mutations. Again, there appeared to be greater benefit to the pembrolizumab arm, but subgroup analysis showed OS was mainly improved in those with PD-L1 levels of 50% or more, while those with PD-L1 tumor proportion score (TPS) of 1%-49% had similar OS to the chemotherapy group. However, this trial has since been updated with data in favor of pembrolizumab over chemotherapy.

The patients were divided according to PD-L1 TPSs of 50% or greater, 20% or greater, and 1% or greater with the median OS for pembrolizumab compared to chemotherapy 20.0 versus 12.2 months, 17.7 versus 13.0 months, and 16.7 versus 12.1 months, respectively. The HR was 0.82 in favor of pembrolizumab in all 3 subgroups. The pembrolizumab groups also had better objective response rates and median DOR.[97] The investigators concluded that single-agent pembrolizumab can be extended to include those without targetable mutations and with PD-L1 of 1% or greater in the first-line setting. However, this is still a category 2B according to the NCCN guidelines, with the only category 1 recommendation for single-agent pembrolizumab being in those with PD-L1 50% or greater.

> **CLINICAL PEARL:** Single-agent pembrolizumab can be used for PD-L1 of 1-49% but this is currently a category 2B recommendation according to the NCCN guidelines.

Combination Chemoimmunotherapy

Using pembrolizumab alone for patients with PD-L1 greater than or equal to 50% is applicable to both squamous and non-squamous histology. For those with PD-L1 of

49% or less, however, the recommended treatments now actually consist of immunotherapy in combination with chemotherapy; regimen selection is based on histologic subtype.

NON-SQUAMOUS HISTOLOGY

KEYNOTE-021 was a phase 2 trial that ultimately changed the landscape of treatment for advanced NSCLC. It randomly assigned untreated patients with stage IIIB/IV non-squamous NSCLC without an EGFR or ALK mutation to receive carboplatin/pemetrexed with or without pembrolizumab. The primary endpoint of overall response rate (ORR) showed superiority with the triple regimen compared to the doublet carboplatin/pemetrexed (55% vs. 26%; p = .0016).[98] This trial was followed up with the phase 3 KEYNOTE-189 trial, which permanently entrenched this regimen into the algorithm for treating metastatic non-squamous NSCLC.

The study involved 616 previously untreated patients with metastatic non-squamous cancer without sensitizing EGFR or ALK mutations. They were randomized to receive platinum and pemetrexed along with either pembrolizumab or placebo every 3 weeks for 4 cycles, followed by pemetrexed plus either pembrolizumab or placebo for up to 35 cycles. At the median follow-up of 10.5 months, the estimated rate of OS was an overwhelming 69.2% in the pembrolizumab arm compared to 49.4% in the placebo arm. OS improvements were seen in all subgroups regardless of PD-L1 status. The median PFS in the pembrolizumab group compared to the placebo was 8.8 months versus 4.9 months, respectively. The rate of grade 3 and above adverse events (AEs) was similar, if not slightly higher, in the triple-regimen group compared to the placebo (67.2% vs. 65.8%, respectively).[99] Still, these findings resulted in approval by the Food and Drug Administration (FDA) of platinum/pemetrexed/pembrolizumab as first-line treatment in patients with non-squamous NSCLC without sensitizing EGFR or ALK mutations who otherwise have no contraindication to immunotherapy.

> **CLINICAL PEARL:** The platinum/pemetrexed/pembrolizumab combination is approved in the first-line setting for metastatic non-squamous NSCLC without targetable mutations.

With the success of this combination, many looked for other chemoimmunotherapy combinations that could be used in this patient population. IMpower150 was another phase 3 trial that looked at immunotherapy in addition to chemotherapy in patients with untreated metastatic non-squamous NSCLC. It differed from the KEYNOTE studies in that it used atezolizumab as the immunotherapeutic agent instead of pembrolizumab and also added bevacizumab. Patients were randomized to receive atezolizumab plus carboplatin/paclitaxel (ACP), bevacizumab plus carboplatin/paclitaxel (BCP), or atezolizumab plus bevacizumab with carboplatin/paclitaxel (ABCP). Treatments were given every 3 weeks for 4-6 cycles, followed by maintenance therapy with atezolizumab, bevacizumab, or both. Median PFS was longer in the four-drug regimen (ABCP) compared to the BCP group (8.3 vs. 6.8 months; HR 0.62, 95% CI 0.52-0.74, p < .001). PFS and median OS were also longer in this group compared to BCP regardless of PD-L1

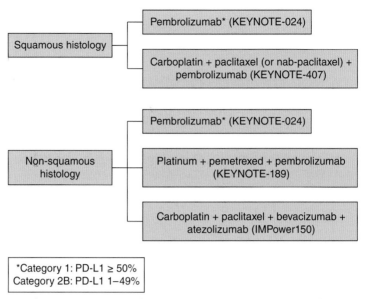

Figure 15-6. First-line treatment options for metastatic NSCLC without targetable mutations.

status, thus making ABCP another viable option for metastatic non-squamous NSCLC (**Figure 15-6**).[100]

CLINICAL PEARL: Atezolizumab/bevacizumab/carboplatin/paclitaxel combination is also approved in the first-line setting for metastatic non-squamous NSCLC without targetable mutations.

SQUAMOUS HISTOLOGY

Immunotherapy can still be used in combination with chemotherapy for metastatic squamous NSCLC, but special consideration has to be given when selecting chemotherapy agents due to the limitations of chemotherapy in this histology, as described previously.

Investigators again added pembrolizumab to chemotherapy but could not use pemetrexed in this population. Instead, in KEYNOTE-407, these patients were randomized to receive carboplatin with either paclitaxel or nab-paclitaxel for the first 4 cycles in addition to either pembrolizumab or placebo for up to 35 cycles. The median OS was 15.9 months in the pembrolizumab arm compared to 11.3 months in the placebo arm. Again, this was seen regardless of the PD-L1 expression. Median PFS was also improved at 6.4 months in the pembrolizumab group versus 4.8 months in the placebo group.[101]

CLINICAL PEARL: The combination carboplatin/paclitaxel or nab-paclitaxel/pembrolizumab is approved in the first-line setting for metastatic squamous NSCLC.

Similar to the trajectory of research regarding chemoimmunotherapy in non-squamous NSCLC, many also looked at the addition of atezolizumab to standard chemotherapy in squamous NSCLC. The IMpower131 study evaluated atezolizumab with carboplatin and paclitaxel or nab-paclitaxel in stage IV squamous NSCLC. Interim analysis showed improved PFS in the immunotherapy arm, and investigators presented an update at the European Society for Medical Oncology Conference in 2018, showing comparable OS. Data from this study are still maturing, and this regimen is currently awaiting FDA approval.[102]

CHEMOTHERAPY

We have discussed the benefits of adding immunotherapy, but what options exist if the patient has an active autoimmune disorder, for example, and is unable to be treated with immunotherapy? Chemotherapy alone still remains a reliable option.

Platinum Agents

Data have shown that a platinum-containing regimen is superior to BSC in patients with incurable disease. Some studies have compared cisplatin to carboplatin in NSCLC and found cisplatin had a slightly better objective response rate and survival benefit (**Table 15-2**).[103,104]

However, cisplatin is generally a tougher regimen, with common adverse effects including, but not limited to, neurotoxicity, usually in the form of peripheral neuropathy, nephrotoxicity, ototoxicity, and myelosuppression. Cisplatin also requires fluid administration before, during, and after treatment, with higher doses requiring more aggressive hydration. This poses a challenge in patients who are prone to fluid overload.

> **CLINICAL PEARL:** Cisplatin can cause peripheral neuropathy, nephrotoxicity, ototoxicity, nausea/vomiting, and myelosuppression.

Carboplatin is another platinum agent that is generally better tolerated than cisplatin. Its metabolism is 100-fold slower, as is its elimination. The dose of carboplatin is usually

TABLE 15-2 Trials Comparing Cisplatin Versus Carboplatin in Advanced NSCLC

AUTHOR	REGIMEN	NO. OF PATIENTS	RR	MEDIAN SURVIVAL	1-YEAR SURVIVAL
Rosell et al.[146]	Cisplatin/ paclitaxel	309	28%	9.8 mo	38%
	Carboplatin/ paclitaxel	309	25%	8.5 mo	33%
Fossella et al.[112]	Cisplatin/ docetaxel	408	32%	11.3 mo	46%
	Carboplatin/ docetaxel	406	24%	9.4 mo	38%

RR, response rate.

calculated to a target area under the curve (AUC) based on glomerular filtration rate (GFR). It can also cause peripheral neuropathy, renal toxicity, nausea/vomiting, and myelosuppression, but often to a lesser degree than cisplatin. For this reason, carboplatin is recommended for patients with multiple comorbidities or those who are unlikely to tolerate cisplatin.

> **CLINICAL PEARL:** Carboplatin is milder than cisplatin and should be given to patients with multiple comorbidities and those who cannot tolerate cisplatin.

Standard Regimens

Combining a third-generation agent such as vinorelbine, paclitaxel, docetaxel, gemcitabine, and pemetrexed with a platinum agent improves survival rates compared to the same third-generation drug used alone (**Table 15-3**).[9-11] Interestingly, this combination also showed better responses and improved survival compared to single-agent cisplatin alone (**Table 15-4**).[12-14]

Thus, combining multiple drugs with different mechanisms of action and non-overlapping toxicities would improve the cytotoxic effects in theory. Numerous studies have demonstrated the feasibility of triplet combinations, with some showing good tolerability and activity, but most randomized trials have not shown a survival advantage with this regimen. Triplets also carry greater toxicity, so they are not routinely recommended for advanced NSCLC.

Effective doublets in advanced NSCLC consist of a platinum agent in combination with paclitaxel or albumin-bound paclitaxel, docetaxel, gemcitabine, etoposide, or vinorelbine. Non-squamous NSCLC has the option of combining with pemetrexed.

The ECOG 4599 trial mentioned previously found better medial survival with BCP compared to carboplatin/paclitaxel alone, but this improvement was only seen with the

TABLE 15-3   Trials Comparing Third-Generation Doublets Versus Single Agents

AUTHOR	REGIMEN	NO. OF PATIENTS	RR	MEDIAN SURVIVAL	1-YEAR SURVIVAL
Georgoulias et al.[9]	Cisplatin/docetaxel	167	36%	10.5 mo	44%
	Docetaxel	152	22%	8.0 mo	43%
Lilenbaum et al.[118]	Carboplatin/paclitaxel	284	30%	8.8 mo	37%
	Paclitaxel	277	17%	6.7 mo	32%
Sederholm et al.[11]	Carboplatin/gemcitabine	164	30%	10.0 mo	40%
	Gemcitabine	170	11%	8.6 mo	32%

RR, response rate.

TABLE 15-4   Trials Comparing Third-Generation Doublets Versus Single-Agent Cisplatin

AUTHOR	REGIMEN	NO. OF PATIENTS	RR	MEDIAN SURVIVAL	1-YEAR SURVIVAL
Wozniak et al.[227]	Cisplatin/ vinorelbine	209	26%	8.0 mo	36%
	Cisplatin	206	12%	6.0 mo	20%
Gatzemeier et al.[228]	Cisplatin/ paclitaxel	207	26%	8.1 mo	30%
	Cisplatin	207	17%	8.6 mo	36%
Sandler et al.[92]	Cisplatin/ gemcitabine	260	30%	9.1 mo	39%
	Cisplatin	262	11%	7.6 mo	28%

RR, response rate.

adenocarcinoma histology; overall, there were more significant toxicities in the bevacizumab arm.[92] Another trial compared cisplatin/pemetrexed to cisplatin/gemcitabine in patients with stage IIIB or IV NSCLC. Those with adenocarcinoma or large cell carcinoma had improved survival with cisplatin/pemetrexed, while those with squamous cell carcinoma had improved survival with cisplatin/gemcitabine.[105]

COMMON PLATINUM-CONTAINING DOUBLETS

Platinum Agent	Second Agent	Third Agent
Cisplatin	Pemetrexed[a]	Bevacizumab[a]
Carboplatin	Paclitaxel/nab-paclitaxel	
	Docetaxel	
	Gemcitabine	
	Etoposide	
	Vinorelbine	

[a]Only for use in non-squamous histology.

Doublets not containing platinum may also be used, such as gemcitabine with docetaxel or vinorelbine. In patients with performance status 2 or greater, single-agent chemotherapy is also an option. These include single-agent paclitaxel, nab-paclitaxel, pemetrexed, docetaxel, or gemcitabine.

Nab-paclitaxel

Nab-paclitaxel is an albumin-bound form of paclitaxel whose active moiety is paclitaxel. It can be substituted for paclitaxel or docetaxel in patients who have hypersensitivity to either of these agents despite premedication or those who cannot receive premedications due to contraindications or other reasons. A trial comparing nab-paclitaxel/

carboplatin to normal paclitaxel/carboplatin showed the former had less neurotoxicity and an improved response rate, leading to its FDA approval.[106]

> **CLINICAL PEARL:** Nab-paclitaxel can be substituted for paclitaxel in patients with hypersensitivity to paclitaxel or docetaxel despite premedications.

MAINTENANCE THERAPY

Initial randomized studies did not show a survival difference with prolonged exposure to chemotherapy. One study randomized patients with advanced NSCLC to either 3 or 6 cycles of cisplatin, vinblastine, and mitomycin and found the median survival (6 months vs. 7 moths) and 1-year survival rates (22% vs. 25%, $p = .2$) were essentially the same.[15] Not surprisingly, the patients randomized to a shorter course of chemotherapy also had less fatigue, nausea, and vomiting. Another study also had similar median survival and 1-year survival data using a carboplatin/vinorelbine doublet (**Table 15-5**).[16]

However, more recent trials have challenged this and have shown a benefit with prolonged duration of therapy.

Maintenance therapy refers to continued systemic therapy for advanced NSCLC after the initial 4-6 cycles of first-line chemotherapy. Patients may only receive maintenance therapy if their disease has remained stable or responded to treatment. There are 2 kinds of maintenance therapy: continuation and switch.

Continuation maintenance refers to continuing with an agent that was already given in the first-line setting, for example, if a patient received cisplatin/pemetrexed initially for 4-6 cycles, then was continued on pemetrexed. This treatment is given until progression of disease or unacceptable toxicities. Both single-agent bevacizumab and single-agent pemetrexed are approved as maintenance therapies if used in the initial regimen.[107-109] The combination of bevacizumab/pemetrexed is also an option but is currently a category 2A recommendation according to NCCN guidelines. Patients who

TABLE 15-5	**Select Trials of Duration of Therapy for Advanced NSCLC**				
AUTHOR	REGIMEN	NO. OF PATIENTS	RR	MEDIAN SURVIVAL	1-YEAR SURVIVAL
Smith et al.[38]	MVP × 3 cycles	155	32%	6.0 mo	22%
	MVP × 6 cycles	153	38%	7.0 mo	25%
von Plessen et al.[229]	Carboplatin/ vinorelbine × 3 cycles	150	NR	6.5 mo	25%
	Carboplatin/ vinorelbine × 6 cycles	147	NR	7.4 mo	25%

MVP, mitomycin, vinblastine, cisplatin; NR, not reported; RR, response rate.

TABLE 15-6	Selected Trials of Maintenance Therapy for Advanced NSCLC			
AUTHOR	REGIMEN	TRIAL TYPE	MEDIAN SURVIVAL	*P* VALUE
Fidias et al.[111]	Carboplatin/gemcitabine × 4 cycles, followed by docetaxel when disease progression	Switch maintenance	9.1 mo	Not significant
	Carboplatin/gemcitabine × 4 cycles, followed by docetaxel immediately × 6 cycles		11.9 mo	
Ciuleanu et al.[110]	Platinum-based regimen × 4 cycles, followed placebo	Switch maintenance	10.6 mo	.012
	Platinum-based regimen × 4 cycles, followed by pemetrexed		13 mo	
Paz-Ares et al.[109]	Cisplatin/pemetrexed × 4 cycles, followed by placebo	Continuation maintenance	11 mo	.0195
	Cisplatin/pemetrexed × 4 cycles followed by pemetrexed		13.9 mo	

received the 4-drug regimen of ABCP may be continued on atezolizumab, bevacizumab, or both.[100] Similarly, patients who received platinum/pemetrexed/pembrolizumab may be continued on pembrolizumab/pemetrexed for maintenance (**Table 15-6**).[99]

Switch maintenance refers to starting a different agent that was not included in the first-line regimen after completing the initial cycles. Trials had shown improved PFS and OS when pemetrexed was started as switch maintenance after 4-6 cycles of initial therapy in patients with non-squamous NSCLC, leading to FDA approval of maintenance pemetrexed.[110] This is currently a category 2A recommendation for non-squamous histology, and docetaxel is a category 2B as switch maintenance in squamous cell carcinoma.[111]

> **CLINICAL PEARL:** In light of these trials, the FDA has approved switch maintenance therapy with pemetrexed or erlotinib and continuation maintenance with pemetrexed.

SUBSEQUENT THERAPY

Subsequent therapy for those with driver mutations is discussed in another section of this book. For all others, immune checkpoint inhibitors are preferred. These include nivolumab, pembrolizumab, or atezolizumab. If the patient still has progression of

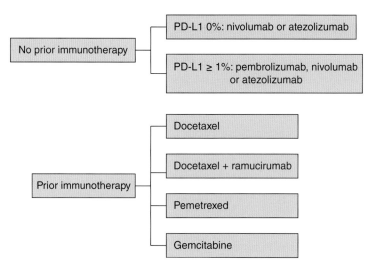

Figure 15-7. Subsequent treatment options in metastatic NSCLC without targetable mutations.

disease, however, switching to another immune checkpoint inhibitor is not routinely recommended.

For patients who progressed on first-line therapy with pembrolizumab, subsequent treatment with a platinum-based doublet such as carboplatin/paclitaxel is recommended. For those who progressed on PD-1/PD-L1 inhibitors or chemotherapy, subsequent therapy is with chemotherapy.

Docetaxel has shown improved survival and quality of life when compared to vinorelbine, ifosfamide, and BSC.[112,113] It can be used alone or in combination with ramucirumab, which is a recombinant monoclonal antibody targeting VEGF. The REVEL trial compared ramucirumab/docetaxel to docetaxel alone in patients with metastatic NSCLC who had progressed. The combination showed a slight increase in medial OS (10.5 vs. 9.1 months; HR 0.86, 95% CI 0.75-0.98, $p < .023$) and was approved in the second-line setting for progression on or after platinum-based chemotherapy.[114] Given its similarity to bevacizumab, ramucirumab also carries a risk of severe hemorrhage, gastrointestinal bleeding, gastrointestinal perforation or fistula, impaired wound healing, and poorly controlled hypertension. Last, gemcitabine and pemetrexed are also approved single-agent options for subsequent therapy (**Figure 15-7**).

TREATMENT OPTIONS AFTER PROGRESSION ON FIRST-LINE THERAPY	
Immune Checkpoint Inhibitors	**Chemotherapy**
Nivolumab	Docetaxel
Pembrolizumab	Docetaxel/ramucirumab
Atezolizumab	Gemcitabine
Pemetrexed	

ELDERLY PATIENTS

Treatment of elderly patients is challenging due to their multiple comorbidities, but studies have shown they derive similar benefits from chemotherapy as younger patients. A phase 3 study randomly assigned patients older than 70 years to either BSC or weekly vinorelbine and found that those in the vinorelbine cohort scored better on quality-of-life scales and had fewer symptoms from their lung cancer.[115] However, they also had more toxicity-related symptoms.

Still, there was a significant median survival of 28 weeks for the chemotherapy group vs. 21 weeks for the other. An international panel for treatment guidelines in elderly patients with NSCLC had recommended single-agent chemotherapy with a third-generation drug, but more recently, studies have shown that a platinum-based doublet was still superior to single-agent regimens in fit elderly patients despite the increased toxicities.[116]

The Francophone de Cancerologie Thoracique conducted a study with patients ages 70 to 89 with ECOG performance status of 0 to 2 who were randomly assigned to either carboplatin/paclitaxel or single-agent vinorelbine or gemcitabine.[117] Median OS was 10.3 months in the doublet arm compared to 6.2 months in the monotherapy arm (HR 0.64, 95% CI 0.62-0.78, $p < .0001$). Several subset analyses of other randomized trials found that older patients who received a platinum-based regimen had more treatment-related toxicities but overall had similar response rates and survival as compared to those for younger patients. Thus, age alone should not preclude patients from receiving appropriate treatment regimens.

> **CLINICAL PEARL:** Chemotherapy should still be offered to fit elderly patients who are able to tolerate treatment.

POOR PERFORMANCE STATUS

Patients with poor performance status (ECOG 2, 3, or 4) generally are less tolerant of treatment and have significantly shorter survival rates. Nevertheless, subset analyses suggest that patients with a performance status of 2 may still have a modest benefit from treatment, with studies favoring a doublet over a single agent if possible. The Cancer and Leukemia Group B (CALGB) 9730 trial randomized patients to single-agent paclitaxel versus carboplatin/paclitaxel.[118] Patients with performance status (PS) of 2 did significantly worse than those with PS of 0 or 1, but of the patients with PS of 2, those treated with the doublet had a better survival rate than those treated with paclitaxel alone (median survival 4.7 months vs .2.4 months; 1-year survival = 18% vs. 10%; $p = .0016$). Another trial involving patients with Zubrod performance status of 2 compared carboplatin (AUC 5)/pemetrexed to pemetrexed alone and found improved median OS with the doublet compared to monotherapy (9.3 months vs. 5.3 months; $p = .001$).[119] Thus, patients with ECOG 2 may still derive benefit from a doublet regimen, though treatment will depend on clinical judgment.

IMMUNOTHERAPY FOR METASTATIC NON–SMALL CELL LUNG CANCER

Moises Harari Turquie, MD, Jose Pinto Llerena, MD, Gil Bazo, MD, Edgardo S. Santos, MD

One year after receiving treatment for a stage III adenocarcinoma of the lung, a 70-year-old male is found to have liver nodules. Core biopsy of one of the nodules was positive for adenocarcinoma of the lung primary. Next-generation sequencing revealed no actionable biomarkers. Immunohistochemistry (IHC) of the patient's tumor expressed a PD-L1 TPS of greater than 50%.

Learning Objectives:

1. Describe the role of PD-L1 TPS and tumor mutation burden in the treatment selection for patients with advanced NSCLC.
2. Compare the tolerability of immunotherapy versus systemic chemotherapy for patients with metastatic NSCLC.
3. Study the current first-line immunotherapy treatment options for patients with metastatic NSCLC

Monoclonal antibodies against PD-1 and PD-L1 have changed the treatment paradigm in NSCLC since their first approval in 2015 by the USFDA, when nivolumab received granted approval for patients with metastatic NSCLC after progression on or after platinum-based chemotherapy.[120]

PD-1 is an inducible protein through T-cell receptors and cytokine receptors; it is expressed on the surface of all activated T cells, B cells, and natural killer cells. PD-1 regulates lymphocyte activation in lymphoid tissue, thereby controlling the magnitude of T-cell response during initiation and reactivation of the immune response, functioning as checkpoints to protect against self-reactivity.[121] PD-L1 is expressed on antigen-presenting cells (APCs), induced by pro-inflammatory cytokines, including interferon 1 and 2, tumor necrosis factor α, and VEGF. Another ligand, PD-L2, is expressed on dendritic cells and macrophages induced by previous cytokines.[122]

Checkpoint inhibitors such as anti–PD-1 and PD-L1 antibodies have shown OS in both common lung cancer histologies adenocarcinoma and squamous cell carcinoma. This section of the chapter is dedicated to discussing and analyzing the evolution of these novel agents in the metastatic setting and how much we have to learn from monotherapy in second-line to single-agent or combo chemoimmunotherapy in first-line treatment for NSCLC. Due to improved OS over conventional cytotoxic chemotherapy as well as their relatively low-toxicity profile other than immune-related adverse events (ir-AEs), currently the immune-oncology approach has displaced chemotherapy to a place further down in the treatment algorithm of NSCLC. To make it easier for the reader, we start our review based on approval granted by the US FDA for each individual compound, and we discuss the initial clinical trials that granted approval by regulatory entities followed by the latest clinical trial in first-line therapy for patients with metastatic NSCLC.

NIVOLUMAB

Nivolumab was the first drug to be approved by the US FDA for the treatment of metastatic NSCLC with progression of disease after platinum-based chemotherapy. Nivolumab is an immunoglobulin (Ig) G4 monoclonal antibody that has high affinity for the PD-1 receptor, blocking its interaction between ligands (PDL-1 and PDL-2), preventing T-cell inhibition. Nivolumab has been involved in multiple trials as first-line therapy in patients with metastatic NSCLC and as second- or third-line treatments following platinum-based chemotherapy (**Table 15-7**).

Second- or Third-Line Treatment: CheckMate 057 Trial

The CheckMate 057 phase 3 randomized controlled trial (RCT) involved patients with advanced NSCLC who progressed during or after platinum-based chemotherapy.[123] Patients were randomized to receive either nivolumab or docetaxel, a chemotherapy still used as a "control arm" in second-line treatment for NSCLC. Patients with documented stage IIIB or IV and recurrent NSCLC following chemotherapy or radiotherapy and good ECOG performance status (0-1) were included in this trial. A total of 582 patients underwent randomization; 292 received nivolumab (3 mg/kg) and 290 docetaxel (75 mg/m^2). Median age was 62 years, and minimum follow-up for OS was 13.2 months. Seventy-nine percent of patients reported current or former smoking status. PD-L1 protein expression was evaluated retrospectively and was further subclassified regarding specific expression levels in 1%, 5%, and 10% or higher. This study met its primary endpoint: OS.

TABLE 15-7	Randomized Clinical Trials Comparing Nivolumab in Patients With Stage IV NSCLC as Either First-Line Treatment or Second or Third Lines					
RTC	N	DESIGN	ORR %	MEDIAN PFS (MONTHS)	AE (GRADE 3 OR 4)
Brahmer et al. Checkmate 017[124]	272	Nivolumab 3 mg/kg every 2 weeks vs. docetaxel 75 mg/m^2 every 3 weeks	20% (95% CI 14-28) vs. 9% (95% CI 5-15)	3.5 (95% CI 2.1-4.9) vs. 2.8 (95% CI 2.1-3.5)	7% vs. 55%
Carbone et al. Checkmate 026[126]	423	Nivolumab 3 mg/kg IV every 2 weeks vs. PDC every 3 weeks	26% vs. 33%	4.2 vs. 5.9 (95% CI 0.91-1.45)	18 % vs. 51%
Borghaei et al. Checkmate 057[123]	582	Nivolumab 3 mg/kg every 2 weeks vs. docetaxel 75 mg/m^2 every 3 weeks	19% (95% CI 15-24) vs. 12% (95% CI 9-17)	2.3 (95% CI 2.2-3.3) vs. 4.2 (95% CI 3.5-4.9)	10% vs. 54%
Hellman et al. Checkmate 227[127]	1,739	Nivolumab 3 mg/kg every 2 weeks plus ipilimumab 1 mg/kg every 6 weeks vs. PDC	45.3% vs. 26.9%	7.2 (95% CI 5.5-13.2) vs. 5.5 (95% CI 4.4-5.8)	31.2% vs. 36.1%

The OS was significantly longer during interim analysis, reporting a median OS of 12.2 months (95% CI 9.7-15) in the nivolumab group, in contrast to 9.4 months (95% CI 8.1-10.7) with docetaxel. The OS rate at 12 months was 51% (95% CI 45-56) with nivolumab versus 39% (95% CI 33-45) in the docetaxel group, and at 18 months, it was 39% (95% CI 34-45) with nivolumab and 23% (95% CI 19-28) with docetaxel. In a subgroup analysis, nivolumab was not favored in third-line therapy, CNS metastases, never-smoked status, and EGFR-positive status. The ORR was higher with nivolumab in comparison with docetaxel, 19% versus 12%, $p = .002$. PFS was 2.3 months (95% CI 2.2-3.3) with nivolumab and 4.2 months (95% CI 3.5-4.9) in the docetaxel group. Regarding PD-L1 expression, 78% of the patients ($n = 455$) had PD-L1 expression; nivolumab was associated with longer PFS, OS, and higher ORR than docetaxel, with PDL-1 expression levels of 1%, 5%, and 10% or higher.[123]

In terms of TRAEs, including grades 3 and 4, they were less prevalent in the nivolumab group than in the docetaxel group (7% to 20% any grade adverse effect, 5% to 18% grade 3 to 4) with median time of onset from 0.9 to 31.1 weeks in the nivolumab group. Eleven percent to 70% of ir-AEs were treated with glucocorticoids. Pneumonitis was the most common treatment-related serious adverse events (TRSAEs), which led to discontinuation of therapy in the nivolumab group.

CheckMate 017 Trial

The CheckMate 017 phase 3, open-label trial compared nivolumab monotherapy with docetaxel single-agent therapy in patients with advanced squamous cell NSCLC after progression with platinum chemotherapy.[5] Inclusion criteria were patients with stage IIIB or IV squamous cell NSCLC histology, disease recurrence after 1 prior platinum-containing regimen, and stable brain metastatic disease. A total of 227 patients underwent randomization; 135 patients were randomly assigned to receive nivolumab (3 mg/kg) every 2 weeks, and 137 patients were to receive docetaxel (75 mg/m^2) every 3 weeks. PD-L1 expression was evaluated retrospectively and categorized in levels of 1%, 5%, or 10% of cells. The median age of the patients was 63 years; most patients had ECOG performance status score 1, stage IV, and were current or former smokers. Median follow-up was 11 months. The median OS was 9.2 months (95% CI 7.3-13.3) in the nivolumab group, in contrast to 6.0 months (95% CI 5.1-7.3) in the docetaxel group. OS was significantly better in favor of nivolumab, with a risk of death of 41% (HR 0.59, $p < .001$). The OS rate at 1 year was 42% (95% CI 34-50) in the nivolumab group versus 24% (95% CI 17-31) in the docetaxel group. HRs for death favored nivolumab across all subgroups except in the rest of the world region (Argentina, Australia, Chile, Mexico, and Peru) and in those 75 years or older. The ORR was significantly higher with nivolumab versus docetaxel (20% vs., 9%, $p = .008$). The PFS was 3.5 months (95% CI 2.1-4.9) in the nivolumab group and 2.8 months (95% CI 2.1-3.5) in the docetaxel group. The HR for death or disease progression was 0.62 ($p < .001$). The rate of PFS at 1 year in the nivolumab group was 21% versus 6% in the docetaxel group. Regarding PD-L1 expression, it was quantifiable in 83% of the patients and across the prespecified expression levels (1%, 5%, and 10%). PD-L1 was neither prognostic nor predictive of OS and PFS.

The TRAEs were less frequent with nivolumab than with docetaxel. Grades 3 and 4 were less prevalent in the nivolumab group than for docetaxel (58% vs. 86% any grade

AE, 7% to 55% grade 3 to 4). The most frequently reported TRAEs of any grade were hypothyroidism (4% nivolumab vs. 0% docetaxel), diarrhea (8% vs. 20%), pneumonitis (5% vs. 0%), and rash (4% to 6%).

The TRAEs that led to discontinuation of treatment were less frequent in the nivolumab group than in the docetaxel group (3% vs. 10%, respectively); the most common AE per group was pneumonitis in the nivolumab group and fatigue in the docetaxel group.[124]

Recently, investigators of CheckMate 057 and 017 reported a 3-year follow-up on these studies. After a 40.3-month follow-up, nivolumab continued to show an OS benefit versus docetaxel: estimated 3-year OS rates were 17% (95% CI 14%-21%) versus 8% (95% CI 6%-11%) in the pooled population with non-squamous or squamous NSCLC. It is noteworthy that there were no new safety concerns identified. A total of 193 patients of 854 randomized patients across both studies had baseline liver metastases; nivolumab improved OS compared with docetaxel in patients with liver metastases (HR 0.68, 95% CI 0.50-0.91). This finding is consistent with the OS reported from the overall pooled study population (HR 0.70, 95% CI 0.61-0.81).[125]

NIVOLUMAB AS FRONT-LINE THERAPY

CheckMate 026 Trial

In the CheckMate 026 clinical trial, 423 patients with untreated stage IV or recurrent NSCLC with PD-L1 tumor expression greater than 1% were randomized to receive either nivolumab- or platinum-based chemotherapy. Nivolumab was not associated with significantly longer PFS than chemotherapy among patients with a PD-L1 expression level of 5% or more. OS was similar between groups.[126]

CheckMate 227 Trial

The CheckMate 227 study is very important and innovative as it brought to the table a novel and potential biomarker: TMB.[127] The CheckMate 227 trial has shown that the combination of nivolumab plus ipilimumab, a cytotoxic T-lymphocyte–associated protein 4 (CTLA4) inhibitor, significantly prolonged PFS versus chemotherapy among untreated patients with stage IV or recurrent NSCLC with high TMB regardless of PD-L1 expression. The analysis included 139 patients treated with nivolumab/ipilimumab (nivolumab 3 mg/kg every 2 weeks plus ipilimumab 1 mg/kg every 6 weeks) and 160 patients who received chemotherapy; randomization in 2 groups of TMB, < 10 and ≥ 10 mutations/megabase. As mentioned, these patients were treatment-naïve and negative for sensitizing *EGFR* or *ALK* mutations.

Chemotherapy consisted of pemetrexed plus cisplatin or carboplatin, with optional pemetrexed maintenance in patients with non-squamous histology and gemcitabine plus cisplatin or carboplatin in patients with squamous histology. Those patients with a level of PD-L1 expression of at least 1% or above were randomly assigned in a 1:1:1 ratio to receive nivolumab plus ipilimumab, nivolumab monotherapy, or chemotherapy; those with a tumor PD-L1 expression level of less than 1% were randomly assigned in a 1:1:1 ratio to receive nivolumab plus ipilimumab, nivolumab plus chemotherapy, or chemotherapy. Co-primary endpoints were PFS and OS. Minimum follow-up was

11.2 months. Median PFS was 7.2 months in the nivolumab/ipilimumab group versus 5.5 months in the chemotherapy group (HR 0.58, p < .001), with 12-month rates of 42.6% versus 13.2%, respectively. Among 213 patients with PD-L1 expression of 1% or greater, the HR was 0.62 (95% CI 0.44-0.88). Among 86 patients with PD-L1 expression less than 1%, the HR was 0.48 (95% CI 0.27-0.85). Among 101 patients with squamous histology, the HR was 0.63 (95% CI 0.39-1.04). For those patients with non-squamous histology (n = 199), the HR was 0.55 (95% CI 0.38-0.80). The ORR was 45.3% in the nivolumab/ipilimumab group versus 26.9% for the chemotherapy group. Median DOR was not reached versus 5.4 months, with an ongoing response of more than 1 year observed in 68% of the nivolumab/ipilimumab group versus 25% in the chemotherapy patients. Among 380 patients with low TMB (<10 mutations/megabase) receiving either treatment in the trial, median PFS was 3.2 months in the nivolumab/ipilimumab patients versus 5.5 months in the chemotherapy group (HR 1.07, 95% CI 0.84-1.35).[127]

In terms of the safety profile, grade 3 or 4 TRAEs occurred in 31.2% of the nivolumab/ipilimumab group (n = 576 patients) versus 36.1% of the chemotherapy group (n = 570 patients), and TRSAEs occurred in 24.0% versus 13.9%, respectively. The most common ir-AEs in the nivolumab/ipilimumab group were skin reactions (32.4%), with the most common grade 3 or 4 events being hepatic events (8.0%). TRAEs led to discontinuation of treatment in 17.4% versus 8.9% of the patients, respectively. AEs led to death in 7 patients (1.2%) in the nivolumab/ipilimumab group (due to pneumonitis in 3 and 1 each with myocarditis, acute tubular necrosis, circulatory collapse, and cardiac tamponade) and in 6 patients (1.1%) in the chemotherapy group (due to sepsis in 2 and 1 each with multiple brain infarctions, interstitial lung disease, thrombocytopenia, and febrile neutropenia with sepsis).[127]

The other co-primary endpoint of this trial, OS, is not mature and is eagerly awaited. The current data of CheckMate 227 demonstrated that the nivolumab plus ipilimumab combination is superior than combination chemotherapy in terms of PFS in patients with TMB of more than 10 mutations/megabase.

PEMBROLIZUMAB

The second checkpoint inhibitor approved by the US FDA for lung cancer was pembrolizumab on October 2015. The initial approval was for patients with advanced/metastatic NSCLC whose disease had progressed after other treatments and with tumors that expressed PD-L1 analyzed via its companion diagnostic test, IHC 22C3. Pembrolizumab is a highly selective IgG4 monoclonal antibody against PD-1 that binds to the PD-1 receptor and inhibits its interaction with ligands PD-L1 and PD-L2, resulting in tumor recognition by T cells.

PEMBROLIZUMAB AS SECOND-LINE THERAPY OR BEYOND
KEYNOTE-001 Trial

The KEYNOTE-001 trial evaluated the safety, antitumor activity, and side effects of pembrolizumab in patients with advanced NSCLC.[128] Inclusion criteria included patients who had locally advanced or metastatic NSCLC and ECOG performance status of 0-1. The study also looked to evaluate efficacy in patients with previously treated NSCLC with high expression of PD-L1 levels. A total of 495 patients were assigned to receive pembrolizumab at a dose of 2 mg/kg or 10 mg/kg every 3 weeks or 10 mg/kg every 2 weeks in the training group (182 patients) or validation group (313 patients). PD-L1 positivity was defined as staining in at least 1% (TPS) of cells within tumor nests or a distinctive staining pattern. Tumor response was assessed every 9 weeks via imaging. PD-L1 expression in at least 50% of tumor cells was selected as a cutoff for the training group.[128]

The ORR was 19.4% (95 CI% 16-23.2), including a response rate of 18% (95% CI 14.4-22.2) in 394 previously treated patients and 24.8% (95% CI 16.7-34.3) in the 101 previously untreated patients. The response rate was similar regardless of dose, schedule, and histologic analysis. At the time of analysis, 84.4% patients had no disease progression, with a median DOR of 12.5 months in all patients.[128] Median PFS was 3.7 months (95% CI 2.9-4.1), and median OS was 12 months (95% CI 9.3-14.7) for all patients. The response rate was 45.2% (95% CI 33.5-57.3) in 73 patients with a TPS of at least 50%, and among all patients with a TPS of at least 50%, median PFS was 6.3 months. The median OS was not reached (**Table 15-7**).

Treatment-related adverse events occurred in 351 patients (70.9%) with no clear difference according to dose or schedule; the most common AEs included fatigue, pruritus, and decreased appetite. Grade 3 or higher AEs were reported in 9.5% of patients. Ir-AEs occurred in more than 2% of patients and presented as infusion-related reaction (3%), hypothyroidism (6.9%), and pneumonitis (3.6%).

KEYNOTE-010 Trial

The KEYNOTE-010 trial was a multicenter, open-label, phase 2/3 trial that evaluated pembrolizumab at a dose of 2 mg/kg or 10 mg/kg every 3 weeks versus docetaxel 75 mg/m^2 every 3 weeks for PD-L1-positive NSCLC that progressed after platinum-based chemotherapy.[129] Patients enrolled in this trial were at least 18 years old with progression of disease after 2 or more cycles of platinum-doublet chemotherapy and appropriate TKI on patients with *EGFR* mutation or *ALK* gene rearrangement, ECOG performance status 0-1, and PD-L1 expression of at least 1% TPS. Patients with previous treatment with PD-L1 inhibitor, brain metastases or carcinomatous meningitis, autoimmune disease on glucocorticoid treatment, and interstitial lung disease history of pneumonitis were excluded. Radiographic imaging was performed every 9 weeks, and response was assessed as per response criteria in solid tumors (RECIST) version 1.1. Primary outcomes were OS and PFS in the intent-to-treat (ITT) population and in patients with TPS of 50% or more. A total of 1,034 patients were enrolled; 345 received pembrolizumab at 2 mg/kg, 346 received pembrolizumab at 10 mg/kg, and 343 were allocated to a docetaxel arm. Most patients were current or former smokers, had non-squamous histology, and received one line of previous systemic treatment; few patients had *EGFR*-mutant or *ALK*-translocated tumors. PD-L1 TPS was referred as 1%-49% or more than 50% and evenly divided in the previous patient groups. Median follow-up was 13.1 months at the time of cutoff. At cutoff, median OS was 10.4 months with pembrolizumab at 2 mg/kg, 12.7 months with pembrolizumab at 10 mg/kg, and 8.5 months with docetaxel. The HR for pembrolizumab at 2 mg/kg versus docetaxel was 0.71 (95% CI 0.58-0.88, p = .0008), and the HR comparing pembrolizumab at 10 mg/kg versus docetaxel was 0.61 (95% CI 0.49-0.75, p < .0001). OS was similar in the 2 pembrolizumab groups in patients with PD-L1 TPS of 50% or higher (2 mg/kg vs. 10 mg/kg; HR 1.12, 95% CI 0.77-1.62). The PFS was longer with pembrolizumab at 2 mg/kg compared to docetaxel in patients with TPS of 50% or greater with a HR 0.59 (95% CI 0.44-0.78, p = .0001) and pembrolizumab at 10 mg/kg (95% CI 0.45-0.78, p < .0001) versus docetaxel. For the entire population, PFS was not statistically significant and did not differ by tumor histology (Table 15-7).[129]

Among patients with TPS of 50% or greater, median OS was significantly longer with pembrolizumab at 2 mg/kg than with docetaxel (14.9 months vs. 8.2 months, p = .0002) and pembrolizumab at 10 mg/kg than with docetaxel (17.3 months vs. 8.2 months, p < .0001). Grade 3-5 AEs occurred in 43 (13%) patients in the pembrolizumab group at 2 mg/kg, in 55(16%) patients in the pembrolizumab group at 10 mg/kg, and in 109 (35%) patients assigned to the docetaxel group. In the setting of ir-AEs, the most common ones were hypothyroidism, hyperthyroidism, and pneumonitis.[129]

PEMBROLIZUMAB AS FRONT-LINE THERAPY
Pembrolizumab as Monotherapy
KEYNOTE-024 Trial

KEYNOTE-010 was the platform to launch the KEYNOTE-024 trial; it included only patients with TPS ≥ 50%; this open-label, randomized, phase 3 trial compared pembrolizumab at 200 mg (flat dose) every 3 weeks with the investigator's choice of platinum-based chemotherapy as first-line treatment for patients with NSCLC with high-expression PD-L1, defined by a TPS score of 50% or greater.[96] Patients enrolled in this trial were 18 years or older, had histological or cytological confirmation of stage IV NSCLC with no *EGFR* mutations or *ALK* translocations, were naïve to systemic therapy for metastatic disease, had an ECOG PS of 0-1, and had a life expectancy of at least 3 months. Patients receiving systemic glucocorticoids or immunosuppressive therapy, untreated brain metastases, interstitial lung disease, or history of pneumonitis were excluded. Patients were randomly assigned in a 1:1 ratio to receive either pembrolizumab at 200 mg every 3 weeks for 35 cycles or the investigator's choice of 1 of 5 platinum-based chemotherapy regimens for 4-6 cycles (carboplatin plus pemetrexed, cisplatin plus pemetrexed, carboplatin plus gemcitabine, cisplatin plus gemcitabine, or carboplatin plus paclitaxel). Pemetrexed regimens were permitted only for patients who had non-squamous tumors. Those patients who did undergo chemotherapy, at disease progression could cross over to receive pembrolizumab. Imaging studies were obtained every 9 weeks, and response to treatment was assessed according to RECIST. The primary endpoint was PFS; OS, ORR, and safety were secondary endpoints. Median duration of follow-up was 11.2 months. In the chemotherapy group, 66 patients (43.7%) crossed over to pembrolizumab after disease progression.

Median PFS was 10.3 months (95% CI 6.7-not reached) in the pembrolizumab group and 6.0 months (95% CI 4.2-6.2) in the chemotherapy group. PFS was significantly longer in the pembrolizumab group than in the chemotherapy group (HR 0.50, p < .001). Regarding OS, there was a 40% decrease in mortality in favor of the pembrolizumab group (HR 0.60, p = .0050).[96] The ORR was 44.8% (95% CI 36.-53.0) in the pembroli-zumab group and 27.8% (95% CI 20.8-35.7) in the chemotherapy group, with a median time of response of 2.2 months in both groups. Median DOR was not reached in the pembrolizumab group and was 6.3 months in the chemotherapy group. In terms of tox-icity, TRAEs occurred in 73.4% of patients in the pembrolizumab group and 90.0% in the chemotherapy group; grade 3 to 5 AEs were reported as much as twice as often in the chemotherapy group versus the pembrolizumab group (53.3% vs. 26.6%, respectively). The most common grade 3, 4, or 5 AEs reported in the pembrolizumab group were diarrhea (3.9%) and pneumonitis (2.6%). ir-AEs occurred in 29.2% of the patients in the pembrolizumab group versus 4.7% in the chemotherapy group; grade 3 to 4 ir-AES were severe skin reactions (3.9%), pneumonitis (2.6%), and colitis (1.3%) (**Table 15-8**).[96]

> **CLINICAL PEARL:** KEYNOTE-024 became a change in practice in 2016 after its presentation at the European Society of Medical Oncology (ESMO) Congress. For the first time ever, patients with NSCLC had an opportunity to receive immunotherapy as a first-line treatment if their tumors expressed TPS ≥ 50%; clinicians were able to discuss with patients 3 potential therapeutic options, depending on their tumors' phenotype in the front-line setting: targeted therapy, immunotherapy, or systemic chemotherapy.

KEYNOTE-042 Trial

In an attempt to offer an immunotherapy front line as monotherapy for patients whose tumors have a PD-L1 TPS of 50% greater, the KEYNOTE-042 study was designed. By the time this study was presented, there were 2 standards of care already established for non-squamous NSCLC histology: (1) single-agent pembrolizumab if PD-L1 TPS was 50% or greater and (2) pembrolizumab plus carboplatin/pemetrexed for all non-squamous NSCLC regardless of PD-L1 TPS. In June 2018, at the American Society of Clinical Oncology (ASCO) annual meeting, Lopes et al. presented the data for patients who had TPS of 1% or greater treated with pembrolizumab alone versus systemic chemo-therapy in this randomized clinical trial. Eligible patients (n = 1,274) were randomized 1:1 to 35 or fewer cycles of pembrolizumab at 200 mg every 3 weeks or the investigator's choice of 6 or fewer cycles of carboplatin/paclitaxel or carboplatin/pemetrexed dou-blet with optional pemetrexed maintenance in non-squamous histology only.[130] One of the stratification factors was TPS (≥50% vs. 1%-49%). Primary endpoints were OS in patients with TPS of 50% or greater, 20% or greater, and 1% or greater.

The OS differences were assessed sequentially using the stratified log-rank test. Dis-tribution of the TPS group was as follows: 599 (47.0%) patients had TPS of 50% or greater, 818 (64.2%) of patients had a TPS of 20% or greater. After a 12.8-month median follow-up, 13.7% were still on pembrolizumab, and 4.9% were receiving pemetrexed maintenance. Pembrolizumab significantly improved OS in patients with TPS of 50% or greater (HR = 0.69), TPS of 20% or greater (HR = 0.77), and TPS of 1% or greater (HR= 0.81).[131] In terms of toxicity, grade 3 to 5 TRAEs were less frequent with pembrolizumab (17.8% vs. 41.0%).

TABLE 15-8 Randomized Controlled Trials Comparing Pembrolizumab in Patients With Stage IV

RCT	N	DESIGN	ORR %	MEDIAN PFS (MONTHS)	MEDIAN OS (MONTHS)	AE (GRADE 3 OR 4)
Garon et al. KEYNOTE 001[128]	495	Pembrolizumab 2 mg/kg or 10 mg/kg every 3 weeks or 10 mg/kg every 2 weeks	19.4% (95 CI% 16-23.2)	3.7 (95% CI 2.9-4.1)	12 (95% CI 9.3-14.7)	9.5%
Herbst et al. KEYNOTE 10[129]	1,034	Pembrolizumab 2mg/kg[+] or 10 mg/kg[^] q3w vs docetaxel 75 mg/m² [~]q3w	[+]18% (95% CI 14.1-22.5) [^]18.5% (95% CI 14.5-23) [~]9.3% (95% CI 6.5-12.9)	[+]3.9 (95% CI 3.1-4.1) [^]4.0 (95% CI 2.7-4.3) [~]4.0 (95% CI 3.1-4.2)	[+]10.4 (95% CI 9.4-11.9) [^]12.7 (95% CI 10.0-17.3) [~]8.5 (95% CI 7.5-9.8)	[+]13%, [^]16%, [~]35%.
Mok et al. KEYNOTE 042[97]	1,274	Pembrolizumab 200 mg q3w vs PDC		7.1 (95 CI 5.9-9.0) vs 6.4 (6.1-6.9)	**TPS 50%** 20.0 (95% CI 4-24.9) vs 12.2 (95% CI 10.4-14.2) **TPS 20%** 17.7 (95% CI 15.3- 22.1) vs 13 (11.6-15.3)	18% vs 41%
Reck et al. KEYNOTE 024[96]	305	Pembrolizumab 200 mg q3w vs investigator's choice platinum-base chemotherapy	44.8% (95% CI 36.8-53.0) vs 27.8% (95% CI 20.8-35.7)	10.3 (95% CI 6.7-not reached) vs 6.0 (95% CI 4.2-6.2)	80.2 (95% CI 72.9-85.7) 72.4 (95% CI 64.5-78.9)	26.6 % vs 53.3%
Borghaei et al. KEYNOTE 021 (G)[132]	123	Pembrolizumab 200 mg q3w +/– Carboplatin 5 mg/mL + pemetrexed 500 mg/m² q3w	56.7% vs 30.2%	24.0 (8.5-NR) vs 9.3 (6.2-14.9)	NR (24.5-NR) vs 21.1 (14.9-NR)	27.4% vs 40.7%
Gandhi et al. KEYNOTE 189[99]	616	PDC + Pembrolizumab vs PDC + Placebo	69.2% (95% CI 64.1-73.8) vs 49.4% (95% CI 42.1-56.2)	8.8 (95% CI 7.6-9.2) vs 4.9 (95% CI 4.7-5.5)	Not reached vs 11.3 (95% CI 8.7-15.1)	67.2% vs 65.8%
Paz-Ares et al. KEYNOTE 407[101]	559	Pembrolizumab 200 mg q3w + carboplatin/ Placlitaxel vs carboplatin/ nab-paclitaxel	57.9% (95% CI 51.9-63.8) vs 38.4% (95% CI 32.7-44.4)	6.4 (95% CI 9.5-14.8) vs 4.8 (95% CI 4.3-5.7)	15.9 (95% CI 13.2-NR) vs 11.3 (95% CI 9.5-14.8)	69.8% vs 68.2%

Although authors of KEYNOTE-042 concluded that this study is the first one demonstrating superiority in OS using pembrolizumab monotherapy over platinum-based chemotherapy in chemo-naïve patients without *EGFR* or *ALK* alterations and PDL-1 of 1% or greater, their exploratory analysis in patients with TPS 1%-49% showed a median OS of 13.4 months for pembrolizumab monotherapy versus 12.1 months for the chemotherapy group (HR = 0.92, CI 0.77-1.11); this is of concern because it raises the possibility that clinical gain seen in this trial for patients with TPS of 1% or greater was driven by those patients whose TPS was 50% or greater. Moreover, results from this last group underperformed those results seen in KEYNOTE-024 and KEYNOTE-189 clinical trials, which are described in the next section.[131]

On April 11, 2019, the US FDA approved pembrolizumab for the first-line treatment of patients with stage III NSCLC who were not candidates for surgical resection or definitive chemoradiation or metastatic NSCLC meanwhile their tumors do not harbor *EGFR* or *ALK* genomic aberrations and express PD-L1 TPS of 1% or greater based on the data from the KEYNOTE-042 trial.

Pembrolizumab in Combination With Chemotherapy
KEYNOTE-021 Cohort G

Prior to the approval of pembrolizumab in combination with a platinum-based doublet using pemetrexed for non-squamous NSCLC, the US FDA granted conditional approval for this therapeutic approach in May 2017 based on the results presented from the KEYNOTE-021 Cohort G, a phase 1/2 clinical trial.[98] The KEYNOTE-021 study (NCT02039674) evaluated pembrolizumab plus carboplatin and pemetrexed versus carboplatin/pemetrexed doublet in first-line therapy for advanced non-squamous NSCLC. Patients with previously untreated stage IIIB/IV non-squamous NSCLC without *EGFR* mutation or *ALK* translocation were randomized 1:1 to receive either 4 cycles of carboplatin AUC 5 mg/mL/min plus pemetrexed at 500 mg/m^2 every 3 weeks with or without pembrolizumab at 200 mg flat doses every 3 weeks for 2 years (maintenance pemetrexed was allowed in both arms). Eligible patients with radiologic disease progression could cross over from carboplatin/pemetrexed to pembrolizumab monotherapy. The response was assessed by blinded independent central review (BICR) per RECIST. The primary endpoint was ORR; PFS and OS were secondary endpoints. In a recent update by Borghaei et al., the triplet combination of chemoimmunotherapy significantly improved PFS and ORR with pembrolizumab plus carboplatin/pemetrexed versus carboplatin/pemetrexed alone; hence, the primary analyses observed previously were maintained. The HR for OS with a 24-month median follow-up was 0.56, favoring the chemoimmunotherapy group.[132] To dissect the results of this important trial, as of December 1, 2017, the median follow-up time was 23.9 months. The ORR was 56.7% with chemoimmunotherapy versus 30.2% with carboplatin/pemetrexed alone (estimated difference 26.4% [95% CI 8.9%-42.4%, *p* = .0016]). The PFS was also significantly improved with the embrolizumab/carboplatin/pemetrexed triplet over chemotherapy alone (HR 0.53, 95% CI 0.33-0.86, *p* = .0049).[132]

KEYNOTE-189 Trial

Clinicians were allowed to use the pembrolizumab plus a carboplatin/pemetrexed combo in the United States based on KEYNOTE-021 Cohort G results, while the KEYNOTE-189 clinical trial was still enrolling. In the 2018 American Association for Cancer Research (AACR) congress held in Chicago, Illinois, Dr. Gandhi et al. presented the final results of this double-blind, placebo-controlled, phase 3 trial.[99] Randomization was at a 2:1 ratio; 616 patients with metastatic non-squamous NSCLC without sensitizing *EGFR* or *ALK* mutations and no prior therapy for metastatic disease were randomized to receive either carboplatin/pemetrexed doublet therapy plus either 200 mg of pembrolizumab or placebo every 3 weeks for 4 cycles, followed by pembrolizumab or placebo for up to a total of 35 cycles plus pemetrexed maintenance therapy. Crossover was allowed for those patients who progressed on placebo. The primary endpoints were OS and PFS, which were assessed by BICR. At 12 months, the estimated OS was 69.2% (95% CI 64.1-73.8) in the pembrolizumab/carboplatin/pemetrexed triplet group versus 49.4% (95% CI 42.1-56.2) in the placebo-combination group ("chemotherapy" alone). The HR for death was 0.49 (95% CI 0.38-0.64, $p < .001$). It is noteworthy that the OS improved across all PD-L1 categories (<1%, 1%-49%, >50%). The median PFS was 8.8 months (95% CI 7.6-9.2) in the chemoimmunotherapy group and 4.9 months (95% CI 4.7-5.5) in the chemotherapy-alone arm. The HR for the PFS was 0.52 (95% CI 0.43-0.64, $p < .001$).[99] AEs of grade 3 or higher were similar in both groups (67.2% and 65.8% for the chemoimmunotherapy and chemotherapy arms, respectively).

> **CLINICAL PEARL:** KEYNOTE-189 established a new standard of care, and a change in clinical practice was rapidly adopted by regulatory entities. For previously untreated metastatic non-squamous NSCLC and the absence of *EGFR* and *ALK* mutations, the triplet of pembrolizumab/carboplatin/pemetrexed followed by maintenance therapy with pemetrexed/pembrolizumab can be given to all patients regardless of PD-L1 TPS as this approach improves OS, PFS, and ORR.[99]

KEYNOTE-407 Clinical Trial

Until the 2018 ASCO annual meeting, pembrolizumab in combination with chemotherapy was only approved for non-squamous NSCLC histology. Paz-Ares et al. presented the results of the landmark KEYNOTE-407 study, which investigated the efficacy and impact of combining pembrolizumab with conventional chemotherapy in patients with squamous NSCLC histology. Pembrolizumab was combined with carboplatin/paclitaxel or carboplatin/nab-paclitaxel and compared against these 2 regimens themselves. A total of 559 patients with metastatic squamous NSCLC and not previously treated with systemic therapy were randomized. The dual primary endpoints were PFS and OS, and secondary endpoints included ORR and DOR.[101]

In this study, the pembrolizumab plus chemotherapy significantly improved OS, reducing the risk of death by 36% compared to chemotherapy alone (HR 0.64, 95% CI 0.49-0.85, $p = .008$). That was the first time that a combination of an anti–PD-1 therapy and chemotherapy significantly extended OS in the first-line treatment of patients with squamous NSCLC. The median OS was 15.9 months in the pembrolizumab/chemo combo group (95% CI 13.2–not estimable) and 11.3 months in the chemotherapy-alone group (95% CI 9.5-14.8). Of the 42.8% of patients ($n = 89$) randomly assigned to the chemotherapy-alone group who discontinued chemotherapy crossed over to receive subsequent anti–PD-1 or anti–PD-L1 therapy.

Prespecified exploratory analyses showed an OS benefit regardless of PD-L1 expression as follows: patients whose tumors did not express PD-L1 (HR 0.61, 95% CI 0.38-0.98); patients whose tumors had PD-L1 TPS of 1%-49% (HR 0.57, 95% CI 0.36-0.90); and patients who had a TPS of 50% or more (HR 0.64, 95% CI 0.37-1.10). The addition of pembrolizumab to carboplatin/paclitaxel or nab-paclitaxel significantly improved PFS, with a reduction in the risk of progression or death of nearly half for patients in the pembrolizumab combo group (HR 0.56, 95% CI 0.45–0.70, $p < .0001$). Interestingly, improvement in PFS was also seen in patients whose tumors did not express PD-L1 (HR 0.68, 95% CI 0.47-0.98); patients with a TPS of 1%-49% (HR 0.56, 95% CI 0.39-0.80); and patients with a TPS of 50% or greater (HR 0.37, 95% CI 0.24-0.58).[101]

In terms of ORR, pembrolizumab plus carboplatin/paclitaxel or nab-paclitaxel was superior to the chemotherapy-alone group: 57.9% (95% CI 51.9%-63.8%) and 38.4% (95% CI 32.7%-44.4%), respectively. The safety of pembrolizumab in combination with chemotherapy was consistent with the safety profiles of pembrolizumab and chemotherapy in previous trials among patients with metastatic NSCLC, with no new safety signals identified. Grade 3 to 5 AEs from any cause occurred in 69.8% of patients in the pembrolizumab plus carboplatin and paclitaxel or nab-paclitaxel group and 68.2% in the chemotherapy-alone group. The most common ir-AEs of any grade in patients in the pembrolizumab plus chemotherapy combo were hypothyroidism (7.9%), hyperthyroidism (7.2%), pneumonitis (6.5%), colitis (2.5%), hepatitis (1.8%), severe skin reactions (1.8%), hypophysitis (1.1%), thyroiditis (1.1%), and nephritis (0.7%) (Table 15-7).[101]

ATEZOLIZUMAB

Atezolizumab is an IgG1 monoclonal antibody against PD-L1 that inhibits its interaction with PD-L1 and B7.1 (CD28) receptors. An additional block on CD28 might inhibit downregulation of the immune response. Atezolizumab was the first anti–PD-L1 antibody approved by the US FDA for treatment of advanced NSCLC as a second-line treatment after progression following platinum-based chemotherapy.

Atezolizumab for Second- or Third-Line Therapy
POPLAR Trial

The POPLAR trial was a multicenter, open-label, phase 2 RCT that compared the efficacy and safety of atezolizumab (at a fixed dose of 1,200 mg) versus docetaxel (75 mg/m²) every 3 weeks, as second- or third-line treatment of NSCLC.[17] Inclusion criteria involved patients 18 years or older, ECOG PS 0 or 1, acceptable end-organ function, and biopsy-proven PD-L1 before enrollment. Patients with untreated or active CNS metastases, history of pneumonitis or autoimmune disorders, previous treatment with docetaxel, anti-CTLA4 or anti–PD-L1 agents were excluded from this trial. A total of 287 patients were randomized (1:1) according to PD-L1 expression, previous chemotherapy lines, and histology (non-squamous vs. squamous) to receive either atezolizumab ($n = 144$ patients) or docetaxel ($n = 143$ patients). No crossover between groups was allowed. Disease was assessed every 6 weeks, with imaging for 36 weeks and every 9 weeks thereafter. PD-L1 was scored in 2 modalities, first as a percentage of tumor cell (TC) area (>50% [TC3], >5% and <50% [TC2], <5% [TC1], and <1% [TC0]) and second as tumor-infiltrating immune cell (IC) score (>10% [IC3], >5% and <10% [IC2], <5% and >1% [IC1], and <1% [IC0]). PD-1, PD-L1, and B7.1 gene expressions were also analyzed. The primary endpoints included OS in the ITT group (population and PD-L1 subgroups). Secondary endpoints included PFS, ORR, and DOR.[133]

During minimum follow-up, atezolizumab improved OS as compared to docetaxel (12.6 vs. 9.7 months; HR 0.73, 95% CI 0.53-0.99, $p = .04$). The PFS was similar for atezolizumab and docetaxel (2.7 months vs. 3.0 months, HR 0.94, 95% CI 0.72-1.23). The OS was noted to increase simultaneously with PD-L1 expression in both TC and IC subgroups. Statistical significance was described in the atezolizumab group in TC3/IC3 (HR 0.49, 95% CI 0.22-1.07, $p = .068$); TC2/3 or IC2/3 (HR 0.54, CI 0.33-0.89, $p = .14$); TC 1/2/3 or ICI 1/2/3 (HR 0.59, 95% CI 0.40-0.85, $p = .005$); TC0 and IC0 (HR 1.04, 95% CI 0.62-1.75. $p = .871$) when compared with the docetaxel group. Although patients underwent longer median treatment duration in the atezolizumab group as compared with the docetaxel group (3.7 months vs. 2.1 months), patients in the atezolizumab group reported fewer grade 3-4 AEs (40% vs. 53%). The ir-AEs of any grade included elevated aspartate and alanine aminotransferase (4% respectively), pneumonitis (3%), colitis (1%), and hepatitis (1%) (Table 15-8).[133]

OAK Trial

The OAK trial was the confirmatory, open-label, multicenter, phase 3 RCT that compared intravenous atezolizumab at a fixed dose of 1,200 mg every 3 weeks versus docetaxel 75 mg/m² every 3 weeks in previously treated metastatic or locally advanced NSCLC.[134] Inclusion criteria were patients 18 years or older, ECOG performance status 0 or 1, prior 1-2 chemotherapy regimens for stage IIIB or IV or TKI in patients with *EGFR* mutation or *ALK* translocation. Importantly, the OAK trial also included patients with treated asymptomatic supratentorial CNS metastases. OAK is one of the largest phase 3 RCTs done for NSCLC; 1,225 patients were enrolled to receive either atezolizumab ($n = 613$) or docetaxel ($n = 612$). No crossover to atezolizumab was allowed.[18] Disease was assessed at baseline, then every 6 weeks until 36 weeks, and afterward every 9 weeks. The primary endpoint was OS compared between treatment groups within ITT and PD-L1 stratification. Secondary endpoints included PFS, ORR, and duration and safety of response. The OS improved in the ITT population in the atezolizumab group (13.8 months, 95% CI 11.8-15.7) in contrast with the docetaxel group (9.6 months; 95% CI 8.6-11.2, HR 0.73, $p = .0003$). The OS was also significantly increased in the TC 1/2/3 or IC 1/2/3 population with atezolizumab versus docetaxel: 15.7 months (95% CI 12.6-18) versus 10.3 months (95% CI 8.8-12.0, HR 0.74, $p = 0.0102$. The OS was improved regardless of PD-L1 expression levels, the TC0 and IC0 subgroups favored atezolizumab over docetaxel (12.6 months [95% CI 9.6-15.2] vs. 8.9 months [95% CI 7.7-11.5]; HR 0.75 [95% CI 0.59-0.96]). Patients with elevated PD-L1 expression (TC3 or IC3) had more benefit from atezolizumab

(20.5 months; 95% CI 17.5-not evaluable) compared with docetaxel (8.9 months; 95% CI 5.6-11.6, HR 0.41, 95% CI 0.27-0.64). The OS benefit was observed regardless of NSCLC histology: squamous (HR 0.73, 95% CI 0.54-0.98) or non-squamous histology (HR 0.73, 95% CI 0.60-0.89]). The PFS was similar in both treatment arms in the PD-L1 subgroups except for the TC3 or IC3 group, which was consistent with the improved benefit of atezolizumab over docetaxel (HR 0.63, 95% CI 0.43-0.91) (Table 15-8).[134]

Regarding AEs, there were fewer TRAEs in the atezolizumab group versus the docetaxel group (15% vs. 43%, respectively). The most common TRAEs in the atezolizumab group included fatigue, nausea, decreased appetite, and asthenia. For any grade, ir-AEs secondary to atezolizumab included pneumonitis (1%), hepatitis (<1%), and colitis (<1%).[18] The OAK trial made the US FDA grant approval to allow atezolizumab in the second-line setting regardless of PD-L1 expression.

ATEZOLIZUMAB IN COMBINATION WITH CHEMOTHERAPY
Atezolizumab as Front-Line Therapy for Non-squamous NSCLC
IMpower150 Trial

The IMpower150 was a phase 3 RCT where 3 arms were compared. Atezolizumab was added to the ECOG 4599 backbone (quadruplet therapy; ABCP); atezolizumab was added to ACP (triplet therapy); and the original triplet BCP.[100] Patients were treated every 3 weeks for 4 or 6 cycles, followed by maintenance therapy with atezolizumab, bevacizumab, or both. The two primary endpoints were investigator-assessed PFS both among patients in the ITT who had a wild-type genotype (WT population; patients with *EGFR* or *ALK* genetic alterations were excluded) and among patients in the WT population who had high expression of an effector T-cell gene signature in the tumor and OS in the WT population. The ABCP group was compared with the BCP group before the ACP group was compared with the BCP group. In the WT population, 356 patients were assigned to the ABCP group and 336 to the BCP group. Median PFS was longer in the ABCP group than in the BCP group (8.3 months vs. 6.8 months; HR 0.62, 95% CI 0.52-0.74, *p* < .001); the corresponding values in the T effector-high WT population were 11.3 months (for the ABCP group) and 6.8 months (for the BCP arm; HR 0.51, 95% CI 0.38-0.68, *p* < .001).[100]

In addition, PFS was longer in the ABCP group than in the BCP group in the entire ITT population (including those with *EGFR* or *ALK* genetic alterations) and among patients with low or negative PD-L1 expression, those with low T-effector gene signature expression, and those with liver metastases. Among patients in the WT population, median OS was longer in the ABCP group than in the BCP group (19.2 months vs. 14.7 months; HR 0.78, 95% CI 0.64-0.96, *p* = .02). No red flag signals were seen in this trial; the safety profile of the ABCP regimen was consistent with previously reported information for these drugs.

> **CLINICAL PEARL:** Adding a PD-L1 inhibitor (atezolizumab) to an antiangiogenic agent (bevacizumab) and systemic cytotoxic chemotherapy significantly improved PFS and OS among patients with metastatic non-squamous NSCLC, regardless of PD-L1 expression and the presence or absence of EGFR or ALK genetic alterations (**Table 15-9**).[100]

TABLE 15-9		Randomized Controlled Trials Comparing Atezolizumab in Patients With Stage IV NSCLC as Either First-Line Treatment or Second or Third Lines					
RCT	N	DESIGN	ORR %	MEDIAN PFS (MONTHS)	MEDIAN OS (MONTHS)	AE (GRADE 3 OR 4)
Fehrenbacher et al. POPLAR[133]	287	Atezolizumab 1,200 mg q3w vs Docetaxel 75 mg/m² q3w	15% vs 15%	2.7 vs 3 (95% CI 0.72-1.23)	12.6 vs 9.7 (95% CI 0.52-0.92) p = .01	40% vs 53%
Rittmeyer et al. OAK[134]	1,225	Atezolizumab 1,200 mg q3w vs Docetaxel 75 mg/m² q3w	13.6% vs 13.4%	2.8 (95% CI 2.6-3.0) vs 4.0 (95% CI 0.82-1.10) p = .49	13.8 (95% CI 11.8-15.7) vs 9.6 (95% CI 8.6-11.2) p = .0003	37% vs 54%
Socinski et al. IMpower150[100]	1,202	Atezolizumab 1,200 mg + Bevacizumab 15 mg/kg + paclitaxel 200 mg/m² and Carboplatin AUC (ABCP) vs Bevacizumab + Paclitaxel + Carboplatin (BCP)	63.5% vs 48.0%	8.3 vs 6.8	19.2 vs 14.7 (95% CI 0.64-0.96)	25.4% vs 19.3%
Socinski et al. IMpower131[106]	1,021	Atezolizumab + Carboplatin/ Paclitaxel (Arm A) Atezolizumab + Carboplatin/Nab-paclitaxel) (Arm B) vs Carboplatin/Nab-paclitaxel (Arm C)	Pending	6.3 (Arm B) vs 5.6 (Arm C)	Pending	68% (Arm A/B) vs 57% (Arm C)

Although benefit to OS was seen in patients with liver metastases and driver mutations (*EGFR* or *ALK*) in the subgroup analyses, to date the IMpower150 trial data is the only objective data that we have to add immunotherapy for patients who are refractory to EGFR or ALK TKIs and who have not seen systemic chemotherapy yet.

Atezolizumab as Front-Line Therapy for Squamous NSCLC
IMpower131 Trial

In the IMpower131 trial, 1,021 chemotherapy-naïve patients with stage IV squamous NSCLC with any level of PD-L1 expression were enrolled. Patients were randomized 1:1:1 to 1 of 3 arms: arm A (atezolizumab + carboplatin/paclitaxel); arm B (atezolizumab + carboplatin/nab-paclitaxel); arm C (control arm: carboplatin/nab-paclitaxel).[102] Treatment in each arm was for 4 or 6 cycles. Arms A and B received atezolizumab maintenance until disease progression or loss of clinical benefit. Arm C was followed with BSC.

Arm C was not included in the analysis presented until now. Co-primary endpoints were investigator-assessed PFS and OS. Regardless of the level of PD-L1 expression, 29% of all patients had a reduced risk of PFS or death with the chemoimmunotherapy combo arm compared with chemotherapy alone. Twelve-month landmark PFS was 24.7% with the chemoimmunotherapy regimen versus 12.0% with chemotherapy alone. The median PFS was 6.3 months in arm B versus 5.6 months in arm C (p = .0001). The PFS was improved in the atezolizumab plus chemotherapy arm in all PD-L1–positive subgroups, with greater benefit observed in subgroups with higher PD-L1 expression. A trend toward improved PFS was observed in patients with PD-L1–negative tumors. The group with high PD-L1 expression had the best outcome with atezolizumab/chemotherapy versus chemotherapy alone, but those who had low or negative PD-L1 expression also benefited from the chemoimmunotherapy combo compared with chemotherapy alone (Table 15-8).[102]

The confirmed ORR and the DOR were better in all patients as well as in the PD-L1–high and PD-L1–low subgroups who did receive atezolizumab/chemotherapy versus those who only received chemotherapy alone. Among all patients, the ORR was 49% for chemoimmunotherapy combo versus 41% for chemotherapy alone. This was different for those patients with high PD-L1 expression, where the ORR was 60% versus 33% for those who received chemotherapy alone. Among patients with PD-L1 low expression, the ORR was 52% versus 44% for those who did receive a chemoimmunotherapy combo and chemotherapy alone, respectively.[102]

At the first interim analysis, the median OS was 14.0 months for the atezolizumab plus chemotherapy arm versus 13.9 months for chemotherapy alone. The OS data are not yet mature. In terms of safety profile, there were no red flag signals seen in this trial. The rate of grade 3 or 4 side effects was higher with the chemoimmunotherapy combo versus chemotherapy alone (68% vs. 57%, respectively). The most common side effects thought to be related to atezolizumab were skin rash, hepatitis, colitis, and low thyroid hormone levels.[102]

DURVALUMAB

Durvalumab is a high-affinity IgG1 monoclonal antibody that blocks PD-L1 binding to PD-1 and CD80, allowing T-cell–mediated immune activity. Durvalumab received approval by the US FDA for consolidation therapy for stage III NSCLC (all histologies) after concurrent chemoradiation-proven lack of the patient's progressed.[135] Other efforts have been done to prove the efficacy of this PD-L1 inhibitor in the metastatic setting.

Durvalumab as Front-Line Therapy
NCT01693562 Clinical Trial

The NCT01693562 phase 1/2, expansion trial for durvalumab at dose of 10 mg/kg every 2 weeks for up to 12 months included patients with diagnosis of NSCLC stage III/IV, ECOG performance status 0-1. PD-L1 testing was performed via fresh biopsy or archival results with a definition of high PD-L1 as greater than 25% membrane staining. Patients excluded from this trial were those with symptomatic or untreated CNS metastases, prior exposure to immune checkpoint therapy, any concurrent chemotherapy, and documented autoimmune disease for the past 2 years. During the first data cut-off, 59 patients of 1,022 total enrolled patients received first-line durvalumab. Median duration of follow-up was 17.3 months, and 49 patients had high PD-L1 expression; on this subpopulation, ORR was 28.6% (95% CI 16.6-43.3), median PFS was 4 months (95% CI 2.3-9.1), and OS was 21.0 months (95% CI 14.5-not estimated). The TRAEs reported during this trial, established grade 3/4 occurred in 10%. Overall, durvalumab has shown encouraging results, but the results can be biased the since final trial has not yet concluded.[136]

AVELUMAB

Avelumab is the first fully human anti–PD-L1 IgG1 monoclonal antibody. Avelumab exerts its mechanism of action by inhibiting the PD-1 signal pathway in addition to retaining a native Fc region, achieving potential restoration of immune function via activation of cytotoxic T-cell lymphocytes and enabling antibody-dependent cellular cytotoxic response to PD-L1 tumor expression cells.[137]

Avelumab as Second-Line Therapy
JAVELIN Solid Tumor Clinical Trial

The JAVELIN Solid Tumor clinical trial is a phase 1, multicenter, ongoing, international RCT that includes dose escalation (part 1a) and dose expansion (1b) of use of avelumab 10 mg/kg every 2 weeks in patients with confirmed squamous or non-squamous stage IIIB or IV NSCLC who had progression of disease after treatment with platinum-based dou-blet chemotherapy.[137] Inclusion criteria were age 18 years or older, ECOG performance status 0-1, no history or active CNS metastases, life expectancy of at least 3 months, and normal hepatic, renal, and hematological function. Patients were not selected according to PD-L1 expression, *EGFR* or *KRAS* mutation, or *ALK* translocation. Among the exclu-sion criteria were the presence of a second malignancy, CNS disease, rapid progression of disease, or autoimmune disorders. Disease was measured by CT or MRI scan using RECIST version 1.1 and were performed at baseline and every 6 weeks. PD-L1 expres-sion was based on proportion of tumor cells, establishing different thresholds, 1% and 5% of PD-L1 with any stain intensity, 25% of positive PD-L1 with moderate-to-high intensity. Primary outcome of this trial was dose limiting toxicity (DLTs) in the first part of the trial; secondary endpoints included overall response, duration, PFS, OS, safety, and TRAEs. A total of 184 patients were eligible to receive avelumab; the median age was 65 years. PD-L1 expression was evaluated in 142 patients; 122 (86%) were positive based on a 1% threshold. A median of 6 doses of avelumab were administered in a median of 12.2 weeks. Median follow-up was 8.8 months.

Confirmed objective response was attained in 22 of 184 patients, including 1 com-plete response and 21 partial responses. From the 22 patients, response was maintained in 83% of patients (95% CI 54-94) for 24 weeks or longer. Median PFS was 11.6 weeks (95% CI 8.4-13.7), median OS was 8.4 months (95% CI 7.3-10.6), and OS at 12 months was 36%. OS and ORR outcomes did not differ between patients who were PD-L1 pos-itive or negative or between any PD-L1 expression subset. However, PFS was longer (HR 0.45, 95% CI 0.27-0.75) in patients with positive PD-L1 versus negative PD-L1 expression. Grade 3 or worse TRAEs were reported in 23 patients (13%), the most common were infusion-related reaction and an increased lipase level. Ir-AEs of any grade occurred in 36 (20%) patients; the most common reported were hypothyroidism, adrenal insufficiency, and radiation pneumonitis.[137]

To date, avelumab is approved by the US FDA for patients with metastatic Merkel cell carcinoma and for patients with locally advanced or metastatic urothelial carcinoma whose disease progressed during or following platinum-based chemotherapy or within 12 months of neoadjuvant or adjuvant platinum-based chemotherapy. Avelumab is currently not approved in the setting of lung cancer.

BEYOND PROGRESSION ON PD-1 AND PD-L1 INHIBITORS: THE NEW CHALLENGE

With the clinical trials KEYNOTE-024, KEYNOTE-189, KEYNOTE-407, and IMpower150, almost all patients with NSCLC will see either immunotherapy alone, or chemoimmunotherapy, or chemo/anti-VEGF/immunotherapy in the first-line setting or after EGFR or ALK TKI resistance. This leaves us with the question: What is next after immunotherapy-based regimen progression? This is a difficult question to answer thus far. To date, there is no standard approach for these patients. Efforts are underway to rescue these patients by combining with other immune cycle pathways.

A combination of anti–PD-1 and PD-L1 antibodies with HDAC inhibitors (eg, entinostat, vorinostat); vaccines (eg, CV-301 [a poxviral-based vaccine comprising a prime-boost strategy with modified vaccinia Ankara prime and fowlpox boost], cytokines that stimulate survival and expansion of intratumoral, antigen-activated CD8+ T cells [eg, pegilodecakin], or others that expand tumor-killing cells [eg, NKTR-214 cytokine designed to target CD122, interleukin 2Rβ]); and others are in development. The goal here is to rescue those patients who have progressed on immuno-oncology (IO) agents or to increase the clinical benefit seen with them on second- or third-line therapy.

ONCOGENE INHIBITION FOR METASTATIC NON–SMALL CELL LUNG CANCER

Cesar Perez, MD, Jennifer Cudris, MD

A 48-year-old female, non-smoker, presented to the emergency department with shortness of breath and was found to have a large lung mass with associated pleural effusion. Pathology was positive for adenocarcinoma of lung origin, and next-generation sequencing revealed an L858R missense mutation on exon 21 of EGFR. What is the current recommended therapy?

Learning Objectives:
1. To study the current data for treatment of patients with EGFR-mutated NSCLC.
2. To describe the most effective agent for the treatment of lung cancer with ALK genomic alterations.
3. To understand the current molecular-targeted therapeutic strategies for uncommon molecular alterations in non–small cell lung cancer.

In the year 2001, imatinib, a multikinase inhibitor with activity against the *BCR-ABL* gene, revolutionized the modern therapeutic management of cancer when it proved to be highly effective in the treatment of chronic myeloid leukemia.[138,139] This finding also exemplified the role of molecular medicine in cancer therapy and the value of identifying a specific target. Since then, many other targeted therapies have been developed in other malignant diseases, including lung cancer. Given the variability and genetic abnormalities seen in lung cancer cells, it was initially difficult to develop effective targeted therapies. However, in 2004 investigators discovered that the *EGFR* gene could carry somatic mutations in different exons, mainly 19 and 21, which correlated with increased response rates to EGFR kinase inhibitors. This was the first driver mutation described with strong therapeutic implications in non–small cell lung cancer. Thereafter, several other driver mutations have been revealed, many of them with approved therapeutic agents used now in the clinical setting (Table 15-1). Testing for these molecular markers is discussed in Chapter 11 of this book, and we focus on the data available for the molecular targeted agents available for this population.

EPIDERMAL GROWTH FACTOR RECEPTOR INHIBITORS

The EGFR is a type I receptor tyrosine kinase (TK) of the ERBB family to which natural ligands (EGF, TGFb) bind and subsequently cause homo-/heterodimerization and cascade activation involving the RAS, RAF, MEK, and MAPK pathways or the PI3K pathways. Activation of these pathways led to cell cycle progression, inhibition of apoptosis, angiogenesis, tumor cell motility, invasion, and metastasis.[140-142] The receptor is composed of 3 major domains: an extracellular ligand-binding domain, a transmembrane lipophilic segment, and a cytoplasmic protein TK domain.[140] Mutations in the TK domain (adenosine triphosphate [ATP]–binding pocket domain involving exons 18-21) lead to constitutive activation. Approximately 85% of all drug-sensitive mutations involve the L858R mutation or small internal deletions of exon 19. Exon 20 insertions are in general resistant to EGFR TKIs.[143-145] L861Q and G719X mutations are less common and are thought to be intermediate in sensitivity to EGFR TKIs.[143,144] Drug-resistant mutations can be categorized as either primary or secondary, with the mutation T790M a cause of 60% of resistant cases.[144,145]

These mutations in the *EGFR* kinase domain were the first driver mutations with a therapeutic implication discovered in patients with NSCLC. The clinical significance in terms of RR, PFS, and OS was initially established by several large phase 3 randomized clinical trials performed with the first-generation inhibitors gefitinib and erlotinib.[146,147] These small molecules inhibit the dimerization of the intracellular EGFR domain, thereby shutting down the signal transduction downstream. The EGFR inhibitors have now established themselves as the preferred option for first-line treatment in patients with advanced NSCLC whose tumors harbor an *EGFR* mutation. Their use, however, is now restricted to these populations. The earlier BR.21 trial led to the initial approval of erlotinib as second- and third-line therapy for all patients with NSCLC. However, the most recent IUNO trial compared erlotinib to placebo after initial induction chemotherapy, excluding patients with EGFR mutations; it demonstrated no benefit of erlotinib against placebo on either PFS or OS, therefore confirming the restrictive benefit of these agents only for patients with activating EGFR mutations.

FIRST-LINE THERAPY OF PATIENTS WITH EGFR-ACTIVATING MUTATIONS

Before the introduction of EGFR kinase inhibitors, systemic chemotherapy was considered the mainstay of first-line therapy for patients with metastatic NSCLC. However, randomized phase 3 trials have demonstrated an improvement of PFS and in some cases OS of EGFR kinase inhibitors when compared with systemic chemotherapy. The Iressa Pan-Asia Study (IPASS trial) is a randomized phase 3 study that enrolled patients from Asia with NSCLC who were non-smokers or light smokers to receive first-line gefitinib, a first-generation EGFR inhibitor, against carboplatin plus paclitaxel. Of the patients enrolled, 261 had activating EGFR mutations; the PFS was significantly longer among those who received gefitinib than among those who received carboplatin-paclitaxel (HR for progression or death 0.48).[147] These findings were supported by the IFUM (IRESSA Follow-Up Measure) trial, a single-arm, phase 4 study that included 106 Caucasian treatment-naïve patients with *EGFR*-positive NSCLC, reporting an ORR of 50% median DOR of 6 months.[148]

Erlotinib, another first-generation EGFR inhibitor, was evaluated in the EURopean TArceva versus Chemotherapy (EURTAC) study, the first trial with a EGFR kinase inhibitor addressed to a European population affected by advanced NSCLC harboring activating EGFR mutations (exon 19 deletion or L858R mutation in exon 21). In this trial, erlotinib 150 mg daily was compared with platinum-based doublets (cisplatin or carboplatin plus gemcitabine or docetaxel) in 174 eligible patients. Patients on the erlotinib arm had a significantly better outcome than the patients on the chemotherapy arm in terms of PFS, the main endpoint of the trial, with 9.7 versus 5.2 months, respectively (HR 0.37, 95% CI 0.25-0.54); the ORRs were 58% and 15%, respectively. Importantly, 6% of the patients on erlotinib had treatment-related severe AEs compared with 20% on chemotherapy. One patient in the erlotinib group and 2 in the standard chemotherapy group died from treatment-related causes.[146]

Afatinib, a second-generation EGFR inhibitor, was developed as an irreversible EGFR/HER2 inhibitor designed to covalently bind to Cys 773 on the *EGFR* TK domain, with improved inhibition of EGFR T790M in preclinical models. It was also evaluated in a first-line setting for patients with *EGFR* mutant NSCLC in the phase 3 LUX-Lung 3 trial, a randomized study where 345 patients were randomly assigned afatinib 40 mg orally daily versus systemic chemotherapy with cisplatin plus pemetrexed. Afatinib demonstrated an improved median PFS (11.1 months for afatinib and 6.9 months for chemotherapy) with higher benefit for patients with exon 19 deletions, showing a median OS in this subset of patients of 33.3 months in the afatinib arm versus 21.1 months in the chemotherapy arm.[149] Similar benefit was also seen in the LUX-Lung 6 study that compared afatinib versus cisplatin plus gemcitabine in Asian patients with *EGFR* mutations, reporting an improved PFS with afatinib (11.0 vs. 5.6 months).[150]

The trials mentioned, therefore, demonstrated the superiority of the EGFR inhibitors gefitinib, erlotinib, and afatinib in the first-line treatment of patients with EGFR driver mutations when compared with chemotherapy in regard to response rate, PFS, and toxicity. The question then remains concerning which inhibitor is more effective. The LUX-Lung 7 trial, a phase 2b randomized study, addressed this concern. It enrolled patients with stage IIIb/IV, treatment-naïve NSCLC and a common *EGFR* muta-tion (exon 19 deletion/L858R) to be treated with afatinib 40 mg/day versus gefitinib 250 mg/day. The trial, however, failed to demonstrate a significant difference in OS. An improved response rate (ORR) was seen with afatinib, but this was met with more fre-quent treatment-related grade 3 or greater AEs and included diarrhea (13.1% vs. 1.3%), rash (9.4% vs. 3.1%), and fatigue (5.6% vs. 0%).[151]

Approximately 50%-60% of the cases of resistance to EGFR inhibitors are mediated by a secondary T790M mutation exon 20. The T790M mutation can induce steric hin-drance to EGFR TKIs and increase the affinity of the receptor to ATP, relative to its affinity to EGFR TKIs, which abolishes the effect of EGFR kinase inhibitors. Osimer-tinib, a third-generation EGFR-inhibitor, has demonstrated clinical activity in patients with these acquired T790M *EGFR* mutations as per the AURA3 trial. The trial was a randomized phase 3 study that included 410 patients with *EGFR* T790M mutations after progression to first-line EGFR inhibitors. Osimertinib 80 mg once daily was com-pared to a platinum-pemetrexed doublet, reporting a significantly improved PFS (10.1 vs. 4.4 months) and ORR (71% vs. 31%). This trial led to the approval of osimertinib in this setting.[152]

In the first-line setting, osimertinib was then compared to gefitinib in the FLAURA trial, a double-blind, phase 3 trial where 556 patients with previously untreated, *EGFR* mutation–positive (exon 19 deletion or L858R) advanced NSCLC were randomized in a 1:1 ratio to receive either osimertinib or the option of gefitinib or erlotinib. The trial demonstrated an impressive superiority of osimertinib in the first-line setting, report-ing a median PFS of 18.9 months versus 10.2 months with the first-generation kinase inhibitor gefitinib or erlotinib, despite a similar ORR in the groups (80% vs. 76%). The improvement in the outcome was likely based on the remarkably long DOR with osim-ertinib of 17.2 months, compared to 8.5 months with the first-generation EGFR inhib-itors. Even more interestingly, the patients in the osimertinib arm had fewer severe AEs than with standard EGFR TKIs (34% vs. 45%).[153] The trial led to the approval of osimertinib for use in first-line treatment of patients with metastatic NSCLC whose tumors have EGFR exon 19 deletions or exon 21 L858R mutations. These data of increased efficacy and decreased toxicity compared to the other first-generation EGFR inhibitors, together with the activity against the T790M resistance mutation, have made osimertinib the preferred agent in the first-line setting of patients with EGFR mutations.

Dacomitinib is another second-generation EGFR inhibitor that is currently in devel-opment, but not commercially available. It was tested against gefitinib in the first-line treatment of patients with advanced or metastatic exon 19 deletion or Leu858Arg EGFR mutations in the randomized ARCHER 1050 trial. It also demonstrated a significantly improved median PFS (14.7 vs. 9.2) compared to gefitinib. Grade 3-4 rash and diarrhea were more common with dacomitinib than with gefitinib. TRSAEs were reported in 9% of patients given dacomitinib and in 4% of patients given gefitinib. Based on these results, dacomitinib was approved by the FDA in September 2018 for the first-line treat-ment patients with metastatic NSCLC with EGFR exon 19 deletion or exon 21 L858R substitution mutations as detected by an FDA-approved test.[152]

There are currently 5 EGFR kinase inhibitors commercially available for the first-line treatment of patients with EGFR mutations.

> **CLINICAL PEARL:** The only agent that has been shown clearly superior in terms of efficacy and less toxicity is osimertinib, possibly because its activity against such acquired resistant EGFR mutations as T790M.

Patients with such driver mutations as EGFR have been excluded by most of the trials with checkpoint inhibitors. Also, it is thought that because of the lower tumor mutation burden, patients with EGFR mutations have less benefit from checkpoint inhibitors than patients with no driver mutations.

> **CLINICAL PEARL**: EGFR inhibitors remain as the agents of choice in the first-line setting for patients with these genomic abnormalities, regardless of their PD-L1 status.

SECOND-LINE THERAPY OF PATIENTS WITH EGFR-ACTIVATING MUTATIONS

The choice of second-line therapy for patients with advanced NSCLC is based on the first-line therapy received and the type of progression, characterized by localized versus multiple and only in the CNS versus systemic. For patients with localized progression, localized therapy (either radiation therapy or surgical resection) should be considered and continuing the EGFR inhibitor the patient was receiving. A similar approach is done for patients with good systemic control but CNS relapse as a single lesion or small lesions that could be targeted with stereotactic radiation therapy surgical resection.

For patients with multiple progressing systemic lesions, the systemic therapy should be switched. In these cases, if patients were receiving first- or second-generation EGFR inhibitors (**Table 15-10**), the molecular testing should be repeated via either a biopsy or blood-based testing, also known as circulating free DNA (cfDNA) of the tumor. If the testing revealed there is development of an acquired T790M *EGFR* mutation, osimertinib will be recommended based on the data of the AURA3 trial.[152] For patients who have disease progression on osimertinib or testing does not reveal the presence of a T790M resistance mutation, cytotoxic chemotherapy or checkpoint inhibitors should be considered.

TABLE 15-10 Commercially Available EGFR Kinase Inhibitors by Generation	
EGFR INHIBITOR	**GENERATION**
Gefitinib	First
Erlotinib	First
Afatinib	Second
Dacomitinib	Second
Osimertinib	Third

ANAPLASTIC LYMPHOMA KINASE INHIBITORS

After the success of inhibiting the EGFR genomic abnormalities in NSCLC, efforts were aimed to the inhibition of the ALK fusion protein, which became the next triumph of molecular targeted therapy for the disease. ALK is a receptor TK originally identified in a subset of anaplastic large cell lymphomas. However, is now known that approximately 2%-7% of patients with NSCLC can have an inversion of the short arm of chromosome 2, which results in the fusion of a protein encoded by echinoderm microtubule-associated-protein-like 4 (EML4) gene with ALK receptor TK resulting in EML4-ALK translocation.

The initial landmark study that demonstrated the activity of ALK inhibition in NSCLC was published by Kwak and colleagues in 2010. This was an expanded cohort of the phase 1 dose escalation trial of crizotinib in patients with NSCLC with ALK rearrangements; 82 patients received a crizotinib dose of 250 mg twice daily in 28-day cycles.[154] The study reported an ORR for the novel agent of 57% (47 of 82 patients, with 46 confirmed partial responses and 1 confirmed complete response) and stable disease for 33%. Crizotinib was found to be well tolerated, with the most common AEs grade 1 or 2 gastrointestinal side effects. This trial led to the initial approval of crizotinib for patients with advanced *ALK*-rearranged NSCLC, becoming the first inhibitor approved for this indication.

However, most patients treated with crizotinib developed progression of disease within the first year of therapy. Several mechanisms of resistance have been proposed to explain the de novo as well as acquired resistance to the drug. An intrinsic resistance to crizotinib has been described in approximately 30% of treatment-naïve individuals, with acquired resistance demonstrated in the remainder of the population.[155] The proposed mechanisms of resistance to crizotinib include a resistant target mutation, gene amplification of the kinase domain of ALK, and target bypassing. A common and well-demonstrated mechanism includes the development of mutations on the ALK TK domain, which have been reported to account for up to 22% of the crizotinib-resistant cases. Although many different potential mutations have been identified, the most recognized have been found to cluster around the ATP-binding pocket of ALK.[156,157] The gatekeeper mutation L1196M inhibits steric binding and is similar to the EGFR and BCR-ABL gatekeeper mutations, leading to resistance to its targeting agents. Two other mutations (G1202R, S1206Y) that resulted in decreased affinity of crizotinib to its binding site on the mutant ALK and the C1156Y mutation increased the catalytic kinase activity. Other mutations have been described to decrease the affinity of ALK to ATP as the 1151Tins mutation.[156] Last, mutations proposed to confer resistance to second-generation ALK inhibitors include as G1202R, F1174C, V118L, and I1171T.[158,159]

Development of inhibitors for the ALK rearrangement has progressed rapidly during the last decade. As of 2018, 5 ALK inhibitors were commercially available, with several others currently being developed.

First-Line Therapy of Patients With ALK-Rearranged NSCLC

Crizotinib was the first agent approved by the regulatory authorities for the treatment of the disease. The first question was if treatment with these agents leads to improved outcomes when compared with standard-of-care cytotoxic chemotherapy in the second-line setting. The phase 3 PROFILE 1007 trial compared the efficacy of crizotinib (250 mg twice daily) versus standard chemotherapy (docetaxel or pemetrexed) after failure of first-line platinum-based therapy in ALK-positive NSCLC (detected by fluorescence in situ hybridization [FISH]). Crossover was allowed for those not responding to chemotherapy.[160] The study demonstrated the superiority of crizotinib in its primary endpoint of PFS, with a PFS benefit of 4.7 months. There was a significantly higher ORR in the crizotinib arm compared to standard chemotherapy (65% vs 20%, $p < .001$). These findings led to the regulatory approval of crizotinib for the treatment of this patient population.

The second and most important question, then, was if cizotinib was better in the first-line setting. The phase 3 PROFILE 1014 trial studied this question and demonstrated the superiority of crizotinib compared to pemetrexed plus cisplatin or carboplatin.[161] There was an advantage in the primary endpoint, with a median PFS of 10.9 months for crizotinib versus 7.0 months for chemotherapy (HR = 0.45, $p < .0001$). The treatment benefit of crizotinib on the PFS was seen in all subgroups analyzed, also reporting an improved ORR of 74% with crizotinib versus 45% in the control arm ($p < .0001$). It is noteworthy that crossover to crizotinib was allowed for those patients receiving the platinum doublet after progression of their disease.

The OS of the PROFILE 1014 trial was updated in 2018.[162] After a median follow-up duration of 46 months in both arms, the median OS was not reached for crizotinib and was 47.5 months with first-line chemotherapy. After crossover adjustment, there was an improvement in OS that favored crizotinib (HR 0.346, CI 0.081-0.718), with the longest OS benefit observed in crizotinib-treated patients who received a subsequent ALK kinase inhibitor.

Despite the efficacy of crizotinib compared to cytotoxic chemotherapy in patients with ALK rearrangements, most of the patients demonstrated disease progression within 11 months, with CNS progression becoming a common failure site. This precipitated the development of second-generation inhibitors, which could improve the systemic and CNS efficacy as well as decrease the toxicity.

Ceritinib is a second-generation–highly selective ALK inhibitor with preclinical data that showed activity against many ALK mutations that conferred resistance to crizotinib, including the gatekeeper mutation L1196M. The ASCEND-4 trial was a randomized, open-label, phase 3 study for patients with untreated stage IIIB/IV ALK-rearranged NSCLC that randomized 376 patients between ceritinib and chemotherapy with platinum plus pemetrexed.[163] Ceritinib improved the mPFS compared to chemotherapy (16.6 vs. 8.1 months, HR 0.55, $p < .00001$) as well as intracranial response rate (73% vs. 27%). The most common AEs for ceritinib were gastrointestinal, including diarrhea in 85% of the patients, nausea in 69%, and vomiting in 66%. Also, 60% of the patients in the ceritinib arm of the ASCEND-4 trial developed an increase in alanine aminotransferase. The trial led to the approval of ceritinib in the first-line setting for this population. Ceritinib was not directly compared to crizotinib in the first-line setting; however, a retrospective comparative analysis from the single-arm trial of ceritinib compared with the crizotinib-treated patients from the PROFILE studies reported an improve OS with ceritinib.[164]

Alectinib, another highly selective second-generation ALK inhibitor, was developed simultaneously to ceritinib. Preclinical data confirmed that it inhibits several ALK mutations that confer resistance to crizotinib as the L1196 the gatekeeper mutation as well as the C1156Y, F1174L, and G1269A mutated clones. Similar to ceritinib, alectinib had better CNS penetration than ceritinib because it is not a substrate of P-glycoprotein.

Two large randomized trials were developed comparing alectinib versus crizotinib in the first-line treatment of patients with ALK-rearranged NSCLC. The J-ALEX trial is an open–label, phase 3 trial from 41 centers in Japan. The study enrolled 207 treatment-naïve patients (or had received one previous chemotherapy regimen) with ALK-positive NSCLC and randomized them to crizotinib versus alectinib.[165] Alectinib improved the median PFS compared to crizotinib (PFS not reached for alectinib vs. 10.2 months for crizotinib. Importantly, alectinib demonstrated better toleration than crizotinib, with grade 3 or 4 AEs occurring at a greater frequency with crizotinib compared to alectinib (52% vs. 26%, respectively). Also, patients in the crizotinib arm had more frequent dose interruptions compared to patients in the alectinib arm (74% vs. 20%, respectively).

The second study was the alectinib versus crizotinib in untreated ALK-positive non-small-cell lung cancer (ALEX) trial, a global phase 3 trial that included 303 previously untreated, ALK-positive NSCLC patients also randomized to receive alectinib versus crizotinib.[166] The trial confirmed the results of its Japanese version, with a 12-month event-free survival of 68.4% versus 48.7% for patients on the alectinib versus crizotinib, respectively. The superiority of alectinib was also noted in terms of improved CNS disease control (12% vs. 45% CNS failures), improved response rates (82.9% vs. 75.5%), and fewer grade 3 to 5 AEs. These trials confirmed the superiority of alectinib when directly compared to crizotinib and led to the approval by the regulatory authorities.

Brigatinib, another second-generation ALK inhibitor is also currently commercially available for this population. Brigatinib has 12-fold more potency inhibiting ALK than crizotinib and also has activity against ROS1- and EGFR-mutant NSCLC cells. Initial trials reported early onset pulmonary events, which is why brigatinib is dosed with step-up dosing over a period of 7 days, initially at 90 mg and then up to 180 mg once daily. Phase 3 study of brigatinib versus crizotinib in anaplastic lymphoma kinase (ALK)-positive advanced non-small cell lung cancer (NSCLC) participants (ALTA-1L) was a randomized between brigatinib and crizotinib.[167] Brigatinib demonstrated an improvement in the PFS when compared to crizotinib, with an estimated 12-month PFS of 67% versus 43%, respectively (HR 0.49, 95% CI 0.33-0.74, $p < .001$). The ORR was also better with brigatinib (71% vs. 60%), as was the intracranial response rate (78% vs. 29%). Toxicity, however, was not noted improved with brigatinib when compared to crizotinib, with grade 3 to 5 AEs in 61% of the patients in the brigatinib group versus 55% in the crizotinib group.[167] An investigator- or protocol-mandated dose reduction for any AEs occurred in 29% of treated patients in the brigatinib group and 21% of treated patients in the crizotinib group. Based on the results of the ALTA trial, brigatinib was approved by the FDA and is currently commercially available.

Therefore, 4 agents are currently commercially available for the first-line treatment of ALK-positive NSLC: crizotinib, alectinib, ceritinib, and brigatinib. Both alectinib and brigatinib have been shown in a randomized trial to have superior PFS when compared to crizotinib.

Second-Line Therapy of Patients With ALK-Rearranged NSCLC

As with many other scenarios in the treatment of advanced NSCLC, the choice of second-line therapy for patients with advanced NSCLC is based on the first-line therapy received and the type of progression, characterized by localized versus multiple and only in the CNS versus systemic. As is the case of EGFR-mutated disease in patients with localized progression, localized therapy and continuing the current ALK inhibitor should be considered. For patients with good systemic control but CNS relapse, local therapy with stereotactic radiation therapy surgical resection should be offered. However, if patients received crizotinib in the first-line setting and had disease progression in the central nervous system (CNS), switching therapy should be considered because of the demonstrated improved CNS activity of second- and third-generation inhibitors.

In the ASCEND-5 trial, ceritinib demonstrated an improved outcome when compared with chemotherapy with docetaxel or pemetrexed for patients with ALK-rearranged NSCLC who had previously received a platinum doublet and crizotinib and had subsequent disease progression (PFS 5.4 vs. 1.6 months, ORR 39.1% vs. 6.9%).[168] Alectinib demonstrated similar results in the ALUR study, where 107 previously treated patients with ALK-positive NSCLC were randomized between alectinib and chemotherapy.[169] An independent review committee–assessed PFS was significantly longer with alectinib compared to chemotherapy (7.1 months vs. 1.6 months with chemotherapy). The CNS response in assessable patients was also improved with alectinib (ORR 54% vs. 0%), and grade 3 or greater AEs were fewer with alectinib (27.1% vs. 41.2%). Therefore, for patients with ALK-positive advanced NSCLC with disease progression on first-line crizotinib, therapy with second-generation ALK inhibitors alectinib and ceritinib is recommended.

However, since second-generation ALK inhibitors have currently moved to the first-line setting, the most common scenario that will be encountered in the near future will be disease progression after using second generation ALK inhibitors in the first-line setting.

Lorlatinib, a novel highly potent and selective third-generation inhibitor of ALK and ROS1, was developed to overcome the resistance to second- and third-generation ALK inhibitors. A phase 2 study enrolled patients with ALK- or ROS1-positive NSCLC in 6 different cohorts treated with lorlatinib 100 mg orally once daily.[170] The cohorts included ALK-positive patients previously treated with crizotinib, patients treated with 1 non-crizotinib ALK inhibitor, and another cohort of patients previously treated with 2 or 3 with 2 previous ALK inhibitors. The ORR of the 215 patients evaluable for response was 48% (95% CI 42%-55%), with a median DOR of 12.5 months. For the 198 ALK-positive patients treated with at least 1 ALK inhibitor, the ORR was seen in 47%, including objective intracranial response in 70% of the patients. For patients previously treated with 1 non-crizotinib ALK inhibitor, the ORR was 32%, and for the group treated with 2 or more previous inhibitors, it was 38.7%.[170] The most common TRAE was hypercholesterolemia in 81%. However, serious TRAEs were only seen in 7% of the patients, with 3% discontinuing treatment because of TRAEs; there were no treatment-related deaths in the 275 evaluable patients. The trial led to accelerated approval by the FDA of lorlatinib for patients with advanced ALK-positive NSCLC who had progressed on crizotinib and at least 1 other ALK inhibitor.

Therefore, for patients who demonstrate disease progression on treatment with crizotinib in the first-line metastatic setting, a second-generation ALK inhibitor is recommended. However, for patients with disease progression on a second-generation ALK inhibitor such as ceritinib or alectinib, lorlatinib is currently the agent of choice.

ROS1 REARRANGEMENT

Genetics and Preclinical Data

The *ROS1* gene was discovered as the human homolog of the avian sarcoma virus oncogene c-ROS in 1986.[171] It encodes for a transmembrane receptor with TK activity. WT ROS1 is expressed in several normal tissues, including the kidney, cerebellum, and stomach, but not in the lung.[172] The function of WT ROS1 is not entirely clear, mostly because investigation has been hampered by the lack of identification of this receptor's ligand. Indirect activation through chimeric fusion proteins has shown possible downstream effects in the PI3K/AKT, STAT3, VAV3, and MAPK/ERK pathways.[173]

The *ROS1* gene has been found to be rearranged in different malignancies, giving origin to fusion proteins with enhanced TK activity in tumors like glioblastoma, ovarian, cholangiocarcinoma, gastric, colorectal, and myofibroblastic tumors and angiosarcoma. Several fusion partners have been documented. The first fusion protein that was described was FIG-ROS1 in a glioblastoma.[174] In NSCLC, at least 8 fusion partners have been identified: SLC34A2, CD74, TPM3, SDC4, EZR, LRIG3, KDELR2, CCDC6(4). These ROS1 fusion proteins have been shown to induce tumorigenicity. Modified fibroblasts that express ROS1 fusion proteins can induce subcutaneous tumors in nude mice.[175]

Blockade of ROS1 fusion protein TK activity induced cell death in preclinical models.[176] Given the structural similarity of about 77% between the TK domain of ROS1 and of ALK within the ATP-binding sites, it was hypothesized that ALK inhibitors would also block ROS1 activity, making it a suitable target for TK inhibition.

Clinicopathological Features

The frequency of these rearrangements in NSCLC is quite low. In one large series of 1,528 non-small cell carcinomas based on an Asian population, ROS1 rearrangements were found in 0.9% of the carcinomas and in 1.2% of the adenocarcinomas. In a second series of 1,073 tumors in a mostly non-Asian cohort, 1.7% were found to have ROS1 rearrangement, and all of them were adenocarcinomas.[177] In these series, it was also noted that ROS1-positive patients were younger and more frequently never smokers. ROS1 rearrangements do not overlap with other molecular markers like EGFR, ALK, or BRAF.

Targeted Treatment Efficacy

Initially, case reports of patients with ROS1 rearrangement that responded to the ALK inhibitor crizotinib supported the hypothesis of the targeting of ROS1 by ALK inhibitors. One patient with bronchoalveolar carcinoma had a brisk clinical response to treatment with crizotinib, and a 2nd patient had a response of 57% shrinkage within 2 cycles of treatment.[177]

The activity of crizotinib was confirmed in the expansion cohort of the phase 1 study of crizotinib for ALK-rearranged NSCLC.[178] This study was amended after the early reports of possible efficacy of crizotinib in ROS1 NSCLC, and the expansion cohort was added. This cohort consisted of 50 patients, mostly previously treated (86%) and a few treatment naïve (14%) patients. The response rate was 72%, the median PFS was 19 months, and OS at 12 months was 85%. The most common side effects seen were visual impairment (82%), diarrhea (44%), nausea (40%), edema (40%), constipation (34%), vomiting, and elevated liver enzymes. Although the low incidence of ROS1 rearrangements precludes randomized trials with chemotherapy, this response rate and DOR is clearly an improvement from cytotoxic chemotherapy, for which the median PFS has been between 6 and 7 months in retrospective reviews focused on ROS1-positive patients.[41]

Crizotinib is currently FDA approved for treatment of ROS1-rearranged NSCLC.

NEW THERAPIES

Among promising therapies that are not yet approved is ceritinib, a second-generation ALK inhibitor currently approved for treatment of crizotinib-resistant ALK-positive NSCLC and treatment-naïve ALK-positive NSCLC. It has been shown to also have inhibitory activity against ROS1 fusion proteins.[179] Its clinical activity against ROS1 was demonstrated in a phase 2 trial in an Asian population, where 32 patients with ROS1 rearrangement were treated. Only 2 of them had been previously treated with crizotinib. There was a response rate of 62%, with a median PFS of 9.3 months in the overall population and 19 months in crizotinib-naïve patients.[180] Common toxicities included diarrhea (78%), nausea (59%), and anorexia (56%), which were more frequent than with crizotinib. Prophylactic antiemetics were usually required with this therapy.

Brain metastases are a common site of relapse in patients with ROS1-positive NSCLC.[181] Therefore, blood-brain barrier penetration plays an important role in controlling CNS relapse. Ceritinib has better CNS penetration than crizotinib, allowing improved control of brain disease. In the mentioned phase 2 trial, there were 8 patients with brain metastasis; the response rate in CNS was 35%, and CNS disease control was 63%.

Entrectinib, a 30 times more potent inhibitor of ROS1 than crizotinib that was designed to penetrate the blood-brain barrier, has demonstrated in a phase I trial a response of 86% in ROS1-positive tumors, mostly NSCLC and 1 melanoma, as first-line therapy. Updated results of the expanded phase 2 of the STARTRK-2 trial in NSCLC reported an impressive median DOR of 28 months.[182] The CNS response rate was 83%. The medication was generally well tolerated, with serious adverse reactions seen in 9% of patients. The most common toxicities were dysgeusia (38%), fatigue (29%), constipation (23%), dizziness (23%), weight gain (19%), diarrhea (17%), and nausea (16%). The FDA has granted the breakthrough designation to entrectinib and approval is being processed.

Despite an initial good response with TKIs, resistance invariably develops, frequently associated with mutations in the TK-binding site. Three mutations in the ATP-binding site have been described: G2032R, which is an analog to the G1201R mutation in ALK-positive tumors; D2033N; and S1986.[183,184] Non-ROS1–dependent resistance mechanisms, like activation of the EGFR pathway, have also been documented to induce TKI failure.[185] Although the similarity between ALK and ROS1 ATP-binding sites has made possible the use of ALK inhibitors as a treatment for ROS1-mutated tumors, it has been noted that the affinity to ROS1 is variable among different ALK inhibitors. In vitro profiling has detected cabozantinib and foretinib to be ROS1 selective with enough potency to overcome G2032R-mutated tumors, but with no activity against ALK.[179] Like crizotinib, other ALK inhibitors, like brigatinib, ceritinib, entrectinib, and lorlatinib, also have activity against ROS1. Alectinib is an ALK-selective TKI with no anti-ROS1 activity.

Lorlatinib, a dual ALK and ROS1 inhibitor, demonstrated in preclinical studies it was a more potent ROS1 inhibitor than crizotinib and remained active in cases positive for the resistant mutation G2032R.[186] In a phase 1 trial with lorlatinib that included both naïve and pretreated patients with ALK/ROS1 rearrangement, 11 patients with ROS1 rearrangement were included.[187] Six of these patients had been previously treated with crizotinib and/or ceritinib. In total, 6 patients had a partial response, and 3 had stable disease. Of the 6 previously treated patients, 2 had a partial response. The onset of response was 1.4 months, and the DOR was 12 months. The medication was well tolerated at a dose of 100 mg once a day; the most common AEs were hypercholesterolemia (59%), hypertriglyceridemia (33%), peripheral edema (39%), cognitive effects (22%), speech effects (19%), and increased lipase (13%). Also, 23% of the patients required a temporary interruption of treatment, but none of the patients stopped permanently due to adverse effects. These data are encouraging for patients with resistant mutations who did not have other targeted options until now. A phase 2 study of lorlatinib that included ROS1- and ALK-positive lung cancer is in progress. The FDA approval of lorlatinib for ALK-rearranged NSCLC is currently being processed.

Cell lines with ROS1 rearrangement positive for the G2013R mutation have been found to be sensitive to cabozantinib[188] and has shown activity in one patient with acquired crizotinib resistance due to development of a D2033N mutation. A response of 92% shrinkage was seen and lasted for 8 months.[189] Clinical trials to test its efficacy are currently underway.

BRAF Mutations

Genetics and Preclinical Data

BRAF is a signal transducer kinase that is part of the MAPK/ERK pathway and intervenes in cell growth and differentiation. BRAF mutations in cancer were one of the first actionable findings of the human cancer genome project.[190] BRAF mutations are most frequent in melanoma, where it is found in 50% of the cases. It is also found in NSCLC, papillary thyroid carcinoma, and ovarian and colorectal carcinomas. In NSCLC, BRAF mutation incidence in a large series has been in the range of 1% to 3%.[191] The most common mutation found in melanoma is the c.1799T>A, which translates into a valine-to-glutamate substitution at codon 600 (V600E). This exchange increases its kinase activity and independence from RAS activation, inducing tumorigenicity.[192] Non-V600E mutations are rare in melanoma, but much more frequent in NSCLC, where roughly half the

BRAF mutations are V600E, and the rest are non-V600E mutations, like G469A and D594G.[193] BRAF mutations are mutually exclusive with other molecular alterations seen in NSCLC, although concurrent EGFR mutation can be seen very occasionally.[194]

Clinicopathological Features

Pathologically, the vast majority of BRAF mutations in NSCLC are seen in adenocarcinomas, and they are more frequently associated with a micropapillary growth pattern. However, it has also been seen in sarcomatous and large cell NOS variants.[191]

Clinically, most patients with BRAF mutations have some smoking history, but never-smokers with V600E mutations are more frequent than among non-V600E mutant cases, where all have been found to be current or former smokers. Women are also more commonly found in the V600E group.

In a large series collected prior to the availability of anti-BRAF therapy, the prognosis of BRAF-mutated NSCLC was similar to those without molecular alterations and therefore worse than for cases with EGFR, ALK, or ROS mutations.[194]

Targeted Treatment Efficacy

Following the success of BRAF inhibitors in melanoma, the use of vemurafenib and dabrafenib in V600E BRAF-mutated NSCLC was documented.[195] Retrospective studies showed a response rate in the range of 53% and median PFS of 25 months when used as first-line therapy.

Soon after that, it was learned that the BRAF and MEK inhibitor combination in melanoma was more effective than BRAF inhibition alone, and this principle was subsequently transferred to BRAF-mutated NSCLC. In a phase 2 study, 57 patients with stage IV NSCLC with the V600E mutation who had previously received systemic chemotherapy were treated with the dabrafenib/trametinib combination at the same doses used for melanoma: oral dabrafenib 150 mg twice daily plus trametinib orally at 2 mg once a day continuously until disease progression or unacceptable toxicity. This trial showed a response rate of 63% and median PFS of 9.6 months.[196] Treatment discontinuation due to adverse effects was necessary in 12% of patients. Common AEs included pyrexia (46%), nausea (40%), vomiting (35%), diarrhea (32%), asthenia (28%), and decreased appetite (30%). Development of squamous cell carcinoma of the skin was seen in 4% of the patients. Severe side effects included neutropenia, hyponatremia, and anemia.

In a second cohort that included treatment-naïve patients, the response rate was 64%, with a disease control rate of 75% and median PFS of 10.9 months.[197]

This combination is currently FDA approved for the treatment of BRAF V600E–mutant NSCLC. Evaluation of left ventricular ejection fraction (LVEF) is required prior to initiation of therapy and should be monitored during treatment every 3 months due to the incidence of a decrease in LVEF of more than 10% in 6% of the patients in the clinical trial. These changes, however, are reversible, and the treatment can be restarted once the ejection fraction has recovered.

New BRAF Therapies

New BRAF inhibitors are being tested in clinical trials in combination with ERK inhibitors. No results are available yet.

RET REARRANGEMENTS

Genetics and Preclinical Data

RET (REarranged during Transfection) is a transmembrane receptor with TK activity. Its ligands are growth factors derived from the glial cell line–derived neurotropic factor (GDNF family ligands or GFL). It leads to downstream activation of several pathways involved in cell growth and differentiation of multiple tissue types, including the neural crest, kidneys, and germ cells. It functions by interacting with the MAPK, PI3K/AKT, and RAS/ERK pathways. RET germline mutations are responsible for inherited forms of medullary thyroid cancer in multiple endocrine neoplasia type 2 (MEN-2) syndrome, and somatic mutations are associated with sporadic cases of medullary carcinoma.[198] RET gene rearrangements like RET-CCDC6 and RET-NCOA4 generate fusion proteins that cause constant unregulated activation of RET and have been involved in the development of papillary thyroid carcinoma.

The RET rearrangements were discovered in a subset of cases of non–small cell carcinoma[199]; the most common rearrangement seen is KIF5B-RET, but other fusion partners like CCDC6 NCOA4 and TRIM33 have also been identified.[200] RET fusion proteins have transforming capabilities in cell lines, and they demonstrate sensitivity to RET inhibitors.[199]

Clinicopathological Features

The RET rearrangements have been found only in adenocarcinomas. A frequency of 1.4% has been established in 2 large series.[175] The patients affected have minimal-to-any tobacco exposure and do not have overlap with other molecular markers.

Targeted Treatment Efficacy

After finding RET rearrangements in NSCLC, cabozantinib, a multikinase inhibitor with activity against RET, was tested in this patient population.[201] In a phase 2 study, 26 patients with RET rearrangements documented by FISH or polymerase chain reaction, some of which were treatment naïve, received cabozantinib at a dose of 60 mg (tablet form) daily continuously until disease progression or unacceptable toxicity. A response rate of 28% was seen; responses were fast, with the majority seen in the first 4 weeks of treatment, but they were all partial responses, and no complete responses were seen. The median DOR was 7 months. Median PFS was 5.5 months. It was hypothesized that responses may be related to the fusion partner involved in the rearrangement, but the sample size did not allow for this kind of assessment. Common side effects were transaminitis (81%), hypothyroidism (15%), diarrhea (46%), palmar-plantar erythrodysesthesia (35%), thrombocytopenia (31%), and mucositis (42%). Serious AEs included lipase elevation, thrombocytopenia, and elevation of liver enzymes. Dose reduction to 40 mg and sometimes 20 mg was necessary in 73% of the patients, and interruption occurred in 8%. Cabozantinib is currently FDA approved for the treatment of renal cell carcinoma and medullary thyroid carcinoma.

Vandetanib, another multikinase inhibitor with activity against VEGF, EGFR, and RET, was tested in 18 previously treated patients with RET rearrangements.[202] The response rate was 18%, all partial responses, with a disease control rate (Partial Response Rate and Stable Disease [PR+SD]) of 65%. Median PFS was 4.5 months, and median OS was 11.6 months. Frequent adverse reactions included hypertension (89%), skin rash (72%), diarrhea (44%), acne (28%), xerosis (22%), abdominal discomfort (17%), and nail changes (17%). Serious AEs were hypertension, QTc prolongation, and transaminitis.

Lenvatinib, another multikinase inhibitor, was tested in a phase 2 trial in which 25 patients positive for RET rearrangement were enrolled.[203] The dose used was 24 mg given continuously until disease progression or unacceptable toxicity. The ORR was 16%, without complete responses; the disease control rate was 76% (PR+SD). The median duration of treatment was only 16 weeks. Side effects were frequent, and there was one fatal pneumonia attributed to lenvatinib. Dose reductions were necessary in 68% of patients. The most common side effects were hypertension (68%), nausea (60%), hyporexia (52%), diarrhea (52%), proteinuria (48%), and vomiting (44%).

Overall, these responses were much less impressive when compared with treatment of EGFR mutations or ALK or ROS1 rearrangements. The reason for this low efficacy is not clear, and it was thought that a more selective RET inhibitor could have a more favorable efficacy with less toxicity.

Very early data with the use of selective RET inhibitors has been promising. BLU667, an investigational agent that is a more potent and selective RET inhibitor, has shown partial responses in 3 patients with NSCLC and medullary thyroid cancer with RET rearrangements, with very limited toxicity.[204] LOXO-292, another potent and selective RET inhibitor, has shown clinical activity in a phase 1 trial where 57 patients with RET-mutated or rearranged tumors, including 27 with NSCLC, showed an ORR of 69%, including patients with disease resistant to prior multikinase inhibitors. Toxicity was mild, with the most frequent being fatigue, diarrhea, and dyspnea. Further development of these compounds is in progress.[205]

NTRK REARRANGEMENTS

Genetics and Preclinical Data

Neurotrophic receptor tyrosine kinase 1 (*NTRK1*), *NTRK2*, and *NTRK3* genes encode for the tropomyosin receptor kinases (TRK) TRKA, TRKB, and TRKC. These receptors were initially described in 1991, but their role in cancer treatment is just now being explored.[206] They are found frequently not only in the CNS but also in other organs, like bone, lung, monocytes, and pancreatic beta cells. Known ligands are nerve growth factor (NGF), brain-derived neurotropic factor (BDNF), and neurotropin 3 (NT-3) involved in developmental neuronal pathways.[207] Their phosphorylation activates downstream pathways PI3K/MAPK/RAS/AKT or PLC-Y/PKC, mediating cell proliferation, synaptic plasticity, and prevention of neurodegeneration or apoptosis.[208]

Mutations in the NTRK genes have been reported in multiple malignancies but were found to be oncogenic only in AML and neuroblastoma.[208] On the other hand, NTRK fusion proteins, products of gene rearrangements, have been identified in a number of malignancies, and the oncogenic potential of these fusion proteins has been well documented. They have been found to use the downstream RAS/RAF/MAPK pathway. Several possible fusion partners have been identified: TPM3, ETV6, TPR, TFG, and MPRIP. The disseminated use of NGS techniques allowed for the finding of these infrequent but recurrent alterations in different malignancies. Examples of frequencies seen in different series are NTRK1 and NTRK2 fusions, found in intrahepatic cholangiocarcinoma (3.6%), papillary thyroid carcinoma (12%), glioblastoma (1.1%), sarcoma (1%), and astrocytoma (3.1%). NTRK3 fusions have been found to be dominant in some rare malignancies, like congenital fibrosarcomas, where it is present in 100% of cases; congenital mesoblastic nephroma (83%); and mammary analogue secretory carcinoma (100%).[209]

Clinicopathological Features

The NTRK1 rearrangements are rare events in NSCLC, found in 3% of a cohort of patients who were negative for other actionable markers,[210] and found to be at 0.1% in an unselected cohort of patients.[211] Clinical and pathological characteristics have not been well defined.

Targeted Treatment Efficacy

The NTRK inhibitors are currently under investigation for the treatment of NRTK-associated malignancies. The first report of a patient with lung adenocarcinoma positive for SQSTM1-NTRK1 rearrangement and advanced refractory disease—including brain metastasis that was treated with the TKI entrectinib, which targets ALK, ROS1, and NTRKA—had a partial response of 6 months' duration, including resolution of brain metastasis.[44] Preliminary data on a phase 1 trial that includes solid tumors of any location with NTRK gene fusions treated with larotrectinib, a selective TRKA/B/C inhibitor, at a dose of 100 mg orally twice a day continuously, has reported an ORR of 78% in 46 patients enrolled so far, with DOR greater than 12 months in 8 patients.[212] Secondary resistance has already developed in some cases, with a finding of de novo mutations, as had also been documented in preclinical studies,[213] demonstrating the challenges ahead. Several NTRK inhibitors are currently being tested in clinical trials.

HER2 MUTATIONS

Genetics and Preclinical Data

HER2 (ERBB2) is a member of the ERBB family of receptors that include ERBB1 (EGFR), ERBB3, and ERBB4. HER2 does not have a specific ligand, but it plays a major role in regulation of downstream signaling when dimerization occurs with any of the other ERBB receptors,[214] executing its effect through the MAPK pathway. HER2 amplification was found to be a predictor of poor prognosis in breast cancer 30 years ago,[215] a finding that eventually led to significant improvements in outcomes with the use of the HER2-targeted monoclonal antibody trastuzumab and later with small molecules with anti-HER2 activity. In NSCLC, 2+ or 3+ overexpression by IHC is seen in 20%-30% of the cases, but strong expression (+3) and gene amplification are seen in only 4% of cases.[216] Initial trials targeting HER2 overexpression in a similar manner as in breast cancer had disappointing results. Trastuzumab was ineffective in a phase 2 trial where only 1 of 22 patients with HER2 overexpression had a partial response to the treatment,[217] stalling the development of anti-HER2 treatment in lung cancer.

   Attention was then shifted to oncogenic-driving mutations. In-frame exon 20 insertions in the HER2 gene were found to have oncogenic effects[218] and downstream activity through the mTOR pathway, suggesting an inhibitory effect by blocking the mTOR activity in preclinical models.

Clinicopathological Features

Large series screening for HER2 mutations in NSCLC have documented a prevalence between 0.5% and 4%.[219] These mutations have been found predominantly in adenocarcinomas and more frequently in non-smokers. Prevalence of up to 6% has been seen when only adenocarcinomas are screened.[220] There is very little overlap with other known driving genetic alterations, with a finding of concomitant mutation in EGFR in 7% of cases and ROS1 and ALK rearrangements in 1% of cases.[221]

Targeted Treatment Efficacy

Small molecules with activity against HER2 have been tested in early clinical trials that included a small number of patients, signaling mild activity. Afatinib, an ERBB family inhibitor, showed clinical activity in 3 cases reported of patients with HER2 mutations.[222]

Neratinib, another dual HER2 and EGFR inhibitor, was tested in a phase 2 trial in combination with the mTOR inhibitor temsirolimus. Preliminary results showed 3 partial responses and 6 patients with stable disease in a cohort of 14. Median PFS was 4 months.[223]

Similarly, dacomitinib, also a pan Her inhibitor, was tried in a phase 2 study where patients with HER2 exon 20 mutations and HER2 amplification were included; responses were seen in 3 of 26 patients with mutations, and no responses were seen in patients with amplification.[224]

These results overall show modest activity of anti-HER2 therapy, except for a recently published phase 2 trial of ado-trastuzumab emtansine (T-DM1), a monoclonal antibody-drug conjugate currently approved for treatment of HER2–positive metastatic breast cancer that was tested in patients with HER2–mutated NSCLC.[225] Eighteen patients were enrolled and received T-DM1 at 3.6 mg/kg IV every 21 days until disease progression or unacceptable toxicity. Overall response was 44%, and median PFS was 5 months. Responses were seen in both pretreated and treatment-naïve patients. AEs were mild; the most frequent ones were infusion reactions, increased transaminases, and thrombocytopenia.

Attempts at improving response by altering the dosing schedule of afatinib with pulse weekly doses have shown a very early signal of improved efficacy, with 3 patients showing partial response. This approach warrants further investigation.[226]

A large retrospective study looking into the efficacy of anti-HER2 therapy in NSCLC in real practice showed a response rate of 50% and disease control (PR+SD) of 75%, with a median PFS of 4.8 months when trastuzumab was used in combination with chemotherapy. Albeit no direct comparison was possible, these results were similar to platinum doublet without trastuzumab in the same cohort, where the response rate was 43%, and disease control was 70%, with a median PFS of 6 months.[221] Small molecules had lower response rates. So far, no anti-HER2 therapy has been FDA approved for NSCLC; the most promising results seen so far have been with the use of T-DM1.

REFERENCES

1. David EA, JM, Cooke DT, Melnikow J, Kelly K, Canter RJ. The role of thoracic surgery in the therapeutic management of metastatic non-small cell lung cancer. *J Thorac Oncol.* 2017;12(11):1636-1645.

2. Congedo MT, Cesario A, Lococo F, et al. Surgery for oligometastatic non-small cell lung cancer: long-term results from a single center experience. *J Thorac Cardiovasc Surg.* 2012;144(2):444-452.

3. Hellman S, Weichselbaum RR. Oligometastases. *J Clin Oncol.* 1995;13(1):8-10.

4. Ashworth AB, Senan S, Palma DA, et al. An individual patient data metaanalysis of outcomes and prognostic factors after treatment of oligometastatic non-small-cell lung cancer. *Clin Lung Cancer.* 2014;15(5):346-355.

5. Ashworth A, Rodrigues G, Boldt G, Palma D. Is there an oligometastatic state in non-small cell lung cancer? A systematic review of the literature. *Lung Cancer.* 2013;82(2):197-203.

6. Lussier YA, Xing HR, Salama JK, et al. MicroRNA expression characterizes oligometastasis(es). *PLoS One.* 2011;6(12):e28650.

7. Lussier YA, Khodarev NN, Regan K, et al. Oligo- and polymetastatic progression in lung metastasis(es) patients is associated with specific microRNAs. *PLoS One.* 2012;7(12):e50141.

8. Patrini D, Panagiotopoulos N, Bedetti B, et al. Surgical approach in oligometastatic non-small cell lung cancer. *Ann Transl Med.* 2018;6(5):93.

9. Bae MK, Yu WS, Byun GE, et al. Prognostic factors for cases with no extracranial metastasis in whom brain metastasis is detected after resection of non-small cell lung cancer. *Lung Cancer.* 2015;88(2):195-200.

10. Xu Q, Wang Y, Liu H, et al. Treatment outcome for patients with primary NSCLC and synchronous solitary metastasis. *Clin Transl Oncol.* 2013;15(10):802-809.

11. Abdel-Rahman O. Outcomes of surgery as part of the management of metastatic non-small-cell lung cancer: a surveillance, epidemiology and end results database analysis. *Cancer Invest.* 2018;36(4):238-245.

12. Billing PS, Miller DL, Allen MS, Deschamps C, Trastek VF, Pairolero PC. Surgical treatment of primary lung cancer with synchronous brain metastases. *J Thorac Cardiovasc Surg.* 2001;122(3):548-553.

13. Kozower BD, Larner JM, Detterbeck FC, Jones DR. Special treatment issues in non-small cell lung cancer: diagnosis and management of lung cancer, 3rd ed: American College of Chest Physicians evidence-based clinical practice guidelines. *Chest.* 2013;143(5 Suppl):e369S-e399S.

14. Tanvetyanon T, Robinson LA, Schell MJ, et al. Outcomes of adrenalectomy for isolated synchronous versus metachronous adrenal metastases in non-small-cell lung cancer: a systematic review and pooled analysis. *J Clin Oncol.* 2008;26(7):1142-1147.

15. Barone M, Di Nuzzo D, Cipollone G, Camplese P, Mucilli F. Oligometastatic non-small cell lung cancer (NSCLC): adrenal metastases. Experience in a single institution. *Updates Surg.* 2015;67(4):383-387.

16. Tamura T, Kurishima K, Watanabe H, et al. Characteristics of clinical N0 metastatic non-small cell lung cancer. *Lung Cancer.* 2015;89(1):71-75.

17. Mordant P, Arame A, De Dominicis F, et al. Which metastasis management allows long-term survival of synchronous solitary M1b non-small cell lung cancer? *Eur J Cardiothorac Surg.* 2012;41(3):617-622.

18. Tonnies M, Pfannschmidt J, Bauer TT, Kollmeier J, Tönnies S, Kaiser D. Metastasectomy for synchronous solitary non-small cell lung cancer metastases. *Ann Thorac Surg.* 2014;98(1):249-256.

19. Kim YH, Lee KS, Primack SL, et al. Small pulmonary nodules on CT accompanying surgically resectable lung cancer: likelihood of malignancy. *J Thorac Imaging.* 2002;17(1):40-46.

20. Gould MK, Donington J, Lynch WR, et al. Evaluation of individuals with pulmonary nodules: when is it lung cancer? Diagnosis and management of lung cancer, 3rd ed: American College of Chest Physicians evidence-based clinical practice guidelines. *Chest.* 2013;143(5 Suppl):e93S-e120S.

21. Martini N, Melamed MR. Multiple primary lung cancers. *J Thorac Cardiovasc Surg.* 1975;70(4):606-612.

22. Girard N, Deshpande C, Lau C, et al. Comprehensive histologic assessment helps to differentiate multiple lung primary nonsmall cell carcinomas from metastases. *Am J Surg Pathol.* 2009;33(12):1752-1764.

23. Girard N, Ostrovnaya I, Lau C, et al. Genomic and mutational profiling to assess clonal relationships between multiple non-small-cell lung cancers. *Clin Cancer Res.* 2009;15(16):5184-5190.

24. Liu Y, Zhang J, Li L, et al. Genomic heterogeneity of multiple synchronous lung cancer. *Nat Commun.* 2016;7:13200.

25. Chang YL, Wu C-T, Lin S-C, Hsiao C-F, Jou Y-S, Lee Y-C. Clonality and prognostic implications of p53 and epidermal growth factor receptor somatic aberrations in multiple primary lung cancers. *Clin Cancer Res.* 2007;13(1):52-58.

26. Sequist LV, Waltman BA, Dias-Santagata D, et al. Genotypic and histological evolution of lung cancers acquiring resistance to EGFR inhibitors. *Sci Transl Med.* 2011;3(75):75ra26.

27. Grob TJ, Hoenig T, Clauditz TC, et al. Frequent intratumoral heterogeneity of EGFR gene copy gain in non-small cell lung cancer. *Lung Cancer.* 2013;79(3):221-7.

28. Detterbeck FC, Jones DR, Kernstine KH, Naunheim KS; American College of Physicians. Lung cancer. Special treatment issues. *Chest*. 2003;123(1 Suppl):244s-258s.

29. Shen KR, Meyers BF, Larner JM, Jones DR; American College of Chest Physicians. Special treatment issues in lung cancer: ACCP evidence-based clinical practice guidelines (2nd edition). *Chest*. 2007;132 (3 Suppl):290s-305s.

30. Hamaji M, Ali SO, Burt BM. A meta-analysis of resected metachronous second non-small cell lung cancer. *Ann Thorac Surg*. 2015;99(4):1470-1478.

31. Hamaji M, Allen MS, Cassivi SD, et al. Surgical treatment of metachronous second primary lung cancer after complete resection of non-small cell lung cancer. *J Thorac Cardiovasc Surg*. 2013;145(3):683-690; discussion 690-691.

32. Lee BE, Port JL, Stiles BM, et al. TNM stage is the most important determinant of survival in metachronous lung cancer. *Ann Thorac Surg*. 2009;88(4):1100-1105.

33. Muranishi Y, Sonobe M, Hamaji M, et al. Surgery for metachronous second primary lung cancer versus surgery for primary lung cancer: a propensity score-matched comparison of postoperative complications and survival outcomes. *Interact Cardiovasc Thorac Surg*. 2018;26(4):631-637.

34. Yang J, Liu M, Fan J, et al. Surgical treatment of metachronous second primary lung cancer. *Ann Thorac Surg*. 2014;98(4):1192-1198.

35. Bae MK, Byun CS, Lee CY, et al. Clinical outcomes and prognostic factors for surgically resected second primary lung cancer. *Thorac Cardiovasc Surg*. 2012;60(8):525-532.

36. Ginsberg RJ, Rubinstein LV. Randomized trial of lobectomy versus limited resection for T1 N0 non-small cell lung cancer. Lung Cancer Study Group. *Ann Thorac Surg*. 1995;60(3):615-622; discussion 622-623.

37. Sienel W, Dango S, Kirschbaum A, et al. Sublobar resections in stage IA non-small cell lung cancer: segmentectomies result in significantly better cancer-related survival than wedge resections. *Eur J Cardiothorac Surg*. 2008;33(4):728-734.

38. Smith CB, Swanson SJ, Mhango G, Wisnivesky JP. Survival after segmentectomy and wedge resection in stage I non-small-cell lung cancer. *J Thorac Oncol*. 2013;8(1):73-78.

39. Shin J, Keam B, Kim M, et al. Prognostic impact of newly proposed M descriptors in TNM classification of non-small cell lung cancer. *J Thorac Oncol*. 2017;12(3):520-528.

40. Morris ZS, Cannon DM, Morris BA, Bentzen SM, Kozak KR. Impact of a contralateral tumor nodule on survival in non-small-cell lung cancer. *J Thorac Oncol*. 2015;10(11):1608-1615.

41. Nagai K, Sohara Y, Tsuchiya R, et al. Prognosis of resected non-small cell lung cancer patients with intrapulmonary metastases. *J Thorac Oncol*. 2007;2(4):282-286.

42. De Leyn P, Dooms C, Kuzdzal J, et al. Preoperative mediastinal lymph node staging for non-small cell lung cancer: 2014 update of the 2007 ESTS guidelines. *Transl Lung Cancer Res*. 2014;3(4):225-233.

43. De Leyn P, Moons J, Vansteenkiste J, et al. Survival after resection of synchronous bilateral lung cancer. *Eur J Cardiothorac Surg*. 2008;34(6):1215-1222.

44. Detterbeck FC, Jantz MA, Wallace M, Vansteenkiste J, Silvestri GA, American College of Chest Physicians. Invasive mediastinal staging of lung cancer: ACCP evidence-based clinical practice guidelines (2nd edition). *Chest*. 2007;132(3 Suppl):202s-220s.

45. Asamura H, Chansky K, Crowley J, et al. The International Association for the Study of Lung Cancer Lung Cancer Staging Project: Proposals for the Revision of the N Descriptors in the Forthcoming 8th Edition of the TNM Classification for Lung Cancer. *J Thorac Oncol*. 2015;10(12):1675-1684.

46. Yoo C, Yoon S, Lee DH, et al. Prognostic significance of the number of metastatic pN2 lymph nodes in stage IIIA-N2 non-small-cell lung cancer after curative resection. *Clin Lung Cancer*. 2015;16(6):e203-e212.

47. Hsieh CP, Hsieh M-J, Wu C-F, et al. Prognostic factors in non-small cell lung cancer patients who received neoadjuvant therapy and curative resection. *J Thorac Dis*. 2016;8(7):1477-1486.

48. Villaruz LC, Kubicek GJ, Socinski MA. Management of non-small cell lung cancer with oligometastasis. *Curr Oncol Rep*. 2012;14(4):333-341.

49. Novoa NM, Varela G, Jimenez MF. Surgical management of oligometastatic non-small cell lung cancer. *J Thorac Dis*. 2016;8(Suppl 11):S895-S900.

50. Jack S, West MA, Raw D, et al. The effect of neoadjuvant chemotherapy on physical fitness and survival in patients undergoing oesophagogastric cancer surgery. *Eur J Surg Oncol*. 2014;40(10):1313-1320.

51. van Meerbeeck JP, Kramer GW, Van Schil PE, et al. Randomized controlled trial of resection versus radiotherapy after induction chemotherapy in stage IIIA-N2 non-small-cell lung cancer. *J Natl Cancer Inst*. 2007;99(6):442-450.

52. Albain KS, Swann RS, Rusch VW, et al. Radiotherapy plus chemotherapy with or without surgical resection for stage III non-small-cell lung cancer: a phase III randomised controlled trial. *Lancet*. 2009;374(9687):379-386.

53. Eberhardt WEE, Pöttgen C, Gauler TC, et al. Phase III study of surgery versus definitive concurrent chemoradiotherapy boost in patients with resectable stage IIIA(N2) and selected IIIB non-small-cell lung cancer after induction chemotherapy and concurrent chemoradiotherapy (ESPATUE). *J Clin Oncol.* 2015;33(35):4194-4201.

54. Van Schil PE, Berzenji L, Yogeswaran SK, Hendriks JM, Lauwers P. Surgical management of stage IIIA non-small cell lung cancer. *Front Oncol.* 2017;7:249.

55. McElnay PJ, Choong A, Jordan E, Song F, Lim E. Outcome of surgery versus radiotherapy after induction treatment in patients with N2 disease: systematic review and meta-analysis of randomised trials. *Thorax.* 2015;70(8):764-768.

56. Boffa DJ, Hancock JG, Yao X, et al. Now or later: evaluating the importance of chemotherapy timing in resectable stage III (N2) lung cancer in the National Cancer Database. *Ann Thorac Surg.* 2015;99(1):200-208.

57. Yang CF, Kumar A, Gulack BC, et al. Long-term outcomes after lobectomy for non-small cell lung cancer when unsuspected pN2 disease is found: a National Cancer Data Base analysis. *J Thorac Cardiovasc Surg.* 2016;151(5):1380-1388.

58. Thomas DC, Arnold BN, Rosen JE, et al. The significance of upfront knowledge of N2 disease in non-small cell lung cancer. *World J Surg.* 2018;42(1):161-171.

59. Cetin K, Christiansen CF, Jacobsen JB, Nørgaard M, Sørensen HT. Bone metastasis, skeletal-related events, and mortality in lung cancer patients: a Danish population-based cohort study. *Lung Cancer.* 2014;86(2):247-254.

60. Bayard LG, Buzón MDCS, Paín EA, Barón LI. Radiation therapy for the management of painful bone metastases: results from a randomized trial. *Rep Pract Oncol Radiother.* 2014;19(6):405-411.

61. Chow E, Zeng L, Salvo N, Dennis K, Tsao M, Lutz S. Update on the systematic review of palliative radiotherapy trials for bone metastases. *Clin Oncol (R Coll Radiol).* 2012;24(2):112-124.

62. Howell DD, James JL, Hartsell WF, et al. Single-fraction radiotherapy versus multifraction radiotherapy for palliation of painful vertebral bone metastases-equivalent efficacy, less toxicity, more convenient: a subset analysis of Radiation Therapy Oncology Group trial 97-14. *Cancer.* 2013;119(4):888-896.

63. Meeuse JJ, van der Linden YM, van Tienhoven G, et al. Efficacy of radiotherapy for painful bone metastases during the last 12 weeks of life: results from the Dutch Bone Metastasis Study. *Cancer.* 2010;116(11):2716-2725.

64. Majumder D, Chatterjee D, Bandyopadhyay A, Mallick SK, Sarkar SK, Majumdar A. Single fraction versus multiple fraction radiotherapy for palliation of painful vertebral bone metastases: a prospective study. *Indian J Palliat Care.* 2012;18(3):202-206.

65. Hird A, Chow E, Zhang L, et al. Determining the incidence of pain flare following palliative radiotherapy for symptomatic bone metastases: results from three canadian cancer centers. *Int J Radiat Oncol Biol Phys.* 2009;75(1):193-197.

66. Chow E, Meyer RM, Ding K, et al. Dexamethasone in the prophylaxis of radiation-induced pain flare after palliative radiotherapy for bone metastases: a double-blind, randomised placebo-controlled, phase 3 trial. *The Lancet Oncology.* 2015;16(15):1463-1472.

67. Niglas M, Raman S, Rodin D, et al. Should dexamethasone be standard in the prophylaxis of pain flare after palliative radiotherapy for bone metastases?—a debate. *Ann Palliat Med.* 2017;7(2):279-283.

68. Lutz S, Balboni T, Jones J, et al. Palliative radiation therapy for bone metastases: update of an ASTRO evidence-based guideline. *Pract Radiat Oncol.* 2017;7(1):4-12.

69. Huisman M, van den Bosch MAAJ, Wijlemans JW, van Vulpen M, van der Linden YM, Verkooijen HM. Effectiveness of reirradiation for painful bone metastases: a systematic review and meta-analysis. *Int J Radiat Oncol Biol Phys.* 2012;84(1):8-14.

70. Laufer I, Rubin DG, Lis E, et al. The NOMS framework: approach to the treatment of spinal metastatic tumors. *Oncologist.* 2013;18(6):744-751.

71. Bilsky MH, Laufer I, Fourney DR, et al. Reliability analysis of the epidural spinal cord compression scale. *J Neurosurg Spine.* 2010;13(3):324-328.

72. Fisher CG, DiPaola CP, Ryken TC, et al. A novel classification system for spinal instability in neoplastic disease: an evidence-based approach and expert consensus from the Spine Oncology Study Group. *Spine (Phila Pa 1976).* 2010;35(22):E1221-E1229.

73. Fisher CG, Schouten R, Versteeg AL, et al. Reliability of the Spinal Instability Neoplastic Score (SINS) among radiation oncologists: an assessment of instability secondary to spinal metastases. *Radiat Oncol.* 2014;9:69.

74. Ryu S, Pugh SL, Gerszten PC, et al. RTOG 0631 Phase II/III Study of Image-Guided Stereotactic Radiosurgery for Localized (1-3) Spine Metastases: Phase II Results. *Pract Radiat Oncol.* 2014;4(2):76-81.

75. Tseng CL, Soliman H, Myrehaug S, et al. Imaging-based outcomes for 24 Gy in 2 daily fractions for patients with de novo spinal metastases treated with spine stereotactic body radiotherapy (SBRT). *Int J Radiat Oncol Biol Phys.* 2018;102(3):499-507.

76. Sprave T, Verma V, Förster R, et al. Randomized phase II trial evaluating pain response in patients with spinal metastases following stereotactic body radiotherapy versus three-dimensional conformal radiotherapy. *Radiother Oncol.* 2018;128(2):274-282.

77. Cox BW, Spratt DE, Lovelock M, et al. International spine radiosurgery consortium consensus guidelines for target volume definition in spinal stereotactic radiosurgery. *Int J Radiat Oncol Biol Phys.* 2012;83(5): e597-e605.

78. Redmond KJ, Robertson S, Lo SS, et al. Consensus contouring guidelines for postoperative stereotactic body radiation therapy for metastatic solid tumor malignancies to the spine. *Int J Radiat Oncol Biol Phys.* 2017;97(1):64-74.

79. Sheu T, Heymach JV, Swisher SG, et al. Propensity score-matched analysis of comprehensive local therapy for oligometastatic non-small cell lung cancer that did not progress after front-line chemotherapy. *Int J Radiat Oncol Biol Phys.* 2014;90(4):850-857.

80. Gomez DR, Blumenschein GR, Jr., Lee JJ, et al. Local consolidative therapy versus maintenance therapy or observation for patients with oligometastatic non-small-cell lung cancer without progression after first-line systemic therapy: a multicentre, randomised, controlled, phase 2 study. *Lancet Oncol.* 2016;17(12):1672-1682.

81. Mole RH. Whole body irradiation—radiobiology or medicine? *Br J Radiol.* 1953;26(305):234-241.

82. Waqar SN, Samson PP, Robinson CG, et al. Non-small-cell lung cancer with brain metastasis at presentation. *Clin Lung Cancer.* 2018;19(4):e373-e379.

83. Li L, Luo S, Lin H, et al. Correlation between EGFR mutation status and the incidence of brain metastases in patients with non-small cell lung cancer. *J Thorac Dis.* 2017;9(8):2510-2520.

84. Hsu F, De Caluwe A, Anderson D, et al. EGFR mutation status on brain metastases from non-small cell lung cancer. *Lung Cancer.* 2016;96:101-107.

85. Sperduto PW, Yang TJ, Beal K, et al. Estimating survival in patients with lung cancer and brain metastases: an update of the graded prognostic assessment for lung cancer using molecular markers (Lung-molGPA). *JAMA Oncol.* 2017;3(6):827-831.

86. Soffietti R, Abacioglu U, Baumert B, et al. Diagnosis and treatment of brain metastases from solid tumors: guidelines from the European Association of Neuro-Oncology (EANO). *Neuro Oncol.* 2017;19(2):162-174.

87. Mahajan A, Ahmed S, McAleer MF, et al. Post-operative stereotactic radiosurgery versus observation for completely resected brain metastases: a single-centre, randomised, controlled, phase 3 trial. *Lancet Oncol.* 2017;18(8):1040-1048.

88. Mulvenna P, Lee C, Waite K, et al. Dexamethasone and supportive care with or without whole brain radiotherapy in treating patients with non-small cell lung cancer with brain metastases unsuitable for resection or stereotactic radiotherapy (QUARTZ): results from a phase 3, non-inferiority, randomised trial. *Lancet.* 2016;388(10055):2004-2014.

89. Magnuson WJ, Lester-Coll NH, Wu AJ, et al. Management of brain metastases in tyrosine kinase inhibitor-naive epidermal growth factor receptor-mutant non-small-cell lung cancer: a retrospective multi-institutional analysis. *J Clin Oncol.* 2017;35(10):1070-1077.

90. Scagliotti GV, Parikh P, von Pawel J, et al. Phase III study comparing cisplatin plus gemcitabine with cisplatin plus pemetrexed in chemotherapy-naive patients with advanced-stage non-small-cell lung cancer. *J Clin Oncol.* 2008;26(21):3543-3551.

91. Sigmond J, Backus HHJ, Wouters D, Temmink OH, Jansen G, Peters GJ. Induction of resistance to the multi-targeted antifolate pemetrexed (ALIMTA) in WiDr human colon cancer cells is associated with thymidylate synthase overexpression. *Biochem Pharmacol.* 2003;66(3):431-438.

92. Sandler A, Gray R, Perry MC, et al. Paclitaxel-carboplatin alone or with bevacizumab for non-small-cell lung cancer. *N Engl J Med.* 2006;355(24):2542-2550.

93. Reck M, von Pawel J, Zatloukal P, et al. Phase III trial of cisplatin plus gemcitabine with either placebo or bevacizumab as first-line therapy for nonsquamous non-small-cell lung cancer: AVAiL. *J Clin Oncol.* 2009;27(8):1227-1234.

94. Leighl NB, Bennouna J, Yi J, Moore N, Hambleton J, Hurwitz H. Bleeding events in bevacizumab-treated cancer patients who received full-dose anticoagulation and remained on study. *Br J Cancer.* 2011;104(3):413-418.

95. Socinski MA, Langer CJ, Huang JE, et al. Safety of bevacizumab in patients with non-small-cell lung cancer and brain metastases. *J Clin Oncol.* 2009;27(31):5255-5261.

96. Reck M, Rodríguez-Abreu D, Robinson AG, et al. Pembrolizumab versus chemotherapy for PD-L1-positive non-small-cell lung cancer. *N Engl J Med.* 2016;375(19):1823-1833.

97. Mok TSK, Wu Y-L, Kudaba I, et al. Pembrolizumab versus chemotherapy for previously untreated, PD-L1-expressing, locally advanced or metastatic non-small-cell lung cancer (KEYNOTE-042): a randomised, open-label, controlled, phase 3 trial. *Lancet.* 2019;393(10183):1819-1830.

98. Langer CJ, Gadgeel SM, Borghaei H, et al. Carboplatin and pemetrexed with or without pembrolizumab for advanced, non-squamous non-small-cell lung cancer: a randomised, phase 2 cohort of the open-label KEYNOTE-021 study. *Lancet Oncol.* 2016;17(11):1497-1508.

99. Gandhi L, Rodríguez-Abreu D, Gadgeel S, et al. Pembrolizumab plus chemotherapy in metastatic non-small-cell lung cancer. *N Engl J Med.* 2018;378(22):2078-2092.

100. Socinski MA, Jotte RM, Cappuzzo F, et al. Atezolizumab for first-line treatment of metastatic nonsquamous NSCLC. *N Engl J Med.* 2018;378(24):2288-2301.

101. Paz-Ares L, Luft A, Vicente D, et al. Pembrolizumab plus chemotherapy for squamous non-small-cell lung cancer. *N Engl J Med.* 2018;379(21):2040-2051.

102. Jotte RM, Cappuzzo F, Vynnychenko I, et al. IMpower131: Primary PFS and safety analysis of a randomized phase III study of atezolizumab + carboplatin + paclitaxel or nab-paclitaxel vs carboplatin + nab-paclitaxel as 1L therapy in advanced squamous NSCLC. *J Clin Oncol.* 2018;36(18_suppl):LBA9000-LBA9000.

103. Hotta K, Matsuo K, Ueoka H, Kiura K, Tabata M, Tanimoto M. Meta-analysis of randomized clinical trials comparing cisplatin to carboplatin in patients with advanced non-small-cell lung cancer. *J Clin Oncol.* 2004;22(19):3852-3859.

104. Ardizzoni A, Boni L, Tiseo M, et al. Cisplatin- versus carboplatin-based chemotherapy in first-line treatment of advanced non-small-cell lung cancer: an individual patient data meta-analysis. *J Natl Cancer Inst.* 2007;99(11):847-857.

105. Scagliotti G, Brodowicz T, Shepherd FA, et al. Treatment-by-histology interaction analyses in three phase III trials show superiority of pemetrexed in nonsquamous non-small cell lung cancer. *J Thorac Oncol.* 2011;6(1):64-70.

106. Socinski MA, Bondarenko I, Karaseva NA, et al. Weekly nab-paclitaxel in combination with carboplatin versus solvent-based paclitaxel plus carboplatin as first-line therapy in patients with advanced non-small-cell lung cancer: final results of a phase III trial. *J Clin Oncol.* 2012;30(17):2055-2062.

107. Patel JD, Hensing TA, Rademaker A, et al. Phase II study of pemetrexed and carboplatin plus bevacizumab with maintenance pemetrexed and bevacizumab as first-line therapy for nonsquamous non-small-cell lung cancer. *J Clin Oncol.* 2009;27(20):3284-3289.

108. Nadler E, Yu E, Ravelo A, Sing A, Forsyth M, Gruschkus S. Bevacizumab treatment to progression after chemotherapy: outcomes from a U.S. community practice network. *Oncologist.* 2011;16(4):486-496.

109. Paz-Ares L, de Marinis F, Dediu M, et al. Maintenance therapy with pemetrexed plus best supportive care versus placebo plus best supportive care after induction therapy with pemetrexed plus cisplatin for advanced non-squamous non-small-cell lung cancer (PARAMOUNT): a double-blind, phase 3, randomised controlled trial. *Lancet Oncol.* 2012;13(3):247-255.

110. Ciuleanu T, Brodowicz T, Zielinski C, et al. Maintenance pemetrexed plus best supportive care versus placebo plus best supportive care for non-small-cell lung cancer: a randomised, double-blind, phase 3 study. *Lancet.* 2009;374(9699):1432-1440.

111. Fidias PM, Dakhil SR, Lyss AP, et al. Phase III study of immediate compared with delayed docetaxel after front-line therapy with gemcitabine plus carboplatin in advanced non-small-cell lung cancer. *J Clin Oncol.* 2009;27(4):591-598.

112. Fossella FV, DeVore R, Kerr RN, et al. Randomized phase III trial of docetaxel versus vinorelbine or ifosfamide in patients with advanced non-small-cell lung cancer previously treated with platinum-containing chemotherapy regimens. The TAX 320 Non-Small Cell Lung Cancer Study Group. *J Clin Oncol.* 2000;18(12):2354-2362.

113. Shepherd FA, Dancey J, Ramlau R, et al. Prospective randomized trial of docetaxel versus best supportive care in patients with non-small-cell lung cancer previously treated with platinum-based chemotherapy. *J Clin Oncol.* 2000;18(10):2095-2103.

114. Garon EB, Ciuleanu T-E, Arrieta O, et al. Ramucirumab plus docetaxel versus placebo plus docetaxel for second-line treatment of stage IV non-small-cell lung cancer after disease progression on platinum-based therapy (REVEL): a multicentre, double-blind, randomised phase 3 trial. *Lancet.* 2014;384(9944):665-673.

115. ELCVISG, Effects of vinorelbine on quality of life and survival of elderly patients with advanced non-small-cell lung cancer. The Elderly Lung Cancer Vinorelbine Italian Study Group. *J Natl Cancer Inst.* 1999;91(1):66-72.

116. Gridelli C, Aapro M, Ardizzoni A, et al. Treatment of advanced non-small-cell lung cancer in the elderly: results of an international expert panel. *J Clin Oncol.* 2005;23(13):3125-3137.

117. Quoix E, Zalcman G, Oster J-P, et al. Carboplatin and weekly paclitaxel doublet chemotherapy compared with monotherapy in elderly patients with advanced non-small-cell lung cancer: IFCT-0501 randomised, phase 3 trial. *Lancet.* 2011;378(9796):1079-1088.

118. Lilenbaum RC, Herndon JE 2nd, List MA, et al. Single-agent versus combination chemotherapy in advanced non-small-cell lung cancer: the cancer and leukemia group B (study 9730). *J Clin Oncol.* 2005;23(1):190-196.

119. Zukin M, Barrios CH, Pereira JR, et al. Randomized phase III trial of single-agent pemetrexed versus car-boplatin and pemetrexed in patients with advanced non-small-cell lung cancer and Eastern Cooperative Oncology Group performance status of 2. *J Clin Oncol.* 2013;31(23):2849-2853.

120. Kazandjian D, Suzman DL, Blumenthal G, et al. FDA approval summary: nivolumab for the treatment of metastatic non-small cell lung cancer with progression on or after platinum-based chemotherapy. *Oncologist.* 2016;21(5):634-642.

121. Saresella M, Rainone V, Al-Daghri NM, Clerici M, Trabattoni D. The PD-1/PD-L1 pathway in human pathol-ogy. *Curr Mol Med.* 2012;12(3):259-267.

122. Boussiotis VA. Molecular and biochemical aspects of the PD-1 checkpoint pathway. *N Engl J Med.* 2016;375(18):1767-1778.

123. Borghaei H, Paz-Ares L, Horn L, et al. Nivolumab versus docetaxel in advanced nonsquamous non-small-cell lung cancer. *N Engl J Med.* 2015;373(17):1627-1639.

124. Brahmer J, Reckamp KL, Baas P, et al. Nivolumab versus docetaxel in advanced squamous-cell non-small-cell lung cancer. *N Engl J Med.* 2015;373(2):123-135.

125. Vokes EE, Ready N, Felip E, et al. Nivolumab versus docetaxel in previously treated advanced non-small-cell lung cancer (CheckMate 017 and CheckMate 057): 3-year update and outcomes in patients with liver metas-tases. *Ann Oncol.* 2018;29(4):959-965.

126. Carbone DP, Reck M, Paz-Ares L, et al. First-line nivolumab in stage IV or recurrent non-small-cell lung cancer. *N Engl J Med.* 2017;376(25):2415-2426.

127. Hellmann MD, Ciuleanu T-E, Pluzanski A, et al. Nivolumab plus Ipilimumab in lung cancer with a high tumor mutational burden. *N Engl J Med.* 2018;378(22):2093-2104.

128. Garon EB, Rizvi NA, Hui R, et al. Pembrolizumab for the treatment of non-small-cell lung cancer. *N Engl J Med.* 2015;372(21):2018-2028.

129. Herbst RS, Baas P, Kim D-W, et al. Pembrolizumab versus docetaxel for previously treated, PD-L1-positive, advanced non-small-cell lung cancer (KEYNOTE-010): a randomised controlled trial. *Lancet.* 2016;387(10027):1540-1550.

130. De Lima Lopes G, Wu Y-L, Sadowski S, et al. P2.43: Pembrolizumab vs Platinum-Based Chemotherapy for PD-L1+ NSCLC: Phase 3, Randomized, Open-Label KEYNOTE-042 (NCT02220894): Track: Immunotherapy. *J Thorac Oncol.* 2016;11(10S):S244-S245.

131. Lopes G, Wu Y-L, Kudaba I, et al. Pembrolizumab (pembro) versus platinum-based chemotherapy (chemo) as first-line therapy for advanced/metastatic NSCLC with a PD-L1 tumor proportion score (TPS) ≥ 1%: Open-label, phase 3 KEYNOTE-042 study. *J Clin Oncol.* 2018;36(18_suppl):LBA4-LBA4.

132. Borghaei H, Langer CJ, Gadgeel S, et al. 24-month overall survival from KEYNOTE-021 Cohort G: peme-trexed and carboplatin with or without pembrolizumab as first-line therapy for advanced nonsquamous non-small cell lung cancer. *J Thorac Oncol.* 2019;14(1):124-129.

133. Fehrenbacher L, Spira A, Ballinger M, et al. Atezolizumab versus docetaxel for patients with previously treated non-small-cell lung cancer (POPLAR): a multicentre, open-label, phase 2 randomised controlled trial. *Lancet.* 2016;387(10030):1837-1846.

134. Rittmeyer A, Barlesi F, Waterkamp D, et al. Atezolizumab versus docetaxel in patients with previously treated non-small-cell lung cancer (OAK): a phase 3, open-label, multicentre randomised controlled trial. *Lancet.* 2017;389(10066):255-265.

135. Antonia SJ, Villegas A, Daniel D, et al. Durvalumab after chemoradiotherapy in stage III non-small-cell lung cancer. *N Engl J Med.* 2017;377(20):1919-1929.

136. Antonia SJ, Brahmer JR, Balmanoukian AS, et al. Safety and clinical activity of first-line durval-umab in advanced NSCLC: updated results from a phase 1/2 study. *J Clin Oncol.* 2017;35(15_suppl):e20504-e20504.

137. Gulley JL, Rajan A, Spigel DR, et al. Avelumab for patients with previously treated metastatic or recurrent non-small-cell lung cancer (JAVELIN Solid Tumor): dose-expansion cohort of a multicentre, open-label, phase 1b trial. *Lancet Oncol.* 2017;18(5):599-610.

138. Druker BJ, Tamura S, Buchdunger E, et al. Effects of a selective inhibitor of the Abl tyrosine kinase on the growth of Bcr-Abl positive cells. *Nat Med.* 1996;2(5):561-566.

139. Druker BJ, Talpaz M, Resta DJ, et al. Efficacy and safety of a specific inhibitor of the BCR-ABL tyrosine kinase in chronic myeloid leukemia. *N Engl J Med.* 2001;344(14):1031-1037.

140. Ullrich A, Schlessinger J. Signal transduction by receptors with tyrosine kinase activity. *Cell.* 1990;61(2):203-212.

141. Carpenter G, Cohen S. Epidermal growth factor. *J Biol Chem.* 1990;265(14):7709-7712.

142. Wikstrand CJ, Bigner DD. Prognostic applications of the epidermal growth factor receptor and its ligand, transforming growth factor-alpha. *J Natl Cancer Inst.* 1998;90(11):799-801.

143. Karachaliou N, Molina-Vila MA, Rosell R. The impact of rare EGFR mutations on the treatment response of patients with non-small cell lung cancer. *Expert Rev Respir Med.* 2015;9(3):241-244.

144. Arrieta O, Cardona AF, Corrales L, et al. The impact of common and rare EGFR mutations in response to EGFR tyrosine kinase inhibitors and platinum-based chemotherapy in patients with non-small cell lung cancer. *Lung Cancer.* 2015;87(2):169-175.

145. Ohashi K, Maruvka YE, Michor F, Pao W, et al. Epidermal growth factor receptor tyrosine kinase inhibitor-resistant disease. *J Clin Oncol.* 2013;31(8):1070-1080.

146. Rosell R, Carcereny E, Gervais R, et al. Erlotinib versus standard chemotherapy as first-line treatment for European patients with advanced EGFR mutation-positive non-small-cell lung cancer (EURTAC): a multi-centre, open-label, randomised phase 3 trial. *Lancet Oncol.* 2012;13(3):239-246.

147. Mok TS, Wu YL, Thongprasert S, et al. Gefitinib or carboplatin-paclitaxel in pulmonary adenocarcinoma. *N Engl J Med.* 2009;361(10):947-957.

148. Douillard JY, Ostoros G, Cobo M, et al. First-line gefitinib in Caucasian EGFR mutation-positive NSCLC patients: a phase-IV, open-label, single-arm study. *Br J Cancer.* 2014;110(1):55-62.

149. Sequist LV, Yang JC, Yamamoto N, et al. Phase III study of afatinib or cisplatin plus pemetrexed in patients with metastatic lung adenocarcinoma with EGFR mutations. *J Clin Oncol.* 2013;31(27):3327-3334.

150. Wu YL, Zhou C, Hu C-P, et al. Afatinib versus cisplatin plus gemcitabine for first-line treatment of Asian patients with advanced non-small-cell lung cancer harbouring EGFR mutations (LUX-Lung 6): an open-label, randomised phase 3 trial. *Lancet Oncol.* 2014;15(2):213-222.

151. Paz-Ares L, Tan E-H, O'Byrne K, et al. Afatinib versus gefitinib in patients with EGFR mutation-positive advanced non-small-cell lung cancer: overall survival data from the phase IIb LUX-Lung 7 trial. *Ann Oncol.* 2017;28(2):270-277.

152. Wu YL, Cheng Y, Zhou X, et al. Dacomitinib versus gefitinib as first-line treatment for patients with EGFR-mutation-positive non-small-cell lung cancer (ARCHER 1050): a randomised, open-label, phase 3 trial. *Lancet Oncol.* 2017;18(11):1454-1466.

153. Soria JC, Ohe Y, Vansteenkiste J, et al. Osimertinib in untreated EGFR-mutated advanced non-small-cell lung cancer. *N Engl J Med.* 2018;378(2):113-125.

154. Kwak EL, Bang Y-J, Camidge DR, et al. Anaplastic lymphoma kinase inhibition in non-small-cell lung cancer. *N Engl J Med.* 2010;363(18):1693-1703.

155. Hamilton G, Rath B, Burghuber O. Pharmacokinetics of crizotinib in NSCLC patients. *Expert Opin Drug Metab Toxicol.* 2015;11(5):835-842.

156. Katayama R, Shaw AT, Khan TM, et al. Mechanisms of acquired crizotinib resistance in ALK-rearranged lung cancers. *Sci Transl Med.* 2012;4(120):120ra17.

157. Doebele RC, Pilling AB, Aisner DL, et al. Mechanisms of resistance to crizotinib in patients with ALK gene rearranged non-small cell lung cancer. *Clin Cancer Res.* 2012;18(5):1472-1482.

158. Katayama R, Friboulet L, Koike S, et al. Two novel ALK mutations mediate acquired resistance to the next-generation ALK inhibitor alectinib. *Clin Cancer Res.* 2014;20(22):5686-5696.

159. Friboulet L, Li N, Katayama R, et al. The ALK inhibitor ceritinib overcomes crizotinib resistance in non-small cell lung cancer. *Cancer Discov.* 2014;4(6):662-673.

160. Shaw AT, Kim D-W, Nakagawa K, et al. Crizotinib versus chemotherapy in advanced ALK-positive lung cancer. *N Engl J Med.* 2013;368(25):2385-2394.

161. Solomon BJ, Mok T, Kim D-W, et al. First-line crizotinib versus chemotherapy in ALK-positive lung cancer. *N Engl J Med.* 2014;371(23):2167-2177.

162. Solomon BJ, Kim D-W, Wu Y-L, et al. Final overall survival analysis from a study comparing first-line crizotinib versus chemotherapy in ALK-mutation-positive non-small-cell lung cancer. *J Clin Oncol.* 2018;36(22):2251-2258.

163. Soria JC, Tan DSW, Chiari R, et al. First-line ceritinib versus platinum-based chemotherapy in advanced ALK-rearranged non-small-cell lung cancer (ASCEND-4): a randomised, open-label, phase 3 study. *Lancet.* 2017;389(10072):917-929.

164. Tan DS, Araújo A, Zhang J, et al. Comparative efficacy of ceritinib and crizotinib as initial ALK-targeted therapies in previously treated advanced NSCLC: an adjusted comparison with external controls. *J Thorac Oncol.* 2016;11(9):1550-1557.

165. Hida T, Nokihara H, Kondo M, et al. Alectinib versus crizotinib in patients with ALK-positive non-small-cell lung cancer (J-ALEX): an open-label, randomised phase 3 trial. *Lancet.* 2017;390(10089):29-39.

166. Peters S, Camidge DR, Shaw AT, et al. Alectinib versus crizotinib in untreated ALK-positive non-small-cell lung cancer. *N Engl J Med.* 2017;377(9):829-838.

167. Camidge DR, Kim HR, Ahn M-J, et al. Brigatinib versus crizotinib in ALK-positive non-small-cell lung cancer. *N Engl J Med*. 2018;379(21):2027-2039.

168. Shaw AT, Kim TM, Crinò L, et al. Ceritinib versus chemotherapy in patients with ALK-rearranged non-small-cell lung cancer previously given chemotherapy and crizotinib (ASCEND-5): a randomised, controlled, open-label, phase 3 trial. *Lancet Oncol*. 2017;18(7):874-886.

169. Novello S, Mazières J, Oh I-J, et al. Alectinib versus chemotherapy in crizotinib-pretreated anaplastic lymphoma kinase (ALK)-positive non-small-cell lung cancer: results from the phase III ALUR study. *Ann Oncol*. 2018;29(6):1409-1416.

170. Solomon BJ, Besse B, Bauer TM, et al. Lorlatinib in patients with ALK-positive non-small-cell lung cancer: results from a global phase 2 study. *Lancet Oncol*. 2018;19(12):1654-1667.

171. Matsushime H, Wang L, Shibuya M. Human c-ros-1 gene homologous to the v-ros sequence of UR2 sarcoma virus encodes for a transmembrane receptorlike molecule. *Mol Cell Biol*. 1986;6(8):3000-3004.

172. Rimkunas V, Crosby KE, Li D, et al. Analysis of receptor tyrosine kinase ROS1-positive tumors in non-small cell lung cancer: identification of a FIG-ROS1 fusion. *Clin Cancer Res*. 2012;18(16):4449-4457.

173. Nguyen K, Zong CS, Uttamsingh S, et al. The role of phosphatidylinositol 3-kinase, rho family GTPases, and STAT3 in Ros-induced cell transformation. *J Biol Chem*. 2002;277(13):11107-11115.

174. Birchmeier C, Sharma S, Wigler M. Expression and rearrangement of the ROS1 gene in human glioblastoma cells. *Proc Natl Acad Sci U S A*. 1987;84(24):9270-9274.

175. Takeuchi K, Soda M, Togashi Y, et al. RET, ROS1 and ALK fusions in lung cancer. *Nat Med*. 2012;18(3):378-381.

176. Rikova K, Guo A, Zeng Q, et al. Global survey of phosphotyrosine signaling identifies oncogenic kinases in lung cancer. *Cell*. 2007;131(6):1190-1203.

177. Bergethon K, Shaw AT, Ou S-H I, et al. ROS1 rearrangements define a unique molecular class of lung cancers. *J Clin Oncol*. 2012;30(8):863-870.

178. Shaw A, Ou S-H I, Bang Y-B, et al. Crizotinib in ROS1-rearranged non-small-cell lung cancer. *N Engl J Med*. 2014;371(21):1963-1971.

179. Davare M, Vellore NA, Wagner JP, et al. Structural insight into selectivity and resistance profiles of ROS1 tyrosine kinase inhibitors. *Proc Natl Acad Sci U S A*. 2015;112(39):E5381-E5390.

180. Lim S, Kim HR, Lee J-S, et al. Open-label, multicenter, phase II study of ceritinib in patients with non-small-cell lung cancer harboring ROS1 rearrangement. *J Clin Oncol*. 2017;35(23):2613-2618.

181. Park S, Ahn B-C, Lim SW, et al. Characteristics and outcome of ROS1-positive non-small cell lung cancer patients in routine clinical practice. *J Thorac Oncol*. 2018;13(9):1373-1382.

182. Ahn M, Cho BC, Siena S, et al. OA 14.06 Entrectinib in Patients with Locally Advanced or Metastatic ROS1 Fusion-Positive Non-Small Cell Lung Cancer (NSCLC). *J Thorac Oncol*. 2017;12(11):S1783.

183. Facchinetti F, Loriot Y, Kuo M-S, et al. Crizotinib-resistant ROS1 mutations reveal a predictive kinase inhibitor sensitivity model for ROS1- and ALK-rearranged lung cancers. *Clin Cancer Res*. 2016;22(24):5983-5991.

184. Awad M, Engelman JA, Shaw AT. Acquired resistance to crizotinib from a mutation in CD74-ROS1. *N Engl J Med*. 2013;368(25):2395-2401.

185. Davies K, Mahale S, Astling DP, et al. Resistance to ROS1 inhibition mediated by EGFR pathway activation in non-small cell lung cancer. *PLoS One*. 2013;8(12):e82236.

186. Zou H, Li Q, Engstrom LD, et al. PF-06463922 is a potent and selective next-generation ROS1/ALK inhibitor capable of blocking crizotinib-resistant ROS1 mutations. *Proc Natl Acad Sci U S A*. 2015;112(11):3493-3498.

187. Shaw A, Felip E, Bauer TM, et al. Lorlatinib in non-small-cell lung cancer with ALK or ROS1 rearrangement: an international, multicentre, open-label, single-arm first-in-man phase 1 trial. *Lancet Oncol*. 2017;18(12):1590-1599.

188. Katayama, R, Kobayashi Y, Friboulet L, et al. Cabozantinib overcomes crizotinib resistance in ROS1 fusion-positive cancer. *Clin Cancer Res*. 2015;21(1):166-174.

189. Drilon A, Somwar R, Wagner JP, et al. A novel crizotinib-resistant solvent-front mutation responsive to cabozantinib therapy in a patient with ROS1-rearranged lung cancer. *Clin Cancer Res*. 2016;22(10):2351-2358.

190. Davies H, Bignell GR, Cox C, et al. Mutations of the BRAF gene in human cancer. *Nature*. 2002;417(6892):949-954.

191. Marchetti A, Felicioni L, Malatesta S, et al. Clinical features and outcome of patients with non-small-cell lung cancer harboring BRAF mutations. *J Clin Oncol*. 2011;29(26):3574-3579.

192. Wan P, Garnett MJ, Roe SM, et al. Mechanism of activation of the RAF-ERK signaling pathway by oncogenic mutations of B-RAF. *Cell*. 2004;116(6):855-867.

193. Paik P, Arcila ME, Fara M, et al. Clinical characteristics of patients with lung adenocarcinomas harboring BRAF mutations. *J Clin Oncol*. 2011;29(15):2046-2051.

194. Barlesi F, Mazieres J, Merlio J-P, et al. Routine molecular profiling of patients with advanced non-small-cell lung cancer: results of a 1-year nationwide programme of the French Cooperative Thoracic Intergroup (IFCT). *Lancet*. 2016;387(10026):1415-1426.

195. Gautschi O, Milia J, Cabarrou B, et al. Targeted therapy for patients with BRAF-mutant lung cancer: results from the European EURAF cohort. *J Thorac Oncol*. 2015;10:1451-1457.

196. Planchard D, Besse B, Groen HJM, et al. Dabrafenib plus trametinib in patients with previously treated BRAF(V600E)-mutant metastatic non-small cell lung cancer: an open-label, multicentre phase 2 trial. *Lancet Oncol*. 2016;17(7):984-993.

197. Planchard D, Smit EF, Groen HJM, et al. Dabrafenib plus trametinib in patients with previously untreated BRAF^V600E-mutant metastatic non-small-cell lung cancer: an open-label, phase 2 trial. *Lancet Oncol*. 2017;18(10):1307-1316.

198. Eng C. RET proto-oncogene in the development of human cancer. *J Clin Oncol*. 1999;17(1):380-393.

199. Kohno T, Ichikawa H, Totoki Y, et al. KIF5B-RET fusions in lung adenocarcinoma. *Nat Med*. 2012;18(3):375-377.

200. Wang R, Hu H, Pan Y, et al. RET fusions define a unique molecular and clinicopathologic subtype of non-small-cell lung cancer. *J Clin Oncol*. 2012;30(35):4352-4359.

201. Drilon A, Rekhtman N, Arcila M, et al. Cabozantinib in patients with advanced RET-rearranged non-small-cell lung cancer: an open-label, single-centre, phase 2, single-arm trial. *Lancet Oncol*. 2016;17(12):1653-1660.

202. Lee S-H, Lee J-K, Ahn M-J, et al. Vandetanib in pretreated patients with advanced non-small cell lung cancer-harboring RET rearrangement: a phase II clinical trial. *Ann Oncol*. 2017;28(2):292-297.

203. Velcheti V, Hida T, Reckamp KL, et al. Phase 2 study of lenvatinib (LN) in patients (Pts) with RET fusion-positive adenocarcinoma of the lung. *Ann Oncol*. 2016;27(6):416-445.

204. Subbiah V, Justin F Gainor JF, Rahal R, et al. Precision targeted therapy with BLU-667 for RET-driven cancers. *Cancer Discov*. 2018;8(7):836-849.

205. Drilon A, Subbiah V, Oxnard L, Bauer TM. A phase 1 study of LOXO-292, a potent and highly selective RET inhibitor, in patients with RE-altered cancers. *J Clin Oncol*. 2018;36(15 suppl.):102.

206. Soppet D, Escandon E, Maragos J, et al. The neurotrophic factors brain-derived neurotrophic factor and neurotrophin-3 are ligands for the trkB tyrosine kinase receptor. *Cell*. 1991;65(5):895-903.

207. Kaplan D, Martin-Zanca D, Parada L. Tyrosine phosphorylation and tyrosine kinase activity of the trk proto-oncogene product induced by NGF. *Nature*. 1991;350(6314):158-160.

208. Miranda C, Fumagalli T, Anania MC, et al. Role of STAT3 in in vitro transformation triggered by TRK onco-genes. *PLoS One*. 2010;5(3):e9446.

209. Farago A, Azzoli C. Beyond ALK and ROS1: RET, NTRK, EGFR and BRAF gene rearrangements in non-small cell lung cancer. *Transl Lung Cancer Res*. 2017;6(5):550-559.

210. Vaishnavi A, Capelletti M, Le AT, et al. Oncogenic and drug-sensitive NTRK1 rearrangements in lung cancer. *Nat Med*. 2013;19(11):1469-1472.

211. Farago A, Le LP, Zheng Z, et al. Durable clinical response to entrectinib in NTRK1-rearranged non-small cell lung cancer. *J Thorac Oncol*. 2015;10(12):1670-1674.

212. Hyman DM, Laetsch TW, Kummar S, et al. The efficacy of larotrectinib (LOXO-101), a selective tro-pomyosin receptor kinase (TRK) inhibitor, in adult and pediatric TRK fusion cancers. *J Clin Oncol*. 2017;35(18_suppl):LBA2501-LBA2501.

213. Fuse M, Okada K, Oh-Hara T, Ogura H, Fujita N, Katayama R. Mechanisms of resistance to NTRK inhibitors and therapeutic strategies in NTRK1-rearranged cancers. *Mol Cancer Ther*. 2017;16(10):2130-2143.

214. Klapper L, Glathe S, Vaisman N, et al. The ErbB-2/HER2 oncoprotein of human carcinomas may func-tion solely as a shared coreceptor for multiple stroma-derived growth factors. *Proc Natl Acad Sci U S A*. 1999;96(9):4995-5000.

215. Slamon D, Clark GM, Wong SG, Levin WJ, Ullrich A, McGuire WL. Human breast cancer: correlation of relapse and survival with amplification of the HER-2/neu oncogene. *Science*. 1987;235(4785):177-182.

216. Hirsch F, Varella-Garcia M, Franklin WA, et al. Evaluation of HER-2/neu gene amplification and protein expression in non-small cell lung carcinomas. *Br J Cancer*. 2002;86(9):1449-1456.

217. Clamon G, Herndon J, Kern J, et al. Lack of trastuzumab activity in nonsmall cell lung carcinoma with over-expression of erb-B2: 39810: a phase II trial of cancer and Leukemia Group B. *Cancer*. 2005;103(8):1670-1675.

218. Perera SA, Li D, Shimamura T, et al. HER2YVMA drives rapid development of adenosquamous lung tumors in mice that are sensitive to BIBW2992 and rapamycin combination therapy. *Proc Natl Acad Sci U S A*. 2009;106(2):474-479.

219. Stephens P, Hunter C, Bignell G, et al. Lung cancer: intragenic ERBB2 kinase mutations in tumours. *Nature*. 2004;431(7008):525-526.

220. Arcila M, Chaft JE, Nafa K, et al. Prevalence, clinicopathologic associations, and molecular spectrum of ERBB2 (HER2) tyrosine kinase mutations in lung adenocarcinomas. *Clin Cancer Res.* 2012;18:4910-4918.
221. Mazières J, Barlesi F, Filleron T, et al. Lung cancer patients with HER2 mutations treated with chemotherapy and HER2-targeted drugs: results from the European EUHER2 cohort. *Ann Oncol.* 2016;27(2):281-286.
222. De Grève J, Teugels E, Geers C, et al. Clinical activity of afatinib (BIBW 2992) in patients with lung adenocarcinoma with mutations in the kinase domain of HER2/neu. *Lung Cancer.* 2012;76(1):123-127.
223. Gandhi L, et al. MA04.02 neratinib ± temsirolimus in HER2-mutant lung cancers: an international, randomized phase II study. *J Thorac Oncol.* 2017;12(1):S358-S359.
224. Kris M, Camidge DR, Giaccone G, et al. Targeting HER2 aberrations as actionable drivers in lung cancers: phase II trial of the pan-HER tyrosine kinase inhibitor dacomitinib in patients with HER2-mutant or amplified tumors. *Ann Oncol.* 2015;26(7):1421-1427.
225. Li BT, Shen R, Buonocore D, et al. Ado-Trastuzumab Emtansine for patients with HER2-mutant lung cancers: results from a phase II basket trial. *J Clin Oncol.* 2018:JCO2018779777.
226. Costa DB, Jorge SE, Moran JP, et al. Pulse afatinib for ERBB2 Exon 20 insertion-mutated lung adenocarcinomas. *J Thorac Oncol.* 2016;11(6):918-923.
227. Wozniak AJ, Crowley JJ, Balcerzak SP, et al. Livingston randomized trial comparing cisplatin with cisplatin plus vinorelbine in the treatment of advanced non-small-cell lung cancer: a Southwest Oncology Group study. *J Clin Oncol.* 1998 Jul;16(7):2459-2465.
228. Gatzemeier U, von Pawel J, Gottfried M, et al. Phase III comparative study of high-dose cisplatin versus a combination of paclitaxel and cisplatin in patients with advanced non-small-cell lung cancer. *J Clin Oncol.* 2000 Oct 1;18(19):3390-3399.
229. von Plessen C, Bergman B, Andresen O, et al. Palliative chemotherapy beyond three courses conveys no survival or consistent quality-of-life benefits in advanced non-small-cell lung cancer. *Br J Cancer.* 2006 Oct 23;95(8):966-973.

16

SMALL CELL LUNG CANCER TREATMENT: EARLY STAGE

Victor van Berkel, MD, PhD • Neal E. Dunlap, MD • Matthew Fox, MD • Alden Klarer, MD, PhD
• Kate Alyse Marino, MD • Phuong T. Ngo, MD • William M. Whited, MD • Mehran Yusuf, MD

SURGERY FOR EARLY STAGE SMALL CELL LUNG CANCER

William M. Whited, MD, Kate Alyse Marino, MD, Matthew Fox, MD, Victor van Berkel, MD, PhD

A 73-year-old gentleman with a past medical history of chronic obstructive pulmonary disease (COPD), hypertension (HTN), and a 50 pack-year cigarette smoking history presents to your office after a screening computed tomographic (CT) scan found a 1-cm mass in the right lung lower lobe. His primary care physician orders a percutaneous biopsy, which returns as small cell lung cancer (SCLC). What further workup does this patient need? Which subgroup of patients would be surgical candidates?

Learning Objectives:
1. Understand the diagnostic workup for patients with SCLC.
2. How is SCLC staged, and what are the recent changes to the staging system?
3. What is the ideal treatment approach to patients with early stage SCLC?

In the United States, there are approximately 234,000 patients diagnosed with lung cancer annually, with only 10%-15% of cases being SCLC.[1] Despite SCLC being less common, it is a particularly deadly and aggressive type of lung cancer, with patients often having metastatic disease at the time of diagnosis.[2] SCLC has been traditionally staged as extensive stage (ES) or as limited stage (LS) disease; the purpose of this simple dichotomous staging system is to identify patients who may be candidates for local control of disease.[3] The cornerstone of treatment for SCLC has been chemotherapy due to the majority of patients having ES disease at the time of diagnosis.[4] The focus of this chapter is on patients with LS disease and what role surgery plays in the treatment of SCLC.

PRESENTATION

Unfortunately, for patients diagnosed with SCLC over two-thirds will have metastatic disease at the time of diagnosis.[5] Symptoms of SCLC are typically broken down into either local or distant symptoms. Symptoms of local disease include shortness of breath, cough, hemoptysis, and chest pain. Symptoms of metastatic or advanced disease include weight loss, weakness, lymphadenopathy, and anorexia. In addition to the traditional symptoms mentioned, SCLC can present with a variety of paraneoplastic syndromes.[6]

Over two-thirds of patients with SCLC will have metastatic disease at the time of diagnosis.

- *Syndrome of Inappropriate Antidiuretic Hormone Secretion (SIADH):* Affects approximately 15% of patients with SCLC. SIADH is characterized by hyponatremia along with high urine osmolality. This is caused by ectopic production of antidiuretic hormone. Symptoms and laboratory values typically improve with treatment of SCLC.[6,7]
- *Cushing Syndrome:* Present in less than 5% of patients with SCLC, Cushing syndrome is caused by ectopic production of corticotropin.[6] Symptoms can include obesity, hirsutism, glucose intolerance, and acne.
- *Lambert-Eaton Syndrome:* Results in proximal muscle weakness and is caused by antibodies that target calcium channels.[6]

Screening CT scans have become increasingly more prevalent after the conclusion of the National Lung Screening Trial demonstrated a reduction of lung cancer mortality with the implementation of screening CT scans in at-risk patients.[8] Recent reports demonstrated a shift toward earlier detection in SCLC patients undergoing screening CT compared to traditional means of detection, with approximately one-third of patients with SCLC detected on screening CT scan having IA disease.[9]

> **CLINICAL PEARL:** With the widespread utilization of CT scans, there has been a shift toward earlier detection of SCLC.

DIAGNOSTIC WORKUP

The diagnostic workup for patients with suspected SCLC is similar to the workup for other types of lung cancer and will include standard thorough history and physical and laboratory evaluation (complete blood count, complete metabolic panel, and serum lactate dehydrogenase). The majority of patients presenting with SCLC often have advanced stage disease at the time of diagnosis, which makes accurately staging patients critically important. High-quality imaging is required to rule out distant metastatic disease; imaging includes CT scan of chest, CT scan of the abdomen, brain magnetic resonance imaging (MRI)/CT scan, in addition to a positron emission tomographic (PET) scan.

High-quality imagining of the chest, abdomen, and brain is required in the workup of SCLC due to the majority of patients having metastatic disease at the time of diagnosis.

Tissue evaluation confirms the diagnosis, with the classic "small blue cells" on light microscopy. Histologic confirmation is required to rule out other neuroendocrine malignancies, such as carcinoid. In patients with LS disease, there is often mediastinal lymph node involvement at time of diagnosis. Invasive mediastinal sampling of suspicious lymph nodes can be performed with mediastinoscopy or endobronchial ultrasound-guided biopsy. Routine bone marrow biopsy is not recommended without evidence of leukopenia or thrombocytopenia.[10]

STAGING

In the past, SCLC has been staged differently from other types of lung cancers, which are staged using the tumor, node, metastasis (TNM) system. Defining characteristics of SCLC are its rapid spread and aggressive nature. This resulted in the Veterans Administration Lung Cancer Study Group (VALSG) to propose a simplified dichotomous staging system that classified disease as either ES or LS.[3] Originally, patients with LS disease were those with disease limited to 1 hemithorax and which could be included in a single field of radiation. This included mediastinal and ipsilateral supraclavicular lymph node disease along with locally advanced disease, including laryngeal nerve and superior vena cava involvement. Patients with evidence of metastatic disease, including contralateral hilar or supraclavicular lymph node involvement, along with malignant pleural or pericardial effusion were classified as ES. The International Association for the Study of Lung Cancer (IASLC) subsequently updated the VALSG staging system to define LS as all non-metastatic disease.

In 2009, the IASLC published a report in which 349 patients with SCLC were analyzed based on the current TNM staging system and found differences in survival based on the TNM groupings, which resulted in the recommendation for the seventh edition of the American Joint Committee on Cancer (AJCC) TNM staging to include SCLC.[11] The IASLC again recommended the continued use of the TNM staging system when the 8th edition was released and is what is currently used to stage SCLC.[12]

> **CLINICAL PEARL:** SCLC was previously staged as either limited stage or extended stage. However, this has recently changed with the adoption of the TMN staging system.

RESECTION OF EARLY STAGE

Small cell lung cancer is an aggressive type of lung cancer, often with metastatic disease at the time of presentation. Patients with metastatic disease are often treated with 4-6 cycles of cisplatin or carboplatin and etoposide, in addition to thoracic radiation and cranial radiation in select groups of patients.[4] The focus of this section is to highlight the treatment of patients with non-metastatic disease and the role of surgery in these patients.

The advanced nature of SCLC undoubtedly limits the use of surgical therapies in newly diagnosed patients. However, even in patients with earlier stage disease, the mainstay of treatment is chemotherapy (cisplatin and etoposide) in addition to thoracic radiation. The role of surgery in patients with LS disease after undergoing induction chemotherapy has been studied previously in a randomized prospective trial, which demonstrated no survival benefit to patients undergoing resection compared to chemotherapy followed by thoracic radiation.[13] One of the biggest flaws of this study is

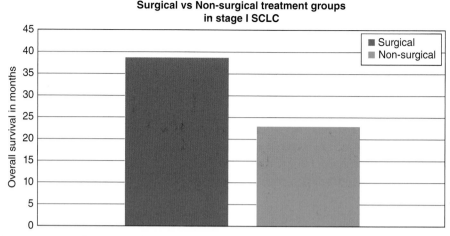

Figure 16-1. Overall survival in the surgical treatment group versus non-surgical treatment group in patients with stage I SCLC. (Data from Wakeam E, Acuna SA, Leighl NB, et al. Surgery versus chemotherapy and radiotherapy for early and locally advanced small cell lung cancer: a propensity-matched analysis of survival. *Lung Cancer.* 2017;109:78-88.)

only 19% of enrolled patients had stage I disease, a group that would arguably benefit most from surgery. Despite this limitation, many cite this paper to advocate for the non-surgical treatment of SCLC.

A recent analysis by Wakeman et al. using the National Cancer Database (NCDB) demonstrated a significant improvement in survival in patients with early stage SCLC undergoing surgical resection.[14] Patients with stage I disease undergoing resection had an overall survival of 38.6 months compared to 22.9 months in the non-surgical group (**Figure 16-1**). An additional subgroup analysis found that patients with stage I and II disease who underwent adjuvant chemotherapy with or without radiation with lobectomy had a median overall survival of 48 months compared to a matched group receiving chemotherapy and thoracic radiation alone. Two recent publications by Yang et al. evaluated the role of surgery followed by adjuvant chemotherapy compared to concurrent chemoradiation using NCDB data.[15,16] The authors found improved overall 5-year survival in the patients with N0 disease undergoing surgery followed by adjuvant chemotherapy compared to concurrent chemoradiation (49.2% vs. 32.5%, $p < .03$).[15] Patients with N1 SCLC undergoing surgery followed by adjuvant therapy had less of a survival advantage compared with those undergoing concurrent chemoradiation.[16] This trial, in addition to other retrospective studies,[17-19] would support the role of surgery in selected patients with SCLC, particularly with early stage N0 disease. Despite increasing evidence in support of surgery, only one-third of patients potentially eligible for surgery undergo resection.[20]

> **CLINICAL PEARL:** There is increasing evidence that in patients with early stage SCLC surgery provides a survival benefit compared to non-surgical treatment groups. Despite these new findings, only one-third of patients with early stage SCLC will undergo resection.

There continues to be growing evidence for the role of surgical resection in patients with SCLC. As with other surgical procedures, patient selection is important. When considering surgical resection, accurately staging the disease is critically important. In otherwise appropriate patients with small (T1-2) tumors without any evidence of nodal involvement, surgical resection is appropriate treatment.[21] Lobectomy with mediastinal lymph node dissection, in an otherwise appropriate patient, should be consider based on recent National Comprehensive Cancer Network (NCCN) guidelines.[22] There have been additional reports of when resection would be appropriate in patients with SCLC.[10,11] These include tumors with a component of NSCLC and stage III disease with mediastinal lymph node involvement if the patient has regression of mediastinal disease after chemotherapy and radiation.

> **CLINICAL PEARL:** The ideal surgical candidate would be a patient with a T1-T2 tumor without any evidence of nodal or metastatic disease. These patients should undergo lobectomy with mediastinal lymph node dissection.

INCREASING ROLE OF SURGERY IN SMALL CELL LUNG CANCER

Small cell lung cancer is an aggressive neuroendocrine tumor of the lung, often with advanced-stage disease at the time of diagnosis. Chemotherapy and radiation have been the mainstay of treatment for the past several decades; however, there is a role for surgical resection in the appropriately selected and accurately staged patient. With the increasing use of screening CT scans and the detection of earlier stage disease, surgery is likely to be an expanding component in the treatment of SCLC.

CHEMOTHERAPY FOR EARLY STAGE SMALL CELL LUNG CANCER

Phuong Ngo, MD

A 64-year-old Caucasian male with a 40 pack-year smoking history was referred by his primary care physician for routine low-dose chest CT given his tobacco use. Imaging showed a 0.9-cm right lower lobe lesion with enlarged left hilar lymphadenopathy. Biopsy of the hilar lymph node returned with evidence of SCLC. PET/CT showed hypermetabolic activity in these lesions without any other disease in the abdomen or pelvis. Brain MRI was negative for metastatic disease. What treatment options are available for this patient?

Learning Objectives:
1. How common is LS SCLC?
2. To what treatment modality is SCLC most sensitive?
3. What are common adjuvant regimens for early stage SCLC?

Only about one-third of SCLC patients present with disease confined to the chest, and only about 5% of patients present with stage I-IIA (T1-2,N0M0). Those with very early disease benefit from surgical resection followed by adjuvant systemic chemotherapy.

> **CLINICAL PEARL:** Small cell lung cancer is the fastest growing solid malignancy.

Small cell lung cancer is initially very sensitive to chemotherapy, with LS patients having response rates of 70%-90% after chemotherapy and radiation. Unfortunately, despite these initial responses, the median survival in these patients is only 14 to 20 months, and most eventually die of recurrent disease.

For patients with very limited disease, adjuvant chemotherapy is recommended after surgical resection. For those with inoperable disease or patients who do not wish to proceed with surgery, the mass be can treated with stereotactic ablative radiotherapy (SABR) followed by adjuvant systemic therapy. Concurrent chemoradiation is the standard of care and is preferred over sequential chemotherapy/radiotherapy.

> **CLINICAL PEARL:** Small cell lung cancer is initially very sensitive to chemotherapy.

COMBINATION CHEMOTHERAPY

Randomized clinical trials in the 1970s found that combination chemotherapy was superior to single-agent therapy. SCLC used to be treated with cyclophosphamide-based regimens such as CAV (cyclophosphamide, doxorubicin, and vincristine); CAE (cyclophosphamide, doxorubicin, and etoposide); and CEV (cyclophosphamide, etoposide, and vincristine). These alkylator/anthracycline regimens were later replaced by cisplatin based on superior efficacy and toxicity.[23,24] A meta-analysis of 36 trials involving cisplatin with or without etoposide showed overall survival benefits in SCLC patients.[25]

> **CLINICAL PEARL:** Small cell lung cancer is typically treated with a platinum-containing doublet as primary or adjuvant therapy.

CISPLATIN VERSUS CARBOPLATIN

Cisplatin/etoposide has since become the most commonly used first-line combination chemotherapy regimen for SCLC. Carboplatin is frequently used in place of cisplatin for its better toxicity profile, including reduced risk of emesis, neuropathy, and renal dysfunction. Carboplatin does, however, carry a higher risk of myelosuppression. Small randomized trials and retrospective analyses have shown similar efficacy for cisplatin and carboplatin in SCLC patients.[26-28]

A small meta-analysis consisting of 4 randomized trials and 663 total patients compared cisplatin-based versus carboplatin-based regimens in SCLC patients, of whom 32% had limited disease and 68% had extensive disease.[29] There was no significant difference in response rate (67% vs. 66%), progression-free survival (5.5 months vs. 5.3 months), and overall survival (9.6 months vs. 9.4 months). Thus, in clinical practice, carboplatin is sometimes substituted for cisplatin based on toxicity profiles since studies have suggested similar efficacy in SCLC.

> **CLINICAL PEARL:** Carboplatin can be substituted for cisplatin based on toxicity profiles.

BEVACIZUMAB

The benefits of bevacizumab in SCLC is unclear. A phase 2 study used carboplatin, irinotecan, and bevacizumab with concurrent radiation followed by maintenance bevacizumab in patients with LS SCLC but found a high incidence of tracheoesophageal fistulas.[30] As a result, the study was terminated early.

> **CLINICAL PEARL:** Current guidelines do not recommend using bevacizumab in SCLC.

ELDERLY PATIENTS

The incidence of lung cancer increases with age, but elderly patients are unfortunately underrepresented in clinical trials. Though being older does portend more adverse reactions with treatment, age alone should not be a factor in deciding treatment options. A retrospective analysis of 8,367 elderly patients with LS SCLC found that chemoradiation still improved survival compared to chemotherapy alone.[31] Elderly patients are more likely to have fatigue and myelosuppression with treatment, but they overall have similar prognosis to younger, stage-matched patients.

RADIATION THERAPY FOR EARLY STAGE SMALL CELL LUNG CANCER

Neal Dunlap, MD, Mehran Yusuf, MD, Alden Klarer, MD

A 60-year-old white female had a 4-cm lung mass on PET that was biopsied by core needle. She smoked 2 packs of cigarettes per day. The pathology shows SCLC. The mass is resected after a good response to chemotherapy. Pathology sees an almost complete response and no involved lymph nodes.

Learning Objective:

1. What is the role of radiation in early stage SCLC?

Early stage SCLC is a relatively rare phenomenon. The traditional Veterans Administration two-stage definition (LS and ES) is the most widely accepted classification system to dictate treatment approaches.[32] TNM classification according to the AJCC becomes useful in patients diagnosed with T1-2N0 SCLC. Although SCLC is widely thought to be a systemic disease, patients with true early stage disease are eligible for local therapy, including surgery or radiation.[33] The NCCN and other expert consensus typically favor surgery in this patient group, but radiation can be considered in medically inoperable patients.

STEREOTACTIC BODY RADIATION THERAPY

Extrapolating from the results using stereotactic body radiation therapy (SBRT) for early-stage NSCLC,[34-37] SBRT has excellent local control and lobar control that are comparable to surgical resection in many cases. These same principles, in theory, can be

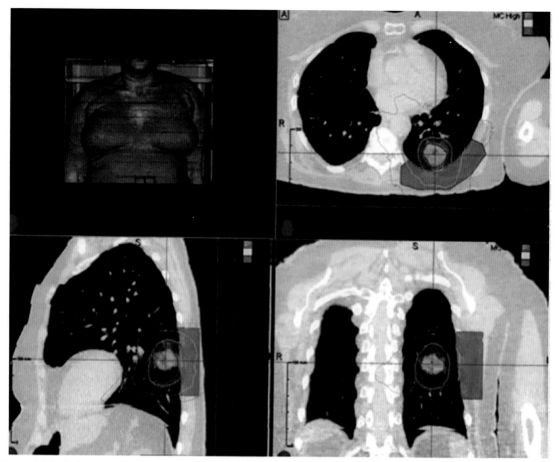

Figure 16-2. Early stage SCLC treated with SBRT using the Cyberknife radiosurgery system.

applied to early stage (T1-2N0) SCLC patients (refer to previous chapters discussing SBRT for NSCLC). Following local therapy, patients still require systemic therapy to address micrometastatic disease (**Figure 16-2**).

CHEST CONSOLIDATION RADIATION

In patients who are medically operable, radiation may still play a role in sterilizing mediastinal and hilar lymph nodes, especially in patients with occult nodal metastases. The Lung Cancer Study Group conducted the only prospective randomized trial evaluating surgery in patients with limited disease.[13] Patients showing a response to 5 cycles of systemic chemotherapy were then randomized to surgery followed by thoracic radiation versus thoracic radiation alone. Unfortunately, only 19% of enrolled patients had T1-2N0 disease; therefore, conclusions from this study are limited. Using elective nodal radiation in SCLC is currently controversial and most commonly not recommended.[38] Current NCCN guidelines recommend limiting thoracic radiation after surgery, only in the setting of node-positive disease.[39,40]

CENTRAL NERVOUS SYSTEM RADIATION

Brain metastases occur commonly for patients with SCLC, with the incidence of intracranial disease as high as 10% at presentation, and more than half of patients developing brain metastases within 2 years of diagnosis.[41,42] Central nervous system (CNS) relapses are a common site of failure for patients with limited SCLC who respond to systemic therapy and thoracic radiation and is the rationale underlying prophylactic cranial irradiation (PCI). Compared to surveillance alone, PCI has been demonstrated to decrease the incidence of brain metastasis vs observation development (3-year cumulative brain metastasis incidence 33.3% vs. 58.6%, $p < .001$) as well as increase survival (3 year overall survival 20.7% vs. 15.3%, $p = .01$) and disease-free survival (3-year disease-free survival 22.3% vs. 13.5%, $p < .001$) for patients with limited SCLC in complete remission.[43] PCI with hippocampal avoidance is an area of active interest[44] and is the current subject of an ongoing NRG Oncology trial (NCT02635009) but is not currently standard of care pending these results.

The role of PCI in patients with locally advanced or extensive SCLC is more controversial. Slotman et al. demonstrated a 1.3-month overall survival benefit with PCI for patients with extensive SCLC with any response to CT.[45] However, CT or MRI of the brain was not routinely performed as part of staging for these patients, and patients with small, asymptomatic brain metastases may have been included in the arm receiving PCI. A recently reported Japanese randomized trial did not find a statistically significant benefit in survival with PCI for a population of extensive SCLC patients well screened with brain MRIs.[46] The cumulative incidence of brain metastases at 18 months was significantly higher for patients who did not receive PCI (64% vs. 40%, $p < .0001$). Additionally, 83% of patients in the observation group subsequently received radiotherapy for brain metastases. Extrapolating these findings to non-Japanese populations with SCLC may be difficult given data suggesting differences in response to treatment between ethnic populations.[47,48] Retrospective analysis of a large US national database of patients with extensive SCLC suggested a significant survival benefit with PCI (13. 9 months vs. 11.1 months, $p < .0001$), although these findings are limited by biases inherent to retrospective analysis. Pending further clarification, NCCN guidelines recommend considering either PCI or close surveillance with serial CNS imaging for patients with extensive SCLC with response to systemic therapy.[49]

REFERENCES

1. Society AC. Key Statistics for Small Cell Lung Cancer. 2018. https://www.cancer.org/cancer/small-cell-lung-cancer/about/key-statistics.html. Accessed October 29, 2018.
2. Janssen-Heijnen ML, Coebergh JW. Trends in incidence and prognosis of the histological subtypes of lung cancer in North America, Australia, New Zealand and Europe. *Lung Cancer.* 2001;31(2-3):123-137.
3. Zelen M. Keynote address on biostatistics and data retrieval. *Cancer Chemother Rep 3.* 1973;4(2):31-42.
4. Morabito A, Carillio G, Daniele G, et al. Treatment of small cell lung cancer. *Crit Rev Oncol Hematol.* 2014;91(3):257-270.
5. Veronesi G, Bottoni E, Finocchiaro G, Alloisio M. When is surgery indicated for small-cell lung cancer? *Lung Cancer.* 2015;90(3):582-589.
6. Jackman DM, Johnson BE. Small-cell lung cancer. *Lancet.* 2005;366(9494):1385-1396.
7. Kanaji N, Watanabe N, Kita N, et al. Paraneoplastic syndromes associated with lung cancer. *World J Clin Oncol.* 2014;5(3):197-223.
8. National Lung Screening Trial Research T, Aberle DR, Adams AM, et al. Reduced lung-cancer mortality with low-dose computed tomographic screening. *N Engl J Med.* 2011;365(5):395-409.

9. Austin JH, Yip R, D'Souza BM, Yankelevitz DF, Henschke CI, International Early Lung Cancer Action Program I. Small-cell carcinoma of the lung detected by CT screening: stage distribution and curability. *Lung Cancer.* 2012;76(3):339-343.

10. de Hoyos A, DeCamp MM. Surgery for small cell lung cancer. *Thorac Surg Clin.* 2014;24(4):399-409.

11. Vallieres E, Shepherd FA, Crowley J, et al. The IASLC Lung Cancer Staging Project: proposals regarding the relevance of TNM in the pathologic staging of small cell lung cancer in the forthcoming (seventh) edition of the TNM classification for lung cancer. *J Thorac Oncol.* 2009;4(9):1049-1059.

12. Nicholson AG, Chansky K, Crowley J, et al. The International Association for the Study of Lung Cancer Lung Cancer Staging Project: proposals for the revision of the clinical and pathologic staging of small cell lung cancer in the forthcoming eighth edition of the TNM classification for lung cancer. *J Thorac Oncol.* 2016;11(3):300-311.

13. Lad T, Piantadosi S, Thomas P, Payne D, Ruckdeschel J, Giaccone G. A prospective randomized trial to determine the benefit of surgical resection of residual disease following response of small cell lung cancer to combination chemotherapy. *Chest.* 1994;106(6 Suppl):320S-323S.

14. Wakeam E, Acuna SA, Leighl NB, et al. Surgery versus chemotherapy and radiotherapy for early and locally advanced small cell lung cancer: a propensity-matched analysis of survival. *Lung Cancer.* 2017;109:78-88.

15. Yang CJ, Chan DY, Shah SA, et al. Long-term survival after surgery compared with concurrent chemoradiation for node-negative small cell lung cancer. *Ann Surg.* 2018;268(6):1105-1112.

16. Yang CJ, Chan DY, Speicher PJ, et al. Surgery versus optimal medical management for N1 small cell lung cancer. *Ann Thorac Surg.* 2017;103(6):1767-1772.

17. Shepherd FA, Ginsberg RJ, Patterson GA, Evans WK, Feld R. A prospective study of adjuvant surgical resection after chemotherapy for limited small cell lung cancer. A University of Toronto Lung Oncology Group study. *J Thorac Cardiovasc Surg.* 1989;97(2):177-186.

18. Fujimori K, Yokoyama A, Kurita Y, Terashima M. A pilot phase 2 study of surgical treatment after induction chemotherapy for resectable stage I to IIIA small cell lung cancer. *Chest.* 1997;111(4):1089-1093.

19. Varlotto JM, Recht A, Flickinger JC, Medford-Davis LN, Dyer AM, DeCamp MM. Lobectomy leads to optimal survival in early-stage small cell lung cancer: a retrospective analysis. *J Thorac Cardiovasc Surg.* 2011;142(3):538-546.

20. Wakeam E, Varghese TK, Jr., Leighl NB, Giuliani M, Finlayson SRG, Darling GE. Trends, practice patterns and underuse of surgery in the treatment of early stage small cell lung cancer. *Lung Cancer.* 2017;109:117-123.

21. Del Sole A, Cinquetti S, Fedato C, et al. Management of women at high risk of hereditary breast cancer in the Veneto Regional Program for Prevention. *Epidemiol Prev.* 2015;39(4 Suppl 1):99-101.

22. Network NCC. *NCCN Guidelines for Small Cell Lung Cancer. Version 1.2019.* 11/08/2018 2018.

23. Fukuoka M, Furuse K, Saijo N, et al. Randomized trial of cyclophosphamide, doxorubicin, and vincristine versus cisplatin and etoposide versus alternation of these regimens in small-cell lung cancer. *J Natl Cancer Inst.* 1991;83(12):855-861.

24. Roth BJ, Johnson DH, Einhorn LH, et al. Randomized study of cyclophosphamide, doxorubicin, and vincristine versus etoposide and cisplatin versus alternation of these two regimens in extensive small-cell lung cancer: a phase III trial of the Southeastern Cancer Study Group. *J Clin Oncol.* 1992;10(2):282-291.

25. Mascaux C, Paesmans M, Berghmans T, et al. A systematic review of the role of etoposide and cisplatin in the chemotherapy of small cell lung cancer with methodology assessment and meta-analysis. *Lung Cancer.* 2000;30(1):23-36.

26. Hatfield LA, Huskamp HA, Lamont EB. Survival and toxicity after cisplatin plus etoposide versus carboplatin plus etoposide for extensive-stage small-cell lung cancer in elderly patients. *J Oncol Pract.* 2016;12(7):666-673.

27. Skarlos DV, Samantas E, Kosmidis P, et al. Randomized comparison of etoposide-cisplatin vs. etoposide-carboplatin and irradiation in small-cell lung cancer. A Hellenic Co-operative Oncology Group study. *Ann Oncol.* 1994;5(7):601-607.

28. Okamoto H, Watanabe K, Kunikane H, et al. Randomised phase III trial of carboplatin plus etoposide vs split doses of cisplatin plus etoposide in elderly or poor-risk patients with extensive disease small-cell lung cancer: JCOG 9702. *Br J Cancer.* 2007;97(2):162-169.

29. Rossi A, Di Maio M, Chiodini P, et al. Carboplatin- or cisplatin-based chemotherapy in first-line treatment of small-cell lung cancer: the COCIS meta-analysis of individual patient data. *J Clin Oncol.* 2012;30(14):1692-1698.

30. Spigel DR, Hainsworth JD, Yardley DA, et al. Tracheoesophageal fistula formation in patients with lung cancer treated with chemoradiation and bevacizumab. *J Clin Oncol.* 2010;28(1):43-48.

31. Corso CD, Rutter CE, Park HS, et al. Role of chemoradiotherapy in elderly patients with limited-stage small-cell lung cancer. *J Clin Oncol.* 2015;33(36):4240-4246.

32. Jett JR, Schild SE, Kesler KA, Kalemkerian GP. Treatment of small cell lung cancer: diagnosis and management of lung cancer, 3rd ed: American College of Chest Physicians evidence-based clinical practice guidelines. *Chest.* 2013;143(5 Suppl):e400S-e419S.

33. Kalemkerian GP, Gadgeel SM. Modern staging of small cell lung cancer. *J Natl Compr Canc Netw.* 2013;11(1):99-104.
34. Videtic GMM, Donington J, Giuliani M, et al. Stereotactic body radiation therapy for early-stage non-small cell lung cancer: executive summary of an ASTRO evidence-based guideline. *Pract Radiat Oncol.* 2017;7(5):295-301.
35. Maquilan G, Timmerman R. Stereotactic body radiation therapy for early-stage lung cancer. *Cancer J.* 2016;22(4):274-279.
36. Timmerman RD, Fernando HC. From the guest editors: treatment of early-stage lung cancer. *Cancer J.* 2011;17(1):1-2.
37. Timmerman R, Paulus R, Galvin J, et al. Stereotactic body radiation therapy for inoperable early stage lung cancer. *JAMA.* 2010;303(11):1070-1076.
38. Stinchcombe TE, Gore EM. Limited-stage small cell lung cancer: current chemoradiotherapy treatment paradigms. *Oncologist.* 2010;15(2):187-195.
39. Yang CF, Chan DY, Speicher PJ, et al. Role of adjuvant therapy in a population-based cohort of patients with early-stage small-cell lung cancer. *J Clin Oncol.* 2016;34(10):1057-1064.
40. Brock MV, Hooker CM, Syphard JE, et al. Surgical resection of limited disease small cell lung cancer in the new era of platinum chemotherapy: its time has come. *J Thorac Cardiovasc Surg.* 2005;129(1):64-72.
41. Komaki R, Byhardt RW, Anderson T, et al. What is the lowest effective biologic dose for prophylactic cranial irradiation? *Am J Clin Oncol.* 1985;8(6):523-527.
42. Arriagada R, Le Chevalier T, Borie F, et al. Prophylactic cranial irradiation for patients with small-cell lung cancer in complete remission. *J Natl Cancer Inst.* 1995;87(3):183-190.
43. Auperin A, Arriagada R, Pignon JP, et al. Prophylactic cranial irradiation for patients with small-cell lung cancer in complete remission. Prophylactic Cranial Irradiation Overview Collaborative Group. *N Engl J Med.* 1999;341(7):476-484.
44. Rodriguez de Dios N, Counago F, Lopez JL, et al. Treatment design and rationale for a randomized trial of prophylactic cranial irradiation with or without hippocampal avoidance for SCLC: PREMER Trial on behalf of the Oncologic Group for the Study of Lung Cancer/Spanish Radiation Oncology Group-Radiation Oncology Clinical Research Group. *Clin Lung Cancer.* 2018;19(5):e693-e697.
45. Slotman B, Faivre-Finn C, Kramer G, et al. Prophylactic cranial irradiation in extensive small-cell lung cancer. *N Engl J Med.* 2007;357(7):664-672.
46. Takahashi T, Yamanaka T, Seto T, et al. Prophylactic cranial irradiation versus observation in patients with extensive-disease small-cell lung cancer: a multicentre, randomised, open-label, phase 3 trial. *Lancet Oncol.* 2017;18(5):663-71.
47. Noda K, Nishiwaki Y, Kawahara M, et al. Irinotecan plus cisplatin compared with etoposide plus cisplatin for extensive small-cell lung cancer. *N Engl J Med.* 2002;346(2):85-91.
48. Hanna N, Bunn PA, Jr., Langer C, et al. Randomized phase III trial comparing irinotecan/cisplatin with etoposide/cisplatin in patients with previously untreated extensive-stage disease small-cell lung cancer. *J Clin Oncol.* 2006;24(13):2038-2043.
49. Ettinger DS, Aisner DL, Wood DE, et al. NCCN Guidelines Insights: Non-Small Cell Lung Cancer, Version 5.2018. *J Natl Compr Canc Netw.* 2018;16(7):807-821.

SMALL CELL LUNG CANCER TREATMENT: LOCALLY ADVANCED

Neal E. Dunlap, MD • Phuong T. Ngo, MD • Cesar A. Perez, MD • Diana Saravia, MD • Mehran Yusuf, MD

CHEMOTHERAPY FOR LOCALLY ADVANCED SMALL CELL LUNG CANCER

Phuong Ngo, MD

A 65-year-old male had a 4-cm lung mass found on positron emission tomography (PET); it was biopsied by core needle. The patient smoked 2 packs of cigarettes per day and has chronic obstructive pulmonary disease (COPD) and hypertension (HTN). The PET reveals positive mediastinal lymph nodes. Magnetic resonance imaging (MRI) of the brain is normal. The pathology shows small cell lung cancer (SCLC). The patient's performance status is good, and his basic laboratory tests are normal.

Learning Objectives:

1. What is the most common chemotherapy doublet for locally advanced SCLC?
2. What is the difference between cisplatin and carboplatin in regard to treatment for SCLC?
3. What treatment options are available for SCLC other than cisplatin or carboplatin plus etoposide?
4. How often should locally advanced patients be scanned during treatment?
5. How are disease relapses classified in SCLC?

Small cell lung cancer (SCLC) is the fastest growing solid malignancy so it is not surprising very few patients present with early stage disease. More often, they are diagnosed at the locally advanced or metastatic stage. These patients typically present with cough and dyspnea, but depending on the extent of disease, they can also have weight loss, bony pain, debility, or even neurologic deficits. Imaging usually reveals a large hilar mass and bulky mediastinal lymphadenopathy. Though SCLC is very sensitive to chemotherapy with rapid initial response, the disease most likely will recur.

The incidence of SCLC overall has been decreasing, but the incidence in women has been rising. It is often centrally located and strongly associated with smoking, so smoking cessation should always be discussed with patients. Those already diagnosed with SCLC who continue to smoke are at risk for greater toxicities with treatment and shorter overall survival.[1]

> **CLINICAL PEARL:** Small cell lung cancer is often centrally located and strongly associated with smoking.

CLASSIFICATION

Unlike other solid malignancies, SCLC often is not classified using the traditional American Joint Committee on Cancer (AJCC) tumor, node, metastasis (TNM) staging. Instead, it is described by the Veterans Administration (VA) scheme in which SCLC is separated into only two groups: (1) limited stage, in which disease is only present in the ipsilateral hemithorax, and (2) extensive stage, wherein it has spread beyond the ipsilateral hemithorax.

However, classifying patients using the TNM staging helps to define those who would be candidates for surgery and radiation, such as those with T1-2,N0. For the purpose of this book, SCLC is described as early stage, locally advanced, and metastatic. Locally advanced in this case refers to stages IIB-IIIC (T3-4,N0,M0; T1-4,N1-3,M0).

PERFORMANCE STATUS

Due to the aggressive nature of SCLC, many patients present with extensive disease and subsequent disease-related debility. When deciding treatment regimens in general, performance status is a key factor for consideration as it predicts how well the patient will tolerate treatment. However, SCLC patients are the exception to this rule.

As mentioned, SCLC is very sensitive to chemotherapy. Patients often have some response after 1-2 cycles, in terms of not only disease response but also improvements in symptoms and functionality. A retrospective study found that 21% of patients with performance status 2 had improved performance status and prolonged survival with salvage topotecan.[2] Another study showed patients with performance status of 3 or 4 who received chemotherapy had improved median survival compared to the large majority of patients who did not receive treatment (67%).[3]

> **CLINICAL PEARL:** Patients with SCLC with poor performance status should still be offered treatment if their debility is thought to be disease related.

CHEMOTHERAPY REGIMENS

Systemic therapy is a key component of treatment for all stages of SCLC. For patients with locally advanced disease, treatment is often with concurrent chemoradiation.

Cisplatin/etoposide is the most commonly used doublet for treating SCLC, which used to be treated with alkylator/anthracycline-based regimens until the current regimen was proven to be superior. A meta-analysis of trials using a cisplatin-containing regimen versus a regimen without it found that the groups treated with cisplatin had an increased objective response rate and overall survival.[4] Another study directly compared cisplatin/etoposide to cyclophosphamide/epirubicin/vincristine and found the doublet improved 2- and 5-year survival rates in limited-stage SCLC.[5]

CISPLATIN VERSUS CARBOPLATIN

Carboplatin is often substituted for cisplatin due to a better toxicity profile, but some wonder if it is as efficacious as cisplatin for SCLC.

A study in 1994 randomized patients to receive cisplatin/etoposide and carboplatin/etoposide for 6 total cycles. Limited-stage patients who had response to treatment and extensive-stage patients who had complete response also received thoracic radiation and prophylactic cranial irradiation with the third cycle. The cisplatin group had more adverse effects, including nausea, vomiting, neutropenic infections, and neurotoxicity, but the median survivals for the cisplatin versus carboplatin groups were 12.5 and 11.8 months, respectively. The complete response rates were also similar at 57% for the cisplatin group and 58% for the carboplatin group.[6]

A more recent study using the Surveillance, Epidemiology, and End Results (SEER)–Medicare database looked at whether patients 67 years and older with extensive-stage SCLC had a non-inferior survival with carboplatin/etoposide compared to cisplatin/etoposide. The results were reassuring, with both groups having nearly identical survival (35.7 weeks for cisplatin/etoposide vs. 35.9 weeks for carboplatin/etoposide). The carboplatin group also had fewer hospitalizations, emergency department visits, and intensive care unit stays.

To further drive the point home, there was a meta-analysis consisting of 4 trials comparing cisplatin versus carboplatin, each combined with etoposide. The median overall survival was 9.6 months for the cisplatin patients and 9.4 months for the carboplatin patients (hazard ratio [HR] 1.08, 95% CI 0.92-1.27, $p = .37$). The objective response rate was 67.1% for the cisplatin group and 66% for the carboplatin group. Median progression-free survival was also similar at 5.5 months for the cisplatin group and 5.3 months for the carboplatin group.[7] The main differences between these groups were the adverse effects. Carboplatin had greater hematologic toxicities, while cisplatin had more non-hematologic toxicities.

> **CLINICAL PEARL:** Cisplatin and carboplatin have similar efficacy when used in combination with etoposide for the treatment of SCLC.

Cisplatin side effects include, but are not limited to, nephrotoxicity, neurotoxicity (mainly as peripheral neuropathy), ototoxicity, nausea, vomiting, myelosuppression, metallic taste, transient elevations in liver enzymes and bilirubin, and alopecia.

> **CLINICAL PEARL:** Carboplatin side effects include, but are not limited to, myelosuppression, nausea, vomiting, peripheral neuropathy, renal toxicity, hypersensitivity reaction, transient elevations in liver enzymes, and alopecia.

GROWTH FACTOR

Myelosuppression is often a dose-limiting factor when treating SCLC patients, but growth factors are not recommended for routine use. A meta-analysis looked at a variety of chemotherapy regimens involving higher doses and accelerated schedules. Given the anticipated worsened myelosuppression with more intensive chemotherapy, these patients received growth factor, but the study found that growth factor actually had a detrimental effect on the response rate in patients on maintenance high-dose chemotherapy with no improvement in survival. Growth factor also did not have an impact on response rate in the accelerated group, and these patients actually had reduced survival. These findings were most likely due to the intensity of chemotherapy itself, but the addition of growth factor had no effect.[8]

> **CLINICAL PEARL:** The use of growth factor is not recommended during concurrent systemic therapy plus radiation.

OTHER TREATMENT OPTIONS

Investigators have looked at combinations other than platinum/etoposide for SCLC. Adding irinotecan to cisplatin was briefly thought to be better. A Japanese trial looked at extensive-stage SCLC patients who were treated with cisplatin/irinotecan and found these patients had a median survival of 12.8 months compared to 9.4 months in those treated with the traditional cisplatin/etoposide. The 2-year survival in these patients was also an impressive 19.5% compared to 5.2% in the cisplatin group.[9] The results from this study were very promising. However, they were unable to be replicated in the United States, where 2 follow-up trials failed to show improved response rate and survival with irinotecan.[10,11]

Some studies did find success when comparing irinotecan plus a platinum drug compared with etoposide and cisplatin or carboplatin.[12,13] However, the absolute survival benefits were also met with more toxicities, so guidelines do list carboplatin or cisplatin with irinotecan as an option but only for extensive-stage disease. The recommended regimen still remains cisplatin or carboplatin in combination with etoposide.

Additional studies looking at other combinations were less successful. Three-drug regimens such as cisplatin or carboplatin with etoposide and paclitaxel led to unacceptable toxicities.[14] Ifosfamide with etoposide and epirubicin also increased side effects.[15]

> **CLINICAL PEARL:** The standard-of-care chemotherapy doublet for SCLC is cisplatin or carboplatin with etoposide.

DOSE INTENSIFICATION

Dose intensification in the treatment of SCLC remains controversial. Some studies found a modest improvement in median survival times with higher doses of chemotherapy, but many others did not.[16]

One study randomized untreated patients with extensive-stage SCLC to standard dose versus higher dose cisplatin/etoposide. The standard dose was defined as etoposide 80 mg/m^2 on days 1 to 3 and cisplatin 80 mg/m^2 on day 1 every 3 weeks. The high dose was etoposide 80 mg/m^2 on days 1 to 5 and cisplatin 27 mg/m^2 on days 1 to 5 every 3 weeks. Overall, there were no significant differences in median survival and complete response rates. Furthermore, patients who received higher dose chemotherapy had more toxicities, including leukopenia, thrombocytopenia, febrile neutropenia, and weight loss.

MAINTENANCE CHEMOTHERAPY

Initial treatment is recommended for a total of 4-6 cycles, but additional chemotherapy beyond (eg, for maintenance) that does not appear to significantly prolong survival.

A study treating extensive-stage SCLC patients with 4 cycles of cisplatin/etoposide then randomized those with stable or responding disease to observation or 4 additional cycles of treatment with topotecan. Progression-free survival appeared to be better with topotecan, but there was no difference in overall survival. There was also no difference in quality of life between those who received additional treatment versus observation.[17]

A meta-analysis involving 14 trials also sought to evaluate maintenance therapy versus observation in SCLC patients. The investigators found that compared to observation, maintenance therapy had no effect on 1-year mortality, 2-year mortality, overall survival, or progression-free survival.[18] Subgroup analysis did show that maintenance chemotherapy improved progression-free survival in the extensive stage, but this needs to be weighed with its lack of impact on overall survival and greater risk of cumulative toxicity.

The exception to maintenance therapy is with extensive-stage patients. A recent trial found that initial treatment with carboplatin/etoposide/atezolizumab followed by maintenance atezolizumab significantly improved progression-free survival and overall survival.[19] Immunotherapy, however, does not currently have a role in locally advanced SCLC.

> **CLINICAL PEARL:** Initial chemotherapy should only be given for a maximum of 4-6 cycles.

RESPONSE ASSESSMENT

For patients with locally advanced disease who are receiving systemic therapy alone, response should be evaluated after every 2 cycles of treatment using CT with contrast of the chest, abdomen, and pelvis.

Disease progression during initial treatment is referred to as refractory disease (**Table 17-1**). Disease progression within 3 months after completion of initial treatment is refractory disease. In these cases, response to subsequent treatment is expected to be poor (<10%). Response rates are slightly better if there is disease progression more than 3 months after completing therapy. This is referred to as sensitive relapse.

> **CLINICAL PEARL:** Disease should be evaluated for response after every 2 cycles of treatment with CT chest, abdomen, and pelvis with contrast.

TABLE 17-1	Definitions of Disease Progression in Small Cell Lung Cancer
Sensitive relapse	Tumor progression >3 months after the last day of initial treatment
Resistant relapse	Tumor progression within 3 months after the last day of initial treatment
Refractory disease	Tumor progression during initial treatment or lack of response to initial treatment

PROPHYLACTIC CRANIAL IRRADIATION

Small cell lung cancer has a very high propensity to metastasize to the brain. Unlike the conflicting data regarding whether patients with extensive-stage disease should have prophylactic cranial irradiation (PCI), the data for limited-stage disease patients are reassuring.

A study looking at limited-stage patients who had response to chemoradiation found better median overall survival with PCI compared to observation (26 vs. 14 months, respectively).[20] A meta-analysis showed that PCI may prevent the incidence of brain metastases. The 3-year incidence of brain metastases was 33.3% in the PCI group versus 58.6% in the control group. They also had better 3-year overall survival (20.7%) compared to that in the control (15.3%).[21] One other study showed patients who received PCI had better survival at 2, 5, and 10 years compared to those who did not.[22]

> **CLINICAL PEARL:** All patients with locally advanced SCLC who had a complete or partial response to initial treatment should be evaluated for PCI.

However, PCI does have drawbacks, with the main one being late neurologic complications. Patients over the age of 60 seem to have more chronic neurotoxicity, though effects may be less when PCI is given at a lower dose after completing chemotherapy.

Prophylactic cranial irradiation may cause neurologic complications, especially in elderly patients.

SUBSEQUENT THERAPY

Despite being initially responsive to treatment, SCLC will likely relapse with resistant disease. Subsequent treatment is more for palliation of symptoms since the median survival with additional therapy is less than a year.

If the relapse occurs more than 6 months from the completion of initial treatment, rechallenging the patient with the initial regimen is reasonable. The exception to this is extensive-stage patients initially treated with carboplatin/etoposide/atezolizumab, who then progress while on maintenance atezolizumab even if the relapse occurs more than 6 months after completing initial therapy.

If relapse occurs after 6 months from completion of initial treatment, consider re-treating with the original regimen.

When relapse occurs less than 6 months from initial treatment, options include a clinical trial or another second-line agent. These include the following:

- Second-line agents
  - Nivolumab with or without ipilimumab
  - Pembrolizumab
  - Topotecan
  - Irinotecan
  - Paclitaxel
  - Docetaxel
  - Temozolomide
  - Vinorelbine
  - Oral etoposide
  - Gemcitabine
  - Cyclophosphamide/doxorubicin/vincristine
  - Bendamustine

As with many other malignancies, SCLC has also been evaluated in relation to immunotherapy. CheckMate 032 evaluated nivolumab versus various doses of nivolumab plus ipilimumab in patients with relapsed SCLC and found that 1-year overall survival was 42% in patients treated with the nivolumab/ipilimumab combination and 30% in patients who received nivolumab alone.[23] CheckMate 331 compared nivolumab to topotecan or amrubicin and found similar overall survival but fewer adverse effects in the nivolumab group.[24] Guidelines recommend using either nivolumab alone or with ipilimumab, though adding the second immunotherapy agent also increases side effects.

Pembrolizumab has also been added to guidelines as a viable second-line option after it showed a response rate of 19.3% and a median overall survival of 7.7 months. It is important to note that both endpoints were higher in patients positive for PD-L1 (programmed death ligand 1), whereas the responses with nivolumab with or without ipilimumab were seen regardless of PD-L1 expression.

If a patient progresses on one of these agents, switching to another checkpoint inhibitor is not recommended. Also, though this is not applicable to locally advanced SCLC, patients who progress on atezolizumab should not be switched to another immunotherapy agent.

ELDERLY

Small cell lung cancer is most frequently diagnosed in the elderly, who are unfortunately underrepresented in clinical studies. Many clinicians shy away from aggressively treating the elderly, though performance status is a much better predictor of response to therapy.

A large study evaluated chemoradiation in elderly patients with limited-stage SCLC who received chemoradiation versus chemotherapy alone and found that patients who had the addition of radiation had a survival benefit.[25] The CONVERT trial was a phase III, randomized superiority trial comparing elderly patients, aged 70 and older with younger patients in regard to concurrent once-daily versus twice-daily radiation. The study found that the elderly patients had comparable survival and toxicity.[26]

After response to initial therapy, however, the risks and benefits of PCI should be discussed with patients 60 years or older since they have an increased risk for cognitive decline compared to younger patients.

RADIATION THERAPY FOR LOCALLY ADVANCED SMALL CELL LUNG CANCER

Neal Dunlap, MD, Mehran Yusuf, MD

A 65-year-old male had a 4-cm lung mass observed on PET biopsied by core needle. He smoked 2 packs of cigarettes per day and COPD and HTN. The PET revealed positive mediastinal lymph nodes. The brain MRI is normal. The pathology shows SCLC. His performance status is good, and his basic laboratory tests are normal.

Learning Objectives:
1. How is limited stage defined?
2. What is the best radiation regimen?
3. What is the benefit of PCI?

DEFINITION OF LIMITED STAGE

Prior to more sophisticated staging classification, SCLC was considered to be either limited stage or extensive stage. Criteria for limited-stage SCLC has been defined as disease that is limited to the hemithorax, mediastinum, and supraclavicular lymph nodes, which can be encompassed within a tolerable radiation field. Despite the development of TNM classification, SCLC continues to be discussed based on limited versus early stage, which, at this time, appears to be the most important tumor-related prognostic factor. Currently, only one-third of new cases are considered limited-stage disease at diagnosis, which generally correlates with the most recent AJCC eighth edition stages I, II, or III.[27]

Although surgery was initially thought to be a curative solution to limited-stage disease, the current treatment paradigm for these early stage patients is systemic chemotherapy with radiation to the disease in the chest after 2 studies that surgery did not improve outcomes when compared to non-invasive treatment.[28,29] SCLC is a highly aggressive disease and is most often considered inoperable at the time of diagnosis. Due to the rapid proliferative rate, SCLC was found to be exquisitely sensitive to chemotherapy, and thus this became the mainstay of treatment until the 1980s, when it became clear that the addition of radiation therapy could dramatically improve outcomes. While trials supported the addition of thoracic radiation to chemotherapy in limited-stage SCLC, the most definitive evidence came from Cancer and Leukemia Group B (CALGB) 8083. Almost 400 patients with limited-stage SCLC were randomized to receive radiotherapy with chemotherapy, delayed radiotherapy plus chemotherapy, or chemotherapy alone. Overall survival, progression-free survival, and local control were all improved in the arms that received radiotherapy, at the cost of somewhat increased toxicity.[30]

Two meta-analyses including thousands of patients treated in over a dozen trials later published their findings that combined modality therapy including chemotherapy and radiation was superior to chemotherapy alone in limited-stage disease, with improved local control and an absolute survival benefit of 5.4% at 2-3 years after treatment. Still, the optimal volume, dose, fractionation, and sequencing of thoracic radiation remained to be elucidated.[31]

TREATMENT VOLUME

As mentioned, the definition of limited-stage SCLC was historically based on the ability to cover the disease within a tolerable radiation field, namely, a single radiation port, which typically included the primary tumor as well as regional and ipsilateral supraclavicular lymph nodes if they could be encompassed safely. This definition relied on older radiation therapy techniques that limited the ability to encompass disease more distant from the tumor without a corresponding increase in toxicity. With the more sophisticated techniques that are now available, the definition of limited-stage SCLC has evolved. Many practitioners now even consider some patients with contralateral mediastinal or supraclavicular lymph nodes to have limited-stage SCLC.[32] Treatment of the primary tumor, the ipsilateral hilum, and the bilateral mediastinum has now been replaced with volumes that only include the primary tumor and involved nodal stations based on PET imaging. While elective nodal coverage was often performed including the ipsilateral hilum, mediastinum, and often the supraclavicular nodal regions, there is now evidence that selective nodal radiation based on PET positivity has a very low rate, less than 5%, of isolated nodal failure.[33] For patients who receive chemotherapy prior to treatment, the target volume includes disease from the most current scan as well as the prechemotherapy originally involved lymph node regions based on prechemotherapy PET imaging. An internal target volume is created to encompass the disease as it moves throughout the respiratory cycle, with additional margin added for setup uncertainties. While a 3-dimensional (3-D) conformal radiation delivery technique can be used, more often physicians are choosing intensity-modulated radiation therapy (IMRT) to reduce the dose to surrounding normal structures, with a resultant decrease in toxicity.

DOSE AND FRACTIONATION

While the large majority of lung cancer histologies respond well to conventionally fractionated radiation therapy (eg, 2 Gy per day over the course of several weeks to a total dose of 60-70 Gy), SCLC was found to be exquisitely radiosensitive based on a number of radiobiologic experiments that led to the choice of a lower total dose, hyperfractionated regimen in a large Intergroup (INT) trial. INT 0096 randomized patients to 45 Gy at 180 cGy per fraction delivered daily versus a hyperfractionated regimen delivering 45 Gy at 150 cGy per fraction twice daily. The hyperfractionated treatment arm showed an overall survival benefit, albeit at the cost of increased esophagitis. The 2- and 5-year overall survival in the hyperfractionated arm was 47% and 26% versus 41% and 16% in the daily treatment arm, respectively.[34] There has been some criticism of this randomization as the 45-Gy dose delivered twice daily likely has a higher biologically effective dose (BED), making it difficult to discern whether the improvement was a result of purely the fractionation schedule.

A recent trial attempting to compare more biologically equivalent doses to randomized patients to either a twice-daily treatment to 45 Gy or a once-daily treatment to 66 Gy. At a median follow-up of 45 months, the median overall survival was 30 months in the twice-daily group versus 25 months in the once-daily group (p = .14) and the 2-year overall survival was 56% versus 51% in the twice- versus once-daily groups, respectively, which did not meet the 12% threshold required to deem twice-daily superior to daily treatment. This trial was not powered for equivalence; thus, similar efficacy of the two treatments cannot be included. Somewhat surprisingly, the toxicities of both fractionation regimens were relatively comparable, with no significant difference in the number of patients who developed grade 2 esophagitis (18% vs. 19%) in the twice- versus once-daily treatment arms, respectively, which is lower than seen in the twice-daily treatment arm on INT 0096 of 32%. This is speculated to stem from improved radiation treatment delivery as technology advanced between the two trials, which should support the decision to recommend hyperfractionation even in patients not in the best performance category.[26] Authors from this trial's publication do state that the twice-daily treatment regimen may have several advantages over once-daily treatment; these include improved delivery of radiation treatment that was reported on trial, as well as the ability to halve the total treatment time. More recent trials have determined that dose escalation is feasible, and we are currently awaiting results of several trials, including Radiation Therapy Oncology Group (RTOG) 0538, which is directly conventionally fractionated radiation to a total dose of 70 Gy to hyperfractionated treatment to 45 Gy.[35,36]

> **CLINICAL PEARL:** Currently, a twice-daily fractionation to 45 Gy and a once-daily fractionation to 60-70 Gy are acceptable treatment schemes, and the choice may be made by physician or patient preference.

SEQUENCING

Sequencing of therapy has also been a subject of interest. A large randomized trial by the Japanese Cooperative Oncology Group determined that concurrent treatment was superior to delayed sequential treatment in patients with limited-stage disease. Patients were randomized to receive the standard 45 Gy over 3 weeks twice daily starting with either cycle 1 or delayed until after completion of cycle 4. The 2-, 3-, and 5-year survival rates for patients receiving concurrently early radiation were 54.4%, 29.8%, and 23.7% versus 35.1%, 20.2%, and 18.3% in those receiving delayed sequential radiation, respectively.[37]

Still, it is unclear when radiation should be initiated after a patient starts systemic therapy. Several meta-analyses and reviews have looked at early versus late radiation in relation to initiation of systemic therapy and found that early radiotherapy, variably defined but typically within 9 weeks of the initiation of chemotherapy, appears to have a small but significant survival benefit. It has additionally been shown that an important predictor of survival is the time from the first day of chemotherapy and the last day of radiotherapy, which is postulated to be secondary to the reduced influence of accelerated repopulation during treatment. A large meta-analysis including more than 2,600 patients treated in 12 trials reported that the hazard ratio for overall survival favored "earlier and shorter" radiotherapy when accounting for chemotherapy compliance. Significant toxicities accompany combined treatment, and it appears that the ability to receive all prescribed chemotherapy at the appropriate dose may dictate whether an earlier or shorter treatment will be beneficial as there appears to be a detriment to early treatment if a patient is unable to complete prescribed systemic therapy.[38]

There are some arguments for delaying radiation therapy until chemotherapy has been completed. The toxicities associated with concurrent chemoradiation can unfortunately sometimes make it difficult for a patient to complete treatment as prescribed. This may lead to chemotherapy dose reduction or radiation treatment breaks that could negate the positive effects of combined therapy. In addition, there are some practitioners who like to deliver chemotherapy first in order to allow resistant disease to declare itself and eliminate thoracic radiation in patients who may not be best served by it. In those patients who do exhibit a positive response with tumor shrinkage, there is an accompanying shrinkage of the radiation treatment volume that may allow for a decreased dose to nearby normal structures and thus reduced toxicity associated with treatment. In general, for patients who can tolerate concurrent therapy, it is currently recommended that radiotherapy start with the first or second cycle of chemotherapy as performed in INT 0096.[34] Otherwise, delayed radiotherapy can be considered (**Figures 17-1 and 17-2**).

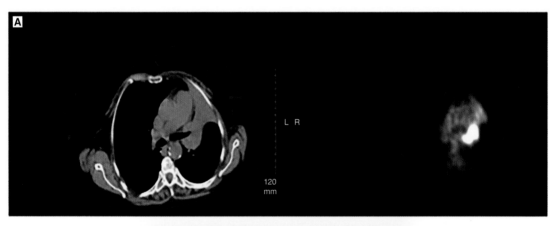

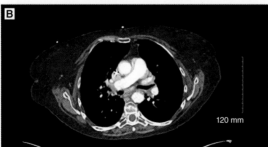

Figure 17-1. A. Prechemotherapy PET/CT showing FDG avid disease. B. Postchemotherapy CT scan used for radiation treatment planning.

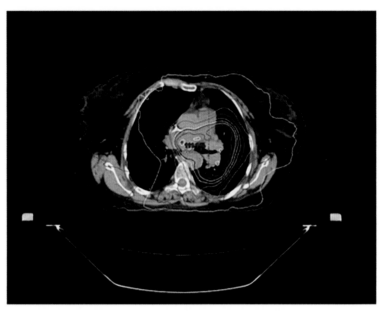

Figure 17-2. Isodose lines from representative IMRT radiation treatment plan using postchemotherapy volumes for treatment planning.

STEREOTACTIC BODY RADIATION THERAPY

With the growing number of pulmonary nodules identified by imaging performed according to new guidelines in the high-risk population, there will likely be an increasing number of stage I SCLC lesions identified. Fortunately, there is now good evidence that stereotactic body radiation therapy (SBRT) can be used successfully in patients with early stage, T1a-T1b lung cancers, including those with SCLC histology. SBRT can deliver high doses of radiation in a small number of fractions to a small treatment volume. Literature in NSCLC (non–small cell lung cancer), mostly inoperable, suggests that this modality can result in local control of more than 80%, which rivals surgical series.[39,40] Despite lack of clinical trials comparing surgery to SBRT in SCLC, a recent review of the literature found 5 publications totaling 108 patients treated with SBRT for early stage SCLC with outcomes similar to those seen for NSCLC.[41] This is encouraging as inherent in these high-risk populations is the coincident incidence of comorbidities that may preclude tissue sampling for both malignant confirmation and determination of NSCLC versus SCLC histology. There are currently ongoing trials evaluating SBRT in early stage SCLC that will further assist in our clinical decision-making.

INTRACRANIAL CONTROL

Brain metastases occur commonly for patients with SCLC, with the incidence of intracranial disease as high as 10% at presentation and more than half of patients developing brain metastases within 2 years of diagnosis.[42,43] Central nervous system relapses are a common site of failure for patients with limited SCLC who respond to systemic therapy and thoracic radiation and are the rationale underlying PCI. PCI has been demonstrated to decrease the incidence of brain metastasis development (3-year cumulative brain metastasis incidence 33.3% vs. 58.6%, $p < .001$) as well as increasing survival (3-year overall survival 20.7 vs. 15.3%, $p = .01$) and disease-free survival (3-years disease-free survival 22.3% vs. 13.5%, $p < .001$) for patients with limited SCLC in complete remission.[20] PCI with hippocampal avoidance is an area of active interest[21] and is the current subject of an ongoing NRG Oncology trial (NCT02635009) but is not currently standard of care pending these results.

In summary, the current paradigm for treatment of early stage SCLC patients is combined chemotherapy and thoracic radiation. It appears that early radiation is preferable to delayed radiation relative to initiation of chemotherapy. With increased screening and improved imaging, there will be more patients diagnosed with stage I SCLC who may be optimally treated with SBRT pending results of current studies. Additionally, due to the high propensity of this subtype of lung cancer to eventually lead to intracranial metastases, prophylactic brain radiation is often recommended.

IMMUNOTHERAPY FOR LOCALLY ADVANCED SMALL CELL LUNG CANCER

Diana Saravia, MD, Cesar Perez, MD

A patient with locally advanced SCLC asks for a second opinion on adjuvant immunotherapy. He has a good partial response (PR) after chemoradiation and is undergoing PCI.

He now wonders if immunotherapy would decrease the risk of recurrence and progression.

Learning Objective:

1. Update on ongoing studies of immunotherapy in SCLC.

Small cell lung cancer is characterized by its rapid growth and early appearance of distant metastases. Patients with advanced SCLC frequently respond to first-line therapy; however, disease inevitably recurs, and few effective options remain available. Extensive research over the past years has been directed at investigating new therapeutic approaches to SCLC. The encouraging data of immune checkpoint inhibitors (ICIs) in NSCLC suggest the potential clinical applicability in SCLC. Although many genetic defects have been detected in SCLC, including *p53* mutations, loss of Rb, and strong expression of cKit, PD-L1 expression of 1% or greater of tumor cells is uncommonly seen.[44] This may account for significantly lower response rates to ICI when compared to NSCLC, where PD-L1 expression approaches an average of 50%.[45]

In the international, multicenter study CheckMate 032 by Antonia et al., the efficacy of PD-1 (programmed cell death protein 1) inhibition as well as combined PD-1 and CTLA4 (T-lymphocyte–associated protein 4) inhibition were investigated.[44]

Patients included had either limited-stage or extensive-stage SCLC and progressive disease after at least one platinum-based chemotherapy regimen. Patients were assigned to treatment with nivolumab or nivolumab plus ipilimumab at 3 different dose combinations. An objective response (determined per investigator-assessed response criteria in solid cancers [RECIST]) was achieved in 10% of patients receiving nivolumab 3 mg/kg alone versus 21% of patients receiving both nivolumab and ipilimumab at any dose combination. Grade 3 or 4 treatment-related adverse events occurred in 13% of patients in the nivolumab cohort versus 24% of those receiving both agents, with the most commonly reported severe toxicities in the combination group being increased lipase and diarrhea. Three patients of 118 who received nivolumab plus ipilimumab died from treatment-related adverse events (myasthenia gravis, worsening renal failure, and treatment-related pneumonitis).

Currently a phase 3 study, CheckMate 331, is ongoing further evaluation of the effectiveness of nivolumab compared to chemotherapy in patients with relapsed SCLC with either limited or extensive disease at initial diagnosis.

Pembrolizumab, a humanized monoclonal antibody against PD-1, has also been studied in patients with PD-L1 expressing ($\geq$1% by immunohistochemistry) SCLC pretreated with platinum-based combination therapy (phase IB study, NCT 02054806). In this study, pembrolizumab was administered at a dose of 10 mg/kg every 2 weeks for 24 months or until disease progression or intolerance occurred. One patient had a complete response, and 7 patients had partial responses, resulting in an objective response rate of 33%. All patients experienced side effects, with the most common being asthenia, fatigue, and cough.

Data suggest that immunotherapy, specifically CTLA4 blockade, may work alongside chemotherapy and radiation to enhance tumor control. This potential synergy may come about as a result of immunogenic tumor antigens that are released by the cytotoxic effects of chemotherapy or by distortion of tumor architecture facilitating the entry of immunotherapeutic agents. Ipilimumab, a fully human anti-CTLA4 monoclonal antibody, has been evaluated in a phase 2 study combined with platinum-based chemotherapy (paclitaxel/carboplatin) in patients with extensive SCLC or stage IV NSCLC.[46] Patients were randomized to 1 of 3 treatment arms: ipilimumab given concurrently with paclitaxel/carboplatin (4 doses of ipilimumab + paclitaxel/carboplatin, followed by 2 doses of placebo + paclitaxel/carboplatin); ipilimumab in a phased schedule with paclitaxel/carboplatin (2 doses of placebo + paclitaxel/carboplatin, followed by 4 doses of ipilimumab + paclitaxel/carboplatin); or a control regimen of placebo plus paclitaxel/carboplatin (up to 6 doses of placebo + paclitaxel/carboplatin). Designated treatment was given every 3 weeks for up to 6 doses. In the SCLC patient cohort, the phased administration of ipilimumab with chemotherapy improved progression-free survival based on immune-related response criteria (HR 0.64, 95% CI 0.40-1.02). There was a non-significant trend toward prolonged overall survival in the phased treatment group that received chemotherapy followed by chemotherapy plus ipilimumab (median overall survival 12.5 vs. 9.1 months for chemotherapy alone).

Another phase III trial by Reck et al. evaluated etoposide plus cisplatin with or without ipilimumab in patients with extensive-disease SCLC.[47] Patients received chemotherapy alone for the first 2 cycles, chemotherapy with or without ipilimumab for the following 2 cycles, and ipilimumab or placebo for the last 2 cycles. No difference was found between chemotherapy plus ipilimumab versus chemotherapy alone in terms of overall survival (11.0 vs. 10.9 months, respectively; HR for death 0.94, 95% CI 0.81-1.09). However, median progression-free survival was improved with addition of ipilimumab (4.6 vs. 4.4 months; HR for progression 0.85, 95% CI 0.75-0.97).

Although a promising and booming field, there are presently many challenges in developing immunotherapeutic treatments for SCLC, including high burden of disease, complex genetic heterogeneity, and lack of prognostic and predictive biomarkers to identify potential responders.[48]

REFERENCES

1. Videtic GM, Stitt LW, Dar AR, et al. Continued cigarette smoking by patients receiving concurrent chemoradiotherapy for limited-stage small-cell lung cancer is associated with decreased survival. *J Clin Oncol.* 2003;21(8):1544-1549.
2. Lilenbaum RC, Huber RM, Treat J, et al. Topotecan therapy in patients with relapsed small-cell lung cancer and poor performance status. *Clin Lung Cancer.* 2006;8(2):130-134.
3. Azam F, Wong H, Green JA, Marshall E. Poor performance status small cell lung cancer: who should we treat? *J Clin Oncol.* 2011;29(15_suppl):e17502.
4. Pujol JL, Carestia L, Daurès JP. Is there a case for cisplatin in the treatment of small-cell lung cancer? A meta-analysis of randomized trials of a cisplatin-containing regimen versus a regimen without this alkylating agent. *Br J Cancer.* 2000;83(1):8-15.
5. Sundstrom S, Bremnes RM, Kaasa S, et al. Cisplatin and etoposide regimen is superior to cyclophosphamide, epirubicin, and vincristine regimen in small-cell lung cancer: results from a randomized phase III trial with 5 years' follow-up. *J Clin Oncol.* 2002;20(24):4665-4672.
6. Skarlos DV, Samantas E, Kosmidis P, et al. Randomized comparison of etoposide-cisplatin vs. etoposide-carboplatin and irradiation in small-cell lung cancer. A Hellenic Co-operative Oncology Group Study. *Ann Oncol.* 1994;5(7):601-607.
7. Rossi A, Di Maio M, Chiodini P, et al. Carboplatin- or cisplatin-based chemotherapy in first-line treatment of small-cell lung cancer: the COCIS meta-analysis of individual patient data. *J Clin Oncol.* 2012;30(14):1692-1698.
8. Berghmans T, Paesmans M, Lafitte JJ, Mascaux C, Meert AP, Sculier JP. Role of granulocyte and granulocyte-macrophage colony-stimulating factors in the treatment of small-cell lung cancer: a systematic review of the literature with methodological assessment and meta-analysis. *Lung Cancer.* 2002;37(2):115-123.
9. Noda K, Nishiwaki Y, Kawahara M, et al. Irinotecan plus cisplatin compared with etoposide plus cisplatin for extensive small-cell lung cancer. *N Engl J Med.* 2002;346(2):85-91.
10. Lara PN, Jr., Natale R, Crowley J, et al. Phase III trial of irinotecan/cisplatin compared with etoposide/cisplatin in extensive-stage small-cell lung cancer: clinical and pharmacogenomic results from SWOG S0124. *J Clin Oncol.* 2009;27(15):2530-2535.
11. Hanna N, Bunn PA, Jr., Langer C, et al. Randomized phase III trial comparing irinotecan/cisplatin with etoposide/cisplatin in patients with previously untreated extensive-stage disease small-cell lung cancer. *J Clin Oncol.* 2006;24(13):2038-2043.
12. Hermes A, Bergman B, Bremnes R, et al. Irinotecan plus carboplatin versus oral etoposide plus carboplatin in extensive small-cell lung cancer: a randomized phase III trial. *J Clin Oncol.* 2008;26(26):4261-4267.
13. Lima JPSN, dos Santos LV, Sasse EC, et al. Camptothecins compared with etoposide in combination with platinum analog in extensive stage small cell lung cancer: systematic review with meta-analysis. *J Thorac Oncol.* 2010;5(12):1986-1993.
14. Niell HB, Herndon JE 2nd, Miller AA, et al. Randomized phase III intergroup trial of etoposide and cisplatin with or without paclitaxel and granulocyte colony-stimulating factor in patients with extensive-stage small-cell lung cancer: cancer and leukemia group B trial 9732. *J Clin Oncol.* 2005;23(16):3752-3759.
15. Berghmans T, Scherpereel A, Meert A-P, et al. A phase III randomized study comparing a chemotherapy with cisplatin and etoposide to a etoposide regimen without cisplatin for patients with extensive small-cell lung cancer. *Front Oncol.* 2017;7:217.
16. Cohen MH, Creaven PJ, Fossieck BE, Jr., et al. Intensive chemotherapy of small cell bronchogenic carcinoma. *Cancer Treat Rep.* 1977;61(3):349-354.
17. Schiller JH, Adak S, Cella D, DeVore RF 3rd, Johnson DH. Topotecan versus observation after cisplatin plus etoposide in extensive-stage small-cell lung cancer: E7593—a phase III trial of the Eastern Cooperative Oncology Group. *J Clin Oncol.* 2001;19(8):2114-2122.
18. Zhou H, Zeng C, Wei Y, Zhou J, Yao W. Duration of chemotherapy for small cell lung cancer: a meta-analysis. *PLoS One.* 2013;8(8):e73805.
19. Horn L, Mansfield AS, Szczęsna A, et al. First-line atezolizumab plus chemotherapy in extensive-stage small-cell lung cancer. *N Engl J Med.* 2018;379(23):2220-2229.

20. Eze C, Roengvoraphoj O, Niyazi M, et al. Treatment response and prophylactic cranial irradiation are prognostic factors in a real-life limited-disease small-cell lung cancer patient cohort comprehensively staged with cranial magnetic resonance imaging. *Clin Lung Cancer*. 2017;18(4):e243-e249.

21. Auperin A, Arriagada R, Pignon JP, et al. Prophylactic cranial irradiation for patients with small-cell lung cancer in complete remission. Prophylactic Cranial Irradiation Overview Collaborative Group. *N Engl J Med*. 1999;341(7):476-484.

22. Patel S, Macdonald OK, Suntharalingam M. Evaluation of the use of prophylactic cranial irradiation in small cell lung cancer. *Cancer*. 2009;115(4):842-850.

23. Hellmann MD, Callahan MK, Awad MM, et al. Tumor mutational burden and efficacy of nivolumab monotherapy and in combination with ipilimumab in small-cell lung cancer. *Cancer Cell*. 2018;33(5):853-861 e4.

24. Reck M, Vicente D, Ciuleanu T, et al. LBA5 Efficacy and safety of nivolumab (nivo) monotherapy versus chemotherapy (chemo) in recurrent small cell lung cancer (SCLC): results from CheckMate 331. *Ann Oncol*. 2018;29(suppl_10).

25. Corso CD, Rutter CE, Park HS, et al. Role of chemoradiotherapy in elderly patients with limited-stage small-cell lung cancer. *J Clin Oncol*. 2015;33(36):4240-4246.

26. Faivre-Finn C, Snee M, Ashcroft L, et al. Concurrent once-daily versus twice-daily chemoradiotherapy in patients with limited-stage small-cell lung cancer (CONVERT): an open-label, phase 3, randomised, superiority trial. *Lancet Oncol*. 2017;18(8):1116-1125.

27. Jemal A, Siegel R, Ward E, et al. Cancer statistics, 2006. *CA Cancer J Clin*. 2006;56(2):106-130.

28. Lad T, Piantadosi S, Thomas P, Payne D, Ruckdeschel J, Giaccone G. A prospective randomized trial to determine the benefit of surgical resection of residual disease following response of small cell lung cancer to combination chemotherapy. *Chest*. 1994;106(6 Suppl):320S-323S.

29. Fox W, Scadding JG. Medical Research Council comparative trial of surgery and radiotherapy for primary treatment of small-celled or oat-celled carcinoma of bronchus. Ten-year follow-up. *Lancet*. 1973;2(7820): 63-65.

30. Perry MC, Eaton WL, Propert KJ, et al. Chemotherapy with or without radiation therapy in limited small-cell carcinoma of the lung. *N Engl J Med*. 1987;316(15):912-918.

31. Pignon JP, Arriagada R, Ihde DC, et al. A meta-analysis of thoracic radiotherapy for small-cell lung cancer. *N Engl J Med*. 1992;327(23):1618-1624.

32. Carter BW, Glisson BS, Truong MT, Erasmus JJ. Small cell lung carcinoma: staging, imaging, and treatment considerations. *Radiographics*. 2014;34(6):1707-1721.

33. van Loon J. De Ruysscher D, Wanders R, et al. Selective nodal irradiation on basis of (18)FDG-PET scans in limited-disease small-cell lung cancer: a prospective study. *Int J Radiat Oncol Biol Phys*. 2010;77(2):329-336.

34. Turrisi AT, Kim K, Blum R, et al. Twice-daily compared with once-daily thoracic radiotherapy in limited small-cell lung cancer treated concurrently with cisplatin and etoposide. *N Engl J Med*. 1999;340(4):265-271.

35. Choi NC, Herndon JE 2nd, Rosenman J, et al. Phase I study to determine the maximum-tolerated dose of radiation in standard daily and hyperfractionated-accelerated twice-daily radiation schedules with concurrent chemotherapy for limited-stage small-cell lung cancer. *J Clin Oncol*. 1998;16(11):3528-3536.

36. Bogart JA, Herndon JE 2nd, Lyss AP, et al. 70 Gy thoracic radiotherapy is feasible concurrent with chemotherapy for limited-stage small-cell lung cancer: analysis of Cancer and Leukemia Group B study 39808. *Int J Radiat Oncol Biol Phys*. 2004;59(2):460-468.

37. Takada M, Fukuoka M, Kawahara M, et al. Phase III study of concurrent versus sequential thoracic radiotherapy in combination with cisplatin and etoposide for limited-stage small-cell lung cancer: results of the Japan Clinical Oncology Group Study 9104. *J Clin Oncol*. 2002;20(14):3054-3060.

38. De Ruysscher D, Lueza B, Le Péchoux C, et al. Impact of thoracic radiotherapy timing in limited-stage small-cell lung cancer: usefulness of the individual patient data meta-analysis. *Ann Oncol*. 2016;27(10):1818-1828.

39. Timmerman R, Paulus R, Galvin J, et al. Stereotactic body radiation therapy for inoperable early stage lung cancer. *JAMA*. 2010;303(11):1070-1076.

40. Onishi H, Araki T, Shirato H, et al. Stereotactic hypofractionated high-dose irradiation for stage I non-small cell lung carcinoma: clinical outcomes in 245 subjects in a Japanese multiinstitutional study. *Cancer*. 2004;101(7):1623-1631.

41. Alongi F, Tebano U, Mazzola R. Stereotactic precision and conventional radiotherapy evaluation (SPACE)-Trial for medically inoperable Stage I NSCLC: a lost opportunity? *Radiother Oncol*. 2017;122(2):319.

42. Komaki R, Byhardt RW, Anderson T, et al. What is the lowest effective biologic dose for prophylactic cranial irradiation? *Am J Clin Oncol*. 1985;8(6):523-527.

43. Arriagada R, Le Chevalier T, Borie F, et al. Prophylactic cranial irradiation for patients with small-cell lung cancer in complete remission. *J Natl Cancer Inst*. 1995;87(3):183-190.

44. Antonia SJ, López-Martin JA, Bendell J, et al. Nivolumab alone and nivolumab plus ipilimumab in recurrent small-cell lung cancer (CheckMate 032): a multicentre, open-label, phase 1/2 trial. *Lancet Oncol.* 2016;17(7):883-895.
45. Borghaei H, Paz-Ares L, Horn L, et al. Nivolumab versus docetaxel in advanced nonsquamous non-small-cell lung cancer. *N Engl J Med.* 2015;373(17):1627-1639.
46. Reck M, Bondarenko I, Luft A, et al. Ipilimumab in combination with paclitaxel and carboplatin as first-line therapy in extensive-disease-small-cell lung cancer: results from a randomized, double-blind, multicenter phase 2 trial. *Ann Oncol.* 2013;24(1):75-83.
47. Reck M, Luft A, Szczesna A, et al. Phase III randomized trial of ipilimumab plus etoposide and platinum versus placebo plus etoposide and platinum in extensive-stage small-cell lung cancer. *J Clin Oncol.* 2016;34(31):3740-3748.
48. Spigel DR, Socinski MA. Rationale for chemotherapy, immunotherapy, and checkpoint blockade in SCLC: beyond traditional treatment approaches. *J Thorac Oncol.* 2013;8(5):587-598.

18

SMALL CELL LUNG CANCER TREATMENT: METASTATIC

Neal E. Dunlap, MD • Muhammad Husnain, MD • Phuong T. Ngo, MD • Cesar A. Perez, MD • Mehran Yusuf, MD

CHEMOTHERAPY FOR METASTATIC SMALL CELL LUNG CANCER
Phuong T. Ngo, MD

A 62-year-old Caucasian male with an 80 pack-year smoking history, chronic obstructive pulmonary disease (COPD), and diabetes presents with progressively worsening shortness of breath over the past week. He is saturating 86% on room air in the emergency room, requiring oxygen at 5 L per nasal cannula and eventually bilevel positive airway pressure (BiPAP). Examination of the arterial blood gas (ABG) shows he is hypoxic and hypercapnic. His breathing becomes more labored, and he is electively intubated. Chest computed tomography (CT) shows bilateral pulmonary nodules with bulky mediastinal and hilar adenopathy. Abdominal/pelvic CT shows multiple hepatic lesions. Brain magnetic resonance imaging (MRI) is negative for brain metastases. Biopsy of a liver lesion returns with presence of small cell carcinoma.

Learning Objectives:
1. When should you expect to see a response in small cell lung cancer (SCLC)?
2. What is a common chemotherapy regimen for SCLC?
3. What is the recommended first line treatment for extensive stage SCLC?

As with early stage SCLC, metastatic SCLC also has a dramatic response initially, with response rates of 60%-70% with chemotherapy alone. However, even with appropriate treatment, the median survival rates are only 9-11 months, and the 2-year survival rate is less than 5% in these patients.[1]

Small cell lung cancer is very sensitive to chemotherapy and often has a dramatic response within 1-2 cycles.

CHEMOTHERAPY DOUBLET

Many chemotherapy combinations have been evaluated for extensive stage SCLC, but none has had consistent benefit when compared to cisplatin/etoposide. A Japanese phase 3 trial showed promising results, with 154 patients randomized to either cisplatin/irinotecan or cisplatin/etoposide.[2] Those treated with cisplatin and irinotecan had a significantly better overall response rate (84.4% vs. 67.5%), median survival (12.8 months vs. 9.4 months), and 1-year survival (58.4% vs. 37.7%) compared to those treated with cisplatin and etoposide, respectively. The irinotecan arm had more grade 3 and 4 diarrhea, while the etoposide arm had higher rates of myelosuppression.

The Southwest Oncology Group (SWOG) tried replicating the trial using the same schema but failed to show a significant difference in response rate or overall survival.[3] However, another phase 3 trial involving 220 patients did find that median overall survival was slightly improved (8.5 months vs. 7.1 months, $p = .04$) with carboplatin/irinotecan compared to carboplatin/oral etoposide.[4] A meta-analysis went on to suggest improved progression-free survival and overall survival with irinotecan plus a platinum drug when compared to etoposide with a platinum drug, but this meta-analysis did not use individual data, and the small absolute survival benefit needed to be balanced with toxicities from irinotecan.[5] Based on these findings, the National Comprehensive Cancer Network (NCCN) guidelines consider carboplatin and irinotecan as an option for extensive-stage SCLC but continue to recommend etoposide plus platinum regimens.

> **CLINICAL PEARL:** The standard doublet for small cell lung cancer is platinum with etoposide.

Many studies have evaluated whether adding a third agent to the current cisplatin/etoposide regimen would improve treatment for extensive-stage SCLC. Two trials added ifosfamide or cyclophosphamide plus an anthracycline to cisplatin/etoposide but only found a modest survival advantage at the cost of significantly increased hematologic toxicities.[6] Adding paclitaxel to a platinum regimen with etoposide had promising results in phase 2 trials but failed to improve survival in phase 3 studies.[7] The Global Analysis of Pemetrexed in SCLC Extensive Stage (GALES) aimed to show non-inferiority of pemetrexed plus carboplatin compared to carboplatin plus etoposide, but the study was terminated prematurely once the pemetrexed arm was found to actually be inferior.[8] The experimental arm had a median progression-free survival of 3.68 months compared to 5.32 months for carboplatin/etoposide and a preliminary overall survival of 7.3 months for pemetrexed/carboplatin compared to 9.6 months for carboplatin/etoposide.

Studies have also looked at the role of immunotherapy as both first-line and maintenance therapy in SCLC. One phase 2 study combined ipilimumab after an initial administration of carboplatin/paclitaxel and found improved immune-related progression-free survival, but a phase 3 trial of ipilimumab added to platinum/etoposide failed to show any difference in progression-free survival or overall survival.[9]

CHEMOIMMUNOTHERAPY COMBINATION

Most recently, the study of carboplatin plus etoposide with or without atezolizumab in participants with untreated extensive-stage (ES) small cell lung cancer (SCLC) (IMpower133) trial met its coprimary endpoints of progression-free survival and overall survival. The phase 4 trial randomized 403 patients to atezolizumab plus carboplatin and etoposide versus carboplatin and etoposide alone. After 4 cycles of treatment, patients[10] went on to receive either atezolizumab or placebo as maintenance until disease progression. The median progression-free survival improved with atezolizumab (5.2 months vs. 4.3 months), as did overall survival (12.3 months vs. 10.3 months) and 1-year survival rate (51.7% vs. 38.2%).[11]

> **CLINICAL PEARL:** The preferred first-line treatment for extensive SCLC is carboplatin/etoposide/atezolizumab followed by maintenance with atezolizumab.

BEVACIZUMAB

The role of bevacizumab in treatment for metastatic SCLC is unclear. Several phase 2 studies have shown improved response and survival outcomes with bevacizumab added to chemotherapy. One study involved 52 patients treated with irinotecan, carboplatin, and bevacizumab for 6 cycles. Patients with no progression went on to receive maintenance bevacizumab. The response rate, time to progression, and survival outcomes were found to be better than chemotherapy alone.[12] Another study of 63 patients involved treatment with bevacizumab plus cisplatin and etoposide followed by bevacizumab alone until disease progression or death. This study found improved progression-free survival and overall survival relative to historical controls who received cisplatin and etoposide with minimal increase in toxicities compared to chemotherapy alone.[13] However, these results have not been consistent.

One phase 3 study also randomized 204 patients to cisplatin/etoposide with or without bevacizumab. Those in the bevacizumab arm who did not have disease progression after 6 cycles of treatment continued on bevacizumab alone until disease progression. At the median follow-up, the median overall survival times for the chemotherapy-alone arm versus chemotherapy plus bevacizumab were 8.9 months and 9.8 months, and 1-year survival rates were 25% and 37% (hazard ratio 0.78, 95% CI 0.58-1.06, $p = .113$), respectively. There was a statistically significant improvement in progression-free survival but not in overall survival.[14] Another study found no difference in response or progression-free survival in patients who received chemotherapy plus bevacizumab versus those who received chemotherapy alone.[15]

> **CLINICAL PEARL:** Bevacizumab is currently not recommended in the treatment of SCLC.

DURATION AND MAINTENANCE THERAPY

Chemotherapy for SCLC has traditionally been given for 4-6 cycles based on randomized trials, but there is no ideal number for treatment cycles. Many have looked at whether maintenance or consolidation treatments are of any benefit to these patients.

The Eastern Cooperative Oncology Group (ECOG) randomized patients who had not progressed after initial therapy to either consolidation or maintenance with topotecan and found the progression-free survival from the treatment arm was significantly better (3.6 months vs. 2.3 months, $p < .001$).[16] However, overall survival for the topotecan versus observation group was not significant (8.9 months vs. 9.3 months, $p = .43$).

A meta-analysis of 14 trials looking at consolidation or maintenance therapy in these patients found that the 1- and 2-year odds ratios for progression-free survival and overall survival favored prolonged treatment.[17] However, these results were not based on individual patient data, and the trials involved not only differed in their designs but also outdated regimens were used by most. As a result, there was still no definitive recommendation for continuing chemotherapy beyond the initial 4 or 6 cycles.

There is currently no role for maintenance chemotherapy. However, immunotherapy may be used after initial treatment based on newer data. A phase 2 trial used pembrolizumab as maintenance after 4-6 cycles of platinum/etoposide but ultimately failed to show improvement in progression-free survival or overall survival.[18] Currently, only atezolizumab is recommended for maintenance therapy based on significant results from IMPower133 as mentioned previously.

SECOND-LINE THERAPY

Despite being very sensitive to treatment initially, most patients with SCLC eventually relapse with relatively resistant disease. Response to subsequent treatment depends on the time from initial therapy to relapse. If this time is less than 3 months, response to second-line therapy is expected to be poor (<10%). If this time is greater than 3 months, response rates are slightly better at about 25%.

> **CLINICAL PEARL:** Sensitive relapse occurs more than 3 months after initial treatment. Resistant relapse occurs within 3 months after initial treatment. Refractory relapse occurs during initial treatment.

> **CLINICAL PEARL:** Time to relapse is often predictive of response to subsequent treatment and dictates treatment choice. If relapse occurs more than 6 months from the initial treatment, consider repeating the original regimen.

Patients with relapse while on atezolizumab maintenance that is more than 6 months from the initial chemotherapy induction can also be treated with the original regimen but without atezolizumab. The exception to this is for patients initially treated with carboplatin/etoposide/atezolizumab who relapse more than 6 months while on atezolizumab maintenance. These patients should receive carboplatin/etoposide without atezolizumab next. For resistant or refractory disease, there is no standard treatment, so when possible, patients should be referred for a clinical trial.

For relapse that occurs within 6 months, treat with a second line regimen.

Single-agent topotecan is approved by the Food and Drug Administration (FDA) as second-line therapy for patients who relapse after initial chemotherapy. An older phase 3 trial compared single-agent intravenous topotecan to CAV (cyclophosphamide, doxorubicin, and vincristine) and found similar response rates but a better toxicity profile with topotecan.[19] Another phase 3 trial compared oral topotecan to best supportive care and found improved overall survival (26 weeks vs. 14 weeks).[20]

Nivolumab with or without ipilimumab was recently added to guidelines, with preliminary data showing a 1-year survival of 42% with nivolumab/ipilimumab together and 30% in those receiving nivolumab alone.[21] Immunotherapy in SCLC is discussed further elsewhere in this book.

There is no optimal duration of subsequent systemic therapy, and it should usually be continued until 2 cycles beyond the best response, progression of disease, or unacceptable toxicities.

Second-line options for extensive stage SCLC are as follows:

- Subsequent therapy options
  - Topotecan
  - Nivolumab with or without ipilimumab
  - Pembrolizumab
  - Irinotecan
  - Paclitaxel
  - Docetaxel
  - Temozolomide
  - Vinorelbine
  - Oral etoposide
  - Gemcitabine
  - CAV
  - Bendamustine

ELDERLY

The incidence of lung cancer increases with age, but elderly patients are unfortunately underrepresented in clinic trials. Though being older does portend more adverse reactions with treatment, age alone should not be a factor in deciding treatment options.

Randomized clinical trials have shown that single-agent chemotherapy is inferior to combination chemotherapy in the elderly patients with good performance status though toxicities including fatigue and myelosuppression were more common. For elderly patients with SCLC, using a smaller area under the curve to dose carboplatin takes into consideration the declining renal function in these patients.[22] Overall, elderly patients appear to have a similar prognosis as younger, stage-matched patients.

CLINICAL PEARL: Standard-of-care treatment should be offered to all fit patients and those whose poor performance status may be due to disease.

POOR PERFORMANCE STATUS

Poor performance status is a universal indicator of poor tolerance to treatment. These patients tend to have more toxicities with treatment and are ineligible for clinical trials. However, given the sensitivity of SCLC to chemotherapy, some patients may have an improvement in their performance status once treated. A retrospective review of 7 trials found that 21% of 152 patients who initially had a performance status of 2 converted to that of 0 or 1 after salvage therapy with topotecan.[23]

A Cancer and Leukemia Group B (CALGB) meta-analysis found that tolerance to therapy was more dependent on dose intensity than performance status.[24] One study randomized patients with poor performance status to either a 4-drug regimen of ECMV (etoposide, cyclophosphamide, methotrexate, and vincristine) or EV (etoposide, vincristine). The two groups had similar response rates, palliation of symptoms, and survival, but not surprisingly, the 4-drug arm had greater toxicities.[25] Oral etoposide was once thought to be more suitable for patients with poor performance status until a study randomized patients with performance status of 2-4 to either oral etoposide or standard chemotherapy with cisplatin/etoposide or CAV.[26] Palliation of symptoms was similar for both groups, but survival was lower in the oral etoposide arm (130 days vs. 183 days). Another trial similarly compared oral etoposide versus CAV or cisplatin/etoposide in patients who were either younger than 75 years old but with poor performance status of 2-3 or older than 75 years with any performance status. The oral etoposide arm again had a lower median survival (4.8 months vs. 5.9 months) and a 1-year survival rate (9.8% vs. 19.3%).[27]

Though a poor performance status typically predicts a patient's inability to tolerate treatment, it may be the result of the disease itself in SCLC patients, so treating the underlying malignancy may improve their functional status.

PARANEOPLASTIC SYNDROMES

Small cell lung cancer is associated with paraneoplastic syndromes, the most common of which is syndrome of inappropriate antidiuretic hormone (SIADH), which is marked by hyponatremia, euvolemia, and confusion. Immediate treatment includes fluid restriction, demeclocyline, vasopressin receptor inhibitors, or hypertonic saline. As with all treatments for hyponatremia, sodium should be corrected slowly to avoid central pontine myelinolysis. Another commonly mentioned paraneoplastic syndrome in SCLC is Lambert-Eaton, in which antibodies attack voltage-gated calcium channels, resulting in proximal leg weakness.

Small cell lung cancer can also produce anti-Hu (ANNA-1) antibodies that cross-react with small cell carcinoma antigens and human neuronal RNA-binding proteins. These patients can develop encephalomyelitis and other severe neurologic deficits.[28] In addition to treating the underlying malignancy, corticosteroids, plasmapheresis, and intravenous immunoglobulin (IVIG) have been used.

> **CLINICAL PEARL:** Anti-Hu antibodies can cause neurologic defects and can be treated with corticosteroids, plasmapheresis, or IVIG.

RADIATION THERAPY FOR METASTATIC SMALL CELL LUNG CANCER

Neal E. Dunlap, MD, Mehran Yusuf, MD

A 60-year-old white female has a central 3-cm lung mass and on positron emission tomography (PET) diffuse osseous metastases. She smoked 2 packs of cigarettes per day and has COPD and coronary artery disease (CAD). The pathology shows SCLC. Her performance status is ECOG 2 due to dyspnea. How will you treat her?

Learning Objective:

1. What is the role of consolidation radiation therapy in metastatic SCLC?

THORACIC RADIATION

The use of thoracic radiation in patients with metastatic SCLC continues to evolve. Initial support of integrating consolidative thoracic radiation into the treatment paradigm was based on the results from the work of Jeremic et al. Patients were only included in the study if they had low-bulk metastatic disease. Only after an initial complete response (CR) or partial response (PR) to systemic chemotherapy were patients randomized to receive sequential thoracic radiation using an accelerated fractionation technique versus further chemotherapy. In patients who received thoracic radiation, the mean survival was increased from 11 months to 17 months.[29] Additionally, our institutional data combine with information from the Kentucky Cancer Registry demonstrated improvements in overall survival in patients with extensive-stage disease who were treated (**Figure 18-1**).

Studies that are more contemporary have attempted to clarify the role of consolidative thoracic radiation in improved survival. The Dutch CREST trial was designed to randomize patients with good performance status and with extensive-stage disease with any response to chemotherapy to either no further treatment or thoracic radiation using 30 Gy in 10 fractions. The primary endpoint of 1-year overall survival was not significant, but secondary analysis of the 2-year survival endpoint showed an overall survival improvement from 3% to 13%. Thoracic progression was also less likely in the group receiving radiation. The authors concluded that patients with a response to systemic chemotherapy should be considered for both prophylactic cranial irradiation (PCI) and consolidative chest radiation.[30,31] In a follow-up report, the authors also stated that the benefit was most pronounced in patients with residual disease after chemotherapy.[30]

The Radiation Therapy Oncology Group (RTOG 0937) attempted to further explore the question of consolidative chest radiation.[32] The premise of the phase 2 randomized trial was to highly select patients with limited extrathoracic metastasis whom were presumed to have more favorable biology. The term *oligometastatic* was applied to this group of patients by limiting enrollment to patients with 1-4 extrathoracic metastases. Eligible patients had to have a PR or CR to 4-6 cycles of platinum-based chemotherapy at a minimum of 1 site of disease and no evidence of progression at any site. Patients were randomized between PCI alone versus PCI plus consolidative radiation of 45 Gy in 15 fractions to all extracranial disease. Metastases were alone treated if residual disease

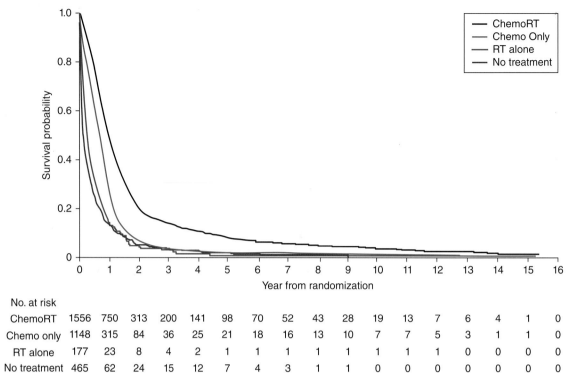

Figure 18-1. Kaplan-Meyer survival curves for patients with extensive-stage SCLC. The data demonstrate the addition of radiation to chemotherapy (ChemoRT, black) leads to a survival benefit over chemotherapy alone (red) or radiation alone (green).

remained after chemotherapy. The study was closed early because of futility at the interim analysis. The median survival was 15.8 months in the PCI arm and 13.8 months in the PCI plus consolidative radiation. Patients who received extracranial radiation had delayed progression compared to the PCI-only group.

Although the RTOG 0937 study failed to confirm a survival advantage as seen in the Jeremic[29] and Slotman[31] studies, important conclusions may be drawn from the results. In highly selected patients with extensive-stage disease, survival rates may approach that of patients with limited-stage disease.[33] The survival advantage compared to historical data evaluated for extensive-stage patients is likely attributable to selection rather than the use of thoracic radiation. Much of this may be from the routine use of PET/CT as part of the staging workup.[34] Radiation therapy may also alter the pattern of failure in patients with extensive-stage disease. RTOG 0937 showed that patients were more likely to fail at sites of initial disease, but those patients receiving extracranial radiation were less likely to have locoregional progression at a site of first failure. Although a possible benefit was seen in controlling locoregional disease, the response was not durable.

> **CLINICAL PEARL:** Consolidative thoracic radiation may improve overall survival in patients with extensive-stage disease with extracranial metastases.

In highly selected patients with good responses to chemotherapy and limited disease, thoracic radiation may be omitted with no detriment to survival for local progression long term. Further work is needed to select which patients may benefit from more aggressive treatment.

CENTRAL NERVOUS SYSTEM RADIATION

Brain metastases occur commonly for patients with SCLC, with the incidence of intracranial disease as high as 10% at presentation and more than half of patients developing brain metastases within 2 years of diagnosis.[35,36] Central nervous system (CNS) relapses are a common site of failure for patients with limited SCLC who respond to systemic therapy and thoracic radiation and is the rationale underlying PCI. PCI has been demonstrated to decrease the incidence of brain metastasis development (3-year cumulative brain metastasis incidence 33.3% vs. 58.6%, $p < .001$) as well as increase survival (3-year overall survival 20.7% vs. 15.3%, $p = .01$) and disease-free survival (3 year disease-free survival 22.3% vs. 13.5%, $p <.001$) for patients with limited SCLC in complete remission.[37] PCI with hippocampal avoidance is an area of active interest[38] and is the current subject of an ongoing NRG oncology trial (NCT02635009) but is not currently standard of care pending these results.

The role of PCI in patients with extensive SCLC is more controversial. Slotman et al. demonstrated a 1.3-month overall survival benefit with PCI for patients with extensive SCLC with any response to CT.[39] However, CT or MRI of the brain was not routinely performed as part of staging for these patients, and patients with small, asymptomatic brain metastases may have been included in the arm receiving PCI.

A recently reported Japanese randomized trial did not find a statistically significant benefit in survival with PCI for a population of extensive SCLC patients well screened with brain MRIs.[40] The cumulative incidence of brain metastases at 18 months was significantly higher for patients who did not receive PCI (64% vs. 40%, $p < .0001$). Additionally, 83% of patients in the observation group subsequently received radiotherapy for brain metastases. Extrapolating these findings to non-Japanese populations with SCLC may be difficult given data suggesting differences in response to treatment between ethnic populations.[2,41]

Retrospective analysis of a large US national database of patients with extensive SCLC suggested a significant survival benefit with PCI (13. 9 months vs. 11.1 months, $p <.0001$), although these findings are limited by biases inherent to retrospective analysis. Pending further clarification, NCCN guidelines recommend considering either PCI or close surveillance with serial CNS imaging for patients with extensive SCLC with response to systemic therapy.[42]

INTRACRANIAL METASTASES

The cumulative incidence of brain metastasis development may be greater than 50%.[8] When determining optimal management for these patients, it is important to consider whether the patient has been previously treated with PCI. For patients with SCLC brain metastases who have not received PCI, the NCCN guidelines currently recommend treatment with whole-brain radiotherapy (WBRT) instead of more focused courses of stereotactic radiation given the tendency of these patients to develop multiple CNS metastases. Retrospective studies, including an analysis of the National Cancer Database (NCDB)[9] have suggested stereotactic radiosurgery (SRS) alone may achieve favorable outcomes in select patients with limited SCLC brain metastases, and results from ongoing prospective trials (NCT03297788) may help clarify if stereotactic radiotherapy is appropriate first-line treatment for select patients with limited SCLC brain metastases.

Radiosurgery may be considered for patients who develop SCLC brain metastases after receiving PCI, particularly in the setting of controlled extracranial disease and a long interval from PCI to subsequent brain metastasis development.[10,11] WBRT after PCI may be considered in carefully selected patients felt to be poor candidates for radiosurgery and may be of particular value for patients with good performance status and controlled systemic disease.[12,13] Best supportive care may be considered for patients with poor performance status, extensive intracranial or systemic disease, or those developing brain metastases shortly after completing PCI (range varies across institutional preference).

IMMUNOTHERAPY FOR METASTATIC SMALL CELL LUNG CANCER

Muhammad Husnain, MD, Cesar A. Perez, MD

After presenting to the emergency department with persistent headache, a 49-year-old female is diagnosed with diffuse brain metastatic disease. CT of the chest revealed a lung mass, and fine-needle aspiration of the mass was compatible with SCLC. The patient is treated with WBRT. What is the recommended systemic therapy for her disease?

Learning Objective:

1. Describe the role of checkpoint inhibitors in the treatment of extensive-stage SCLC?

EARLY TRIALS OF IMMUNOTHERAPY

Systemic chemotherapy with platinum and etoposide has long been the standard of care for metastatic SCLC, with a median survival of 9-11 months and a 2-year survival rate of 5%. Given this poor outcome, there is great interest in the study of the role of immunotherapy for this population. One of the initial trials of checkpoint inhibition in SCLC was a phase 2 study reported by Reck et al. using ipilimumab in combination with paclitaxel and carboplatin as first-line therapy in extensive-stage SCLC. Adding ipilimumab to carboplatin and paclitaxel in a phased sequence (after an initial administration of carboplatin plus paclitaxel) improved immune-related progression-free survival (6.4 vs. 5.3 months; hazard ratio [HR] 0.64, $p = .03$).[9]

However, a phase 3 trial of ipilimumab plus etoposide and platinum in newly diagnosed extensive-stage SCLC failed to show any significant difference in overall survival or progression-free survival, with an overall survival of 11.0 months for the chemotherapy plus ipilimumab arm versus 10.9 months for the chemotherapy plus placebo arm (HR 0.94, 95% CI 0.81-1.09, $p = .37$).[10]

On the maintenance setting, pembrolizumab was studied after of 4-6 cycles of induction chemotherapy with platinum/etoposide in a phase 2 study, also failing to show any significant benefit in terms of overall survival and progression-free survival.[18,43] Thus, so far no trials have demonstrated a strong benefit of checkpoint inhibition in the first-line and maintenance settings. In the second-line setting, the phase 1/2 CheckMate32 trial treated platinum-refractory patients with nivolumab alone or in combination with ipilimumab. The trial showed a response rate for the total population (independent of programmed death ligand 1 [PD-L1] status) of 10% with nivolumab alone and 23% for nivolumab plus ipilimumab.[44]

CheckMate 032 investigators presented their updated data at the International Association for the Study of Lung Cancer (IASLC) 18th World Conference on Lung Cancer in Yokohama, Japan, showing that in a pooled intent-to-treat population of 401 patients the objective response rate was 11% with nivolumab alone and 22% with nivolumab plus ipilimumab. Patients with a high tumor mutation burden (TMB) who received nivolumab plus ipilimumab had an objective response rate of 46%; the objective response rates were 16% and 22% in patients with medium and low levels of TMB, respectively. In patients with high tumor burden who received nivolumab plus ipilimumab, 62% were alive at 1 year. Pembrolizumab was also used in platinum-refractory SCLC patients with a membranous PD-L1 expression in 1% or greater in tumor and associated inflammatory cells. Of the patients screened, only 32% had PD-L1–positive tumors, and 24 patients were treated, demonstrating an overall response rate of 33.3%.[45] These results are really encouraging but merit further study. Based on these preliminary data nivolumab with or without ipilimumab or pembrolizumab is a reasonable option for patients with extensive-stage SCLC who have failed a first- or second-line of chemotherapy.

NEW STANDARD OF CARE

The IMpower133 trial is a double-blind, placebo-controlled, phase 3 trial that added the PD-L1 antibody atezolizumab in combination with carboplatin and etoposide in patients with extensive-stage SCLC who had not previously received treatment versus carboplatin plus etoposide.[11] Patients received 4 cycles of the triplet followed by a maintenance phase of either atezolizumab or placebo, with 404 patients in total randomized between the two groups in a 1:1 ratio. At a median follow-up of 13.9 months, the median overall survival was 12.3 months in the atezolizumab group and 10.3 months in the placebo group (HR for death 0.70, 95% CI 0.54-0.91, $p = .007$). The median progression-free survival was 5.2 months and 4.3 months, respectively (HR for disease progression or death 0.77, 95% CI 0.62-0.96, $P = .02$). The safety profile of atezolizumab plus carboplatin and etoposide was consistent with the previously reported safety profile of the individual agents, with no new findings observed.

> **CLINICAL PEARL:** IMpower133 is the first trial in the first-line setting that demonstrated an overall survival advantage of adding a checkpoint inhibitor to the platinum-etoposide doublet and has changed the treatment landscape for this population.

Other ongoing trials are evaluating the use of checkpoint inhibitor combinations in the first-line setting against platinum-based chemotherapy.[46] The results from the IMpower133 trial have changed the landscape of treatment for SCLC, and together with other agents in development, immunotherapy plus chemotherapy might become the new standard of care for patients with SCLC. Unlike non-SCLC, however, no driver mutations have been revealed to be good therapeutic targets for SCLC.

Research is ongoing to identify pathways and targets against which we can develop therapeutic agents. One such target is Delta-like protein 3 (DLL3). DLL3 is a member of the notch receptor ligand family that, instead of activating, seems to inhibit notch receptor activation. Notch activation in SCLC suppresses tumor growth.[47,48] Hence, DLL3 plays a tumorigenesis role by inhibiting notch receptor. Also, DLL3 appears to be a downstream transcriptional target of the ASCL1 transcription factor.[10,11,42,49] DLL3 protein is expressed in more than 80% of patients. It is expressed on tumor cells but not in normal cells and is thought to be an oncogenic driver in SCLC and high-grade neuroendocrine tumors.[50]

Rovalpituzumab tesirine is a first-in-class antibody drug conjugate directed against DLL3. Its safety and activity were assessed in a phase 1 study enrolling total 82 patients, including 74 patients with SCLC who had progressed after first- or second-line chemotherapy.[51] The drug was well tolerated, with 38% of patients having grade 3 or worse adverse effects. The most frequent grade 3 or worse adverse events were thrombocytopenia (11%), pleural effusion (8%), and increased lipase (7%). Of the patients, 17% achieved a confirmed objective response, and 54% had stable disease. Further trials are ongoing to assess the efficacy of these targeted therapies.

REFERENCES

1. Chute JP, Chen T, Feigal E, Simon R, Johnson BE. Twenty years of phase III trials for patients with extensive-stage small-cell lung cancer: perceptible progress. *J Clin Oncol.* 1999;17(6):1794-1801.
2. Noda K, Nishiwaki Y, Kawahara M, et al. Irinotecan plus cisplatin compared with etoposide plus cisplatin for extensive small-cell lung cancer. *N Engl J Med.* 2002;346(2):85-91.
3. Lara PN, Jr., Natale R, Crowley J, et al. Phase III trial of irinotecan/cisplatin compared with etoposide/cisplatin in extensive-stage small-cell lung cancer: clinical and pharmacogenomic results from SWOG S0124. *J Clin Oncol.* 2009;27(15):2530-2535.
4. Hermes A, Bergman B, Bremnes R, et al. Irinotecan plus carboplatin versus oral etoposide plus carboplatin in extensive small-cell lung cancer: a randomized phase III trial. *J Clin Oncol.* 2008;26(26):4261-4267.
5. Lima JP, dos Santos LV, Sasse EC, Lima CSP, Sasse AD. Camptothecins compared with etoposide in combination with platinum analog in extensive stage small cell lung cancer: systematic review with meta-analysis. *J Thorac Oncol.* 2010;5(12):1986-1993.
6. Miyamoto H, Nakabayashi T, Isobe H, et al. A phase III comparison of etoposide/cisplatin with or without added ifosfamide in small-cell lung cancer. *Oncology.* 1992;49(6):431-435.
7. Niell HB, Herndon JE 2nd, Miller AA, et al. Randomized phase III intergroup trial of etoposide and cisplatin with or without paclitaxel and granulocyte colony-stimulating factor in patients with extensive-stage small-cell lung cancer: Cancer and Leukemia Group B Trial 9732. *J Clin Oncol.* 2005;23(16):3752-3759.
8. Socinski MA, Langer CJ, Huang JE, et al. Safety of bevacizumab in patients with non-small-cell lung cancer and brain metastases. *J Clin Oncol.* 2009;27(31):5255-5261.
9. Reck M, Bondarenko I, Luft A, et al. Ipilimumab in combination with paclitaxel and carboplatin as first-line therapy in extensive-disease-small-cell lung cancer: results from a randomized, double-blind, multicenter phase 2 trial. *Ann Oncol.* 2013;24(1):75-83.
10. Reck M, Luft A, Szczesna A, et al. Phase III randomized trial of ipilimumab plus etoposide and platinum versus placebo plus etoposide and platinum in extensive-stage small-cell lung cancer. *J Clin Oncol.* 2016;34(31):3740-3748.

11. Horn L, Mansfield AS, Szczęsna A, et al. First-line atezolizumab plus chemotherapy in extensive-stage small-cell lung cancer. *N Engl J Med*. 2018;379(23):2220-2229.

12. Spigel DR, Greco FA, Zubkus JD, et al. Phase II trial of irinotecan, carboplatin, and bevacizumab in the treatment of patients with extensive-stage small-cell lung cancer. *J Thorac Oncol*. 2009;4(12):1555-1560.

13. Horn L, Dahlberg SE, Sandler AB, et al. Phase II study of cisplatin plus etoposide and bevacizumab for previously untreated, extensive-stage small-cell lung cancer: Eastern Cooperative Oncology Group Study E3501. *J Clin Oncol*. 2009;27(35):6006-6011.

14. Tiseo M, Boni L, Ambrosio F, et al. Italian, multicenter, phase III, randomized study of cisplatin plus etoposide with or without bevacizumab as first-line treatment in extensive-disease small-cell lung cancer: the GOIRC-AIFA FARM6PMFJM Trial. *J Clin Oncol*. 2017;35(12):1281-1287.

15. Pujol JL, Lavole A, Quoix E, et al. Randomized phase II-III study of bevacizumab in combination with chemotherapy in previously untreated extensive small-cell lung cancer: results from the IFCT-0802 trialdagger. *Ann Oncol*. 2015;26(5):908-914.

16. Schiller JH, Adak S, Cella D, DeVore RF 3rd, Johnson DH. Topotecan versus observation after cisplatin plus etoposide in extensive-stage small-cell lung cancer: E7593—a phase III trial of the Eastern Cooperative Oncology Group. *J Clin Oncol*. 2001;19(8):2114-2122.

17. Bozcuk H, Artac M, Ozdogan M, Savas B. Does maintenance/consolidation chemotherapy have a role in the management of small cell lung cancer (SCLC)? A metaanalysis of the published controlled trials. *Cancer*. 2005;104(12):2650-2657.

18. Gadgeel SM, Ventimiglia J, Kalemkerian GP, et al. Phase II study of maintenance pembrolizumab (pembro) in extensive stage small cell lung cancer (ES-SCLC) patients (pts). *J Clin Oncol*. 2017;35(15_suppl):8504-8504.

19. von Pawel J, Schiller JH, Shepherd FA, et al. Topotecan versus cyclophosphamide, doxorubicin, and vincristine for the treatment of recurrent small-cell lung cancer. *J Clin Oncol*. 1999;17(2):658-667.

20. O'Brien ME, Ciuleanu T-E, Tsekov H, et al. Phase III trial comparing supportive care alone with supportive care with oral topotecan in patients with relapsed small-cell lung cancer. *J Clin Oncol*. 2006;24(34):5441-5447.

21. Hellmann MD, Rizvi NA, Goldman JW, et al. Nivolumab plus ipilimumab as first-line treatment for advanced non-small-cell lung cancer (CheckMate 012): results of an open-label, phase 1, multicohort study. *Lancet Oncol*. 2017;18(1):31-41.

22. Okamoto H, Watanabe K, Nishiwaki Y, et al. Phase II study of area under the plasma-concentration-versus-time curve-based carboplatin plus standard-dose intravenous etoposide in elderly patients with small-cell lung cancer. *J Clin Oncol*. 1999;17(11):3540-3545.

23. Lilenbaum RC, Huber RM, Treat J, et al. Topotecan therapy in patients with relapsed small-cell lung cancer and poor performance status. *Clin Lung Cancer*. 2006;8(2):130-134.

24. Spiegelman D, Maurer LH, Ware JH, et al. Prognostic factors in small-cell carcinoma of the lung: an analysis of 1,521 patients. *J Clin Oncol*. 1989;7(3):344-354.

25. Party M.R.C.L.C.W. Randomised trial of four-drug vs less intensive two-drug chemotherapy in the palliative treatment of patients with small-cell lung cancer (SCLC) and poor prognosis. Medical Research Council Lung Cancer Working Party. *Br J Cancer*. 1996;73(3):406-413.

26. Girling DJ. Comparison of oral etoposide and standard intravenous multidrug chemotherapy for small-cell lung cancer: a stopped multicentre randomised trial. Medical Research Council Lung Cancer Working Party. *Lancet*. 1996;348(9027):563-566.

27. Souhami RL, Spiro SG, Rudd RM, et al. Five-day oral etoposide treatment for advanced small-cell lung cancer: randomized comparison with intravenous chemotherapy. *J Natl Cancer Inst*. 1997;89(8):577-580.

28. Graus F, Keime-Guibert F, Reñe R, et al. Anti-Hu-associated paraneoplastic encephalomyelitis: analysis of 200 patients. *Brain*. 2001;124(Pt 6):1138-1148.

29. Jeremic B, Shibamoto Y, Nikolic N, et al. Role of radiation therapy in the combined-modality treatment of patients with extensive disease small-cell lung cancer: a randomized study. *J Clin Oncol*. 1999;17(7):2092-2099.

30. Slotman BJ, van Tinteren H. Which patients with extensive stage small-cell lung cancer should and should not receive thoracic radiotherapy? *Transl Lung Cancer Res*. 2015;4(3):292-294.

31. Slotman BJ, van Tinteren H, Praag JO, et al. Use of thoracic radiotherapy for extensive stage small-cell lung cancer: a phase 3 randomised controlled trial. *Lancet*. 2015;385(9962):36-42.

32. Gore EM, Hu C, Sun AY, et al. Randomized phase II study comparing prophylactic cranial irradiation alone to prophylactic cranial irradiation and consolidative extracranial irradiation for extensive-disease small cell lung cancer (ED SCLC): NRG Oncology RTOG 0937. *J Thorac Oncol*. 2017;12(10):1561-1570.

33. Pignon JP, Arriagada R, Ihde DC, et al. A meta-analysis of thoracic radiotherapy for small-cell lung cancer. *N Engl J Med*. 1992;327(23):1618-1624.

34. Niho S, Fujii H, Murakami K, et al. Detection of unsuspected distant metastases and/or regional nodes by FDG-PET [corrected] scan in apparent limited-disease small-cell lung cancer. *Lung Cancer*. 2007;57(3):328-333.

35. Komaki R, Byhardt RW, Anderson T, et al. What is the lowest effective biologic dose for prophylactic cranial irradiation? *Am J Clin Oncol*. 1985;8(6):523-527.

36. Arriagada R, Le Chevalier T, Borie F, et al. Prophylactic cranial irradiation for patients with small-cell lung cancer in complete remission. *J Natl Cancer Inst*. 1995;87(3):183-190.

37. Auperin A, Arriagada R, Pignon JP, et al. Prophylactic cranial irradiation for patients with small-cell lung cancer in complete remission. Prophylactic Cranial Irradiation Overview Collaborative Group. *N Engl J Med*. 1999;341(7):476-484.

38. de Dios NR, Couñago F, López JL, et al. Treatment design and rationale for a randomized trial of prophylactic cranial irradiation with or without hippocampal avoidance for SCLC: PREMER trial on behalf of the oncologic group for the study of lung cancer/Spanish Radiation Oncology Group-Radiation Oncology Clinical Research Group. *Clin Lung Cancer*. 2018;19(5):e693-e697.

39. Slotman B, Faivre-Finn C, Kramer G, et al. Prophylactic cranial irradiation in extensive small-cell lung cancer. *N Engl J Med*. 2007;357(7):664-672.

40. Takahashi T, Yamanaka T, Seto T, et al. Prophylactic cranial irradiation versus observation in patients with extensive-disease small-cell lung cancer: a multicentre, randomised, open-label, phase 3 trial. *Lancet Oncol*. 2017;18(5):663-671.

41. Hanna N, Bunn PA, Jr., Langer C, et al. Randomized phase III trial comparing irinotecan/cisplatin with etoposide/cisplatin in patients with previously untreated extensive-stage disease small-cell lung cancer. *J Clin Oncol*. 2006;24(13):2038-2043.

42. Ettinger DS, Aisner DL, Wood DE, et al. NCCN Guidelines Insights: Non-Small Cell Lung Cancer, Version 5.2018. *J Natl Compr Canc Netw*. 2018;16(7):807-821.

43. Gadgeel SM, Pennell NA, Jo Fidler M, et al. Phase II study of maintenance pembrolizumab in patients with extensive-stage small cell lung cancer (SCLC). *J Thorac Oncol*. 2018;13(9):1393-1399.

44. Antonia SJ, López-Martin JA, Bendell J, et al. Nivolumab alone and nivolumab plus ipilimumab in recurrent small-cell lung cancer (CheckMate 032): a multicentre, open-label, phase 1/2 trial. *Lancet Oncol*. 2016;17(7):883-895.

45. Ott PA, Elez E, Hiret S, et al. Pembrolizumab in patients with extensive-stage small-cell lung cancer: results from the phase Ib KEYNOTE-028 study. *J Clin Oncol*. 2017;35(34):3823-3829.

46. Paz-Ares LG, Jiang H, Huang Y, Dennis PA. A phase 3, randomized study of first-line durvalumab (D) ± tremelimumab (T) + platinum-based chemotherapy (CT) vs CT alone in extensive disease small-cell lung cancer (ED-SCLC): caspian. *J Clin Oncol*. 2017;35(15_suppl):TPS8586-TPS8586.

47. Chapman G, Sparrow DB, Kremmer E, Dunwoodie SL. Notch inhibition by the ligand DELTA-LIKE 3 defines the mechanism of abnormal vertebral segmentation in spondylocostal dysostosis. *Hum Mol Genet*. 2011;20(5):905-916.

48. Dunwoodie SL, Henrique D, Harrison SM, Beddington RS. Mouse Dll3: a novel divergent delta gene which may complement the function of other delta homologues during early pattern formation in the mouse embryo. *Development*. 1997;124(16):3065-3076.

49. Henke RM, Meredith DM, Borromeo MD, Savage TK, Johnson JE. Ascl1 and Neurog2 form novel complexes and regulate Delta-like3 (Dll3) expression in the neural tube. *Dev Biol*. 2009;328(2):529-540.

50. Saunders LR, Bankovich AJ, Anderson WC, et al. A DLL3-targeted antibody-drug conjugate eradicates high-grade pulmonary neuroendocrine tumor-initiating cells in vivo. *Sci Transl Med*. 2015;7(302):302ra136.

51. Rudin CM, Pietanza MC, Bauer TM, et al. Rovalpituzumab tesirine, a DLL3-targeted antibody-drug conjugate, in recurrent small-cell lung cancer: a first-in-human, first-in-class, open-label, phase 1 study. *Lancet Oncol*. 2017;18(1):42-51.

19

SUPPORTIVE AND PALLIATIVE CARE IN LUNG CANCER

Shruti Bhandari, MD • Jonathan S. Alexander, MD

A 50-year-old Hispanic male is treated for metastatic adenocarcinoma of the lung. He complains about cough, shortness of air, and severe back pain. He does not tolerate narcotics well and appears very depressed.

Learning Objectives:
1. What are the different types of palliative care available to cancer patients?
2. How are common symptoms in lung cancer patients evaluated and managed?
3. How is pain in cancer patients managed?

Supportive care in cancer is the prevention and management of the symptoms and side effects of cancer and its treatment across the cancer continuum from diagnosis to the end of life. There is mounting evidence in oncology that early and effective supportive care is linked to better quality of life and survival.[1,2]

The delivery of palliative care can be categorized as primary, secondary, and tertiary.

- Primary palliative care is the provision of basic symptom management and psycho-social care by -ology teams and primary care clinicians.
- Secondary palliative care refers to consultation services provided by interdisciplinary specialist palliative care teams.
- Tertiary palliative care denotes the situation when a palliative care team becomes the primary coordinating team.

Patients with advanced cancer have multiple symptoms and require systematic assessment. Patient descriptions of physical symptoms and their severity are the primary data

Edmonton Symptom Assessment System: (revised version) (ESAS-R)	

Please circle the number that best describes how you feel NOW:

No pain	0 1 2 3 4 5 6 7 8 9 10	Worst possible pain
No tiredness (Tiredness = lack of energy)	0 1 2 3 4 5 6 7 8 9 10	Worst possible tiredness
No drowsiness (Drowsiness = feeling sleepy)	0 1 2 3 4 5 6 7 8 9 10	Worst possible drowsiness
No nausea	0 1 2 3 4 5 6 7 8 9 10	Worst possible nausea
No lack of appetite	0 1 2 3 4 5 6 7 8 9 10	Worst possible lack of appetite
No shortness of breath	0 1 2 3 4 5 6 7 8 9 10	Worst possible shortness of breath
No depression (depression = feeling sad)	0 1 2 3 4 5 6 7 8 9 10	Worst possible depression
No anxiety (anxiety = feeling nervous)	0 1 2 3 4 5 6 7 8 9 10	Worst possible anxiety
Best Well-being (Welllbeing = how you feel overall)	0 1 2 3 4 5 6 7 8 9 10	Worst possible well-being
No _____ other problem (for example constipation)	0 1 2 3 4 5 6 7 8 9 10	Worst possible _____

Patient's Name _____

Date _____ Time _____

Completed by (check one):
☐ Patient
☐ Family caregiver
☐ Health care professional caregiver
☐ Caregiver-assisted

ESAS-r   BODY DIAGRAM ON REVERSE SIDE

Figure 19-1. Edmonton Symptom Assessment System: revised. (Reproduced with permission from Watanabe SM, Nekolaichuk C, Beaumont C, et al. A multicenter study comparing two numerical versions of the Edmonton Symptom Assessment System in palliative care patients. *J Pain Symptom Manage.* 2011;41:456. © 2011 U.S. Cancer Pain Relief Committee. Published by Elsevier Inc. All rights reserved.)

for symptom assessment. Formal multiple-symptom assessment tools provide a good overview of symptoms in individual patients. A number of validated multiple-symptom assessment tools are in wide usage in palliative care settings, including

- The revised Edmonton Symptom Assessment Scale[3] (**Figure 19-1**)
- Memorial Symptom Assessment Scale–Short (MSAS) Form

- M. D. Anderson Brief Symptom Inventory
- Rotterdam Symptom Checklist
- Symptom Distress Scale

Multiple-symptom assessment tools are highly effective in recognizing unreported symptoms when combined with further patient interviewing to delineate the details of positive responses. When a specific tool has been chosen, it should be used consistently to ensure reliability in the clinical setting.

This chapter includes a discussion about assessing and treating highly prevalent symptoms in a lung cancer patient.

CACHEXIA AND ANOREXIA

Cancer-related anorexia/cachexia syndrome (CACS) is a debilitating wasting syndrome that affects many patients who are undergoing treatment for a malignancy.

Cachexia is a complex metabolic syndrome associated with underlying illness and characterized by loss of muscle with or without loss of fat mass. The prominent clinical feature of cachexia is weight loss in adults (corrected for fluid retention) or growth failure in children (excluding endocrine disorders). Anorexia, inflammation, insulin resistance, and increased muscle protein breakdown are frequently associated with cachexia. Unlike *wasting*, cachexia is not reversible solely by caloric supplementation.

Its etiology is multifactorial:

1. Physiological burden of the malignancy, which serves to increase basal metabolic energy expenditure
2. Hormonal disruptions
3. Body composition changes
4. Poor intake secondary to anorexia

The effects of CACS are far reaching, with patients reporting increased fatigue, weakness, and poorer qualities of life. Patients also exhibit less favorable responses to chemotherapy agents and suffer shorter survival times. The radical change in physical appearance of the patient and the inability to continue to enjoy family mealtimes are sources of significant psychosocial distress.

Early identification of cachexia is important, as prompt intervention can affect clinical outcomes as well as quality of life. Therefore, it is recommended that all cancer patients should ideally undergo nutritional screening at the time of cancer diagnosis to identify patients with and those at risk for malnutrition or cachexia.

More recently, an international group of researchers developed a definition and classification system for cachexia in cancer[4]: The following are the criteria for cancer cachexia:

- weight loss greater than 5%, or
- weight loss greater than 2% in individuals already showing depletion according to current body weight and height body mass index (BMI) 20 kg/m^2 or less, or
- skeletal muscle mass (sarcopenia) and weight loss greater than 2%.

These experts considered three stages: precachexia, cachexia, and refractory cachexia.

Careful history must be obtained with a focus on nutritional issues, including risk factors that compromise the ability to obtain or take in nutrition, anorexia or reduced food intake, functional and psychosocial impairment. Also evaluate for major contributors to anorexia, such as nausea and vomiting, constipation, taste alterations, xerostomia, mucositis, pain, dyspnea, and depression.

The following interventions are recommended:

Nutritional Counseling: Strategies should be employed that help to increase nutritional intake by focusing on multiple small, caloric-dense, meals throughout the day.

- Alleviate anxiety and improve adherence by helping the patient to identify foods that he or she finds pleasurable and try to incorporate these foods into all mealtimes. Although there are no extensive data on the efficacy of nutritional counseling, most cancer patients will agree that they find it helpful; thus, it is often a good place to begin.

Pharmacological Interventions: Palliating the anorexia aspect of CACS with appetite stimulation has long been considered an important area of focus, with corticosteroids and progesterone analogues successfully used in this capacity for many years.

Corticosteroids: Dexamethasone, prednisolone, and methylprednisolone have all been shown to be effective.

- Long-term side effects: Adrenal suppression, myopathy, decreased bone mineral density, peptic ulcer disease, as well as many others, are common side effects and should be considered on a per patient basis.
- Suggested dosing regimens: Dexamethasone up to 4 mg/day

Progesterone analogues: Megestrol acetate and medroxyprogesterone acetate are the most commonly used.

- Long-term side effects: Progesterone analogues have been shown to increase the risk of prothrombotic events. Additionally, due to mild glucocorticoid-like effects, stress dose steroids may be required in trauma, surgical, or septic patients.
- Suggested dosing regimens: Megestrol acetate 160-800 mg/day (liquid formulation may be tolerated better by patients).
- Note: Considered to be superior to glucocorticoids due to a quick onset of action, a longer lasting effect on appetite stimulation, and a less severe side-effect profile.

Mirtazapine: This tetracyclic antidepressant induces weight gain and increases food intake. The dose is 15-30 mg by mouth daily at bedtime.

Others: Myriad other agents, including androgens, cannabinoids, ghrelin analogues, tumor necrosis factor alpha inhibitors, as well as many others, have been hypothesized to help patients with CACS. To date, however, further information is currently required from randomized trials—many of which are still ongoing—before any recommendations can be made.

FATIGUE

Cancer-related fatigue (CRF) is one of the most common symptoms experienced by patients with malignancies. Eight of 10 cancer patients undergoing cytotoxic chemotherapy, biotherapy, and/or radiation therapy endorse fatigue. Despite its high prevalence, CRF is often underdiagnosed and undertreated.

Cancer-related fatigue is a distressing, persistent, subjective sense of physical, emotional, and/or cognitive tiredness or exhaustion related to cancer and/or cancer treatment that is not proportional to recent activity and interferes with usual functioning.

Its etiology is multifactorial:

1. Increased levels of systemic inflammation
2. Skeletal muscle wasting
3. Metabolic dysregulation
4. Psychological distress
5. Medication side effects
6. Circadian rhythm desynchronization

Unlike everyday fatigue, which is temporary and able to be relieved by rest, CRF is chronic and unrelenting. For these reasons, it is consistently reported to be one of the most distressing symptoms to affect cancer patients. CRF may have ongoing effects for years after remission is achieved or treatment is discontinued. The implications of this are far reaching, with patients suffering from a reduced quality of life at home as well as, at times, an inability to maintain a job.

When should you screen for fatigue?[5]

- Initial visit
- Conclusion of primary therapy
- Yearly during follow-up survivor care appointments
- During each visit in patients with advance disease

The visual analog scale (VAS) can be employed by asking a patient to rate his or her fatigue severity on a scale of 0-10. Mild, moderate, and severe fatigue are represented by scores of 1-3, 4-6, and 7-10, respectively. A score of 4 or above requires a focused evaluation. The Brief Fatigue Inventory (BFI) is an alternate option for quick screening (https://www.mdanderson.org/research/departments-labs-institutes/departments-divisions/symptom-research/symptom-assessment-tools/brief-fatigue-inventory.html).

A common differential for fatigue is

- Disease status: consider recurrence or progression
- Assess for anemia, pain, sleep disturbance, emotional distress: depression or anxiety, medication side effect (drug interaction, over-the-counter [OTC] medications), substance abuse
- Nutritional deficiencies: vitamin status, weight/calorie intake change, electrolyte imbalance
- Endocrine dysfunction: hypothyroidism, hypogonadism, adrenal insufficiency
- Cardiac dysfunction

The following interventions are recommended[5]:

Lifestyle modifications and non-pharmacological interventions[6]:

- Patient education and reassurance: It is important to inform patients that increased levels of fatigue do not necessarily equate to disease progression.

- Establishment of adequate support systems: Delegating daily tasks to friends and family members can allow for patients to conserve what little disposable energy they may have.
- Counseling on good sleep hygiene: Although CRF cannot, by definition, be relieved by rest, insomnia can worsen symptoms.
- Healthy distractions: During waking hours, activities that give meaning and fulfillment to the patient should be prioritized. This has been shown to help decrease fatigue.
- Pain: Reduction in daily pain levels can improve energy levels. Caution must be taken, however, as opioids can obviously worsen fatigue/drowsiness.
- Physical activity: Although it may sound counterintuitive, it is recommended that 150 minutes of moderate aerobic exercise, along with 2-3 strength-training sessions, be performed weekly.[7]
- Mind-body wellness: Randomized control trials have shown yoga, mindfulness, and acupuncture to have utility in relieving fatigue in cancer survivors.
- Psychological counseling/support groups: These help with depression/anxiety, substance abuse issues, and overall coping mechanisms. Cognitive behavioral therapy has also been shown to be of benefit.
- Massage therapy.
- Nutrition consult.
- Consider referral to rehabilitation: physical therapy, occupational therapy, and physical medicine.

Pharmacologic interventions[6]:

- Medication elimination: Before considering what pharmacological agents can be added to help reduce fatigue, drugs already being taken should be evaluated for interactions/side effects. The following are of notable mention: opioids, antidepressants, anxiolytics, beta-blockers.
- Anemia: This is known to be a major contributing factor to CRF. Treatment can vary from simple folic acid and/or vitamin b_{12} supplementation to routinely administered transfusions or erythropoiesis-stimulating agents.
- Antidepressants: These can be of benefit in patients with fatigue and depression.
- Glucocorticoids: These are useful for patients with known adrenal dysfunction; they can also be tried in patients with advanced disease and high symptom burden: dexamethasone 4 mg orally twice a day.
- Levothyroxine: This is given in patients with known thyroid dysfunction.
- Stimulants: For patients who have moderate-to-severe fatigue that persists despite lifestyle modification and medical optimization, a therapeutic trial of a psychostimulant can be considered after other causes have been ruled out. Usually, these are administered during active treatment.[6,8]
  - Drugs and specific dosing regimens:
    - Methylphenidate: 5 mg twice daily (every morning and noon), increase by 10 mg daily every 3 days until a maximum daily dose of 40 mg is reached.
    - Modafinil: 100 mg once daily for 3 days followed by 200 mg once daily.

DYSPNEA

Dyspnea is a subjective experience of breathing discomfort or breathlessness. It is reported in more than 90% of advanced lung cancer patients.[9] Dyspnea is a major detriment to quality of life and has been identified as the most important variable influencing the will to live among terminally ill cancer patients.[10]

A general symptom assessment tool, such as the revised Edmonton Symptom Assessment Scale can be a first step in recognizing the presence of dyspnea. After screening, a careful history is crucial to understand the quality, intensity, and functional impact of dyspnea on a patient. The trajectory and temporal relationship to its evolution can provide important insight to a potential reversible cause.

Physical examination with emphasis on factors that are potentially reversible is important. There is no gold standard clinical tool or scale for dyspnea. Available scales include the Borg scale, modified Medical Research Council Dyspnea Scale, the Dyspnea Exertion Scale, the Cancer Dyspnea Scale, and more.

Investigations help determine the cause of dyspnea and guide the choice of treatment. These include pulse oximetry, arterial blood gases, chest radiographs, pulmonary function tests, echocardiograms, and others.

In patients where an underlying cause of dyspnea is identified,[11] management is based on the cause:

- Pneumonia: antibiotics
- Pneumonitis (immunotherapy or radiation induced): glucocorticoids
- Pleural effusion
  - Thoracentesis
  - If it reaccumulates, indwelling pleural catheter with intermittent drainage
  - Pleurodesis
- Venous thromboembolism
  - Anticoagulation
  - In select cases with massive pulmonary embolism and right heart strain, can consider thrombolysis
- Bronchoconstriction (chronic obstructive pulmonary disease [COPD], asthma): bronchodilators, glucocorticoids
- Airway obstruction by tumor or lymphadenopathy: airway stent, radiation, glucocorticoids
- Excess secretions: anticholinergics (scopolamine patch, glycopyrrolate)
- Heart failure: diuretics, angiotensin-converting enzyme (ACE) inhibitors; cardiology referral
- Superior vena cava syndrome: radiation, stent placement
- Anemia: red blood cell transfusion
- Massive ascites: periodic paracentesis; avoid drains unless in hospice as they have a tendency to become infected and to be clogged
- Pain: opioids

- Anxiety: anxiolytic medication
- Immunotherapy-induced pneumonitis: glucocorticoids (1-2 mg/kg based on grade)

Non-pharmacologic management includes the use of a fan with cool air blowing on the face, relaxation techniques, and psychosocial support.

Pulmonary rehabilitation includes exercise training, psychosocial support, nutrition therapy, and self-management strategies, such as diaphragmatic and pursed lip breathing.

Oxygen[12]: Oxygen is a standard therapy for symptomatic management of patients with hypoxemia on room air. For patients who are not hypoxemic, supplemental oxygen provides no relief of dyspnea when compared to room air.[13]

- Helium/oxygen (Heliox): Studies in non-hypoxemic, exercising patients with lung cancer showed Heliox was superior to room air for exercise tolerance and dyspnea. But due to the cost, uneven availability, and lack of experience, use of Heliox in dyspnea management remains unclear.

Pharmacologic treatment for dyspnea includes

- Opioids[12]: These are a well-established treatment strategy in advanced disease and recommended by National Comprehensive Cancer Network (NCCN) guideline. Morphine is the most widely studied drug, and the systemic route is preferred. Nebulized opioids have been studied, but there are insufficient data to recommend.

COUGH

For patients with advanced lung cancer, cough is reported in up to 90% of the patients.[9] Causes of cough in advanced cancer include intrinsic or extrinsic airway involvement, lymphangitic carcinomatosis, atelectasis, pleural effusion, treatment- (radiation or chemotherapy) induced pneumonitis, aspiration, or pneumonia.

Thorough history and physical examination: Factors are type of cough (productive/non-productive), onset, associated factors, rigor, nocturnal or daytime, severity of cough, and effects on quality of life.

Consider imaging based on differential diagnosis: A chest x-ray or computed tomographic (CT) scan of the chest can look for pneumonia, pleural effusion, worsening lung cancer, or metastasis.

Treat potentially reversible causes such as

- Antimicrobials for infection
- Proton pump inhibitors for cough related to gastroesophageal reflux disease
- Smoking cessation
- Optimizing medications for COPD
- Thoracentesis for pleural effusion

Disease-directed therapy:

- Patients with cough related to extrinsic or intrinsic airway involvement may benefit from palliative radiation or airway stent or dilation. These cases need to be discussed in a multidisciplinary conference followed by appropriate referral to radiation oncology and interventional pulmonology.

Symptom-directed treatment:

- May be used alongside the disease directed therapy
- Also appropriate when a specific cause of cough cannot be identified or when disease-directed therapy is not feasible

SYMPTOM-DIRECTED TREATMENT

For mild severity of cough, consider non-pharmacologic therapies first (cough suppression exercises, breathing exercises). For moderate-to-severe cough (defined as that which impairs sleep), the mainstay of therapy is cough suppression with antitussives. Antitussives suppress the cough reflex.

- *Peripherally acting antitussives:* Benzonatate anesthetizes stretch receptors in the lung and pleura. The recommended dose is 100-200 mg 3 times a day. Side effects are sedation, headache, bronchospasm, and nausea.
- *Centrally acting antitussives:*
  - Non-opioid
    - Gabapentin: initiated at a low dose (300 mg once a day) with gradual increases until cough relief, dose-limiting adverse effects, or a dose of 1,800 mg a day in 2 divided doses is achieved.
    - Pregabalin: Initiated at a low dose and gradually increased over a week to 300 mg/day to minimize sedation and dizziness.
  - Opioid is first-line symptomatic treatment for severe, distressing cough.
    - Codeine: Usual adult dose is 10-20 mg every 4-6 hours. It is available alone or as a combination with guaifenesin.
    - Dextromethorphan: Usual adult dose is 10-20 mg every 4-6 hours. It is available alone or as a combination with guaifenesin.
    - Hydrocodone: Usual dose is 5-10 mg every 4 hours.
    - All opioid analgesics have antitussive activity, and there is no strong evidence that any one opioid has superior efficacy for cough. For patients already taking opioids for pain, it is unclear whether adding a second opioid such as codeine for cough is effective.
- *Expectorants* thin bronchial secretions and ease expectoration. Examples include guaifenesin (200-400 mg every 4 hours) and nebulized acetylcysteine or hypertonic saline.
- *Bronchodilators* may help if there is a bronchoconstrictive component to the cough.
- Corticosteroids (dexamethasone 4-12 mg oral daily) may diminish inflammation and mucus production.

NAUSEA AND VOMITING

Chemotherapy-therapy–induced nausea and vomiting (CINV) can significantly affect a patient's quality of life, leading to poor compliance with further treatment. In addition, nausea and vomiting can result in dehydration, metabolic imbalances, nutrient depletion, anorexia, decline of the patient's performance status, and withdrawal from potentially useful or curative anticancer treatment.

The incidence and severity of nausea and/or vomiting is patients with cancer is affected by the[14]

1. specific chemotherapy agents used;
2. dosage of the agents;
3. schedule and route of administration of the agents;
4. cancer diagnosis and location of metastasis;
5. concomitant administration of chemotherapy and radiation;
6. target of the radiotherapy (eg, whole body, upper abdomen); and
7. individual patient variability (eg, age, sex, prior chemotherapy, history of alcohol use).

Four types of CINV have been defined:

1. Acute-onset CINV: Begins within a few minutes to hours of chemotherapy administration and usually peaks in 4-6 hours. Commonly resolves within the first 24 hours.
2. Delayed-onset CINV: Develops more than 24 hours after chemotherapy administration.
3. Anticipatory CINV: Occurs prior to treatment as a conditioned response in patients who have developed significant nausea and vomiting during previous cycles of chemotherapy.
4. Breakthrough CINV: Refers to nausea and/or vomiting that occurs despite prophylactic treatment and/or requires rescue with antiemetic agents.

The principles of CINV control in cancer patients include prevention based on risk[14]: The main goal is to prevent nausea and vomiting, and this should be achievable in the majority of patients receiving chemotherapy, even with highly emetic agents.

Estimating the risk of CINV: The most important factor in estimation of the risk of CINV is the intrinsic emetogenic potential of the chemotherapy agents. Chemotherapy agents were divided into four categories based on the risk of emesis in the absence of antiemetic prophylaxis (**Table 19-1**):

- Highly emetic: More than 90% risk of emesis
- Moderately emetic: More than 30%-90% risk of emesis
- Low emetogenicity: 10%-30% risk of emesis
- Minimally emetic: Less than 10% risk of emesis

Emetic risk lasts for at least 3 days for high and 2 days for moderate risk after the last dose of chemotherapy. Patients need to be protected throughout the full period of risk. Choose prophylactic and breakthrough antiemetics. The choice of antiemetic(s) used should be based on the emetic risk of the therapy, prior experience with antiemetics, and patient factors.

The following antiemetics are commonly used[14]:

- *5-HT3 receptor antagonists*: All appear equally effective at preventing CINV. Oral formulations of these drugs are as effective as an intravenous formulation. They all have warning about QTc prolongation and potentially fatal cardiac arrhythmias, which occurs in a dose-dependent manner.

TABLE 19-1	Emetogenic Potential of Commonly Used Chemotherapy Agents in Lung Cancer	
LEVEL	AGENT (INTRAVENOUS)	AGENT (ORAL)
High risk (>90% frequency of emesis)	Cisplatin Carboplatin (AUC ≥ 4)	
Moderate risk (>30%-90% frequency of emesis)	Carboplatin (AUC < 4) Irinotecan	Ceritinib Crizotinib
Low emetic risk (10%-30% frequency of emesis)	Docetaxel Etoposide Gemcitabine Paclitaxel Paclitaxel-albumin Pemetrexed Topotecan	Afatinib Axitinib Brigatinib Etoposide Erlotinib Gefitinib Osemeritinib
Minimal emetic risk (<10% frequency of emesis)	Bevacizumab Durvalumab Ipilimumab Nivolumab Pembrolizumab Vinorelbine	

- Ondansetron: Available in intravenous, oral, oral disintegrating tablet; usual is dose 8 mg every 8 hours as needed
- Palonosetron: Available in intravenous and oral formulation
- Dolasetron: Oral only
- Granisetron: Available in intravenous, oral, transdermal patch

- *Neurokinin-1 (NK-1) receptor antagonists*
  - Aprepitant is given for 3 days, while the fosaprepitant usual dose is 150 mg IV once before chemotherapy. Both aprepitant and fosaprepitant are moderate inhibitors of the cytochrome P450 3A4 enzyme; therefore, when given in combination with dexamethasone the dose of dexathesone is decreased.
  - Rolapitant does not inhibit cytochrome P450 3A4; combination includes Akynzeo capsule (netupitant 300 mg plus polanosetron 0.5 mg) and Akynzeo for injection (fosnetupitant 235 mg plus polanosetron 0.25 mg).
- *Glucocorticoids: Dexamethasone:* The dose with NK-1 antagonist at 8-12 mg IV/PO on the day of chemotherapy followed by 8 mg oral daily (usually 4 mg twice a day) on days 2, 3, 4. The dose without NK-1 inhibitors is 8-20 mg IV/PO on the day of chemotherapy followed by 8 mg oral twice a day on days 2, 3, 4 for highly emetogenic chemotherapy and 4 mg oral twice a day on days 2 and 3 for moderate emetogenic chemotherapy.
- *Other agents include the following:* Olanzapine 5-10 mg oral daily for days 1-4 of highly emetogenic chemotherapy; prochlorperazine 5-10 mg IV/PO every 6 hours as needed; and metoclopromide 5-10 mg IV or 5 mg oral every 6 hours as needed.

Prophylaxis for CINV depends on emetogenic risk[14]:

- *Highly emetogenic chemotherapy*
  - Day 1: We recommend antiemetic therapy with a combination of an NK-1 receptor antagonist, a 5-HT3 receptor antagonist, dexamethasone, and olanzapine.
  - Days 2 to 4: We recommend continuing dexamethasone (days 2-4) plus minus olanzapine (days 2-4).
  - If aprepitant is used on day 1, continue aprepitant on days 2 and 3. All other NK-1 receptor antagonists are administered on day 1 only.
  - No further therapy required if palonsetron, granisetron extended-release injection, or granisetron transdermal patch given on day 1.
- *Moderately emetogenic chemotherapy*
  - Day 1: We recommend the combination of a 5-HT3 receptor antagonist plus dexamethasone on day 1 followed by single-agent treatment with dexamethasone on days 2 and 3.
    OR
  - Day 1: We recommend the combination of an NK-1 receptor antagonist, a 5-HT3 receptor antagonist, and dexamethasone on day 1. This may be followed by dexamethasone on days 2 and 3.
- *Low-emetogenic chemotherapy*
  - We recommend single-agent dexamethasone or prochlorperazine or a 5-HT3 receptor antagonist. We usually do not require prophylaxis against delayed emesis.
- *Anticipatory emesis*
  - Benzodiazepines
- *Rescue therapy*: Review history and prophylactic emetic regimen to ensure that there are no other factors responsible for continued emesis and that adequate antiemetic therapy actually was administered for the given chemotherapy regimen.
  - Olanzapine 5 or 10 mg daily for 3 days can be considered as rescue therapy for patients with breakthrough nausea and vomiting who did not receive olanzapine initially. For patients already receiving olanzapine, we suggest trying an agent from a different class than was used for initial prophylaxis, like prochlorperazine.
  - Consider using an H_2 blocker or proton pump inhibitor to prevent dyspepsia, which can mimic nausea.
  - Lifestyle measures may help to alleviate nausea/vomiting, such as eating small, frequent meals, choosing healthful foods, controlling the amount of food consumed, and eating food at room temperature.

DIARRHEA

Diarrhea is defined as 3 or more loose or watery stools in a 24-hour period. In patients with cancer, diarrhea can be caused by number of factors[15]:

- Anticancer treatment–related side effects: including chemotherapy, radiation to abdomen or pelvis, immunotherapy, tyrosine kinase inhibitors
- Surgery related (short bowel syndrome, etc.)

- Infection
- Antibiotic use
- Dietary changes
- Fecal impaction

    A careful and detailed history is a crucial part in the assessment[16]:

- *Ask specific questions* about dizziness, orthostatic hypotension, lethargy, nausea/vomiting, fever. Perform a detailed physical examination to evaluate for dehydration.
- *Assess severity*[17]:
    ○ Grade 1: Increase of less than 4 stools/day over baseline; mild increase in ostomy output
    ○ Grade 2: Increase of 4–6 stools/day over baseline; moderate increase in ostomy output
    ○ Grade 3: Increase of more than 7 stools/day over baseline; incontinence; hospitalization indicated; severe increase in ostomy output; limiting self-care; interferes with activities of daily living (ADLs)
    ○ Grade 4: Life-threatening consequences; urgent intervention indicated
- *Classify based on symptoms:* **Uncomplicated symptoms** include grade 1 or 2 diarrhea with no other signs or symptoms. **Complicated symptoms** include grade 3 or 4 diarrhea or grade 1 or 2 diarrhea with any one of the following risk factors:
    ○ Moderate-to-severe cramping
    ○ Grade 2 or higher nausea/vomiting
    ○ Decreased performance status
    ○ Fever
    ○ Sepsis
    ○ Neutropenia
    ○ Dehydration
- *Assess if patient needs inpatient admission*: Usually for grade 3 and above; also, if patient has concomitant nausea/vomiting and is unable to tolerate oral intake.
- *Rule out other infectious etiology*: Check for *Clostridium difficile* infection and stool cultures, ova/parasite. Laboratory testing should include complete blood count, comprehensive metabolic panel with magnesium level; if febrile consider blood cultures also.
- *Radiographic imaging*: Not typically needed in most patients with diarrhea. Indicated in patients who have fever, peritoneal signs, or bloody diarrhea; use abdominal imaging (most typically CT) to identify potential complications, such as bowel perforation, abscess, or neutropenic enterocolitis or to rule out causes of diarrhea not associated with chemotherapy.
- *Endoscopy*: Should be considered for refractory cases and for patients who develop chronic diarrhea.

    Management is based on grade and etiology of diarrhea[16]:

- *For grade 1 or 2 with no other signs or symptoms (uncomplicated symptoms)*: Management is conservative.

- Provide oral hydration and electrolyte replacement
- Antidiarrheal medications: Loperamide (see next item for dose).
- Initial dose 4 mg (maximum: 16 mg/day)
- If symptoms persist after 12-24 hours (but are not worse or associated with worrisome signs and/or symptoms), the loperamide dose can be increased to 2 mg every 2 hours. If mild-to-moderate diarrhea persists 12-24 hours later despite the higher dose of loperamide, patients should be evaluated in the office.

- *For complicated diarrhea*:
  - This warrants inpatient management with intravenous fluids, serial assessment of electrolytes, and workup.
  - Cultures of stool and diagnostic testing for toxin-producing strains of *C. difficile* should be performed.

Non-pharmacologic measures:

- *Diet modification*[16]:
  - Patient should consume easy-to-digest food until diarrhea resolves.
  - Patient is advised to follow a BRAT diet (ie, bananas, rice, applesauce, and toast).
  - Fresh fruits and vegetables should be avoided, except for bananas.
  - High-osmolar dietary supplements should be avoided.
  - Alcohol and caffeine should be avoided.
  - The patient should follow a lactose-free diet.

Stop other medications that could contribute to diarrhea: stool softeners, laxatives, milk thistle, saw palmetto, high dose of vitamin C, green tea.

- *Withholding chemotherapy/immunotherapy*
  - Anti-epidermal growth factor receptor (EGFR) tyrosine kinase inhibitors (TKIs; afatinib, erlotinib, gefitinib)
    - For grade 2 diarrhea, continue the drug.
    - If the patient does not respond to loperamide by 48 hours, temporarily discontinue the drug until diarrhea returns to grade 1, after which the drug can be resumed with a dose reduction.
    - For grade 3 or 4 diarrhea, withhold the TKI until diarrhea reaches grade 1, then resume, usually with a dose reduction.
    - If the diarrhea does not resolve to grade 1 within 14 days, the drug should be permanently discontinued.
  - For the anaplastic lymphoma kinase (ALK) inhibitor ceritinib, withhold the drug for severe or intolerable diarrhea, despite optimal antidiarrheal therapy, and resume once resolved with a dose reduction.
  - Immunotherapy-related diarrhea: Treatment is dependent on grade and usually consists of glucocorticoids (1-2 mg/kg dose).

Pharmacologic measures:

- *Loperamide*
  - Preferred initially.
  - Usual dose: 4 mg initial dose followed by 2 mg every 4 hours as needed

- For mild-to-moderate uncomplicated diarrhea that persists after 24 hours of loperamide, we suggest high-dose loperamide (4 mg initially, followed by 2 mg every 2 hours).
- Loperamide is not absorbed but is excreted in stool.

- *Diphenoxylate atropine*
  - Usual dose: 5 mg 4 times daily until control achieved (maximum diphenoxylate is 20 mg/day).
  - No data available on use of diphenoxylate atropine in loperamide-refractory diarrhea (ie, persistent diarrhea despite 24-48 hours of loperamide use).
- *Octreotide*
  - Recommend initiating for any patient with chemotherapy-related diarrhea refractory to loperamide.
  - Initial dose: 100-150 µg subcutaneously 3 times a day. Can be escalated to 500 µg subcutaneously 3 times a day if lower dose is not effective.

Refer to gastroenterology for diarrhea that has not resolved after loperamide and higher dose of octreotide.

> **CLINICAL PEARL:** Always rule out infectious etiology of diarrhea before considering chemotherapy- or immunotherapy-related diarrhea and before starting loperamide.

CANCER PAIN

Pain due to cancer is experienced by most patients with advanced disease and affects most aspects of a person's life, including physical functioning, the performance of activities of daily living, psychological and emotional status, and social interactions. Given the high prevalence of pain related to cancer and its potential for profound adverse consequences,[9] all patients with active malignancy should be routinely screened for pain.

Assess pain in patients at each visit or interaction. A patient's self-report of pain is the standard of care. The goal of comprehensive pain assessment is to find the cause of the pain and identify optimal therapies. Individualized pain treatment is based on the etiology and characteristics of pain, the patient's clinical condition, and patient-centered goals of care.

Comprehensive pain assessment should include the following[18]:

1. **Pain**:
   a. For each site of pain, determine intensity level using a 0-10 numeric rating scale (no pain = 0, mild pain = 1-3, moderate pain = 4-6, severe pain = 7-10).
   b. Assess at rest and with activity; location; onset (acute, chronic, acute exacerbation of chronic pain); pathophysiology (somatic, visceral, neuropathic); temporal factors (continuous, intermittent, breakthrough, incidental); etiology (eg, tumor, non–tumor-related, fracture).
   c. Evaluation of medical history includes oncologic or other significant medical illnesses, medication history, relevant imaging and laboratory studies.
   d. Physical examination.
   e. Current use of analgesics and their efficacy and tolerability.

f. Assess for presence of sedation (inpatient setting, consider Richmond Agitation Sedation Scale [RASS]) and other common opioid side effects (nausea/vomiting, constipation).

2. **Function**:
    a. Evaluate patient's ability to ambulate, perform ADL, range of motion (ROM), deep breathing, and coughing.
    b. Assess restrictions related to pain.
    c. Report patient's evaluation of functional ability.

3. **Psychosocial issues**:
    a. Evaluate patient's distress, family support, psychiatric history, patient/family knowledge and beliefs surrounding pain and its management, and risk factors for undertreatment of pain, which include the following: underreporting; prior treatment of pain and response to other pain medications; concerns about addiction to pain medications or side effects; extremes of age; gender; cultural barriers; communication barriers; and prior history of drug abuse.
    b. Report patient's assessment of psychological distress.

4. **Personalized pain goal (PPG)**:
    a. Determine the verbal or written goal stated by the patient describing the desired level/intensity of pain that will allow the patient to achieve comfort in physical, functional, and psychosocial domains.

Pain intensity guides analgesic choices. Opioid tolerance is described as patients who are chronically receiving opioid analgesics, that is, receiving at least 60 mg of morphine daily or an equianalgesic dose of another opioid for a week or longer.

For mild pain (score 1-3)[18]:

- *For patients not previously on opioids:*
  ○ Choose non-opioids (**Table 19-2**): Acetaminophen/NSAIDs (non-steroidal anti-inflammatory drugs) or, if contraindicated, use weak opioids (**Table 19-3**). This may be combined with an adjuvant analgesic that provides additional analgesia, treats a side effect, or manages a coexisting symptom.

- *For patients currently taking opioids:*
  ○ If no side effects, continue current analgesic regimen. For breakthrough pain, prescribe short-acting opioids at 10%-20% of 24-hour opioid dose every 4 hours as needed. If the patient is taking more than 4 breakthrough doses, you may consider adding or increasing scheduled opioids by 20%-30%.

Reassess pain and opioid side effects at the subsequent visit.

For moderate-to-severe pain (score > 4)[18] or PPG not met:

- *For patients not previously on opioids:*
  ○ Prescribe short-acting opioids; choose from weak or strong opioids (see Table 19-3). If pain is expected to be continuous, consider scheduling opioids around the clock **or** long-acting opioids.

- *For patients currently taking opioids:*
  ○ Scheduled opioid: Increase dose by 30%-50% of prior scheduled dose or equal to calculated prior 24-hour opioid dose, whichever is higher. Administer as an around-the-clock regimen of short-acting opioids **or** long-acting opioids.

TABLE 19-2	Non-opioid Pain Medications	
DRUG	**RECOMMENDED STARTING DOSE**	**COMMENTS**
Acetaminophen	500-1,000 mg orally every 6 hours as needed	Available orally and per rectum; at higher doses, can cause hepatotoxicity; does not have anti-inflammatory effect.
Ibuprofen	200-800 mg orally every 6 hours as needed	Inhibits platelet aggregation; can cause gastrointestinal side effects or renal failure; use with caution in patients at high risk
Naproxen	500 mg orally initially, then 250 mg every 4 hours as needed	Inhibits platelet aggregation; can cause gastrointestinal side effects or renal failure
Celecoxib	200-400 mg orally every 12 or 24 hours as needed	Does not affect platelet aggregation; can cause renal insufficiency
Ketorolac	15-30 mg IV or orally every 6 hours as needed	Limit treatment to 5 days; use is contraindicated in patients with advanced renal impairment or patients at risk for renal failure due to volume depletion

TABLE 19-3	Opioid Prescribing Chart				
PAIN INTENSITY	**MEDICATION**	**USUAL STARTING DOSE FOR ADULTS, OPIOID NAÏVE PATIENTS (1/2 DOSE FOR ELDERLY, OR SEVERE RENAL OR LIVER DISEASE)**		**CHRONIC OPIOID ADMINISTRATION EQUIANALGESIC DOSE**	
		Parenteral	Oral	Intravenous Onset 15-30 min	Oral Onset 30-60 min
Mild	Hydrocodone	—	5-10 mg every 6 h		30-45 mg
Moderate	Morphine	2-4 mg every 4 h	5-15 every 4 h	10 mg	30 mg
	Oxycodone	—	IR 5-10 mg q4h ER 10 mg q12h	—	20 mg
Severe	Hydromorphone	0.5 mg every 4 h	IR 2 mg every 4 h ER 8 mg every 24 h	1.5 mg	7.5 mg
	Fentanyl	Not recommended in opioid-naïve patients		—	—

IR: immediate release; ER: extended release.

- Calculate short-acting opioids as 10%-20% of new opioid regimen and administer every 2 hours as needed.
- Manage other side effects if present.
- Consider specialty consultation.

Reassess pain, opioid regimen/side effects, and PPG within 72 hours.

OPIOID DRUGS

Opioids are widely used for treatment of pain in cancer patients because of their effectiveness for all types of pain and multiple routes of administration (Table 19-3).

- *Morphine:* It is considered a standard for comparison. Available in multiple formulations: immediate-release tablets, oral liquid, intravenous, and sustained-release tablets. It is primarily metabolized in the liver and its metabolites are renally excreted. Therefore, morphine should be administered cautiously in the setting of renal insufficiency.

- *Hydrocodone:* The short-acting form is only available in combination with acetaminophen.

- *Oxycodone:* Available in immediate-release and extended-release tablet.

- *Hydromorphone:* Available in oral liquid, immediate-release tablet, extended-release tablet, and solution for intravenous or subcutaneous use. The extended-release form of hydromorphone (Exalgo) is available in 8-, 12-, and 16-mg strengths and is dosed once daily. It is preferable in patients with renal insufficiency.

- *Fentanyl:* Highly lipophilic opioid, available in intravenous, transdermal, and oral transmucosal forms. It is relatively infrequently dosed: every 2-3 days for transdermal fentanyl. It should be avoided in opioid-naïve patients. It may be preferred in patients with renal insufficiency due to lack of active metabolites. Exposing the patch to heat can cause an unintentional increase in systemic fentanyl absorption, so avoid warm compress or a heating pad.

- *Patient-controlled analgesia (PCA):* It allows patients to self-administer parenteral analgesia. It can provide patients with a greater sense of personal control over their pain. Morphine, hydromorphone, and fentanyl can be used for PCA.
  - Indications:
    - For a patient who requires parenteral analgesia (eg, severe pain and/or oral/transdermal/rectal route not usable) and has incident pain or other pain patterns that are not predictable.
    - For a patient in acute severe pain when rapid dose titration and dose finding.
  - Relative contraindications:
    - Do not use with patients who do not have the cognitive ability to understand how to use a PCA device.
    - Do not if there is an anticipated need for parenteral opioids in less than 24 hours.

- *Methadone:* This is a low-cost option with a long duration of action. It should only be initiated and managed by clinicians trained and experienced in pain management.

It can prolong the QTc interval and can predispose to life-threatening cardiac arrhythmias. It is important to check an electrocardiogram (ECG) prior to therapy in most patients, and repeated monitoring is required in those who have significant heart disease and those taking other QTc-prolonging drugs.

It is important to manage the risks of opioid use.

Patients receiving opioids for chronic cancer pain may develop an opioid use disorder and can be at high risk for premature death from opioid overdose. Education about risks of opioid overdose and provision of take-home naloxone should be provided to opioid users and families.[19]

Opioids can slow reaction time and cause drowsiness, which could impair the ability to drive or work safely. For patients initiating opioid therapy or changing doses, driving or operating heavy machinery is unsafe and should be avoided until a stable dose has been reached.

Opioids affect gastrointestinal motility and manifest as constipation. The prevalence of constipation is very high in opioid-treated cancer patients. Prevention is the preferred strategy.[20] All cancer patients should be considered for prophylactic laxative therapy when opioid treatment is initiated. They should be encouraged to increase fluid intake, mobility, and dietary fiber. Senna (2 tablets at bedtime) with or without a stool softener (docusate at 10 mg orally twice a day).

ADJUVANT ANALGESICS

Opioid therapy is the first-line approach for moderate or severe pain in patients with active cancer. If opioid therapy by itself yields a good outcome (satisfactory analgesia and tolerable side effects), additional interventions for pain are not needed.

Should the patient demonstrate a poor response to the opioid, however, therapy must be changed. This common scenario may be addressed in many ways, among which is the addition of another analgesic drug, so-called adjuvant analgesic or coanalgesic.

- *Multipurpose adjuvant analgesic*[18]
  - Glucocorticoids: May be beneficial for a variety of types of pain, including neuropathic and bone pain, pain associated with capsular expansion or duct obstruction, pain caused by lymphedema, and headache caused by increased intracranial pressure.
    - Typical regimen: 1-2 mg dexamethasone orally or parenterally twice daily.
  - Topical therapies: For localized peripheral pain.
    - Transdermal lidocaine 5% patch for 12 hours per day
    - Capsaicin cream
    - Diclofenac (1%) or ibuprofen (5%, 10%) topical gel

Adjuvant Analgesic for Bone Pain

Bone pain is usually related to bone metastasis. Consider evaluation for possible radiation therapy, surgery, or kyphoplasty. When bone pain is limited to a single or limited number of sites, local field external beam radiation therapy to the painful sites can provide pain relief. Therefore, patients should be referred to radiation oncology.

Bone pain can usually be managed with an NSAID (unless there is a specific contraindication to use of these agents) and an opioid, with or without an adjuvant analgesic. Adjuvant analgesics to consider are the following:

- *Osteoclast inhibitors* (zoledronic acid via intravenous infusion; denosumab via subcutaneous injection) are recommended in conjugation with opioids. These drugs prevent skeletal-related events and improve quality of life, although their analgesic effects are only modest.
- *Glucocorticoids* may be useful in patients with opioid-refractory bone pain, especially in patients with a "pain crisis."
- Use of *bone-targeted radiopharmaceuticals*, such as radium 223, is typically reserved for the patient with multifocal bone pain that is refractory to other treatment. Once injected, the drug is taken up at the site of bone metastases and delivers radiation locally. Myelosuppression is a main concern. The majority of the data on efficacy are in patients with metastatic prostate cancer.

Adjuvant Analgesic for Neuropathic Pain

For cancer-related neuropathic pain with depressed mood, we suggest first-line therapy with an antidepressant. Preferred options include

- Duloxetine (oral: initially 30 mg once daily for 1 week, then 60 mg once daily).
- Desipramine.
- Given the positive trial of duloxetine[21] and the negative trials of gabapentin, other anticonvulsants, and tricyclic antidepressants in patients with painful chemotherapy induced peripheral neuropathy (CIPN), we prefer duloxetine in cancer- or cancer-treatment–related neuropathic pain.

For neuropathic pain that is not associated with a depressed mood, we suggest first-line therapy with gabapentin or pregabalin.

- Gabapentin: Initial dosing for immediate release gabapentin is 300-900 mg/day in 1-3 divided doses; increase dose based on response and tolerability to a target dose of 1,200-3,600 mg/day in 3 divided doses. **Note:** An adequate trial with gabapentin may require 2 months or more. It is cleared renally and requires adjustment in kidney disease.
- Pregabalin: Initial oral dose for immediate release pregabalin is 50-75 mg/day, increased to 100-150 mg/day in 2 divided doses after few days based on response and tolerability up to a usual effective dose of 300-600 mg/day in 2 divided doses in 1-2 weeks.

A trial of topical lidocaine is another option for patients who have focal, peripherally generated pain. Interventional therapies like somatic nerve blocks (paravertebral or intercostal blocks) may be valuable options for treatment of cancer pain that is refractory to systemic opioids, non-opioid analgesics, and other non-pharmacologic pain control treatments.

DEPRESSION

Depression is more common in patients with cancer then the general population, with prevalence around 15%-20%.[22]

- **Risk factors include** general medical comorbidity, pain, poor social support, advance cancer, impairment in functioning, and prior history of depression.
- **Implications include** diminished quality of life, poor adherence to treatment, increased all-cause and cancer-related mortality[23]
- **Screening**[24]: All patients with cancer should be screened for depression when the initial diagnosis of cancer is made and periodically thereafter as clinically indicated (eg, post-treatment, recurrence, or progression).[24] Screen with the self-report, 2-item Patient Health Questionnaire (PHQ-2): **Over the past 2 weeks, how often have you been bothered by any of the following problems?**

1. Little interest or pleasure in doing things
   a. Not at all
   b. Several days
   c. More than half the days
   d. Nearly every day
2. Feeling down, depressed, or hopeless
   a. Not at all
   b. Several days
   c. More than half the days
   d. Nearly every day

Patients who screen positive (a single yes response) should be interviewed to diagnose depression; the interview can be facilitated with the self-administered 9-item Patient Health Questionnaire (PHQ-9).

ASSESSMENT

Detailed history and physical examination: This includes psychiatric history, drug abuse history, sleep disruption, pain. Take medication history, including over-the-counter medications and herbal supplements. Assess safety: evaluate for suicidal/homicidal ideation. If there is a concern for safety of self or others, consider hospitalization and psychiatric evaluation. Check laboratory values, including B_{12} level and thyroid function.

MANAGEMENT

Management[25] includes a combination of cognitive behavioral therapy, creative arts therapy, and antidepressants.

Antidepressants are a mainstay of management. They are safe and effective. The choice of antidepressant depends on other medical conditions and the side-effect profile.

- *Selective serotonin reuptake inhibitors*[26]: These are the most widely used and have fewer cardiac and anticholinergic side effects than tricyclic antidepressants. They can increase the blood level of drugs by inhibiting cytochrome P450.
  - Drugs:
    - Citalopram: Usual starting dose 20 mg/day
    - Escitalopram: Usual starting dose 10 mg/day
    - Fluoxetine: Usual starting dose 20 mg/day
    - Paroxetine: Usual starting dose 20 mg/day

- Sertraline: Usual starting dose 20 mg per day; preferred in patients with history of seizures
- *Tricyclic antidepressants:* Can be sedating and cause anticholinergic side effects (dry mouth, blurred vision, urinary retention); therefore should be avoided in elderly, frail patients
  - Drugs:
    - Mirtazapine: Increases appetite and can be sedating; preferred in patient with sleep disruption and poor appetite; usual starting dose 15 mg at bedtime; can be increased 30 mg
    - Trazodone: Sedating; used in patients with sleep disturbance
    - Venlafaxine: Mixed serotonin and norepinephrine uptake inhibitor; also helps with neuropathic pain and hot flashes; usual starting dose 37.5-75 mg daily

> **CLINICAL PEARL:** All patients with cancer should be screened for depression when the initial diagnosis of cancer is made and periodically thereafter as clinically indicated.

INSOMNIA

Insomnia is a common condition that affects more than half of cancer patients, with a prevalence more than double the general population. Although it is a different entity from CRF, the two are often closely intertwined.

Definition

Insomnia is a sleep disorder defined by having difficulty initiating sleep (anticipatory), difficulty maintaining sleep, or having issues with early morning awakenings and/or non-restorative sleep.

Etiology: Multifactorial

- Physiologic effects of cancer
- Psychological effect of serious illness: Most prevalent in early stage cancer diagnosis due to stress and anxiety of prognosis and treatment
- Pain
- Dyspnea
- Side effects of treatment: Glucocorticoids, nausea from chemotherapy, and so on
- Disruption of routine due to hospitalizations

It primarily affects women (patients >65 years old) with a history of insomnia (personal and family) and those suffering from anxiety or depression. Insomnia is more likely to affect breast cancer patients than any others; however, those with lung cancer are also commonly affected.

Insomnia worsens daytime fatigue symptoms. Because of this, patients will often attempt to nap during the day, further disrupting healthy sleep patterns and worsening existent insomnia. This has a cascade effect, serving to exacerbate anxiety and depressive symptoms, as well as making it harder to cope with side effects from treatment.

Screening for insomnia in cancer patients is vital, as prevalence is high and under-treatment remains an ongoing problem. Initially, the clinician can begin by asking his or her patient the following:

1. Do you have problems with your sleep or sleep disturbance on average for 3 or more nights a week? If yes:
2. Does the problem with your sleep negatively affect your daytime functioning?

Answering yes to both answers warrants a more focused assessment. This can include one of the following:

- A sleep diary the patient completes over a week
- The Pittsburgh Sleep Quality Index (PSQI)
- The Epworth Sleepiness Scale
- Insomnia Severity Index

The following interventions for insomnia are recommended. Treated appropriately, a physician is able to significantly improve a patient's quality of life and even help to slow the progression of disease.

- *Non-pharmacologic interventions:* Cognitive behavioral therapy is effective in reducing insomnia in the general population, as well as in cancer patients.[27] Notably, sleep hygiene is an important component of this. This includes
  - Reduce daytime napping as much as possible.
  - Keep time spent in bed to nighttime for sleeping.
  - Caffeine should be kept to a minimum and preferably consumed earlier in the day.
  - TV watching and the use of electronics should be avoided close to bedtime.
  - Exercise and relaxation practices (eg, yoga) are beneficial in treating insomnia, although they should be avoided within 3 hours of bed time.

Also, evaluate and treat for contributing factors: pain, anxiety, depression, and nausea, and consider medication side-effects, for example, corticosteroids and opioids can cause insomnia.

- *Pharmacologic interventions*[15]: Implementing the previously mentioned interventions in cancer patients can be difficult, if not sometimes impossible, thereby introducing the need for medications. The lowest effective dose should be used for the shortest period. Barbiturates should be avoided. Take caution in patients with delirium as benzodiazepines, zolpidem, and diphenhydramine can worsen the condition. Available drugs include the following:
  - Mirtazapine is an atypical antidepressant that is associated with sedating effects (dose 7.5-15 mg at bedtime).
  - Trazodone is a sedating antidepressant that has been shown to have a benefit in hospice patients with insomnia (dose 12.5-50 mg at bedtime).
  - A benzodiazepine can be carefully considered in select patients given the risk of dependence. Examples include lorazepam (dose 0.5-1 mg at bedtime) and zolpidem (dose 5 mg at bedtime as needed).
  - A selective melatonin receptor agonist, such as ramelteon (dose 8 mg, 30 minutes before bedtime), is useful in a patient with sleep onset and sleep phase disruption disorder. It is not habit forming.

ADVANCED CARE PLANNING

All patients with advanced-stage lung cancer should have a discussion about advanced care planning.[15]

Assess decision-making capacity and need for a surrogate decision-maker as early in the course as possible. Ask the patient if he or she has a living will, medical power of attorney, health care proxy, or patient surrogate for health care.

* If not, encourage the patient to prepare one.
* Refer to social worker if available.

Initiate a discussion of personal values, goals of care, and preferences for end-of-life care. Encourage the patients to discuss wishes with the family/proxy. Document patient values and preferences and any decisions in an accessible site in the medical record. Initiate a discussion of palliative care options, including referral to the palliative care team or hospice when appropriate.

REFERENCES

1. Temel JS, Greer JA, Muzikansky A, et al. Early palliative care for patients with metastatic non-small-cell lung cancer. *N Engl J Med.* 2010;363(8):733-742.
2. Zimmermann C, Swami N, Krzyzanowska M, et al. Early palliative care for patients with advanced cancer: a cluster-randomised controlled trial. *Lancet (London, England).* 2014;383(9930):1721-1730.
3. Watanabe SM, Nekolaichuk C, Beaumont C, Johnson L, Myers J, Strasser F. A multicenter study comparing two numerical versions of the Edmonton Symptom Assessment System in palliative care patients. *J Pain Symptom Manage.* 2011;41(2):456-468.
4. Fearon K, Strasser F, Anker SD, et al. Definition and classification of cancer cachexia: an international consensus. *Lancet Oncol.* 2011;12(5):489-495.
5. Bower JE, Bak K, Berger A, et al. Screening, assessment, and management of fatigue in adult survivors of cancer: an American Society of Clinical oncology clinical practice guideline adaptation. *J Clin Oncol.* 2014;32(17):1840-1850.
6. National Comprehensive Cancer Network. Cancer-related Fatigue. 2018; Version 2.2018: https://www.nccn.org/professionals/physician_gls/pdf/fatigue.pdf. Accessed December 1, 2018.
7. Brown JC, Huedo-Medina TB, Pescatello LS, Pescatello SM, Ferrer RA, Johnson BT. Efficacy of exercise interventions in modulating cancer-related fatigue among adult cancer survivors: a meta-analysis. *Cancer Epidemiol Biomarkers Prev.* 2011;20(1):123-133.
8. Minton O, Richardson A, Sharpe M, Hotopf M, Stone P. Drug therapy for the management of cancer-related fatigue. *Cochrane Database Syst Rev.* 2010;(7):CD006704.
9. Iyer S, Roughley A, Rider A, Taylor-Stokes G. The symptom burden of non-small cell lung cancer in the USA: a real-world cross-sectional study. *Support Care Cancer.* 2014;22(1):181-187.
10. Chochinov HM, Tataryn D, Clinch JJ, Dudgeon D. Will to live in the terminally ill. *Lancet (London, England).* 1999;354(9181):816-819.
11. Dy SM, Lorenz KA, Naeim A, Sanati H, Walling A, Asch SM. Evidence-based recommendations for cancer fatigue, anorexia, depression, and dyspnea. *J Clin Oncol.* 2008;26(23):3886-3895.
12. Ben-Aharon I, Gafter-Gvili A, Paul M, Leibovici L, Stemmer SM. Interventions for alleviating cancer-related dyspnea: a systematic review. *J Clin Oncol.* 2008;26(14):2396-2404.
13. Abernethy AP, McDonald CF, Frith PA, et al. Effect of palliative oxygen versus room air in relief of breathlessness in patients with refractory dyspnoea: a double-blind, randomised controlled trial. *Lancet (London, England).* 2010;376(9743):784-793.
14. National Comprehensive Cancer Network. Antiemesis. 2018; Version 3.2018: https://www.nccn.org/professionals/physician_gls/pdf/antiemesis.pdf. Accessed December 1, 2018.
15. National Comprehensive Cancer Network. Palliative Care. 2018; Version 1.2018: https://www.nccn.org/professionals/physician_gls/pdf/palliative.pdf. Accessed December 1, 2018.
16. Benson AB, 3rd, Ajani JA, Catalano RB, et al. Recommended guidelines for the treatment of cancer treatment-induced diarrhea. *J Clin Oncol.* 2004;22(14):2918-2926.

17. U.S. Department of Health and Human Services. Common Terminology Criteria for Adverse Events (CTCAE) Version 5.0. 2017; https://ctep.cancer.gov/protocolDevelopment/electronic_applications/docs/CTCAE_v5_Quick_Reference_5x7.pdf. Accessed July 1, 2018.

18. Bruera E, et al. Cancer Pain—Adult. 2017; https://www.mdanderson.org/documents/for-physicians/algorithms/clinical-management/clin-management-cancer-pain-web-algorithm.pdf.

19. Dowell D, Haegerich TM, Chou R. CDC Guideline for Prescribing Opioids for Chronic Pain—United States, 2016. *JAMA*. 2016;315(15):1624-1645.

20. American Pain Society. *Principles of Analgesic Use in the Treatment of Acute Pain and Cancer Pain*. 5th ed. Glenview, IL: American Pain Society; 2003.

21. Smith EM, Pang H, Cirrincione C, et al. Effect of duloxetine on pain, function, and quality of life among patients with chemotherapy-induced painful peripheral neuropathy: a randomized clinical trial. *JAMA*. 2013;309(13):1359-1367.

22. Mitchell AJ, Chan M, Bhatti H, et al. Prevalence of depression, anxiety, and adjustment disorder in oncological, haematological, and palliative-care settings: a meta-analysis of 94 interview-based studies. *Lancet Oncol*. 2011;12(2):160-174.

23. Pinquart M, Duberstein PR. Depression and cancer mortality: a meta-analysis. *Psychol Med*. 2010;40(11):1797-1810.

24. Andersen BL, DeRubeis RJ, Berman BS, et al. Screening, assessment, and care of anxiety and depressive symptoms in adults with cancer: an American Society of Clinical Oncology guideline adaptation. *J Clin Oncol*. 2014;32(15):1605-1619.

25. Pitman A, Suleman S, Hyde N, Hodgkiss A. Depression and anxiety in patients with cancer. *BMJ*. 2018;361.

26. Fisch MJ, Loehrer PJ, Kristeller J, et al. Fluoxetine versus placebo in advanced cancer outpatients: a double-blinded trial of the Hoosier Oncology Group. *J Clin Oncol*. 2003;21(10):1937-1943.

27. Howell D, Oliver TK, Keller-Olaman S, et al. Sleep disturbance in adults with cancer: a systematic review of evidence for best practices in assessment and management for clinical practice. *Ann Oncol*. 2014;25(4):791-800.

20

INTERVENTIONAL RADIOLOGY IN THE DIAGNOSIS AND TREATMENT OF LUNG CANCER

Douglas M. Coldwell, MD, PhD • Omar Safi Zuberi, DO

A 80-year-old male developed increasing shortness of air (SOA), and a 5-cm left hilar mass is found on computed tomography (CT) compressing the central airway. He has known chronic obstructive pulmonary disease (COPD). A positron emission tomographic (PET) scan identifies SUV-positive mediastinal lymph nodes and contralateral smaller nodules. Magnetic resonance imaging (MRI) of the brain shows a 2.5-cm mass.

The patient does not wish to undergo diagnostic or therapeutic bronchoscopy. Radiation oncology is consulted and asks for a tissue diagnosis before any radiation treatment.

Learning Objectives:
1. What is the role of interventional radiology (IR) in diagnosing lung cancer?
2. Can IR treat lung cancer?
3. Can IR palliate lung cancer symptoms?

DIAGNOSTICS OF LUNG CANCER

Diagnostic radiology has been the mainstay of the diagnosis of lung cancer, with screening chest radiographs and CT. Early detection has led to initiation of therapy at a stage where the disease is still vulnerable to treatment for cure and not palliation. However, the specifics of treatment require pathologic diagnosis of tissue samples.

Interventional radiology started the fluoroscopically guided placement of small needles into both peripheral and central lesions. The first needle biopsy was reported in Germany shortly after the discovery of x-rays, but Martin and Ellis from the Memorial Hospital in New York are credited for the development of the needle aspiration technique in 1930 using an 18-gauge needle.[1] The technique did not gain traction initially because the techniques of cytologic preparation of these small tissue specimens had not been sufficiently developed. It was not until the 1950s that the tissue preparation began to be more sophisticated. With the development of cross-sectional imaging and IR in the 1960s, the use of this technique became standard practice. Today, these needles are typically 22 or 20 gauge. Fine-needle aspirates are utilized to detect the presence of metastatic disease rather than primary lung cancer. The diagnostic accuracy depends on the technique utilized and cooperation and presence of a pathology team at the time of biopsy to evaluate the adequacy of the sample for diagnosis.

The puncture site is obviously determined by the site of the tumor. The most direct and shortest distance is determined, and the skin site is sterilized and anesthetized with lidocaine. Under imaging guidance, the needle is advanced until the tip is seen to move the lesion or to move with the lesion when the fluoroscopy unit is tilted from side to side. A 20-gauge needle can be placed and a 22-gauge needle placed coaxially within it. Multiple biopsies can then be obtained with a single needle placement.

The risks of lung biopsy to the patient include bleeding if a large vessel is crossed or a smaller amount of bleeding due to the extraction of tissue. Minor hemoptysis will likely occur if the lesion becomes more indistinct in appearance. Tumor seeding of the biopsy tract is possible, but only a handful of cases have been reported. The most common and serious complication is pneumothorax, which occurs in about 30% of patients but usually resolves with the patient on oxygen in the immediate postprocedural period. However, about 2%-3% of patients require a chest tube to relieve the air collection. This tube should be placed in the mid-second or third anterior interspace. The skin is sterilized and anesthetized, and an 8-10F catheter inserted over the rib to avoid the intercostal artery lying inferior to the more superior rib. As much air as possible should be aspirated before the Heimlich valve is attached. This valve prevents air from entering through the catheter and expels any collected air on expiration. The patient is then admitted overnight, and a chest x-ray is obtained in the morning. If the pneumothorax is resolved, the Heimlich valve is closed off by a three-way stopcock, and a repeat chest x-ray is repeated in 4-6 hours. If the air does not appear on the second chest radiograph, the chest tube can be removed. If the morning chest imaging shows that the pneumothorax still is present, the catheter and valve are left in place for another 24 hours, and the process repeated.

> **CLINICAL PEARL:** If the pneumothorax cannot be resolved with the small tube, it is likely that a bronchopleural fistula is present, requiring surgical consultation.

With the advent of CT, most lung biopsies are now performed utilizing that modality. In either modality, when the needle crosses the pleura, the patient should be instructed to stop breathing so that the sharp tip of the needle does not cause a rent in the pleura and a likely subsequent pneumothorax. Utilizing either fluoroscopy or CT, the process is the same to place the needle in the lesion.

Since many lung biopsies are now being sent for genetic analysis, the sheer amount of tissue removed with a 17-gauge guiding needle and 18-gauge core biopsy needles results in a higher rate of pneumothoraces and hemorrhage. However, careful choice of patients to minimize crossing of blebs and emphysematous changes of COPD will allow the complications to be as few as possible.

The current role of IR in the diagnosis of lung cancer is that of performing biopsies of peripheral lung lesions. It is absolutely necessary for the IR to coordinate with pathology so that they can be present to determine the adequacy of the specimens. Due to current Joint Commission on the Accreditation of Hospitals rules, the interventional radiology (IR) obtaining the biopsy must be informed of the pathology so that the patient is adequately informed of the results. It is also a quality control to assess the adequacy of the biopsies and personnel (**Figure 20-1**).

THERAPY FOR LUNG CANCER

Since the placement of a needle into a lesion is now standard practice, the use of local therapy has also been developed. The placement of a 14-gauge guiding needle allows a monopolar radio-frequency ablation (RFA) needle to be inserted and the individual tumor to be ablated with accuracy and efficacy. The use of such a technique is limited to those patients who have 1 or 2 lesions so that the number of pleural punctures is lessened. The overall survival rate for those tumors treated solely with RFA in a meta-analysis of about 1,300 patients was 84%, 67%, 62%, 55%, and 43% for the 1-, 2-, 3-, 4-, and 5-year weighted average, respectively. Since these are aggregated numbers, individual stage survival rates are not available.[2] However, three studies demonstrated that in stage 1 non–small cell lung cancer, the local control rates of patients treated with RFA were statistically significantly lower than those treated with stereotactic body radiation, and the overall survival rates were not different. Complications of thermal ablation, whether it is via RFA or microwave ablation, are between 11% and 16%. These include medical intervention for pneumothorax, effusion, hemoptysis, pneumonia, pain, and bronchopleural fistula. There has been no demonstrated difference between the results utilizing RFA and microwave ablative techniques; however, they have been demonstrated to be superior to cryotherapy.

THERAPY FOR ADVERSE EVENTS

One of the presenting symptoms of lung cancer is often massive hemoptysis, as defined as a cup of blood or more in a 24-hour period. This is usually due to bleeding from the bronchial arteries. The bronchial arteries, similar to the hepatic arteries, supply tumor, while the lower pressure pulmonary arteries and portal vein supply normal parenchyma. This is due to the difference in the interstitial pressure of the normal parenchyma and the increased pressure seen in the wall of the malignancy over that of the pulmonary artery but less than the bronchial arteries.[3] These tumors may be embolized

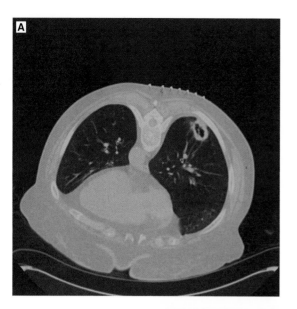
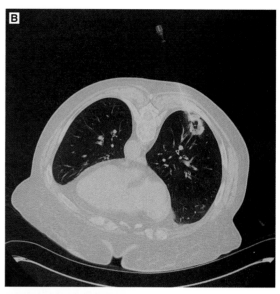

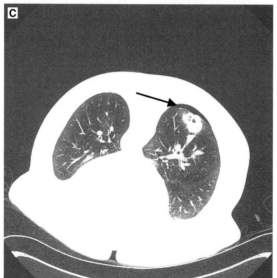

Figure 20-1. A 68-year-old female with posterior necrotizing mass. A. CT demonstrates a small peripherally located mass. Lead grids are placed on the patient's skin to help localize the needle placement. B. A 19-gauge guiding needle is placed within the lung adjacent to the mass. C. Multiple core biopsies were obtained and the needles removed. The mass is noted to be somewhat hazy, indicating that mild hemorrhage has occurred. Even though the biopsy was uneventful, a small left pneumothorax, posterior to the peripheral mass (arrow) occurred, which resolved over the next 2 hours and did not require a chest tube.

with particles, but care needs to be taken to ensure that there are no branches seen supplying midline arteries, which are likely supplying the anterior spinal cord. Additionally, tumors that lie near the spine that have been treated with radiation should be viewed as though there may be small vessels communicating with the spinal cord. By taking care

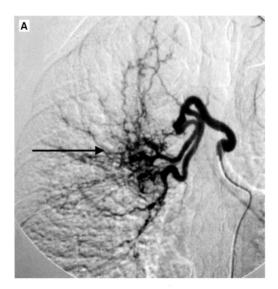

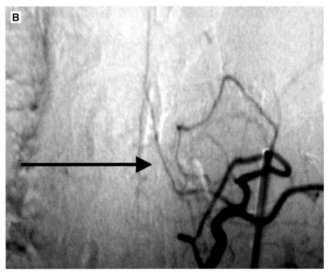

Figure 20-2. A 59-year-old male with non–small cell lung cancer (NSCLC) in the right hilum with significant hemoptysis. A. Selective bronchial arteriogram demonstrates the tumor vascularity (*arrow*). B. This was then embolized with particles measuring 250 μm in diameter (*arrow*) with the halting of his hemoptysis. The anterior spinal artery is noted to originate from the left bronchial artery. It usually originates from the right intercostal bronchial trunk.

to perform high-quality power injected arteriograms, the chances of recognizing these arteries is increased. Use of microcatheters through the usual 5F diagnostic catheters helps to place the particles, which should measure about 100 μm in diameter precisely into the tumor. Smaller particles are more likely to travel to and occlude the smaller arteries, especially those supplying the spinal cord (**Figure 20-2**).[3]

Recurrent malignant effusions are commonplace in patients with lung cancer. A tunneled multi-sideholed catheter can be placed into the effusion, allowing the patients to drain themselves at home with a minimum of instruction and with the aid of home care. A set of 1-L vacuum bottles is supplied to the patients, and they may drain themselves as frequently as twice per week. It should be noted that a trial of thoracenteses is usually performed so that an idea of the frequency of the drainage can be obtained. Once that frequency is about once per week, and enough effusion is present, such a catheter can be placed on an outpatient basis.

Patients having lung cancer centrally are prone to the development of superior vena cava (SVC) syndrome, which is manifested by swelling of the face and neck, inability to lie flat, and shortness of breath due to the compression of the SVC by the tumor. Patients having this syndrome can be easily treated by either a jugular or brachial vein approach and the placement of a stent in the SVC with angioplasty to a minimum of 10 mm. This is one of the few procedures performed in IR that has instantaneous results. Once the stent is dilated, the patient immediately feels relief of the pressure in their head and neck. Balloon-dilated stents are usually utilized from 10- to 14-mm in diameter. Self-expanding stents may be used, but dilation is essential as the tumor is very firm, and the stent would not expand enough to relieve the patient's symptoms. Stents should also be at least 6-8 cm in length so that they are not "squirted" to one side or the other, not landing on the area that needs to be treated (**Figure 20-3**).[4]

Metastatic lung cancer to the osseous structures is a common event. Metastases to the spine, pelvis, and long bones are commonly and reflexively treated with radiation therapy. If these lesions involve only 1 or 2 levels, placement of an 8-gauge guiding trocar under fluoroscopic or CT guidance allows the placement of a bipolar radio-frequency probe that consistently will ablate a 1.8 by 3 cm ovoid lesion. The tumor can usually be ablated from a single transpedicular approach and the lesion then filled with polymethylmethacrylate (PMMA) cement. This procedure is usually well tolerated with few complications. The complications are due to the leakage of the cement from the vertebral body anteriorly into Batson's venous plexus, where it can be delivered to the lungs as PMMA pulmonary emboli. The cement is dense enough so that any leakage with embolic formation can be anticipated and the procedure halted. The major complication that should be avoided is the posterior leakage of the cement into the spinal canal, which may cause an increase in pain and require a surgical procedure to remove the extravasated cement. Since these procedures are usually performed in a biplane fluoroscopy room or angiography suite, lateral as well as anteroposterior visualization of the cement as it is delivered should be enough to stop the flow of cement before it reaches the spinal canal. This procedure may be utilized to immediately relieve the pain of metastatic disease in a single location, which can then allow the patient to undergo a complete course of radiation therapy.

While it may seem that these techniques are in competition, they are actually complementary. This technique has also been applied to almost any other bony structure with good effect.[5] Patients who may benefit from this procedure include those who have radioresistant tumors, who have persistent or recurrent pain after radiation therapy, who have reached their radiation dose limit, who have focal pain that is preventing palliative radiation, and those who cannot undergo other palliative treatments due to current systemic treatments (**Figure 20-4**).

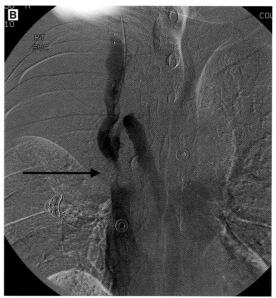

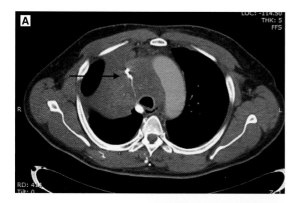

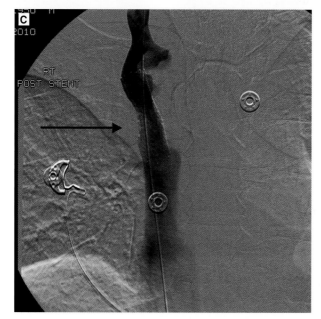

Figure 20-3. A 58-year-old man with NSCLC in the right hilum. **A.** The CT scan demonstrates a large mass narrowing the SVC (*arrow*), collapsing the right upper lobe. **B.** The SVC gram demonstrates the high-grade stenosis of the SVC (*arrow*) and the enlarged collateral azygous vein (*arrowhead*). **C.** After the stent was placed and dilated, there is free flow of contrast beyond the stenosis into the right atrium, with resolution of the patient's symptoms. Note that the azygous vein is no longer filling.

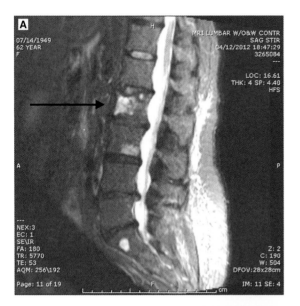
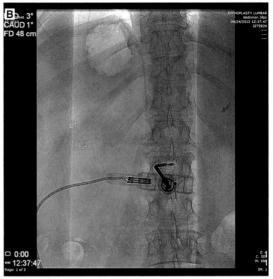
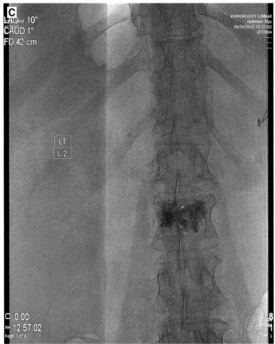

Figure 20-4 A 62-year-old woman with metastatic lung cancer to the lumbar spine with 8/10 pain. A. Sagittal MRI of the lumbar spine demonstrating the destruction of the L2 lumbar vertebral body, which is at the site of her pain (*arrow*). B. The RFA probe was placed via a transpedicular approach into the vertebral body and the tumor heated to 50°C. C. PMMA cement was instilled into the vertebral body, extending across the midline and bridging the superior and inferior end plates. At the end of the procedure, the patient stated that she had no pain.

REFERENCES

1. Martin HE, Ellis EB. Biopsy by needle puncture and aspiration. *Ann Surg.* 1930;92:169-181.

2. Yuan Z, Wang Y, Zhang J, Zheng J, Li W. A meta-analysis of clinical outcomes after radiofrequency ablation and microwave ablation for lung cancer and pulmonary metastases. *J Am Coll Radiol.* 2019;16(3):302-314. doi:10.1016/j.jacr.2018.10.012

3. Schwartz L, Coldwell DM. Is Liver Disease Caused by Increased Pressure? Interstitial Pressure as a Causative Mechanism in Carcinogenesis and in the Differential Blood Supply in Liver Tumors from the Hepatic Artery. *J Liver.* 2015;3(3):156. doi:10.4172/2167-0889.1000156

4. Niu S, Xu YS, Cheng L, Cao C. Stent insertion for malignant superior vena cava syndrome: effectiveness and long-term outcome. *Radiol Med.* 2017;122:633-638.

5. Anchala PR, Hilllen TJ, Irving WD, et al. Treatment of spine metastatic lesions with a navigational bipolar radio-frequency ablation al device: a multi-center retrospective study. *Pain Physician.* 2014;17(4):317-327.

21

IMMUNOTOXICITY

Amitoj Gill, MD • Rahul Gosain, MD

This case involves a 68-year-old man diagnosed with metastatic non–small cell lung cancer (NSCLC) and adenocarcinoma histology with a programmed death ligand 1 (PDL-1) score of 35%. He completed 4 cycles of carboplatin, pemetrexed, and pembrolizumab combination treatment and is currently on pemetrexed and pembrolizumab maintenance treatment. He presented to the hospital with abdominal cramps, 6-8 episodes of bloody diarrhea in a day, and fatigue. An infectious etiology has been ruled out, and immune-related colitis is speculated. What treatment should be offered to this patient?

Learning Objectives:
1. What are common toxicities of immunotherapy?
2. How are the toxicities graded?
3. How are lower and higher grade toxicities of immunotherapy treated?

In the past, limited success from traditional immunotherapy agents for most solid malignancies resulted in a perception that immunotherapy has only a limited role in oncology.[1] However, with a better understanding of genetic patterns, predictive biomarkers such as PD-L1 and tumor mutational load have resulted in promising outcomes with immunotherapy.[2-4]

The development of this novel class of immune-based therapy presents new challenges in recognizing and managing a spectrum of treatment-related toxicities.

The toxicity profiles of these agents, including those that block immune checkpoints, immunostimulatory agents, and adoptive T-cell therapy, are the result of hyperactivated T cells and a surge of cytokines directed against normal tissue.[5,6]

Immunotoxicity management is based on expert consensus, and a majority of the guidelines are obtained from the National Comprehensive Cancer Network (NCCN) with 2a category evidence (based on lower level evidence with a uniform consensus that intervention is appropriate).

A detailed history and physical examination remain the key to approaching any new presenting complaints. Non-inflammatory (including infectious) etiology should be ruled out before considering drug toxicity. Hence, treatment-related toxicity should be a diagnosis of exclusion. An understanding of the timing, likelihood, and presentation of immune toxicity as well as how to manage the toxicity effectively will be a necessity for any health care provider dealing with cancer patients.

GRADING OF SEVERITY

Once the diagnosis of treatment-related toxicity is confirmed, management is based on a patient's presenting grade. Common Terminology Criteria for Adverse Events v4.0 (CTCAE) provides a descriptive terminology that can be utilized for an adverse event (AE) and grading severity scale for each AE term (**Table 21-1**).

HEPATIC ADVERSE EVENTS

Hepatic toxicity is a common immunotoxicity present in about 2%-10% of cases treated with immunotherapy.[7,8] This number increases to 25%-30% in combination immunotherapy, with presentation around 6-12 weeks.[9] It is important to rule out other potential causes of liver dysfunction, including viral hepatitis, disease-related hepatic dysfunction, and drug-induced hepatic dysfunction. Any potential hepatotoxic medication should be discontinued. It is important to obtain an alcohol history. Other workup includes iron studies, liver ultrasound, and imaging for potential liver metastasis. Auto-immune hepatitis should be ruled out if suspicion is high; this can be done by checking serum antinuclear antibody (ANA), antineutrophil cytoplasmic antibody (ANCA), and anti–smooth muscle antibodies. For isolated elevation of transaminases, consider checking creatine kinase (CK) for other etiologies.

In case of hepatotoxicity with total bilirubin (T. Bili) greater than 1.5 the upper limit of normal (ULN) and other causes of hepatic dysfunction ruled out, immunotherapy must be permanently discontinued. The patient should be admitted to the hospital, and prednisone/methylprednisone should be started at 2 mg/kg/day. Hepatology consultation should be obtained, and daily transaminases should be checked. If there is no improvement in 3 days, mycophenolate should be considered. Infliximab should not be used in hepatic AEs.

In patients with hepatotoxicity with transaminitis only and normal bilirubin, management depends on the degree of severity of transaminitis. In Grade 1 (G1) transaminitis (<3 × ULN), immunotherapy should be continued, but liver function should be checked more frequently. For Grade 2 (G2) (3-5 × ULN) toxicity, immunotherapy should be held, and liver function should be assessed every 3-5 days. In case of worsening transaminitis, prednisone should be started at 0.5-1 mg/kg/day. Severe or Grade 3 (G3) toxicity (5-20 × ULN), inpatient care should be considered. Prednisone should be started at 1-2 mg/kg/day. For Grade 4 (G4) toxicity (>20 × ULN/life-threatening disease), prednisone should be started at 2 mg/kg/day. The patient should be treated as an inpatient, and mycophenolate should be considered. Infliximab should not be used due to potential concerns of hepatotoxicity, but there is no evidence to support this.[10]

TABLE 21-1 Grading Severity Scale for Adverse Events

GRADING SCALE	DIARRHEA/COLITIS (GASTROINTESTINAL EVENTS)	CREATININE (Cr) ELEVATION (RENAL EVENTS)	PNEUMONITIS (PULMONARY EVENTS)	LIVER TEST ELEVATION (HEPATIC EVENTS)	RASH (DERMATOLOGY EVENTS)	NEUROLOGICAL SYMPTOMS (CENTRAL NERVOUS SYSTEM EVENTS)
Grade 1	Diarrhea: <4 stools/day over baseline. Colitis: asymptomatic	Cr 1.50 times above the baseline or absolute increase of ≥0.3 mg/dL	Radiographic changes only. Confined to one lobe or <25% of lung parenchyma	AST (aspartate aminotransferase) or ALT (Alanine aminotransferase) <3.0 times ULN and or T. bili <1.5 times ULN.	Covering <30% of BSA; G1 <10%; G2 10%-30%	Asymptomatic or mild symptoms; intervention not indicated
Grade 2	Diarrhea: 4-6 stools/day over baseline; intravenous fluids for <24 hours; not interfering with ADLs. Colitis: abdominal pain; blood in stool	Cr 2-3 times above the baseline. Cr >3 times the baseline or above 4 mg/dL	Mild-to-moderate new symptoms	AST or ALT >3.0-5.0 times ULN and/or T. bili >1.5 to <3.0 times ULN		Moderate symptoms; limiting instrumental ADLs
Grade 3	Diarrhea: >7 stools/day over baseline; incontinence; intravenous fluids for >24 hours; interfering with ADLs. Colitis: severe abdominal pain; medical intervention indicated; peritoneal signs		Severe new symptoms; new/worsening hypoxia. Involvement of all lung lobes or more than 50% of lung parenchyma	AST or ALT >5 times ULN and/or T. bili >3 times ULN	Covering >30% BSA	Severe symptoms; limiting self-care ADLs
Grade 4	Life-threatening situation, perforation	Cr >6 times ULN/dialysis indicated/life threatening	Life threatening	Life threatening	Life threatening consequences	Life threatening

Adapted from CTCAE, with modifications per NCCN.

GASTROINTESTINAL ADVERSE EVENTS

One of the most common toxicities associated with immunotherapy is diarrhea from colitis. With cytotoxic T-lymphocyte–associated protein 4 (CTLA4) inhibitors, the incidence of diarrhea can be as high as 54%, and it is lower with programmed cell death protein 1 (PD1) inhibitors at around less than 19%.[11] Colitis in this setting tends to mimic inflammatory bowel disease, and patients with colitis were more likely to have been prescribed nonsteroidal anti-inflammatory drugs (NSAIDs) as compared to patients without colitis.[12] Appropriate management is necessary to prevent life-threatening complications from this AE.

Mild or G1 colitis is consistent with fewer than 4 bowel movements more than the baseline. It is important to know the baseline rate of bowel movements per day since the grading depends on excess of that. For G1 colitis, immunotherapy can be continued; however, close monitoring is required, and in case of worsening symptoms, it is important to rule out any infectious etiology (stool studies, including testing for *Clostridium difficile* colitis).

Moderate (G2) colitis is defined as 4-6 stools more than baseline not affecting the quality of life, and severe (G3-G4) is defined as more than 6 bowel movements above baseline or symptoms of colitis affecting activities of daily living (ADLs), causing hospitalizations, hemodynamic instability, and other severe complications (toxic megacolon, ischemic bowel disease, perforation). For moderate–severe colitis, it is important to rule out an infectious etiology with stool testing as previously discussed. Other investigations, such as computed tomographic (CT) imaging and esophagogastroduodenoscopy (EGD)/colonoscopy should be considered. If available, stool lactoferrin/calprotectin can be used to distinguish underlying inflammation from infection.

PANCREATIC ADVERSE EVENTS

Pancreatitis is a rare immunotoxicity but has been reported.[13] If there are clinical signs/symptoms of acute pancreatitis and it is suspected, proper workup with CT imaging and laboratory tests should be done. Magnetic resonance cholangiopancreatography (MRCP) should be considered if otherwise radiographically negative but high suspicion is present. Gastrointestinal consultation should be considered. Management depends on the severity of pancreatitis.

When there is elevation of amylase/lipase without signs/symptoms of pancreatitis, workup as mentioned is necessary to diagnose pancreatitis. In the absence of pancreatitis, resuming immunotherapy can be considered. This holds true for G1 or mild acute pancreatitis as well. Acute pancreatitis is considered mild when there are any of the three following present: signs/symptoms of pancreatitis, CT findings consistent with pancreatitis, or pancreatic enzymes (amylase/lipase) greater than three times the ULN.

If two of these parameters are present, it is considered G2 or moderate pancreatitis, which warrants holding immunotherapy. In addition, methylprednisone/prednisone should be used at 0.5-1 mg/kg/day. Immunotherapy can be restarted with no radiographic evidence of pancreatitis and improvement in amylase/lipase. If all of the parameters are present or there is hemodynamic instability, this is considered G3 or severe toxicity, which warrants permanently stopping immunotherapy. Methylprednisone/prednisone at

1-2 mg/kg/day should be used, and mycophenolate mofetil can be considered if symptoms are not improving.

PULMONARY ADVERSE EVENTS

Pneumonitis is an uncommon toxicity but is very challenging to manage, especially in patients with lung cancer. It is hard to diagnose pneumonitis radiographically in patients with lung cancer because of different confounding factors, such as radiation-related changes, lung cancer itself, lymphangitic spread, and more. The incidence of pneumonitis varies with different immunotherapy agents. Incidence ranges between 0% and 10% in anti-PD-1/PDL1 agents with an overall incidence of about 2.7% in anti-PD1 agents.[14-17] The incidence is interestingly less with CTLA4 inhibitors.[18] Pneumonitis is seen more with combination immunotherapy as compared to monotherapy.

Some studies have shown higher odds of pneumonitis in NSCLC as compared to other cancers.[16] Symptoms include cough, dyspnea, chest pain, leading to hypoxia and respiratory failure. Even though pneumonitis can have various manifestations radiographically, commonly seen are ground glass opacities and patchy nodular infiltrates.[19] The timeline of symptoms also helps with diagnosing pneumonitis since it is rarely seen early on, and the median time of presentation is around 3 months.[15] Workup includes proper history, physical examination, and imaging. If the clinical picture, including radiographic findings, is consistent with pneumonitis, treatment should be started. Biopsy is mostly unnecessary but can be done to rule out other etiologies in case of an unclear clinical picture.

Generally, with any suspicion of pneumonitis, immunotherapy should be held. With G1 or mild pneumonitis (described in Table 21-1), the patient should be reassessed in 1-2 weeks, and chest imaging should be repeated in 3-4 weeks. G2 or moderate pneumonitis requires ruling out an infectious etiology with viral panels, cultures, and bronchoscopy and bronchoalveolar lavage (BAL) can be considered as well. Empiric antibiotics can be started if an infectious process is in the differential. Methylprednisone/prednisone at 1-2 mg/kg/day should be started, and close monitoring every 3-7 days is important.

> **CLINICAL PEARL:** If the clinical picture does not improve in 48-72 hours, the patient should be treated as having G3 or severe pneumonitis.

Steroids should be continued until the clinical picture is G1 or less and then tapered slowly over 4-6 weeks. Immunotherapy can be restarted once G1 or less is present with radiographic improvement/resolution.

For G3-G4 pneumonitis, immunotherapy should be permanently withheld. Management should be in an inpatient setting with methylprednisone/prednisone at 1-2 mg/kg/day. Infectious workup as previously mentioned should be done to rule out infectious etiologies. If symptoms do not improve in 48 hours, agents such as infliximab, mycophenolate mofetil, or even intravenous immunoglobulin (IVIG) can be used. Pulmonary consultation should be obtained early in severe pneumonitis.

ENDOCRINE ADVERSE EVENTS

A meta-analysis done recently showed that the incidence of endocrine AEs was around 10% with immune checkpoint inhibitor usage.[20] Common manifestations include diabetes, thyroiditis, hypophysitis, and adrenal insufficiency.

Diabetes

With hyperglycemia (fasting glucose level > 200 mg/dL), it is important to obtain a proper history and rule out underlying type 2 diabetes mellitus (DM). New-onset DM should be worked up with c-peptide levels. Anti-glutamic acid decarboxylase (anti-GAD), anti-islet cell antibodies should be considered, and diabetic ketoacidosis (DKA) workup should be done. In the case of DKA and new-onset DM, the patient should be managed as an inpatient with endocrinology consultation, and immunotherapy should be held. Immunotherapy can be restarted once the DKA is resolved and blood glucose stabilized.

Thyroid

Thyroid abnormalities can manifest as either central hypothyroidism (normal or low thyroid-stimulating hormone [TSH], low free thyroxine [T_4]) or primary hypothyroidism (elevated TSH). Subclinical hypothyroidism is asymptomatic, with elevated TSH levels and normal free T_4 levels. Thyroid hormones should be evaluated every 4-6 weeks. Immunotherapy should be continued with subclinical hypothyroidism; however, levothyroxine can be started with TSH levels above 10.

Even with primary hypothyroidism, immunotherapy can be continued. Endocrinology consultation should be obtained for the management of primary hypothyroidism. Adrenal insufficiency should be ruled out.

Thyrotoxicosis can be rarely seen as well and management requires symptom control with beta-blockers until the thyrotoxicosis resolves. Thyroid function evaluations should be repeated in 4-6 weeks, and if thyrotoxicosis resolves, no further treatment is needed. In case TSH remains low with elevated free T_4/total T_3 (triiodothyronine), a radioiodine uptake scan should be done to differentiate between true hyperthyroidism versus Graves-like etiology. If hypothyroidism develops with TSH greater than 10, levothyroxine should be started.

Adrenal Insufficiency

Primary adrenal insufficiency requires proper workup with morning cortisol levels, cortisol, 30- or 60-minute cortisol test, corticotropin (ACTH) levels, comprehensive metabolic panel (CMP), and renin levels. Immunotherapy should progress, and endocrinology consultation should be obtained. Corticosteroids should be started prior to hormone replacement to avoid adrenal crisis. Steroid replacement should be with either prednisone 7.5 mg/10 mg or hydrocortisone 20 mg in the morning and 10 mg in the evening with a slow taper. In addition, mineralocorticoid, fludrocortisone, should be started at 0.1 mg every other day and as needed titration. Patients with hemodynamic instability should be admitted and managed with intravenous fluids and stress dose steroids.

Hypophysitis

Hypophysitis can present as headaches, fatigue, nausea/vomiting, and low sodium and potassium. Complete workup includes evaluation of ACTH, cortisol, FSH, luteinizing hormone (LH), testosterone/estrogen (male/premenopausal female), free T_4. Brain magnetic resonance imaging (MRI) should be obtained in symptomatic patients. Immunotherapy should be held in these patients. Endocrinology consultation should be obtained, and hormone replacement given as appropriate. Methylprednisone/prednisone at 1-2 mg/kg/day should be started. Immunotherapy can be restarted once symptoms are controlled with a prednisone dose less than 10 mg daily or equivalent.

RENAL ADVERSE EVENTS

Acute kidney injury (AKI) or nephritis is an uncommon AE with an incidence of about 1%-2% in monotherapy and about 4.5% in patients treated with combination immunotherapy.[10] Grade 3 and above toxicity is less than 2%.[21] Median time to onset for grade 3 or above nephritis is around 16.3 weeks.[22]

With any evidence of elevated creatinine, it is important to rule out any other etiologies, such as dehydration, potential nephrotoxic medications, or recent intravenous contrast use. It is also important to obtain a spot urine/creatinine ratio. For proteinuria greater than 3 g/24-hour, check ANA, rheumatoid factor (RF), anti-neutrophil cytoplasmic antibody (ANCA), anti-dsDNA (anti–double-stranded DNA), and serum complement 3 (C3), complement 4 (C4), and total complement (CH50) to rule out other etiologies. With other causes ruled out, management depends on the degree of severity. G1 or mild nephritis requires creatinine monitoring every 3-7 days. Immunotherapy can be held until improvement is seen.

For G2 nephritis, immunotherapy should be held, and nephrology consultation should be obtained. Once other causes are ruled out, treatment should be started with prednisone 0.5-1 mg/kg/day. Creatinine and urine albumin creatinine ratio should be monitored every 3-7 days. If persistent over a week, the steroid dose should be increased to methylprednisone/prednisone 1-2 mg/kg/day. Treatment should be continued until symptoms improve to G1 or less and be tapered over 4-6 weeks. Immunotherapy can be restarted with improvement concomitantly with steroids.

G3 or above nephropathy requires permanently discontinuing immunotherapy. The patient should be treated as an inpatient, and nephrology consultation should be obtained. Renal biopsy can be considered if the diagnosis is unclear. Treatment should be started with methylprednisone/prednisone at 1-2 mg/kg/day. If still greater than G1 after 1 week of steroids, other therapies (eg, azathioprine, cyclophosphamide [monthly], cyclosporine, infliximab, mycophenolate) should be considered.

CUTANEOUS ADVERSE EVENTS

Dermatological toxicities are seen in almost 30%-50% of patients using immunotherapy,[23] with 1%-3% grade 3 toxicities[24] with the CTLA4 inhibitor ipilimumab. The PD-1 inhibitors (pembrolizumab and nivolumab) have a lower incidence of cutaneous toxicity.[17] The presence of cutaneous AEs such as rash and vitiligo have interestingly shown a better prognosis in many studies.[25-28]

The different types of skin AEs include maculopapular rash, pruritus, blistering disorders such as bullous dermatitis, Steven-Johnson syndrome (SJS), and toxic epidermal necrolysis (TEN). It is important to obtain a complete history, including history of underlying dermatological diseases, as well as a full-body dermatological examination. Any atypical features warrant a skin biopsy and dermatological consultation.

Maculopapular Rash

The maculopapular rash is the most common dermatological toxicity observed in patients undergoing treatment with immunotherapy. With grade 1 (<10% body surface area [BSA] involved) presenting dermatologic signs, it is recommended to continue with immunotherapy treatment and proceed with symptomatic management (topical steroids, emollients, or oral antihistamines) of skin symptoms. In the case of grade 2 (10%-30% BSA involvement), consider holding immunotherapy and treating with high-potency topical steroids and/or oral steroids (prednisone 0.5-1 mg/kg/day). High-potency topical steroids for shorter duration are preferred over longer treatment with low-potency steroids. Oral antihistamines and topical emollients can be used for symptomatic control. Once an improvement is noted, taper steroids over at least 1 month. Immunotherapy rechallenge can be done once symptoms become milder (≤G1). For grade 3-4 symptoms, it is recommended to hold the immunotherapy and prescribe prednisone at 0.5-1.0 mg/kg/day. Dosage can be increased if there is no improvement, and urgent dermatology evaluation is recommended. If symptoms improve to grade 1, taper steroids over 4-6 weeks.

Pruritis

Another common AE is pruritis. This can be divided into mild or localized (G1); widespread, causing skin changes from scratching (G2); and G3, which includes intense pruritis limiting ADLs significantly and affecting sleep.

For G1 pruritis, immunotherapy can be continued and symptoms controlled with high-potency topical steroids. Immunotherapy can be held for G2 until symptoms are G1 or less, and treatment is high-grade topical steroids and oral antihistamines. Dermatology consultation is recommended.

G3 pruritis can have significant implications on quality of life; hence, it is recommended to hold immunotherapy. Serum immunoglobulin (Ig) E levels and histamine levels should be checked. Omalizumab can be used in case of elevated IgE levels, and antihistamines can be used in case of elevated histamine. Gabapentin and pregabalin can be used for symptom control, and aprepitant can be considered as well. Urgent dermatology referral should be made. Systemic steroids with prednisone/methylprednisone 0.5-1 mg/kg/day should be used.

Bullous Dermatitis

Bullous dermatitis can be seen as an AE in some cases, although rare. The grading of toxicity mimics maculopapular rash, with G1 less than 10% BSA, G2 10%-30% BSA, and G3 greater than 30% BSA.

> **CLINICAL PEARL:** Immunotherapy should be held with any evidence of bullous disease until symptoms resolve.

Urgent dermatology referral should be made for a skin biopsy. Treatment includes high-potency topical steroids for G1 and systemic steroids with prednisone/methylprednisone 0.5-1 mg/kg/day.

For G3 toxicity, immunotherapy should be permanently held, and the patient should be managed in an inpatient setting. Prednisone/methylprednisone at 1-2 mg/kg/day and urgent dermatology consultation should be obtained. The management mentioned previously is the same in the case of other severe cutaneous AEs, including Stevens-Johnson syndrome (SJS), toxic epidermal necrolysis (TEN), and drug reaction with eosinophilia and systemic symptoms (DRESS). For SJS and TEN, the patient should be managed in a burn unit.

NEUROLOGICAL ADVERSE EVENTS

Neurological AEs seen with immunotherapy include peripheral neuropathies, Guillian-Barré syndrome (GBS), myasthenia gravis (MG), encephalitis, and meningitis. As per an analysis of neurological AEs, patients on CTLA4 inhibitors had an incidence of 3.8%, patients on PD-1 inhibitors had an incidence of 6.1%, and patients on combination immunotherapy had an incidence of about 12%. Most of the neurological AEs are relatively mild, and grade 3-4 AEs are seen in less than 1% of patients.[29]

Peripheral Neuropathy

With the development of peripheral neuropathy, other causes like medications, metabolic, infectious, and endocrine etiologies should be ruled out. Neuraxial imaging should be performed as needed. Mild neuropathy causes no interference in ADLs and no concern to the patient. No intervention is recommended for mild symptoms and management includes monitoring symptoms over a week. Immunotherapy can be held in case of worsening symptoms. Moderate neuropathy is when symptoms have some interference with ADLs. Symptoms can be observed initially; however, prednisone at 0.5-1 mg/kg can be initiated in case of worsening symptoms. This can be increased to 2-4 mg/kg IV methylprednisone in case of symptom progression. Neurology consult, neuraxial imaging, electromyography (EMG), and nerve conduction studies (NCS) should be considered. Gabapentin, pregabalin, or duloxetine can be used for pain control. Severe neuropathy with significant impairment of ADLs with weakness or respiratory issues is managed like GBS.

Guillain-Barré Syndrome

Guillain-Barré syndrome is a life-threatening AE with symptoms of symmetrical ascending muscle weakness with decreased or absent deep tendon reflexes. This can become life threatening with involvement of respiratory muscles. Patients need to be monitored in an inpatient setting in consultation with neurology. Intensive care unit access should be available. Management includes lumbar puncture with cytology (this can also diagnose leptomeningeal disease), serum antibody tests for GBS variants like Miller-Fisher, and pulmonary function testing. Treatment includes pulse dose steroids at 1 g daily for 5 days with IVIG or plasmapheresis. Immunotherapy should be permanently stopped.

Myasthenia Gravis

Another rare AE with immunotherapy includes MG. Symptoms consist of progressive muscle weakness. Ocular symptoms include diplopia and ptosis. Facial muscle weakness, dysphagia, and respiratory muscle weakness can be seen as well. Workup should be done with neurology consultation and includes imaging with brain and spine MRI to rule out metastatic disease. EMG or NCS should be considered as well. Acetylcholine receptor (AChR) antibodies and anti–muscle-specific tyrosine kinase antibodies can be checked, but this is not necessary for diagnosis. Moderate MG includes some symptoms interfering with ADLs. Immunotherapy should be held, and treatment should be with pyridostigmine and low-dose prednisone, which can be slowly increased. Steroids should be tapered slowly with improvement. Severe MG consists of symptoms significantly affecting ADLs. Patients should be treated in an inpatient setting, and immunotherapy should be withheld. Treatment consists of high-dose steroids, IVIG, and plasmapheresis.

Meningitis/Encephalitis

Other uncommon neurological AEs of immunotherapy include meningitis/encephalitis. Workup should be done with neurology consultation and includes imaging and lumbar puncture (with autoimmune and paraneoplastic panel) to rule out metastatic disease. Vasculitis should be excluded as well as cortisol, thyroid functions should be checked. Once bacterial and viral infections have been ruled out, management should be in the hospital with methylprednisone. Dose can be escalated with worsening symptoms. With the presence of oligoclonal bands in encephalitis or with worsening symptoms, pulse dose steroids should be used. In case of encephalitis (with positive autoimmune antibodies or with no improvement in 7-14 days), rituximab should be considered. Immunotherapy should be held if symptoms are mild; however, it should be permanently discontinued in case of moderate-severe symptoms. Transverse myelitis is managed along similar lines, except IVIG/plasmapheresis should be strongly considered.

MUSCULOSKELETAL ADVERSE EVENTS

Musculoskeletal AEs are commonly seen with immunotherapy usage; however, severe inflammatory AEs are not very common.[10] With mild arthritis, immunotherapy can be continued and symptoms managed with NSAIDs; low-dose prednisone can be used if symptoms are not improving. Intra-articular steroid injections should be considered. For moderate arthritis, immunotherapy should be held, and prednisone can be used at a dose of 0.5-1 mg/kg for 4-6 weeks. With severe arthritis (interfering with ADLs/presence of joint erosions), prednisone at 1-2 mg/kg/day should be used. Disease-modifying anti-rheumatic drugs (DMARDs) can be used in case of no improvement with steroids. This should be done in consultation with rheumatology.

Myositis is another uncommon AE that requires checking serial CK levels. Management should be with pain medication for mild myositis and prednisone along with pain medication for moderate-severe disease. Immunotherapy can be continued with mild symptoms; however, it should be held for moderate-severe symptoms. Muscle biopsy should be considered in severe/refractory symptoms.

CARDIAC ADVERSE EVENTS

Cardiac AEs are rarely seen and include myocarditis, pericarditis, arrhythmias, and systolic dysfunction. Immunotherapy should be permanently held in case of severe cardiac AEs (arrhythmias, significant echocardiography findings, elevated cardiac markers).

Management should be in consultation with cardiology, and other etiologies such as viral infection should be ruled out. A severe cardiac AE as just described should be managed in an inpatient setting. Pulse dose steroids should be considered, with a slow taper on achieving baseline cardiac function. Life-threatening cardiac AEs (severe cardiac findings as mentioned plus hemodynamic instability) are treated with pulse dose steroids. If there is no improvement in 24 hours, antithymocyte globulin or infliximab should be considered.

Immune checkpoint inhibitors have shown significant clinical benefit in several malignancies. Based on their unique mechanism of action, drug-related toxicities are unlike the toxicities seen as a result of conventional cytotoxic chemotherapy. Although the profiles of the approved immunotherapy agents may differ slightly, they all share a similar clinical presentation of drug-related toxicity symptoms, and general principles guiding their management are by holding immunotherapy or considering immunosuppressive treatment.[17,24,28,30-34]

It is exceedingly important to make the distinction that immunotherapy is not chemotherapy; the method of action and AEs observed with immunotherapy have a vastly different underlying mechanism compared to that of chemotherapy.[5,6]

Though immunotherapy is overall better tolerated than chemotherapy despite its longer exposure to the patient,[35] selecting the right patient for this treatment is critical.

> **CLINICAL PEARL:** It is important to know that the CTLA4 blocking antibody (ipilimumab) toxicities are dose related,[36] whereas PD-1 blockage (nivolumab or pembrolizumab) have a similar incidence of toxicity even at a higher dose.[6]

AWARENESS AND MANAGEMENT OF IMMUNOTOXICITY

The AEs can present in an insidious and unpredictable manner. Therefore, it is crucial for the clinical team and patient to be educated and aware of the potential toxicities and the manner in which they may present. Earlier reporting and prompt investigation of the symptoms will allow for timely treatment and avoidance of adverse outcomes. A general principle is that differential diagnoses should be diligently evaluated according to standard medical practice. Non-inflammatory etiologies should be considered and appropriately treated. Corticosteroids are a primary therapy for immune-oncology drug-related AEs. High-dose steroids, anti–tumor necrosis factor alpha, and other immunosuppressive therapies such as tacrolimus and mycophenolate mofetil can interfere with the efficacy of immunotherapeutic agents; therefore, these drugs are not used concurrently. However, low-dose steroids (<10 mg prednisone) are speculated to be safe, and restarting immunotherapy for its treatment benefit appears to outweigh side effects.[37] Furthermore, other less common toxicities of immunotherapy treatment such as GBS, encephalitis, or transverse myelitis are rare, but clinicians should be cognizant of these in appropriate settings. Management of these rare events follows the same guidelines with supportive treatment and initiating steroids or immunosuppression in a timely fashion.

Consultation with a medical or surgical specialist, especially prior to an invasive diagnostic or therapeutic procedure, is recommended.

> **CLINICAL PEARL:** Adding adequate prophylactic antibiotics (Bactrim/acyclovir) for an opportunistic infection is also vital for the cohort that requires a long course of steroids or a slow taper.[37]

Newer phase 1/2 studies continue to provide encouraging data, and there are several other immune checkpoint inhibitors in development with promising clinical activity that are likely to be approved by the regulatory agencies. Ongoing phase 2/3 clinical trials such as colitis in melanoma patients treated with immunotherapy (COLIPI) and infliximab-steroid combinations in preventing side effects are imperative.

Immune checkpoint inhibitors have offered an opportunity for the development of effective treatment options for some historically known "chemoresistant" malignancies. With increasing use of such novel agents, it is therefore imperative that the clinical teams, including physicians, first responders, nurses, pharmacists, as well as the patients, become familiar with the AEs and their management.

REFERENCES

1. Yang JC, Childs R. Immunotherapy for renal cell cancer. *J Clin Oncol.* 2006;24(35):5576-5583. doi:10.1200/JCO.2006.08.3774
2. Garon EB, Rizvi NA, Hui R, et al. Pembrolizumab for the treatment of non-small-cell lung cancer. *N Engl J Med.* 2015;372(21):2018-2028. doi:10.1056/NEJMoa1501824
3. Rizvi NA, Hellmann MD, Snyder A, et al. Cancer immunology. Mutational landscape determines sensitivity to PD-1 blockade in non-small cell lung cancer. *Science.* 2015;348(6230):124-128. doi:10.1126/science.aaa1348
4. Van Allen EM, Miao D, Schilling B, et al. Genomic correlates of response to CTLA-4 blockade in metastatic melanoma. *Science.* 2015;350(6257):207-211. doi:10.1126/science.aad0095
5. Messerschmidt JL, Prendergast GC, Messerschmidt GL. How cancers escape immune destruction and mechanisms of action for the new significantly active immune therapies: helping nonimmunologists decipher recent advances. *Oncologist.* 2016;21(2):233-243. doi:10.1634/theoncologist.2015-0282
6. Topalian SL, Hodi FS, Brahmer JR, et al. Safety, activity, and immune correlates of anti-PD-1 antibody in cancer. *N Engl J Med.* 2012;366(26):2443-2454. doi:10.1056/NEJMoa1200690
7. Nanda R, Chow LQ, Dees EC, et al. Pembrolizumab in patients with advanced triple-negative breast cancer: phase Ib KEYNOTE-012 study. *J Clin Oncol.* 2016;34(21):2460-2467. doi:10.1200/JCO.2015.64.8931
8. Weber J. Ipilimumab: controversies in its development, utility and autoimmune adverse events. *Cancer Immunol Immunother.* 2009;58(5):823-830. doi:10.1007/s00262-008-0653-8
9. Ziemer M, Koukoulioti E, Beyer S, Simon JC, Berg T. Managing immune checkpoint-inhibitor-induced severe autoimmune-like hepatitis by liver-directed topical steroids. *J Hepatol.* 2017;66(3):657-659. doi:10.1016/j.jhep.2016.11.015
10. Brahmer JR, Lacchetti C, Schneider BJ, et al. Management of immune-related adverse events in patients treated with immune checkpoint inhibitor therapy: American Society of Clinical Oncology Clinical Practice Guideline. *J Clin Oncol.* 2018;36(17):1714-1768. doi:10.1200/JCO.2017.77.6385
11. Gupta A, De Felice KM, Loftus EV, Jr., Khanna S. Systematic review: colitis associated with anti-CTLA-4 therapy. *Aliment Pharmacol Ther.* 2015;42(4):406-417. doi:10.1111/apt.13281
12. Marthey L, Mateus C, Mussini C, et al. Cancer immunotherapy with anti-CTLA-4 monoclonal antibodies induces an inflammatory bowel disease. *J Crohns Colitis.* 2016;10(4):395-401. doi:10.1093/ecco-jcc/jjv227
13. Cramer P, Bresalier RS. Gastrointestinal and hepatic complications of immune checkpoint inhibitors. *Curr Gastroenterol Rep.* 2017;19(1):3. doi:10.1007/s11894-017-0540-6
14. Naidoo J, Page DB, Li BT, et al. Toxicities of the anti-PD-1 and anti-PD-L1 immune checkpoint antibodies. *Ann Oncol.* 2016;27(7):1362. doi:10.1093/annonc/mdw141
15. Naidoo J, Wang X, Woo KM, et al. Pneumonitis in patients treated with anti-programmed death-1/programmed death ligand 1 therapy. *J Clin Oncol.* 2017;35(7):709-717. doi:10.1200/JCO.2016.68.2005

16. Nishino M, Giobbie-Hurder A, Hatabu H, Ramaiya NH, Hodi FS. Incidence of programmed cell death 1 inhibitor-related pneumonitis in patients with advanced cancer: a systematic review and meta-analysis. *JAMA Oncol.* 2016;2(12):1607-1616. doi:10.1001/jamaoncol.2016.2453

17. Hodi FS, O'Day SJ, McDermott DF, et al. Improved survival with ipilimumab in patients with metastatic melanoma. *N Engl J Med.* 2010;363(8):711-723. doi:10.1056/NEJMoa1003466

18. Chuzi S, Tavora F, Cruz M, et al. Clinical features, diagnostic challenges, and management strategies in checkpoint inhibitor-related pneumonitis. *Cancer Manag Res.* 2017;9:207-213. doi:10.2147/CMAR.S136818

19. O'Kane GM, Labbe C, Doherty MK, Young K, Albaba H, Leighl NB. Monitoring and management of immune-related adverse events associated with programmed cell death protein-1 axis inhibitors in lung cancer. *Oncologist.* 2017;22(1):70-80. doi:10.1634/theoncologist.2016-0164

20. Barroso-Sousa R, Barry WT, Garrido-Castro AC, et al. Incidence of endocrine dysfunction following the use of different immune checkpoint inhibitor regimens: a systematic review and meta-analysis. *JAMA Oncol.* 2018;4(2):173-182. doi:10.1001/jamaoncol.2017.3064

21. Sznol M, Ferrucci PF, Hogg D, et al. Pooled analysis safety profile of nivolumab and ipilimumab combination therapy in patients with advanced melanoma. *J Clin Oncol.* 2017;35(34):3815-3822. doi:10.1200/JCO.2016.72.1167

22. Gettinger SN, Horn L, Gandhi L, et al. Overall survival and long-term safety of nivolumab (anti-programmed death 1 antibody, BMS-936558, ONO-4538) in patients with previously treated advanced non-small-cell lung cancer. *J Clin Oncol.* 2015;33(18):2004-2012. doi:10.1200/JCO.2014.58.3708

23. Villadolid J, Amin A. Immune checkpoint inhibitors in clinical practice: update on management of immune-related toxicities. *Transl Lung Cancer Res.* 2015;4(5):560-575. doi:10.3978/j.issn.2218-6751.2015.06.06

24. Eggermont AM, Chiarion-Sileni V, Grob JJ, et al. Adjuvant ipilimumab versus placebo after complete resection of high-risk stage III melanoma (EORTC 18071): a randomised, double-blind, phase 3 trial. *Lancet Oncol.* 2015;16(5):522-530. doi:10.1016/S1470-2045(15)70122-1

25. Freeman-Keller M, Kim Y, Cronin H, Richards A, Gibney G, Weber JS. Nivolumab in resected and unresectable metastatic melanoma: characteristics of immune-related adverse events and association with outcomes. *Clin Cancer Res.* 2016;22(4):886-894. doi:10.1158/1078-0432.CCR-15-1136

26. Hua C, Boussemart L, Mateus C, et al. Association of vitiligo with tumor response in patients with metastatic melanoma treated with pembrolizumab. *JAMA Dermatol.* 2016;152(1):45-51. doi:10.1001/jamadermatol.2015.2707

27. Teulings HE, Limpens J, Jansen SN, et al. Vitiligo-like depigmentation in patients with stage III-IV melanoma receiving immunotherapy and its association with survival: a systematic review and meta-analysis. *J Clin Oncol.* 2015;33(7):773-781. doi:10.1200/JCO.2014.57.4756

28. Weber JS, D'Angelo SP, Minor D, et al. Nivolumab versus chemotherapy in patients with advanced melanoma who progressed after anti-CTLA-4 treatment (CheckMate 037): a randomised, controlled, open-label, phase 3 trial. *Lancet Oncol.* 2015;16(4):375-384. doi:10.1016/S1470-2045(15)70076-8

29. Cuzzubbo S, Javeri F, Tissier M, et al. Neurological adverse events associated with immune checkpoint inhibitors: review of the literature. *Eur J Cancer.* 2017;73:1-8. doi:10.1016/j.ejca.2016.12.001

30. Hellmann MD, Rizvi NA, Goldman JW, et al. Nivolumab plus ipilimumab as first-line treatment for advanced non-small-cell lung cancer (CheckMate 012): results of an open-label, phase 1, multicohort study. *Lancet Oncol.* 2017;18(1):31-41. doi:10.1016/S1470-2045(16)30624-6

31. Motzer RJ, Escudier B, McDermott DF, et al. Nivolumab versus everolimus in advanced renal-cell carcinoma. *N Engl J Med.* 2015;373(19):1803-1813. doi:10.1056/NEJMoa1510665

32. Postow MA, Chesney J, Pavlick AC, et al. Nivolumab and ipilimumab versus ipilimumab in untreated melanoma. *N Engl J Med.* 2015;372(21):2006-2017. doi:10.1056/NEJMoa1414428

33. Robert C, Schachter J, Long GV, et al. Pembrolizumab versus ipilimumab in advanced melanoma. *N Engl J Med.* 2015;372(26):2521-2532. doi:10.1056/NEJMoa1503093

34. Wolchok JD, Neyns B, Linette G, et al. Ipilimumab monotherapy in patients with pretreated advanced melanoma: a randomised, double-blind, multicentre, phase 2, dose-ranging study. *Lancet Oncol.* 2010;11(2):155-164. doi:10.1016/S1470-2045(09)70334-1

35. Ribas A, Puzanov I, Dummer R, et al. Pembrolizumab versus investigator-choice chemotherapy for ipilimumab-refractory melanoma (KEYNOTE-002): a randomised, controlled, phase 2 trial. *Lancet Oncol.* 2015;16(8):908-918. doi:10.1016/S1470-2045(15)00083-2

36. Wolchok JD, Kluger H, Callahan MK, et al. Nivolumab plus ipilimumab in advanced melanoma. *N Engl J Med.* 2013;369(2):122-133. doi:10.1056/NEJMoa1302369

37. Linardou H, Gogas H. Toxicity management of immunotherapy for patients with metastatic melanoma. *Ann Transl Med.* 2016;4(14):272. doi:10.21037/atm.2016.07.10

PART V

Less Common Cancers of the Lung

22

PULMONARY CARCINOID

Hamza Hashmi, MD

A 65-year-old white man with a past medical history of hypertension (HTN) and chronic obstructive pulmonary disease (COPD) presents with persistent cough for the last 4 months. A chest x-ray reveals a solitary lesion in the right middle lobe. Chest computed tomography (CT) confirms a 4-cm non-spiculated lesion without any associated lymphadenopathy. Endobronchial ultrasound-guided fine-needle aspiration biopsy reveals bronchial carcinoid with no evidence of necrosis or mitosis under a high-powered field (HPF).

Learning Objectives:
1. What are the common presenting features of carcinoid?
2. What is the most sensitive and specific imaging study for carcinoid diagnosis?
3. What are the two characteristic microscopic features that differentiate typical and atypical carcinoid?
4. What is the first line of therapy for metastatic carcinoid?

CLINICAL PRESENTATION

Carcinoids represent 1.2% of all primary lung malignancies. Their incidence in the United States has increased rapidly over the last 30 years and is currently about 6% per year.[1] Typical carcinoids represent 80%-90% of all lung carcinoids and occur more frequently in the fifth and sixth decades of life. Nearly all bronchial neuroendocrine tumors (NETs) are sporadic; however, they can rarely occur in the setting of multiple endocrine neoplasia type 1 (MEN1). No external environmental toxin or other stimulus has been identified as a causative agent for the development of pulmonary carcinoid tumors.

About 60% of the patients with bronchial carcinoid are symptomatic at presentation (**Figure 22-1**). The most common clinical findings are those associated with bronchial obstruction, such as persistent cough, hemoptysis, and recurrent or obstructive pneumonitis. Wheezing, chest pain, and dyspnea also may be noted. Although uncommon,

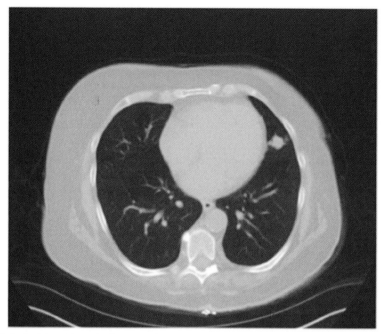

Figure 22-1. Peripheral bronchial carcinoid.

various endocrine or neuroendocrine syndromes can be initial clinical manifestations of either typical or atypical pulmonary carcinoid tumors.[2]

Diagnostics

Chest radiography is abnormal in about 75% of patients with a pulmonary carcinoid tumor. A CT scan provides excellent resolution of tumor extent, location, and the presence or absence of mediastinal adenopathy. Because carcinoid tumors are highly vascular, they show greater enhancement than benign lesions on contrast CT.

Although highly vascular, carcinoid tumors of the lung do not show increased metabolic activity on positron emission tomography (PET) and would be incorrectly designated as benign lesions on the basis of findings from a PET scan.

The overexpression of somastatin receptor (SSTR) is a characteristic feature of bronchial NETs, which can be used to localize the primary tumor and its metastases by imaging with the radiolabeled somastatin (SST) analogues.

> **CLINICAL PEARL:** With regard to somatostatin receptor scintigraphy testing, PET using Ga–DOTATATE/TOC has a sensitivity of 97% and specificity of 92%; hence, it is preferable to Octreoscan in highly aggressive atypical bronchial NETs.

Ga-DOTATATE/TOC scan also provides an estimate of receptor density and evidence of the functionality of receptors, which helps with selection of suitable treatments that act on these receptors.

Serum levels of chromogranin A in bronchial NETs are expressed at a lower rate than other sites of carcinoid tumors. Hence, its measurement is of limited utility in following disease activity in bronchial NETs.

For central tumors, transbronchial tumors, and peripheral tumors, CT-guided percutaneous biopsy is the accepted diagnostic approach. The diagnostic yield of brush cytology is low overall (4%-63%); hence, fine-needle biopsy is preferred.

> **CLINICAL PEARL:** If a suspicion of malignancy exists despite a negative finding on transthoracic biopsy, surgical excision of the nodule and pathologic analysis should be undertaken.

Distinction between typical and atypical carcinoid is made based on the presence of one or more of the following features (**Figure 22-2, Table 22-1**)[3]:

- Increased mitotic activity in a tumor with an identifiable carcinoid cellular arrangement with 2-10 mitotic figures per high-power field (HPF)
- Pleomorphism and irregular nuclei with hyperchromatic and prominent nucleoli
- Areas of increased cellularity; with loss of regular, organized architecture observed in typical carcinoid
- Areas of necrosis within the tumor

A Ki-67 cell proliferation labeling index can be used to distinguish between high-grade lung NETs (>40%) and carcinoids (<20%), particularly in crushed biopsy

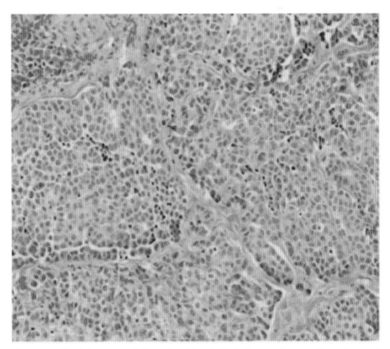

Figure 22-2. Nests of lightly eosinophilic cells with relatively low nuclear grade and granular chromatin.

CARCINOID	TYPICAL	ATYPICAL
Incidence	80%-90%	10%-20%
Size	Smaller	Larger
Location	Central	Peripheral
Number of mitoses	<2 per HPF	2-10 per HPF
Necrosis	Absent	Present
5-year survival	87%-100%	30%-95%
Distant metastases/local recurrence	Less common	More common

TABLE 22-1 Distinguishing Features Between Typical Versus Atypical Carcinoid[3]

specimens, in which carcinoids may be mistaken for small cell lung cancers. However, given overlap in the distribution of the Ki-67 labeling index between typical carcinoids (TCs) (≤5%) and atypical carcinoids (ACs) (≤20%) Ki-67 expression does not reliably distinguish between well-differentiated lung carcinoids.

The number of mitoses per HPF of viable tumor area and the presence or absence of necrosis continue to be the salient features distinguishing typical and atypical bronchial NETs.

TREATMENT

Localized and Resectable Carcinoid

Surgical resection is the treatment of choice for early stage carcinoid. The extent of resection is determined by the tumor size, histology, and location. The standard surgical approach is the minimal anatomic resection (lobectomy, sleeve lobectomy, bi-lobectomy, or pneumonectomy) needed to obtain microscopically negative margins, with an associated mediastinal and hilar lymph node dissection for staging.[4]

> **CLINICAL PEARL:** An adaptive approach must be taken for patients undergoing wedge resection of pulmonary lesions without a known diagnosis. If intraoperative frozen section is consistent with carcinoid and the margins are negative, mediastinal lymph node dissection should be performed. If the patient is node negative, then complete lobectomy is not required. In node-positive patients with adequate pulmonary reserve, lobectomy should be performed regardless of histology. If atypical features are found during pathologic evaluation, then interval completion lobectomy may be used for patients with adequate pulmonary reserve.

Postoperative adjuvant therapy for most resected bronchial NETs even in the setting of positive lymph nodes is generally not recommended. Radiotherapy (RT) is a reasonable option for atypical bronchial NETs if gross residual disease remains after surgery, although whether this improves outcomes is unproven.

Localized and Unresectable Disease

For inoperable patients and for those with surgically unresectable but non-metastatic disease, options for local control of tumor growth include RT with or without concurrent chemotherapy and palliative endobronchial resection of obstructing tumor.

Metastatic Disease[5,6]

Everolimus

Everolimus is currently used as **first-line therapy** for progressive, well-differentiated, non-functional NETs of lung origin that are unresectable, locally advanced, or metastatic.

Somatostatin Analogues

The National Comprehensive Cancer Network (NCCN) and European Neuroendocrine Tumor Society (ENETS) guidelines also recommend the use of somatostatin analogues (SSAs) as a first-line option in patients with

- lung carcinoids exhibiting hormone-related symptoms, and
- slowly progressive TC or AC with a low proliferative index (preferably Ki-67 <10%), provided there is a strongly positive SSTR status.

In cases where metastatic lung NETs are associated with the carcinoid syndrome, initiation of long-acting SSA therapy in combination with everolimus is recommended.

Cytotoxic Chemotherapy

- For patients with highly aggressive atypical bronchial NETs, a combination regimen of platinum and etoposide has shown a better response rate and overall survival data.

The following regimens can be used, but there is limited data for objective responses:

- Temozolomide plus capecitabine
- Fluorouracil plus dacarbazine
- Epirubicin, capecitabine, plus oxaliplatin
- Capecitabine plus liposomal doxorubicin

> **CLINICAL PEARL:** For patients who have a limited, potentially resectable, liver-isolated metastatic NET, surgical resection should be pursued. For more extensive, unresectable liver metastases, treatment options include embolization, radio-frequency ablation (RFA), and cryoablation.

POSTTREATMENT SURVEILLANCE

Posttreatment surveillance is recommended after resection of node-positive typical bronchial NETs and for all atypical tumors. CT scans (including the thorax and abdomen) every 6 months for 2 years followed by annual scans for a total of 5 years represent a reasonable surveillance schedule.

PROGNOSIS

Typical Bronchial NETs

Typical bronchial NETs have an excellent prognosis following surgical resection. Reported 5-year survival rates are 87%-100%. Features associated with negative prognostic significance include lymph node involvement and incomplete resection.

Atypical Bronchial NETs

Atypical bronchial NETs have a worse prognosis than typical tumors. Five-year survival rates range widely, from 30% to 95%. Atypical tumors have a greater tendency to both metastasize (16%-23%) and recur locally (3%-25%). Distant metastases to the liver or bone are more common than local recurrence.

REFERENCES

1. Hauso O, Gustafsson BI, Kidd M, et al. Neuroendocrine tumor epidemiology: contrasting Norway and North America. *Cancer*. 2008;113(10):2655-2664.
2. Fink G, Krelbaum T, Yellin A, et al. Pulmonary carcinoid: presentation, diagnosis, and outcome in 142 cases in Israel and review of 640 cases from the literature. *Chest*. 2001;119(6):1647-1651.
3. Beasley MB, Thunnissen FB, Brambilla E, et al. Pulmonary atypical carcinoid: predictors of survival in 106 cases. *Hum Pathol*. 2000;31(10):1255-1265.
4. Fox M, Van Berkel V, Bousamra M, 2nd, Sloan S, Martin RC, 2nd. Surgical management of pulmonary carcinoid tumors: sublobar resection versus lobectomy. *Am J Surg*. 2013;205(2):200-208.
5. Caplin ME, Baudin E, Ferolla P, et al. Pulmonary neuroendocrine (carcinoid) tumors: European Neuroendocrine Tumor Society expert consensus and recommendations for best practice for typical and atypical pulmonary carcinoids. *Ann Oncol*. 2015;26(8):1604-1620.
6. Oberg K, Hellman P, Ferolla P, Papotti M, Group EGW. Neuroendocrine bronchial and thymic tumors: ESMO Clinical Practice Guidelines for diagnosis, treatment and follow-up. *Ann Oncol*. 2012;23(Suppl 7):vii120-123.

23

MALIGNANT PLEURAL MESOTHELIOMA

Hamza Hashmi, MD

A 70-year-old white man with past medical history of hypertension (HTN) and chronic obstructive pulmonary disease (COPD) presents with a persistent cough for the last 2 months. He has a 60 pack-year smoking history. He worked for 20 years as a coal miner. Chest x-ray reveals a moderate size right-sided pleural effusion. Chest computed tomography (CT) confirms a loculated pleural effusion and pleural-based nodules. On thoracentesis, 500 mL of fluid is removed, and analysis reveals exudative effusion without evidence of malignant cells on cytology. What should be the next step in management of this patient?

Learning Objectives:

1. What are the risk factors associated with malignant pleural mesothelioma?
2. What is the diagnostic modality of choice for malignant pleural mesothelioma?
3. What is the ideal treatment approach for resectable non-metastatic malignant pleural mesothelioma?
4. What is the first line of therapy for metastatic malignant pleural mesothelioma?

INCIDENCE

Malignancies involving mesothelial cells that normally line the body cavities, including the pleura, peritoneum, pericardium, and testis, are known as malignant mesothelioma. Pleural involvement is the most common (85%), followed by peritoneum (15%) and pericardium and tunica vaginalis (1%).

Mesothelioma is a rare malignancy with 2,500 new cases diagnosed annually in the United States. It commonly develops in the fifth to seventh decade of life. The male-to-female ratio is 4:1.

RISK FACTORS

Asbestos, particularly the types of amphibole asbestos known as crocidolite and amosite asbestos, is the principal carcinogen implicated in the pathogenesis of malignant pleural mesothelioma.[1] A substantial proportion of patients with malignant pleural mesothelioma are exposed to asbestos in asbestos mills, mines, shipping yards, paper mills, auto parts (asbestos brake lining), railroad repair, and insulation.

> **CLINICAL PEARL:** Family members of workers exposed to asbestos can also be at risk of exposure if asbestos becomes embedded in the workers' clothing.

Other associations include exposure to **radiotherapy** (RT) and **erionite** (mineral found in sand gravel).

Smoking does not increase the increase of mesothelioma, but together with asbestos exposure does significantly increase the risk of lung carcinoma (adenocarcinoma).

PRESENTATION

Dyspnea and non-pleuritic chest wall pain are the most common presenting symptoms of malignant mesothelioma. Chest discomfort, pleuritic pain, easy fatigability, fever, sweats, and weight loss are the other common accompanying symptoms. Metastatic disease is uncommon at presentation.

> **CLINICAL PEARL:** Contralateral pleural abnormalities are usually secondary to asbestos-related pleural disease rather than to metastatic disease.

DIAGNOSTICS

Biochemical Tests

Several biomarkers are selectively elevated in patients with mesothelioma, including soluble mesothelin-related peptides, fibulin-3, and osteopontin. Of these biomarkers, the circulating serum mesothelin receptor protein level has been reported to be elevated in 84% of patients with malignant mesothelioma and in 2% of patients with lung cancer. Although they are not routinely used for diagnosis, these levels can be used to follow response to treatment.

More than 90% of patients with pleural mesothelioma present with pleural effusion. Cytology findings are diagnostic in only 32% of patients. Diagnosis of mesothelioma by detection of chromosomal aberrations with fluorescence in situ hybridization (FISH) has 79% sensitivity; positive and negative predictive values for detection of mesothelioma were 100% and 72%, respectively.

IMAGING STUDIES

Chest radiographs in malignant pleural mesothelioma show obliteration of the diaphragm, nodular thickening of the pleura, and loculated pleural effusion. A CT or magnetic resonance imaging (MRI) scan of the chest or a positron emission tomographic

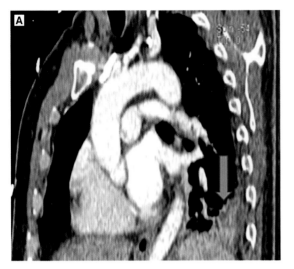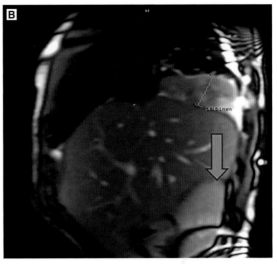

Figure 23-1. A. Chest CT showing malignant pleural mesothelioma with pleural involvement (*arrow*). B. Chest MRI showing malignant pleural mesothelioma with pleural involvement (*arrow*).

(PET) scan can also be used in the diagnosis of mesothelioma (**Figure 23-1**). MRI performed with different pulse sequences and gadolinium-based contrast material can offer more details, with improved detection of tumor extension, especially to the chest wall and diaphragm. Although PET scans can provide metabolic and anatomic information, especially for patients with extrathoracic or mediastinal metastasis, the appropriate role of PET scans in the management of malignant mesothelioma is still undefined.

> **CLINICAL PEARL:** Thoracoscopically guided pleural biopsy is the diagnostic modality of choice. It is positive in 98% of cases.

PATHOLOGY

> **CLINICAL PEARL:** Histological subtypes include
>   a. Epithelioid, 80%
>   b. Sarcomatoid, 10%
>   c. Biphasic or mixed, 10%

> **CLINICAL PEARL:** Sarcomatoid histology is associated with worse prognosis compared to epithelial or mixed.

Useful immunohistochemistry (IHC) markers are noted in **Table 23-1**.

It is important to know that thyroid transcription factor 1 (TTF-1) and carcinoembryonic antigen (CEA), typically positive in lung adenocarcinoma, are negative in mesothelioma.

TABLE 23-1	Immune Histochemical Stains in Mesothelioma
	IHC MARKERS
Positive	Calretinin, WT-1, D2-40, CK 5/6
Negative	TTF-1, CEA

GENETICS

Most malignant mesotheliomas have complex karyotypes, with extensive aneuploidy and the rearrangement of many chromosomes. Loss of 1 copy of chromosome 22 is the single most common karyotypic change in malignant mesothelioma. Other chromosomal changes commonly observed include deletions in the chromosome arms 1p, 3p, 9p, and 6q.

STAGING

For diagnosed cases of pleural mesothelioma, integrated PET-CT is done as the initial staging assessment. For patients in whom imaging suggests resectable disease, surgical staging involving mediastinoscopy or endobronchial ultrasound (EBUS)–mediated staging of mediastinal lymph nodes should be pursued. It typically also includes laparoscopy with peritoneal lavage to detect subdiaphragmatic involvement, which is most useful when there is concern for invasion of the diaphragm.

Four staging categories have been proposed for mesothelioma. Currently, the accepted system is the tumor, node, metastasis (TNM) classification accepted by the International Mesothelioma Interest Group (IMIG). The stages of mesothelioma are as follows:

- **Stage I**: Completely resected within the capsule of the parietal pleura without adenopathy (ie, ipsilateral pleura, lung, pericardium, diaphragm, or chest wall disease limited to previous biopsy sites)
- **Stage II**: All stage I characteristics, with positive resection margins, intrapleural adenopathy, or a combination
- **Stage III**: Local extension of disease into the chest wall or mediastinum, into the heart, through the diaphragm or peritoneum, or extrapleurally to involve the lymph nodes
- **Stage IV**: Distant metastatic disease

TREATMENT

Pretreatment workup includes

a. Pulmonary function testing
b. Perfusion scanning only if the forced expiratory volume in 1 second (FEV_1) is less than 80%
c. Cardiac stress testing to determine if surgical candidates

Trimodality treatment is the goal; however, a high proportion of patients are unable to complete all 3 modalities.[2]

For patients with disease limited to 1 hemithorax, a detailed evaluation is indicated to assess whether the disease is amenable to a macroscopic complete resection (MCR), whether there is adequate cardiopulmonary function to tolerate such a procedure, and whether there are any medical contraindications.

> **CLINICAL PEARL:** For surgical candidates, a combined modality approach that includes chemotherapy (generally a platinum plus pemetrexed), surgery (MCR) with either pleurectomy/decortication (P/D) or radical extrapleural pneumonectomy (EPP), and RT is recommended. For patients who are not surgical candidates, systemic chemotherapy is the treatment of choice. Palliative RT may all have a role in the management of symptoms (from any pleural effusion).

Surgery

There are 2 procedures that can be employed for surgical resection of the tumor for patients who are considered good surgical candidates.

a. **Pleurectomy/decortication**[3] is a more limited procedure and requires less cardiorespiratory reserve. It involves dissection of the parietal pleura, incision of the parietal pleura, and decortication of the visceral pleura, followed by reconstruction. It has a morbidity rate of 25% and a mortality rate of 2%. It is a difficult procedure because the tumor encases the whole pleura, and the local recurrence rate is high.

b. **Extrapleural pneumonectomy** is a more extensive procedure and has a higher mortality rate of 3.8%. The procedure involves dissection of the parietal pleura, division of the pulmonary vessels, and en bloc resection of the lung, pleura, pericardium, and diaphragm, followed by reconstruction. It provides the best local control because it removes the entire pleural sac along with the lung parenchyma.

> **CLINICAL PEARL:** A meta-analysis showed no statistically significant difference in 2-year mortality after pleurectomy with decortication compared with EPP, but pleurectomy with decortication was associated with a significantly lower proportion of short-term deaths (perioperatively and within 30 days) than EPP (1.7% vs. 4.5%).[4]

Radiotherapy

Hemithoracic RT decreases local recurrence after EPP. It can also be used to treat surgical sites prophylactically to decrease tracking through the chest wall and for palliation to areas of chest wall invasion. External beam RT is delivered in a standard fractionation over 5.5-6 weeks.

Chemotherapy

For patients with advanced pleural mesotheliomas who are not candidates for a combined modality approach that incorporates definitive surgery, treatment with combination chemotherapy[5,6] using a platinum-based doublet is recommended. This approach has been shown to significantly prolong overall survival compared with single-agent chemotherapy using cisplatin. The addition of bevacizumab to the pemetrexed-cisplatin regimen improved both progression-free and overall survival compared with pemetrexed plus cisplatin without bevacizumab in a large phase III trial. Prophylactic folic acid and vitamin B_{12} should be used for patients on pemetrexed.

Patients should be appropriately selected to receive this regimen, generally being younger than 75 years of age with a good performance status and without contraindications to bevacizumab.

Maintenance pemetrexed can be administered after 4-6 cycles of the platinum-pemetrexed doublet.

The gemcitabine **plus** cisplatin regimen was evaluated in a multicenter phase 2 trial, in which 106 previously untreated patients were treated with gemcitabine plus cisplatin and randomly assigned to receive either bevacizumab or placebo. The median survival was approximately 15 months on both treatment arms, consistent with the results seen with cisplatin plus pemetrexed.

Cisplatin has also been combined with a number of older chemotherapy agents in phase 2 studies including

- anthracyclines (doxorubicin, epirubicin)
- fluorouracil, mitomycin, and etoposide
- methotrexate plus vinblastine

Progressive and Relapsed Disease

> **CLINICAL PEARL:** For patients who progress on their initial platinum-based regimen or within 6 months of completion of therapy, single-agent chemotherapy with an active agent such as gemcitabine or pemetrexed that was not included in the original chemotherapy regimen can be employed. If disease progression occurs 6 months after completion of therapy, patients can be rechallenged with the same regimen.[6]

Other older agents that also have some activity in malignant pleural mesothelioma include anthracyclines and vinca alkaloids.

PROGNOSIS

The overall prognosis[7] is poor, with high risk of local and distant recurrence. Median survival for patients with malignant mesothelioma is 11 months. It is almost always fatal. Median survival based on histologic type is 9.4 months for sarcomatous, 12.5 months for epithelial, and 11 months for mixed. Without treatment, malignant mesothelioma is fatal within 4-8 months. With trimodality treatment, some patients have survived 16-19 months.

REFERENCES

1. Liu B, van Gerwen M, Bonassi S, Taioli E, International Association for the Study of Lung Cancer Mesothelioma Task Force. Epidemiology of environmental exposure and malignant mesothelioma. *J Thorac Oncol.* 2017;12(7):1031-1045.

 2. Kapeles M, Gensheimer MF, Mart DA, et al. Trimodality treatment of malignant pleural mesothelioma: an institutional review. *Am J Clin Oncol.* 2018;41(1):30-35.
 3. Neragi-Miandoab S, Richards WG, Sugarbaker DJ. Morbidity, mortality, mean survival, and the impact of histology on survival after pleurectomy in 64 patients with malignant pleural mesothelioma. *Int J Surg.* 2008;6(4):293-297.
 4. Taioli E, Wolf AS, Flores RM. Meta-analysis of survival after pleurectomy decortication versus extrapleural pneumonectomy in mesothelioma. *Ann Thorac Surg.* 2015;99(2):472-480.
 5. Patel SC, Dowell JE. Modern management of malignant pleural mesothelioma. *Lung Cancer (Auckl).* 2016;7:63-72.
 6. Disselhorst MMJ, Burgers SJA, Baas P. Optimal therapy of advanced stage mesothelioma. *Curr Treat Options Oncol.* 2017;18(8):48.
 7. Chen Z, Gaudino G, Pass HI, Carbone M, Yang H. Diagnostic and prognostic biomarkers for malignant mesothelioma: an update. *Transl Lung Cancer Res.* 2017;6(3):259-269.

24

THYMIC CANCER

Hamza Hashmi, MD

A 50-year-old white male with no other past medical history presents with gradually worsening shortness of breath for the last 3 months. Chest x-ray reveals a moderate size right-sided pleural effusion. Chest computed tomography (CT) confirms a loculated pleural effusion and pleural-based nodules. A thoracentesis removes 500 mL of fluid and analysis reveals exudative effusion without evidence of malignant cells on cytology. What should be the next step in management of this patient?

Learning Objectives:
1. What are the paraneoplastic syndromes associated with thymoma and thymic cancer?
2. What is the ideal approach for obtaining a tissue biopsy for a thymic mass?
3. What is the ideal treatment approach for unresectable and non-metastatic thymic cancer?
4. What are the two most important prognostic factors for thymic cancer?
5. What are the common malignancies associated with thymic cancer?

Thymic tumors are rare neoplasms that arise in the anterior mediastinum. Thymomas/thymic cancer account for about 20% percent of mediastinal neoplasms. Most patients are between 40 and 60 years of age. There is a slight male predominance. Asian and African individuals are more commonly affected than Caucasians.

ETIOLOGY/RISK FACTORS

> **CLINICAL PEARL:** There are no known risk factors, although there is a strong association with myasthenia gravis and other paraneoplastic syndromes.

PRESENTATION

Approximately 50% of individuals presenting with thymoma are clinically asymptomatic.[1] When present, symptoms may be local or systemic. Chest pain, cough, and shortness of breath are the most commonly identified local symptoms. More severe symptoms, such as superior vena cava syndrome, phrenic nerve paralysis, or recurrent laryngeal nerve involvement resulting in hoarseness, are less common. Constitutional symptoms are associated with thymoma in almost 20% of patients and include weight loss, fever, fatigue, and night sweats.

a. **Myasthenia gravis:** Up to one half of patients with thymoma have symptoms consistent with myasthenia gravis. Myasthenia gravis is common with all types of thymoma, but it is rare in thymic carcinoma. Common symptoms include diplopia, ptosis, dysphagia, weakness, and fatigue. Patients with thymoma and myasthenia gravis usually present with less advanced disease than those without myasthenia gravis, possibly because neuromuscular symptoms may lead to an earlier diagnosis.

b. **Pure red cell aplasia**: Pure red cell aplasia results from an autoimmune-mediated hypoproliferation of erythrocyte precursors in the bone marrow. This paraneoplastic disorder occurs in 5%-15% of patients with thymoma and is more common in older women.

c. **Immunodeficiency**: Hypogammaglobulinemia and pure white blood cell aplasia are present in less than 5% of patients with thymoma, most commonly in older women. Conversely, up to 10% of patients with acquired hypogammaglobulinemia have an associated thymoma (Good syndrome), typically of spindle cell histology. Patients usually have recurrent infections, diarrhea, and lymphadenopathy.

d. **Thymoma-associated multiorgan autoimmunity**: Several case reports have described a syndrome of thymoma-associated multiorgan autoimmunity (TAMA) that is similar to graft-versus-host disease. Patients present with variable combinations of a morbilliform skin eruption, chronic diarrhea, and liver enzyme abnormalities.

DIAGNOSTIC WORKUP

Biochemical Test

Although no biochemical study exists that can be used as a screening test to determine the presence of a thymoma or thymic cancer, laboratory studies can be helpful to identify a syndrome associated with thymoma.

Molecular Biology

- **KIT** overexpression is seen in 86% of thymic cancer. Mutation is rarely seen, only in about 10% of cases.
- **Human epidermal growth receptor 2 (HER2) and B cell leukemia/lymphoma 2 promoting tumorigenesis (BCL2)** overexpression is more commonly seen in thymic cancer than thymoma.
- **Epidermal growth factor receptor (EGFR)** overexpression is commonly seen in thymic cancer, but mutation is seen in only 10% of patients.
- **Cytogenetics**: There are alterations in chromosome 6p21.3 (major histocompatibility complex locus).

- **Karyotype abnormalities** involve gain of chromosome 1q, 17q, 18, and loss of 3p, 6, 16q, 17p.

CHEST RADIOGRAPHY

Most thymic neoplasms are visualized on standard chest radiography. The lateral chest radiograph is very helpful in the determination of the involved compartment of the mediastinum.

COMPUTED TOMOGRAPHY

Computed tomography is the preferred imaging modality to visualize a thymoma. However, thymomas have no absolute diagnostic features; they are usually homogeneous and enhance with contrast. CT scans can reveal evidence of local invasion of adjacent structures by a mass or the presence of intrathoracic metastases (**Figure 24-1**). CT has been found to be able to differentiate stage I/II from stage III/IV and may be useful for predicting the need for neoadjuvant therapy.

Magnetic Resonance Imaging

Magnetic resonance imaging (MRI) is useful in both the initial diagnosis of a mediastinal mass and the follow-up evaluation after treatment. Nevertheless, MRI adds little that CT does not provide and should not be performed except under special circumstances.

Positron Emission Tomography

A high 18-fluorodeoxyglucose (FDG) uptake on positron emission tomography (PET) reflects the invasiveness of the malignant nature of thymic tumors and can be used to differentiate these from benign thymomas.

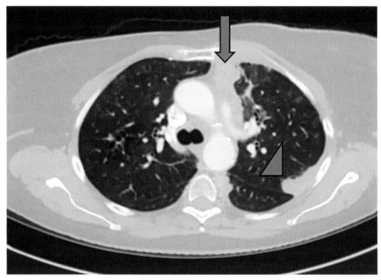

Figure 24-1. Thymic cancer (*arrowhead*) with pleural metastases (*pointer*).

TABLE 24-1 Immune Histochemical Stains in Thymic Cancer	
Epithelial cells	+Keratin, +Leu-7
Thymic lymphocytes	+LCA, +CD 1/3, +CD99
Thymic cancer	+CD 5, +CD 117 (c-kit)

TISSUE BIOPSY

The definitive diagnosis of a thymoma or thymic carcinoma requires a tissue diagnosis.[2]

> **CLINICAL PEARL:** For patients thought to have a thymoma that will be amenable to complete resection, the initial step in management is surgical resection, which can definitively establish the diagnosis. For patients with a tumor that is not considered amenable to complete resection or in whom surgery is contraindicated because of age or comorbidity, a tissue diagnosis with a core needle biopsy or an open biopsy is required prior to therapy.

Besides histological features, immunohistochemistry can be useful for identification on a biopsy specimen (**Table 24-1**).

STAGING

Staging of thymic neoplasms, including both thymomas and thymic carcinoma, is based on the extent of the primary tumor and the presence of invasion into adjacent structures and/or dissemination.

The Masaoka staging system is widely used to stage both thymomas and thymic carcinomas.

- **Stage I**: Completely encapsulated both macroscopically and microscopically; 5e-year survival 94% to 100%.
- **Stage II**: Transcapsular invasion; 5-year survival 86%-95%.
  - Stage IIA: Microscopic transcapsular invasion
  - Stage IIB: Macroscopic invasion into surrounding fatty tissue or grossly adherent to but not through the mediastinal pleura or pericardium
- **Stage III**: Pericardial or lung involvement; 5-year survival 56%-69%.
  - Stage IIIA: Macroscopic invasion into pericardium or lung without great vessel invasion
  - Stage IIIB: Macroscopic invasion into pericardium or lung with great vessel invasion
- **Stage IV**: Disseminated disease; 5-year survival 11%-50%.
  - Stage IVA: Pleural or pericardial dissemination
  - Stage IVB: Lymphatic or hematogenous metastases

TREATMENT

Localized/Non-Metastatic and Resectable Disease Surgical Treatment

Complete surgical resection is the initial treatment approach for all patients when preoperative evaluation suggests that a complete resection will be feasible and there are no medical contraindications to surgery.[3,4]

The current standard of care is an open surgical approach via a median sternotomy. A minimally invasive (thoracoscopic or robotic) approach is not recommended except in the context of specialized centers with experience in these techniques.

> **CLINICAL PEARL:** Surgical intervention often involves resection of phrenic nerve. Preoperative pulmonary function studies should be obtained in all patients so that the extent of respiratory compromise following division of the phrenic nerve can be estimated. If the patient has myasthenia gravis, resection of even one phrenic nerve may lead to significant respiratory problems.

ADJUVANT THERAPY

- For patients with a Masaoka stage I (completely encapsulated) thymoma, postoperative radiation therapy (RT) or adjuvant chemotherapy is *not* recommended given the favorable prognosis and risks and morbidity associated with adjuvant therapy.
- For patients with Masaoka stage II disease who have undergone a complete resection, adjuvant RT is *not* recommended unless other high-risk features (R1 resections, or other high-risk, higher grade, larger tumor size) are present.
- For patients with Masaoka stage III thymoma who have undergone a complete resection, postoperative RT is recommended.

NON-METASTATIC AND UNRESECTABLE DISEASE

For patients with initially unresectable disease (Masaoka stage III or IVA), initial treatment with neoadjuvant chemotherapy should be pursued. If the response to chemotherapy is sufficient to permit surgery and the patient's overall condition permits, surgical resection should be followed by adjuvant RT. RT alone or with chemotherapy is an alternative for patients in whom surgery is not technically feasible or is contraindicated.

METASTATIC AND UNRESECTABLE DISEASE

Chemotherapy

For patients with inoperable recurrent disease or disseminated metastases, systemic chemotherapy with a cisplatin-based regimen is recommended.[5] The following are examples of widely used first-line regimens for the treatment of thymic neoplasms:

- CAP: Cisplatin, doxorubicin, and cyclophosphamide, repeated every 3 weeks. In a US intergroup study, 29 patients with metastatic or progressive thymoma were treated with CAP. The overall and complete response rates were 50% and 10%, respectively, and the median survival was 38 months.

- CP: Carboplatin and paclitaxel every 3 weeks. In a prospective, multicenter study of patients with advanced disease, 3 complete responses and 6 partial responses were observed in 21 patients with thymoma (overall response rate 43%).
- PE: Cisplatin and etoposide repeated every 3 weeks.
- VIP: Etoposide, ifosfamide, and cisplatin repeated every 3 weeks.

Second-Line Therapy

A wide range of agents have been used in the second-line setting, including etoposide, ifosfamide, pemetrexed, octreotide, and 5-fluorouracil plus leucovorin, gemcitabine, and paclitaxel.

TARGETED THERAPY

- **Sunitinib:** A multicenter phase 2 study has evaluated 23 patients with thymic carcinoma after progression of disease on platinum-based therapy. There were 6 partial responses (26%) and 15 with stable disease (65%). Median progression-free survival was 7 months, and median overall survival was 16 months.
- **mTOR inhibitors**: Immunosuppressive agents like tacrolimus and sirolimus, which inhibit the mechanistic target of rapamycin (mTOR), have had activity in a limited number of patients with progressive disease following systemic chemotherapy that included a platinum agent.
- **Octreotide:** Octreotide may have activity in octreotide scan-positive thymoma, with complete response seen in 5% and partial response seen in 25% of the patients.

POSTTREATMENT SURVEILLANCE

For patients who achieve a complete response with either surgery or a combined modality approach, prolonged follow-up is indicated since late relapses are possible. The National Comprehensive Cancer Network recommends CT every 6 months for 2 years, then annually for 5 years for thymic carcinoma, and annually for 10 years for thymoma.

PROGNOSIS

Thymomas usually are slow-growing tumors, and the presence of invasion is an important adverse prognostic marker.

Thymic carcinomas are more aggressive and are associated with a poorer prognosis.

The main factors influencing prognosis are: (1) stage of disease and (2) complete resectability of the tumor.[6]

The prognostic value of tumor histology is more controversial.

- Survival rates associated with tumors that are encapsulated or stage I is 95%-97% at 5 years and 80%-95% at 10 years.
- Invasive or stage II tumors are associated with a reduced 5-year survival rate of 60%-70% and a 10-year survival rate of 40%-50%.
- Survival rates for stage III tumors are reported to be less than 60% at 5 years and 14% at 10 years.

- Survival rates for stage IVA tumors have been reported at 40% for 5 years and 0% at 10 years.

> **CLINICAL PEARL:** Patients with thymoma are at risk (17%-28%) for the development of secondary malignancies like B-cell non-Hodgkin lymphoma, gastrointestinal cancers, and soft tissue sarcomas.

REFERENCES

1. Eng TY, Fuller CD, Jagirdar J, Bains Y, Thomas CR, Jr. Thymic carcinoma: state of the art review. *Int J Radiat Oncol Biol Phys.* 2004;59(3):654-664.
2. Lewis JE, Wick MR, Scheithauer BW, Bernatz PE, Taylor WF. Thymoma. A clinicopathologic review. *Cancer.* 1987;60(11):2727-2743.
3. Falkson CB, Bezjak A, Darling G, et al. The management of thymoma: a systematic review and practice guideline. *J Thorac Oncol.* 2009;4(7):911-919.
4. Paulus A, Sibille A, Bourhaba M, Martin M, Louis R, Duysinx B. Management of thymic epithelial tumors. *Rev Med Liege.* 2015;70(12):623-628.
5. Girard N, Merveilleux du Vignaux C. Systemic treatment for thymic malignancies. *Curr Opin Oncol.* 2017;29(2):112-117.
6. Wilkins KB, Sheikh E, Green R, et al. Clinical and pathologic predictors of survival in patients with thymoma. *Ann Surg.* 1999;230(4):562-572; discussion 572-574.

INDEX

Page numbers followed by *f* or *t* indicate figures or tables, respectively.